Laboratory Exercises for Competency in Respiratory Care

Second Edition

Laboratory Exercises for Competency in Respiratory Care

Second Edition

Thomas J. Butler, PhD, RRT-NPS, RPFT
Professor of Science
Rockland Community College
Suffern, New York
Staff Therapist
Kessler Institute for Rehabilitation
West Orange, New Jersey
NIOSH Approved Spirometry Instructor

F. A. DAVIS COMPANY • Philadelphia

F. A. Davis Company
1915 Arch Street
Philadelphia, PA 19103
www.fadavis.com

Printed in the United States of America

Last digit indicates print number: 10 9 8 7 6 5 4 3 2 1

Senior Acquisitions Editor: Quincy McDonald
Manager of Content Development: George W. Lang
Development and Production Services: Keith Donnellan, Dovetail Content Solutions
Art and Design Manager: Carolyn O'Brien

As new scientific information becomes available through basic and clinical research, recommended treatments and drug therapies undergo changes. The authors and publisher have done everything possible to make this book accurate, up to date, and in accord with accepted standards at the time of publication. The authors, editors, and publisher are not responsible for errors or omissions or for consequences from application of the book, and make no warranty, expressed or implied, in regard to the contents of the book. Any practice described in this book should be applied by the reader in accordance with professional standards of care used in regard to the unique circumstances that may apply in each situation. The reader is advised always to check product information (package inserts) for changes and new information regarding dose and contraindications before administering any drug. Caution is especially urged when using new or infrequently ordered drugs.

ISBN 978-0-8036-1378-2 (pbk. : alk. paper)

This book is dedicated to all the graduates of the Rockland Community College Respiratory Care Program. Thank you for your dedication to the well-being of your patients and for enriching my life.

Contents

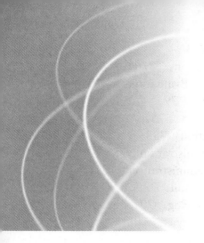

Contributing Authors

Kelly L. Coreas, MSHS, RRT-NPS
Faculty
Respiratory Care Program
Mt. San Antonio College
Walnut, California
Chapter 32

Albert J. Heuer, PhD, MBA, RRT, RPFT
Associate Professor and Program Director; Respiratory Care Program-North
University of Medicine and Dentistry of New Jersey
Newark, New Jersey
Chapters 26, 36, 37, 38, and 46

Ruben D. Restrepo, MD, RRT, FAARC
Associate Professor
Department of Respiratory Care
The University of Texas Health Science Center at San Antonio
San Antonio, Texas
Chapters 25, 27, 28, 29, 30, 34, 39, 40, 41, 42, 44, and 45

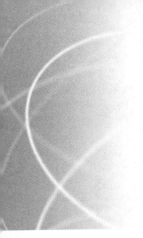

Preface

The second edition of this laboratory manual continues the teaching philosophy outlined in the first edition. Critical thinking skills cannot be taught or achieved by cookbook methodologies that simply have students assemble equipment and follow prescribed steps. These do not achieve any goal except slavish adherence to a procedure that has no variability. Clearly the laboratory setting is the ideal location for the exploration and experimentation with various pieces of equipment.

The exercises contained in the new chapters continue that philosophy. The demands placed on clinical educators in today's health care environment are challenging as well as daunting. Hopefully, a substantially meaningful laboratory experience, where the students are challenged to develop the cognitive, psychomotor and affective skills, will help the students achieve the clinical proficiency necessary for success.

Thomas J. Butler

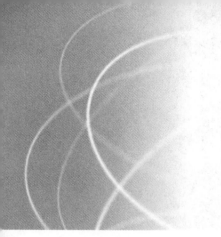

Acknowledgments

The second edition of this manual was no less daunting than the first. It too reflects the work of many individuals. It would be a grave injustice not to thank...

- Janice and Robert Close for their efforts in trying to bring the second edition to press.
- Andy Mc Phee, Quincy McDonald, and the entire F.A. Davis staff for their counsel, commitment, and support.
- Keith Donnellan, the best developmental and production editor anyone could hope for, whose insight and suggestions were invaluable.
- Kelly Coreas, Albert Heuer, and Reuben Restrepo for the contribution of their expertise to the various chapters they revised or wrote.
- Arlene Deas whose organizational skills and tenacity in obtaining and managing the many images used in this edition were indispensible.
- Susan Gilbert, medical illustrator, whose continued dedication and perseverance made the artwork for the second edition consistent and of high caliber.
- The respiratory care programs which have utilized the first edition and have patiently waited for the second edition.

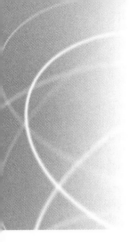

Introduction

PURPOSE AND SCOPE OF THIS BOOK

The evolution of the respiratory care profession continues to present challenges to respiratory care education. Credentialing examinations, added clinical responsibility, and the skills required by potential employers have placed a burden not only on the educational institution, but on the student as well. For most, enrollment in a respiratory care program may represent a student's first exposure to professional education. As in other modes of education, a body of specialized knowledge must be mastered. However, professional health-care education is unique in that it requires the student to skillfully apply this knowledge in practical settings, often with the patient's life in the balance. In addition, specific interpersonal skills and behavioral attributes must be developed for effective professional competence.

Laboratory exercises are an essential and integral part of health professions education. Any laboratory text must include practice of the basic cognitive, psychomotor, and affective principles related to respiratory practice. This text is designed to provide the hands-on and communication skills necessary to integrate theory and clinical practice. Additional chapters have been included to cover the expanded role of the respiratory care practitioner. However, this book is *not* intended to be an all-inclusive compendium of respiratory equipment or tasks or a replacement for the theoretical content found in other respiratory care texts; it is still envisioned to be a complementary tool to be used in conjunction with other resources. It can, however, be used by students and instructors as a teaching, study, and evaluation tool in the preclinical or clinical setting.

The laboratory should be used as a risk-free environment for formative development of respiratory care skills. Students will be asked to assess their "patients," perform procedures, manipulate equipment, and determine settings to observe and experience the resulting consequences. The exercises are designed to promote critical thinking rather than solely to practice psychomotor skills. Some of the exercises are designed for students to *purposely* set up or use equipment incorrectly in order for them to differentiate the right way from the wrong way. It is better to explore these situations in a controlled laboratory setting than in a patient care environment. The text is flexible and general enough to cover these principles without being too specific as to particular brand name products, which may not always be available.

The manual is formatted so that most chapters can be completed in one or more formally scheduled two hour laboratory periods. The longer chapters found in the first edition have been divided into separate chapters in order to make them easier to complete in that time frame. The sequence of chapters is not intended to be rigid and may be assigned to suit curricular needs. The text is, however, detailed enough so that students could perform the exercises with minimal supervision in an independent practice setting as a supplement or replacement for a scheduled laboratory period.

Each chapter includes:

- An introduction
- Objectives
- Key terms
- A list of required equipment
- Exercises appropriate to content
- Tables summarizing normal, abnormal, and critical values where appropriate
- References

- A laboratory report form
- Procedural competency evaluations (PCEs) for each skill assessment
- A performance rating scale form for each PCE

The key terms are not limited to vocabulary found in the text of the chapter. Terms that may be necessary to communicate effectively, understand concepts, or answer chapter questions are also included. All are defined in the glossary. Objectives are not limited to manipulation of equipment, but are geared toward both basic and higher-level cognitive, psychomotor, and affective skills. Troubleshooting exercises and verbal and written communication exercises are included where appropriate. Charting of procedures performed is extensively practiced.

The list of required equipment is provided for each chapter. However, there are materials that should be provided for every activity:

- 50 psi gas source
- Alcohol prep pads
- Flowmeter
- 4x4 gauze
- Gloves, non-sterile, latex-free, and in various sizes
- Goggles or face shields
- Hand sanitizer
- Human patient simulator (if available)
- Large bore corrugated tubing, 6 inch and 6 foot lengths
- Oxygen nipple adapter
- Small bore oxygen tubing

The laboratory report form documents data collection during the exercises. Questions and clinically relevant scenarios are included in the report to enhance critical thinking skills, integrate theory with practice, and focus on the affective domain. The placement of this report allows for easy removal so that it may be submitted to the instructor, leaving the remainder of the manual intact for study, review, and additional practice.

PROCEDURAL COMPETENCY EVALUATIONS

Evaluation is a vital link in the teaching–learning process. A procedural competency evaluation (PCE) involves a demonstration of a specific respiratory care skill in conjunction with an assessment of the student's understanding and ability to apply the related theory. The PCE forms have been revised to make them more user-friendly. A PCE for common performance elements has been added. Certain common elements are required as part of every procedural competency to meet national practice standards and provide quality patient care. Three main categories of common behaviors are Equipment and Patient Preparation, Assessment and Implementation, and Follow-up. These include steps that are common to almost all respiratory care procedures. These common performance elements are:

Patient and Equipment Preparation

1. Verifies, interprets, and evaluates physician's order or protocol
2. Scans chart for any other pertinent data and notes, including diagnosis, medications, therapies, radiographic and other laboratory results
3. Washes hands or applies disinfectant
4. Selects, obtains, assembles equipment correctly, verifies function
5. Trouble shoots equipment and corrects malfunctions if indicated
6. Applies personal protective equipment (PPE); observes standard precautions and transmission-based isolation procedures as appropriate
7. Identifies patient, introduces self and department
8. Explains purpose of the procedure and confirms patient understanding

Assessment and Implementation

9. Positions patient for procedure
10. Assesses patient including, where applicable, vital signs, SpO_2, breath sounds and ventilatory status

Follow-up

11. Reassesses and reinstructs patient as needed
12. Ensures patient comfort and safety
13. Maintains/processes equipment
14. Disposes of infectious waste and washes hands or applies disinfectant
15. Records pertinent data in chart and departmental records
16. Notifies appropriate personnel and makes any necessary recommendations or modifications to the patient care plan

Detailed steps are included for each procedure. The sequence may occasionally vary, but there is usually a critical order for many steps. Legal issues, such as verifying orders or respiratory protocols, patient identification, compliance with OSHA regulations or CDC guidelines for infection control, and documentation, are addressed. In more advance skills these common performance elements have been streamlined into a single step, thus avoiding needless repetition. The procedures are not brand specific regarding equipment, but are intended to verify that the student can select, obtain, assemble, verify function, and correct malfunctions of the required equipment for the procedure. Students should always clean up after the procedure, adhering to infection control guidelines. The manner in which the student interacts with patients or other health care professionals should also be assessed. Students should be able to react appropriately to adverse reactions, notify appropriate personnel, and make recommendations to modify the patient care plan according to patient needs.

The rating scale on the reverse of each PCE has also been revised in order to effect a more objective evaluation of the student's performance of that particular skill. A copy of the PCE for each skill is available in each chapter for laboratory or clinical application. Additional PCEs can be downloaded from Davis*Plus* (http://davisplus.fadavis.com). A complete alphabetical list of all PCEs is included in the front matter for easy reference. The skills included represent the most common entry-level and advanced procedures required of the respiratory care practitioner. The PCEs are intended to be used as study tools as well as evaluation tools. All procedures are in compliance with the AARC Clinical Practice Guidelines (CPGs).

The task to be evaluated is identified on each PCE form. The evaluator may be a peer or an instructor. The PCE form may be used for student review or peer evaluation, preclinical evaluation in the laboratory setting, and for clinical competency evaluation. Multiple copies should be made for these purposes. Each competency evaluation consists of a list of steps in the task or procedure, definitions of acceptable performance, a scoring scheme, and a performance rating form. The student's evaluation of a particular skill now includes objective scoring of the cognitive, psychomotor and affective domains.

When both the student and evaluator believe that a skill has been mastered, an evaluation session may be scheduled. It therefore follows that students should be fully prepared to demonstrate mastery *without assistance of any kind*. If it becomes necessary for the evaluator to intervene either to safeguard the patient's welfare or to expedite completion of the procedure, additional practice, laboratory or clinical, will be required and a repeat evaluation session will be necessary.

The student should fill out his or her complete name and the date of the evaluation, including the year. The conditions should be described, such as the level of patient cooperation; whether the procedure was performed on an infant, child, or adult; unexpected emergencies; if the procedure was simulated on a peer; or any other applicable variables. The equipment used (e.g., a particular brand of ventilator or spirometer) should be identified.

The scoring criteria reflect what the student knows, does, and says. Students should demonstrate knowledge of essential concepts as part of the procedural evaluation. The ability to apply, analyze, and synthesize didactic information in the clinical setting is needed for higher ratings. The procedures must be completed in a reasonable time frame consistent with patient safety and national time frame standards. Performance is rated as independent, minimal supervision required, competent, marginal, and dependent. The scoring guidelines for each level of performance are:

- Independent; near flawless performance; minimal errors; able to perform without supervision; seeks out new learning; shows initiative; A = 4.7–5.0 average

- Minimally Supervised: few errors, able to self-correct; seeks guidance when appropriate; B = 3.7–4.65

- Competent: minimum required level; No critical errors; Able to correct with coaching; Meets expectations; safe; C = 3.0–3.65

- Marginal: below average; critical errors or problem areas noted; would benefit from remediation D = 2.0–2.99

- Dependent: poor; unacceptable performance; unsafe; gross inaccuracies; potentially harmful F = <2.0.

The instructor also has the option of choosing "not applicable" for any step. If the student can correct noncritical errors without endangering patient safety or the validity of data, without prompting from the evaluator, a satisfactory rating should result.

Satisfactory completion of a given PCE requires more than a rigid adherence to the listed steps. The performance criteria include behaviors to be evaluated in addition to the procedural steps. Students are graded on these criteria using the same scale. A rating of 5 represents a near flawless performance while a 1 represents a performance fraught with error or dangerous behavior. Each item should be rated individually and independently, avoiding "middle-of-the-road" ratings.

Student performance should be rated using the score of 3 as the starting point. This represents average or minimal competency and indicates that the student's performance is safe and effective without critical errors. The student is able to self-correct errors, reports information accurately, and demonstrates awareness of his or her own limitations. No directive cues or prompting is needed, but the student may require supportive cues. Some unnecessary energy may be used to complete the activity, and the student may occasionally be anxious and distracted as skills become more complex.

A score of 1 indicates critical errors and unsafe practice, inability to demonstrate the behavior, or potentially harmful behaviors are noted frequently. The student demonstrates a lack of understanding of the basic concepts, inability to apply concepts or adapt to changing situations and is unaware of his or her limitations. The student lacks organization, appears frozen or is nonproductive, and requires continuous directive cues.

A score of 2 is below minimal competency. Performance is marginal or below average, and although the student may perform safely under direct supervision, performance is not always accurate, and some critical errors are noted. Improvement is needed and significant problem areas still exist.

A score of 4, above average or supervised performance, indicates that the student requires no directive prompting or correction, is able to self-correct errors, and is aware of his or her own limitations. Minimal supportive cues may be needed and some unnecessary energy may be used to complete activities.

The highest score of 5 is reserved for flawless performance, far exceeding expected level of performance. This is intended for the student who has superior knowledge, judgment, independence, and initiative. The student contributes to his or her own and the group's learning, spends minimal time on tasks, applies theory and rationale accurately each time, and uses subtle cues to modify his or her own behaviors.

The summary performance evaluation and recommendations section has been expanded to give more recommendations to the student. Therefore the student should have no question as to the result of the performance.

The evaluator should review the completed PCE evaluation with the student, emphasizing positive performance elements as well as areas needing improvement. Both evaluator and student should sign the completed PCE.

LABORATORY REPORT

Efficient use of laboratory time depends on adequate preparation by the student. The assigned chapter should be read before the scheduled laboratory session, and related didactic information should be reviewed. Students are encouraged to practice all skills as frequently as necessary in order to master the art of communication and the performance of psychomotor tasks. This will require additional independent laboratory time outside of scheduled sessions. Students should not realistically expect to be competent after performing a skill once or twice in a laboratory setting or after watching someone else perform the task.

Data collection and observations performed during the laboratory exercises should be documented completely and neatly on the laboratory report form. Each section of exercises and subsets that require documentation of data or observations is correlated with the corresponding number in the chapter. Exercises that do not require any documentation are excluded.

The laboratory session is intended for hands-on practice. Questions and calculations that do not involve direct contact with equipment or performance of procedures should be completed outside of laboratory time. Answers to the Critical Thinking Questions should be written out neatly or word processed and attached to the laboratory report. The question and corresponding number should be included in the attachment to facilitate ease of grading for the instructor.

The questions at the end of each laboratory report are not designed to be answered solely from performing the laboratory exercises and procedures, nor from a single reference source. Students are expected to research a variety of supplemental readings. Keeping current with the literature is an important part of professional development.

Students are expected to complete the laboratory report and all questions. The report should be submitted to the instructor by the assigned date. Deductions for late reports, according to individual programs' policies, are to be expected. The remainder of the laboratory chapter should be kept intact. Students may wish to keep returned graded laboratory reports for further review and study.

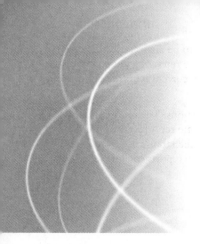

Procedural Competency Evaluations Directory

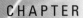

Laboratory and Clinical Safety

INTRODUCTION

Whether in the laboratory or clinical setting, successful and positive experiences can only occur if the student is well-oriented into those environments. Employers spend the necessary time and resources to ensure that employees are informed about safety in the work environment. The same should occur with respiratory care students.

OBJECTIVES

Upon completion of this chapter, the student will be able to:

1. Relate the safety information contained on an MSDS sheet.
2. Perform a scene survey to establish the safety of a setting.
3. Identify potential safety hazards in the laboratory or clinical setting.
4. Safely position a patient in the semi-Fowler's position.

KEY TERMS

hazardous material
MSDS sheet
OSHA

professionalism
prone
safety

semi-Fowler's position
supine
surrogate

Exercises

EQUIPMENT REQUIRED

☐ Call bell
☐ Clinical agency and/or college safety or policy and procedure manual
☐ Hospital bed (or equivalent)
☐ Mannequin
☐ Pillows

EXERCISE 1.1 PROFESSIONALISM

The instructor will review the following with you:

1. Laboratory schedule, availability, hours, open-lab
2. Rules for equipment use, storage and clean-up, eating and drinking in the lab area, oxygen or compressed air usage
3. Reporting mechanisms
4. Punctuality
5. Dress and personal hygiene codes
6. Professional responsibility

The following basic rules should be observed in order to make the laboratory a safe and meaningful experience:

1. Students should read the assignments **before** the start of each laboratory session. It is important that there be a familiarity with terminology, equipment, and the types of exercises before beginning any practice.
2. For any independent practice, students must sign in and out according to laboratory policies.
3. Smoking, eating, and drinking should not be allowed in the laboratory area. Food should not be stored in the laboratory area. "No Smoking" signs should be posted even though most educational and healthcare institutions are "smoke free."
4. Applying cosmetics or contact lenses should not be permitted in the laboratory area.
5. All equipment must be handled with care. Compressed gas cylinders must never be left freestanding. Oil, grease, and any other flammable materials should not be used near oxygen equipment.
6. Equipment should not be handled before instruction in its use is given by the instructor.
7. Any defective or broken equipment must be reported immediately to the laboratory instructor or supervisor. This includes any equipment with frayed wires or loose connections. Immediately report any electrical equipment that is sparking or that causes a shock.
8. Personal protective equipment (PPE) should be used as required in the exercises.
9. Handle all chemicals and disinfecting solutions as instructed. MSDSs should be available for all substances kept in the laboratory.
10. Needles should not be recapped with two hands. All sharps should be disposed of in the puncture-proof containers provided.
11. Any injury or accidental needle stick should be reported immediately to the instructor or laboratory supervisor.
12. All students are responsible for cleaning up after each laboratory session. The laboratory personnel are not substitutes for housekeeping or mothers. Discard any papers or disposable equipment and supplies properly before leaving the laboratory.
13. Make sure all equipment is turned off and returned to its proper place before leaving.
14. Any disposable equipment that is assigned to students for repeated use (such as oxygen devices, noseclips, or mouthpieces) should be stored in a designated container and labeled with the student's name. It is the student's responsibility to maintain this equipment and have it available for the laboratory exercises.
15. Never remove equipment from the laboratory unless instructed to do so.

EXERCISE 1.2 AARC GUIDE TO PROFESSIONALISM MODULE

1. Have the students go to the AARC web site and review the presentation on Professionalism at http://www.aarc.org/resources/professionalism/.
2. The student should read the following statements:
   A. Statement of Ethics and Professional Conduct
   B. Role Model Statement
   C. Position Statement on Diversity
3. Have the students review the following questions from the module:
   A. What behaviors have you observed among healthcare providers that you consider unprofessional?
   B. Are there behaviors that you consider essential to professionalism that were not addressed in the program?
   C. What is the most important attribute of the professional you most admire?
4. Split the students into smaller groups.
   A. Have the students engage in a 10- to 15-minute discussion.
   B. Students should appoint a designated recorder.
5. Have the student group recorders share and discuss their small group conclusions.

EXERCISE 1.3 MEDICAL DIRECTOR OR PHYSICIAN INTERACTION

Have the Medical Director (or designee) prepare a 15- to 30-minute talk on professionalism and the respiratory therapist. Topics to include are therapist–physician interaction; role of the therapist in the physician practice, and the need for clear, unambiguous communication.

EXERCISE 1.4 SAFETY CONSIDERATIONS

EXERCISE 1.4.1 ELECTRICAL SAFETY

Have the students review the clinical agency or college policy and procedure manual regarding electrical safety. **Summarize the policies on your laboratory report.**

EXERCISE 1.4.2 FIRE SAFETY

Have the students review the clinical agency or college policy and procedure manual regarding fire safety. **Summarize the policies on your laboratory report.**

EXERCISE 1.4.3 OSHA STANDARDS

Have the students review the clinical agency or college policy and procedure manual regarding OSHA standards for workplace safety. **Summarize the policies on your laboratory report.**

EXERCISE 1.4.4 HAZARDOUS MATERIALS AND MSDS SHEETS

Have the students locate the MSDS manual and have them compare its contents to the sample MSDS sheet shown in Figure 1.1. **Record health hazard data and special protection and precaution information on your laboratory report.**

The Clorox Company
7200 Johnson Drive
Pleasanton, California 94588
Tel. (510) 847-6100

Material Safety Data Sheet

I Product:	CLOROX BLEACH - FOR INSTITUTIONAL USE
Description:	CLEAR, LIGHT YELLOW LIQUID WITH CHLORINE ODOR

Other Designations	Manufacturer	Emergency Telephone No.
EPA Reg. No. 5813-1 Sodium hypochlorite soultion Liquid chlorine bleach Clorox Liquid Bleach Clorox Germicidal Bleach	The Clorox Company 1221 Broadway Oakland, CA 94612	For Medical Emergencies, call Rocky Mountain Poison Center: 1-800-446-1014 For Transportation Emergencies, call: Chemtrec: 1-800-424-9300

II Health Hazard Data

*Causes substantial but temporary eye injury. May irritate skin. May cause nausea and vomiting if ingested. Exposure to vapor or mist may irritate nose, throat and lungs. The following medical conditions may be aggravated by exposure to high concentrations of vapor or mist; heart conditions or chronic respiratory problems such as asthma, chronic bronchitis or obstructive lung disease. Under normal consumer use conditions the likelihood of any adverse health effects are low.

FIRST AID: EYE CONTACT: Immediately flush eyes with plenty of water. If irritation persists, see a doctor. SKIN CONTACT: Remove contaminated clothing. Wash area with water. INGESTION: Drink a glassful of water and call a physician. INHALATION: If breathing problems develop remove to fresh air.

III Hazardous Ingredients

Ingredients	Concentration	Worker Exposure Limit
Sodium hypochlorite CAS # 7681-52-9	5.25%	not established

None of the ingredients in this product are on the IARC, NTP or OSHA carcinogen list. Occasional clinical reports suggest a low potential for sensitization upon exaggerated exposure to sodium hypochlorite if skin damage (e.g. irritation) occurs during exposure. Routine clinical tests conducted on intact skin with Clorox Liquid Bleach found no sensitization in the test subjects.

IV Special Protection and Precautions

Hygienic Practices: Wear safety glasses. With repeated or prolonged use, wear gloves.

Engineering Controls: Use general ventilation to minimize exposure to vapor or mist.

Work Practices: Avoid eye and skin contact and inhalation of vapor or mist.

Keep out of the reach of children.

V Transportation and Regulatory Data

U.S. DOT Hazard Class: Not restricted

U.S. DOT Proper Shipping Name: Hypochlorite solution with not more than 7% available chlorine. Not Restricted per 49CFR172.101(c)(12)(iv).

EPA CERCLA/SARA TITLE III Superfund Amendment and Reauthorization Act:

	CERLA/304		
	RQ (lbs)	311/312	313
Sodium hypochlorite	100	----	---
Sodium hydroxide	1000	Yes	---

VI Spill or Leak Procedures

Small Spills (<5 gallons)
1) Absorb, containerize, and landfill in accordance with local regulations.
(2) Wash down residual to sanitary sewer.*

Large Spills (>5 gallons)
1) Absorb, containerize, and landfill in accordance with local regulations; wash down residual to sanitary sewer.* - OR - (2) Pump material to waste drum(s) and dispose in accordance with local regulations; wash down residual to sanitary sewer.*

VII Reactivity Data

Stable under normal use and storage conditions. Strong oxidizing agent. Reacts with other household chemicals such as toilet bowl cleaners, rust removers, vinegar, acids or ammonia containing products to produce hazardous gases, such as chlorine and other chlorinated species. Prolonged contact with metal may cause pitting or discoloration.

VIII Fire and Explosion Data

Not flammable or explosive. In a fire, cool containers to prevent rupture and release of sodium chlorate.

IX Physical Data

Boiling point . . . . 212°F/100°C decomposes)
Specific Gravity (H₂O=1) 1.085
Solubility in Water . . . . complete
pH 11.4

Figure 1.1. Material safety data sheet (MSDS) for Clorox. (Courtesy of the Clorox Co., Oakland, CA.)

EXERCISE 1.5 SCENE SURVEY

EXERCISE 1.5.1 IDENTIFICATION OF SAFETY HAZARDS—DIAGRAM

Identify at least 10 safety hazards in Figure 1.2. **Record the list on your laboratory report.**

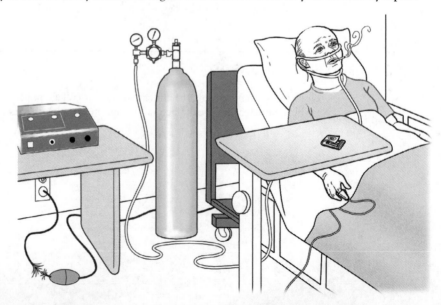

Figure 1.2. Scene survey; identification of safety hazards.

EXERCISE 1.5.2 IDENTIFICATION OF SAFETY HAZARDS—SCENARIO

In this exercise, the instructor uses a mannequin or student to act as a surrogate patient.

With the "patient" in bed, the instructor prepares the scene to include possible safety hazards. The student then performs the following:

1. When entering the "patient" area, quickly observe your surroundings. Look up, down, and all around. Take a maximum of 45 seconds.
2. Turn away from the scene and **record on your laboratory report** all your recollections about the scene for the following factors:
    A. Was the scene safe? List any hazardous conditions.
    B. What equipment did you see in the immediate area?
    C. Were the conditions conducive to patient comfort?
        i. What were the environmental conditions like? Describe the temperature, humidity, lighting, and cleanliness.
        ii. Were the patient's material needs within easy reach?

EXERCISE 1.6 PATIENT POSITIONING

Using a mannequin or fellow student, place him or her in a semi-Fowler's position.

1. Ensure that no peripheral lines or oxygen tubing is taut or caught on the side rails.
2. Lower the side rails and position the "patient" properly in the supine position.
3. Adjust any pillows or blankets as necessary.
4. Elevate the head of the bed to a 45-degree angle.
5. Raise and secure side rails.
6. Ensure that the nurse call bell is within reach.
7. Ensure that all other patient-required materials are in reach.
8. Reinspect the scene before leaving to make sure there are no unsafe conditions.

Laboratory Report

CHAPTER 1: LABORATORY AND CLINICAL SAFETY

Name _____   Date _____

Course/Section _____   Instructor _____

Data Collection

EXERCISE 1.2 AARC Guide to Professionalism

SMALL GROUP DISCUSSION NOTES

Recorder: _____

Group members: _____

Unprofessional behaviors: _____

_____

_____

Essential behaviors: _____

_____

_____

Most important attribute: _____

Professionalism post-test (if asigned by instuctor). **Attach score.** _____

EXERCISE 1.4 Safety Considerations

EXERCISE 1.4.1 ELECTRICAL SAFETY

Summarize policies: _____

_____

_____

_____

EXERCISE 1.4.2 FIRE SAFETY

RACE: _____

PASS: _____

Nearest emergency exits: _____

Fire alarm: _____

Fire extinguisher: Location _____ Type _____

RT responsibilities: _____

EXERCISE 1.4.3 OSHA STANDARDS

OSHA regulation no.: _____

Date of policy manual: _____

Prohibited activities: _____

EXERCISE 1.4.4 HAZARDOUS MATERIALS AND MSDS SHEETS

Attach printout. _____

Name of chemical: _____

Health risk: _____

Flammability: _____

Reactivity: _____

PPE: _____

First aid procedures: _____

Antidote (if any): _____

EXERCISE 1.5.1 SCENE SURVEY (Fig. 1.2)

1. _____ 2. _____

3. _____ 4. _____

5. _____ 6. _____

7. _____ 8. _____

9. _____ 10. _____

EXERCISE 1.5.2 IDENTIFICATION OF SAFETY HAZARDS (SCENARIO)

1. Was the scene safe? List any hazardous conditions.

   A. _____

   B. _____

   C. _____

   D. _____

   E. _____

   F. _____

   G. _____

   H. _____

   I. _____

   J. _____

2. What equipment was seen in the immediate area? _____

3. Were the conditions conducive to patient comfort? _____

4. What were the environmental conditions like? Describe the temperature, humidity, lighting, and cleanliness. _____

   _____

5. Were the patient's material needs within easy reach? _____

Critical Thinking Questions

1. Why is it necessary for hospitals to have special codes for fire, disasters, and cardiac arrests?

2. Scenario: You are asked to enter a patient's room to perform morning vital signs. When you approach the patient, you put the side rail of the bed down to allow better access to the patient. There is an intravenous (IV) pump on the same side on which you are standing. As you grab the IV pump to move it out of the way, you feel a mild tingling sensation in your hand.

    A. What would your next actions be?

    B. Why?

Procedural Competency Evaluation

STUDENT: **DATE:**

CLINICAL ORIENTATION

Evaluator: ☐ Peer ☐ Instructor	**Setting:** ☐ Lab	☐ Clinical Simulation
Equipment Utilized:	**Conditions (Describe):**	

Performance Level:

S or ✓ = Satisfactory, no errors of omission or commission
U = Unsatisfactory Error of Omission or Commission
NA = Not applicable

Performance Rating:

5   **Independent:** Near flawless performance; minimal errors; able to perform without supervision; seeks out new learning; shows initiative; A = 4.7–5.0 average

4   **Minimally Supervised:** Few errors, able to self-correct; seeks guidance when appropriate; B = 3.7–4.65

3   **Competent:** Minimal required level; no critical errors; able to correct with coaching; meets expectations; safe; C = 3.0–3.65

2   **Marginal:** Below average; critical errors or problem areas noted; would benefit from remediation; D = 2.0–2.99

1   **Dependent:** Poor; unacceptable performance; unsafe; gross inaccuracies; potentially harmful; F = < 2.0

Two or more errors of commission or omission of mandatory or essential performance elements will terminate the procedure, and require additional practice and/or remediation and reevaluation. Student is responsible for obtaining additional evaluation forms as needed from the Director of Clinical Education (DCE).

Columns on right: PERFORMANCE RATING | PERFORMANCE LEVEL

STUDENT PREPARATION

	RATING	LEVEL
1. Obtained health clearance		
2. CPR certification verified		
3. Completed OSHA Blood Borne Pathogen training		
4. Completed HIPAA training		
5. Completed any other training as required by the clinical site		
6. Compliant with uniform dress code including: cleanliness of uniform, appropriate length of hair, and hand and fingernail hygiene		
7. Has stethoscope and other appropriate equipment		
8. Has received a clinical policy and procedure manual		
9. Placed in a course appropriate clinical rotation		

CLINICAL SITE

	RATING	LEVEL
10. Introduced to Department Director and other appropriate clinical staff		
11. Given tour of the facility		
12. Instructed on site-specific policies regarding: infection control, fire and safety, cell phone and beeper usage, and other policies		

SIGNATURES   Student: Evaluator: Date:

Clinical Performance Evaluation

PERFORMANCE RATING:

5   **Independent:** Near flawless performance; minimal errors; able to perform without supervision; seeks out new learning; shows initiative; A = 4.7–5.0 average

4   **Minimally Supervised:** Few errors, able to self-correct; seeks guidance when appropriate; B = 3.7–4.65

3   **Competent:** Minimal required level; no critical errors; able to correct with coaching; meets expectations; safe; C = 3.0–3.65

2   **Marginal:** Below average; critical errors or problem areas noted; would benefit from remediation; D = 2.0–2.99

1   **Dependent:** Poor; unacceptable performance; unsafe; gross inaccuracies; potentially harmful; F = < 2.0

Circle the appropriate response below. Please be consistent, objective, and honest in your assessment of the student's clinical performance and ability.

PERFORMANCE CRITERIA	SCORE				
COGNITIVE DOMAIN					
1. Consistently displays knowledge, comprehension, and command of essential concepts	5	4	3	2	1
2. Demonstrates the relationship between theory and clinical practice	5	4	3	2	1
3. Able to select, review, apply, analyze, synthesize, interpret, and evaluate information; makes recommendations to modify care plan	5	4	3	2	1
PSYCHOMOTOR DOMAIN					
4. Minimal errors, no critical errors; able to self-correct; performs all steps safely and accurately	5	4	3	2	1
5. Selects, assembles, and verifies proper function and cleanliness of equipment; assures operation and corrects malfunctions; provides adequate care and maintenance	5	4	3	2	1
6. Exhibits the required manual dexterity	5	4	3	2	1
7. Performs procedure in a reasonable time frame for clinical level	5	4	3	2	1
8. Applies and maintains aseptic technique and PPE as required	5	4	3	2	1
9. Maintains concise and accurate patient and clinical records	5	4	3	2	1
10. Reports promptly on patient status/needs to appropriate personnel	5	4	3	2	1
AFFECTIVE DOMAIN					
11. Exhibits courteous and pleasant demeanor; shows consideration and respect, honesty, and integrity	5	4	3	2	1
12. Communicates verbally and in writing clearly and concisely	5	4	3	2	1
13. Preserves confidentiality and adheres to all policies	5	4	3	2	1
14. Follows directions, exhibits sound judgment, and seeks help when required	5	4	3	2	1
15. Demonstrates initiative, self-direction, responsibility, and accountability	5	4	3	2	1

TOTAL POINTS = _____ /15 = AVERAGE GRADE = _____

ADDITIONAL COMMENTS: IDENTIFY AREAS OF EXCELLENCE; LIST ERRORS OF OMISSION OR COMMISSION, CRITICAL ERRORS

SUMMARY PERFORMANCE EVALUATION AND RECOMMENDATIONS

☐ PASS: Satisfactory Performance

     ☐ Minimal supervision needed, may progress to next level provided specific skills, clinical time completed

     ☐ Minimal supervision needed, able to progress to next level without remediation

☐ FAIL: Unsatisfactory Performance (check all that apply)

     ☐ Minor reevaluation only

     ☐ Needs additional clinical practice before reevaluation

     ☐ Needs additional laboratory practice before skills performed in clinical area

     ☐ Recommend clinical probation

SIGNATURES

Evaluator (print name): _____ Evaluator signature: _____ Date: _____

Student Signature: _____ Date: _____

Student Comments:

Procedural Competency Evaluation

STUDENT: **DATE:**

PATIENT POSITIONING AND SAFETY

		PERFORMANCE RATING	PERFORMANCE LEVEL
Evaluator: ☐ Peer ☐ Instructor **Setting:** ☐ Lab ☐ Clinical Simulation			
Equipment Utilized: **Conditions (Describe):**			

Performance Level:
 	
    S or ✓ = Satisfactory, no errors of omission or commission
    U = Unsatisfactory Error of Omission or Commission
    NA = Not applicable			

Performance Rating:
 	
  5   **Independent:** Near flawless performance; minimal errors; able to perform without supervision; seeks out new learning; shows initiative; A = 4.7–5.0 average
  4   **Minimally Supervised:** Few errors, able to self-correct; seeks guidance when appropriate; B = 3.7–4.65
  3   **Competent:** Minimal required level; no critical errors; able to correct with coaching; meets expectations; safe; C = 3.0–3.65
  2   **Marginal:** Below average; critical errors or problem areas noted; would benefit from remediation; D = 2.0–2.99
  1   **Dependent:** Poor; unacceptable performance; unsafe; gross inaccuracies; potentially harmful; F = < 2.0
 	
    Two or more errors of commission or omission of mandatory or essential performance elements will terminate the procedure, and require additional practice and/or remediation and reevaluation. Student is responsible for obtaining additional evaluation forms as needed from the Director of Clinical Education (DCE).			

EQUIPMENT AND PATIENT PREPARATION			
1. Common Performance Elements Steps 1–8			
2. Reads the medical record for any patient safety precautions identified: cardiac precautions, fall precautions, NPO, and/or fluid restriction			
3. Reads the medical record for any contraindication to position changes: post surgical procedure orders, blood pressure precautions, etc.			
4. Observes the presence and location of any IV line, gastric tubes, arterial lines that would need to be safe guarded during a position change			
5. Lowers side rail			
6. Repositions patient into the desired position using assistance if required			
7. Insures the safety and integrity of any inserted lines			
8. Observes/assesses for any changes in mental status, blood pressure, and pulse oximetry			
9. Asks the patient (if able to respond) if any dizziness, nausea, or other complaints are present			
10. Raises the side rail			
11. Reaffirms patient comfort			
FOLLOW-UP			
12. Common Performance Elements Steps 11–16			

SIGNATURES   Student: Evaluator: Date:

Clinical Performance Evaluation

PERFORMANCE RATING:

5   **Independent:** Near flawless performance; minimal errors; able to perform without supervision; seeks out new learning; shows initiative; A = 4.7–5.0 average

4   **Minimally Supervised:** Few errors, able to self-correct; seeks guidance when appropriate; B = 3.7–4.65

3   **Competent:** Minimal required level; no critical errors; able to correct with coaching; meets expectations; safe; C = 3.0–3.65

2   **Marginal:** Below average; critical errors or problem areas noted; would benefit from remediation; D = 2.0–2.99

1   **Dependent:** Poor; unacceptable performance; unsafe; gross inaccuracies; potentially harmful; F = < 2.0

Circle the appropriate response below. Please be consistent, objective, and honest in your assessment of the student's clinical performance and ability.

PERFORMANCE CRITERIA	SCORE				
COGNITIVE DOMAIN					
1. Consistently displays knowledge, comprehension, and command of essential concepts	5	4	3	2	1
2. Demonstrates the relationship between theory and clinical practice	5	4	3	2	1
3. Able to select, review, apply, analyze, synthesize, interpret, and evaluate information; makes recommendations to modify care plan	5	4	3	2	1
PSYCHOMOTOR DOMAIN					
4. Minimal errors, no critical errors; able to self-correct; performs all steps safely and accurately	5	4	3	2	1
5. Selects, assembles, and verifies proper function and cleanliness of equipment; assures operation and corrects malfunctions; provides adequate care and maintenance	5	4	3	2	1
6. Exhibits the required manual dexterity	5	4	3	2	1
7. Performs procedure in a reasonable time frame for clinical level	5	4	3	2	1
8. Applies and maintains aseptic technique and PPE as required	5	4	3	2	1
9. Maintains concise and accurate patient and clinical records	5	4	3	2	1
10. Reports promptly on patient status/needs to appropriate personnel	5	4	3	2	1
AFFECTIVE DOMAIN					
11. Exhibits courteous and pleasant demeanor; shows consideration and respect, honesty, and integrity	5	4	3	2	1
12. Communicates verbally and in writing clearly and concisely	5	4	3	2	1
13. Preserves confidentiality and adheres to all policies	5	4	3	2	1
14. Follows directions, exhibits sound judgment, and seeks help when required	5	4	3	2	1
15. Demonstrates initiative, self-direction, responsibility, and accountability	5	4	3	2	1

TOTAL POINTS =   /15 = AVERAGE GRADE =

ADDITIONAL COMMENTS: IDENTIFY AREAS OF EXCELLENCE; LIST ERRORS OF OMISSION OR COMMISSION, CRITICAL ERRORS

SUMMARY PERFORMANCE EVALUATION AND RECOMMENDATIONS

☐ PASS: Satisfactory Performance

    ☐ Minimal supervision needed, may progress to next level provided specific skills, clinical time completed

    ☐ Minimal supervision needed, able to progress to next level without remediation

☐ FAIL: Unsatisfactory Performance (check all that apply)

    ☐ Minor reevaluation only

    ☐ Needs additional clinical practice before reevaluation

    ☐ Needs additional laboratory practice before skills performed in clinical area

    ☐ Recommend clinical probation

SIGNATURES

Evaluator (print name):   Evaluator signature: Date:

Student Signature: Date:

Student Comments:

Procedural Competency Evaluation

STUDENT: DATE:

PATIENT AND CAREGIVER TRAINING

Evaluator: ☐ Peer ☐ Instructor	**Setting:** ☐ Lab ☐ Clinical Simulation
Equipment Utilized:	**Conditions (Describe):**

Performance Level:

    S or ✓ = Satisfactory, no errors of omission or commission
    U = Unsatisfactory Error of Omission or Commission
    NA = Not applicable

Performance Rating:

5   **Independent:** Near flawless performance; minimal errors; able to perform without supervision; seeks out new learning; shows initiative; A = 4.7–5.0 average

4   **Minimally Supervised:** Few errors, able to self-correct; seeks guidance when appropriate; B = 3.7–4.65

3   **Competent:** Minimal required level; no critical errors; able to correct with coaching; meets expectations; safe; C = 3.0–3.65

2   **Marginal:** Below average; critical errors or problem areas noted; would benefit from remediation; D = 2.0–2.99

1   **Dependent:** Poor; unacceptable performance; unsafe; gross inaccuracies; potentially harmful; F = < 2.0

Two or more errors of commission or omission of mandatory or essential performance elements will terminate the procedure, and require additional practice and/or remediation and reevaluation. Student is responsible for obtaining additional evaluation forms as needed from the Director of Clinical Education (DCE).

	PERFORMANCE RATING	PERFORMANCE LEVEL
EQUIPMENT AND PATIENT PREPARATION		
1. Common Performance Elements Steps 1–8		
ASSESSMENT AND IMPLEMENTATION		
2. Common Performance Elements Steps 9 and 10		
3. Assesses the patient and/or family members for limitations to training		
A. Language, literacy, or cultural barriers		
B. Motivation and cooperation		
C. Physical impairment (e.g., hypoxia, decreased sensorium, hearing, vision, energy, age-specific, pain, medication side effects)		
D. Psychosocial barriers (e.g., anxiety, depression, substance abuse)		
4. Determines gap between current knowledge and educational goals		
5. Interviews patient or caregiver regarding past experience with topic being taught		
6. Observes patient's or caregiver's performance of skills and determines whether they are adequate for self-care		
7. Arranges convenient time for patient, family, caregiver, and practitioner		
8. Arranges location for training conducive to learning		
9. Prepares/obtains lesson plan and instructional materials		
10. Limits interruptions, distractions, and noise		
11. Conducts educational session using terminology appropriate to audience		
12. Monitors patient or caregiver during training session including verbal and nonverbal responses		
13. Evaluates outcomes by appropriate methods including:		
A. Demonstration of skills		
B. Verbal, non-threatening questioning		
C. Requests patient or caregiver to repeat information in own words		
14. Answers patient or caregiver questions using terminology appropriate to audience		
FOLLOW-UP		
15. Common Performance Elements Steps 11–16		
16. Documents competencies achieved		

SIGNATURES   Student: Evaluator: Date:

Clinical Performance Evaluation

PERFORMANCE RATING:

5   **Independent:** Near flawless performance; minimal errors; able to perform without supervision; seeks out new learning; shows initiative; A = 4.7–5.0 average

4   **Minimally Supervised:** Few errors, able to self-correct; seeks guidance when appropriate; B = 3.7–4.65

3   **Competent:** Minimal required level; no critical errors; able to correct with coaching; meets expectations; safe; C = 3.0–3.65

2   **Marginal:** Below average; critical errors or problem areas noted; would benefit from remediation; D = 2.0–2.99

1   **Dependent:** Poor; unacceptable performance; unsafe; gross inaccuracies; potentially harmful; F = < 2.0

Circle the appropriate response below. Please be consistent, objective, and honest in your assessment of the student's clinical performance and ability.

PERFORMANCE CRITERIA	SCORE				
COGNITIVE DOMAIN					
1. Consistently displays knowledge, comprehension, and command of essential concepts	5	4	3	2	1
2. Demonstrates the relationship between theory and clinical practice	5	4	3	2	1
3. Able to select, review, apply, analyze, synthesize, interpret, and evaluate information; makes recommendations to modify care plan	5	4	3	2	1
PSYCHOMOTOR DOMAIN					
4. Minimal errors, no critical errors; able to self-correct; performs all steps safely and accurately	5	4	3	2	1
5. Selects, assembles, and verifies proper function and cleanliness of equipment; assures operation and corrects malfunctions; provides adequate care and maintenance	5	4	3	2	1
6. Exhibits the required manual dexterity	5	4	3	2	1
7. Performs procedure in a reasonable time frame for clinical level	5	4	3	2	1
8. Applies and maintains aseptic technique and PPE as required	5	4	3	2	1
9. Maintains concise and accurate patient and clinical records	5	4	3	2	1
10. Reports promptly on patient status/needs to appropriate personnel	5	4	3	2	1
AFFECTIVE DOMAIN					
11. Exhibits courteous and pleasant demeanor; shows consideration and respect, honesty, and integrity	5	4	3	2	1
12. Communicates verbally and in writing clearly and concisely	5	4	3	2	1
13. Preserves confidentiality and adheres to all policies	5	4	3	2	1
14. Follows directions, exhibits sound judgment, and seeks help when required	5	4	3	2	1
15. Demonstrates initiative, self-direction, responsibility, and accountability	5	4	3	2	1

TOTAL POINTS =   /15 = AVERAGE GRADE =

ADDITIONAL COMMENTS: IDENTIFY AREAS OF EXCELLENCE; LIST ERRORS OF OMISSION OR COMMISSION, CRITICAL ERRORS

SUMMARY PERFORMANCE EVALUATION AND RECOMMENDATIONS

☐ PASS: Satisfactory Performance

    ☐ Minimal supervision needed, may progress to next level provided specific skills, clinical time completed

    ☐ Minimal supervision needed, able to progress to next level without remediation

☐ FAIL: Unsatisfactory Performance (check all that apply)

    ☐ Minor reevaluation only

    ☐ Needs additional clinical practice before reevaluation

    ☐ Needs additional laboratory practice before skills performed in clinical area

    ☐ Recommend clinical probation

SIGNATURES

Evaluator (print name):   Evaluator signature: Date:

Student Signature: Date:

Student Comments:

2 Communication and Cultural Diversity in Healthcare

INTRODUCTION

Oral and written **communication** is one of the key skills required by all healthcare practitioners. This chapter will address oral communication skills; Chapter 5 will address written skills. The respiratory therapist must communicate orally on several levels. First is peer communication with nurses, fellow therapists, and other members of the healthcare team. Second is communication with physicians and supervisors. Third and most important is communication with the client. While the communication should be clear, **empathetic**, and therapeutic, the practitioner must also be able to communicate with clients of all ages. This age-specific communication competency requires practice. Therefore, each level of communication requires a different approach and skill. In the healthcare setting, many factors influence communication. These are summarized in Table 2.1.

In addition, careful attention must be paid to understand the cultural and religious needs of the client. This requires the cultivation of a **sensitivity** to the **cultural diversity** of the population. Language barriers, inappropriate use of translators, and lack of time frequently are misinterpreted as bias, prejudice, or disrespect.

OBJECTIVES

Upon completion of this chapter, the student will be able to:

1. Relate factors that influence communication.
2. Discuss the impact of culture on healthcare delivery.
3. Use therapeutic communication skills to establish patient rapport.

KEY TERMS

communication
cultural diversity

empathetic
sensitivity

Exercises

EQUIPMENT REQUIRED

None

Table 2.1 Factors Influencing
Communication

	Internal Factors	Sensory/ Emotional Factors	Environmental Factors	Verbal Expression	Nonverbal Expression
Clinician	Previous experiences Attitudes, values Cultural heritage Religion Self-concept Listening habits Preoccupation Feelings Age	Stress Workload Nonwork- related issues	Lighting Noise Privacy Distance	Jargon Technical language Voice tone	Body language Facial expressions Dress Professionalism Warmth Interest
Client	Previous experiences Attitudes, values Cultural heritage Religion Self-concept Listening habits Preoccupation Feelings Illness Age	Fear Pain Anxiety Stress Mental acuity Brain injury Hypoxia Sense impair- ment	Lighting Noise Privacy Distance Temperature	Language barrier Jargon Voice tone	Body language Facial expressions

Adapted from Wilkins, RL, Sheldon, RL, and Krider, SJ: Clinical Assessment in Respiratory Care, ed 2, Mosby-Year Book, St. Louis, 1990.

EXERCISE 2.1 COMMUNICATION EXERCISE

Discuss with your laboratory partner any experiences each of you may have had as patients in a hospital or other setting. Describe your feelings in this situation. Include in your discussion attitudes toward healthcare that are culturally based. Do you feel that the quality of your care was affected by cultural, ethnic, or racial issues? If you and your partner have never had these experiences, describe what concerns would be most important in the event one of you was hospitalized. Have the groups share their experiences with the class.

EXERCISE 2.2 CULTURAL DIVERSITY

EXERCISE 2.2.1 CULTURE-RELATED HEALTHCARE BELIEFS

Divide the students into diverse pairs. Ask each student to identify with which cultural group he or she identifies. Ask the students to list five cultural influences that have an effect on their healthcare beliefs. These may be related to diet, religious practice, or family influences. **Record the beliefs on your laboratory report.** Have students share their culture-related healthcare beliefs with the class. Compare the similarities and contrast the differences.

EXERCISE 2.2.2 CULTURAL CASE STUDY

Scenario

Read the following scenario and critique how the case was handled. What could the caregivers have done to be more culturally aware and sensitive to the needs of the client?

Mr. Rodriguez is a 70-year-old Mexican man recently arrived in the United States, who does not speak English. He is brought to the emergency department (ED) by his 13-year-old granddaughter. The nurse asks him why he is in the ED. He begins to explain in Spanish, but the nurse cuts him off and starts quizzing the girl. Mr. Rodriguez begins to get agitated at the nurse, screams aloud, and clutches his chest. The nurse asks the young girl to leave and shouts at Mr. Rodriguez to shut up. The physician's assistant, who has been in the room the entire time, begins to take vital signs and start an IV in silence. Mr. Rodriguez is still agitated but takes out a religious prayer card and begins praying. The nurse confiscates the card, muttering that this is not the appropriate place for personal property to be kept.

Laboratory Report

CHAPTER 2: Communication and Cultural Diversity in Healthcare

Name _____ Date _____

Course/Section _____ Instructor _____

Data Collection

EXERCISE 2.1 Communication Exercise

_____

_____

_____

_____

_____

EXERCISE 2.2 Cultural Diversity

EXERCISE 2.2.1 CULTURE-RELATED HEALTHCARE BELIEFS

Cultural or ethnic group:

Culture-related healthcare beliefs:

1.

2.

3.

4.

5.

Critical Thinking Questions

1. How might differences in cultural or ethnic background between the practitioner and the client affect the practitioner's ability to perform a patient assessment?

2. How might a respiratory care practitioner better prepare for and understand the cultural needs of the patient when providing care?

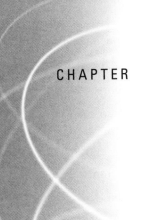

3 Infection Control

For centuries, infectious diseases have been the major cause of death in humans. Until recently, the scientific community believed that advances in the development of vaccines and antibiotic therapy would eliminate many infectious diseases by the 21st century. However, misuse and overuse of antibiotics, lax attitudes regarding the application of these advances, and the remarkable ability of microorganisms to adapt are threatening much of the progress made in the fight against infection. As a result, we now find ourselves faced with a resurgence of diseases that were thought to be no longer a problem, including tuberculosis, measles, cholera, and typhoid.

Resistant strains of microorganisms and the discovery of previously unheard of infectious diseases such as SARS and H5-N1 influenza are appearing in **epidemic** proportions. All are challenging our medical technology and altering the way healthcare is delivered.

The combination of a susceptible host, invasive procedures providing a route of transmission, and the presence of **virulent** and antibiotic-resistant strains of microbial organisms makes healthcare settings the perfect location for the transmission of infectious disease.

Recent concerns center around the protection of healthcare workers from bloodborne pathogens, which include but are not limited to hepatitis B virus, HIV, and related transmissible illnesses such as tuberculosis.[1]

Infection control in the healthcare setting has two primary goals. The first is to protect healthcare workers from transmissible diseases. The second is to reduce the incidence of **nosocomial** infections in susceptible patients. All healthcare personnel must maintain an up-to-date knowledge and compliance with most current guidelines.

We can reduce the risks to healthcare workers and patients by four methods[2]:

1. *Providing barriers to transmission.* This includes understanding the routes of transmission and applying standard precautions and transmission-based isolation procedures to prevent transmission.

2. *Eliminating sources of infectious agents.* This includes decontamination, disinfection, and sterilization of equipment; proper disposal of infectious waste; and, most important, handwashing or hand sanitation before and after patient contact, attending to any personal hygiene activities, and proper handling of dirty and clean equipment.

3. *Reducing host susceptibility.* This includes factors related to the patient's immune status, reducing exposure to sources of infection, appropriate use of antimicrobial agents, and limiting invasive procedures to only those that are essential.

4. *Monitoring and evaluating the effectiveness of infection control procedures.* This includes epidemiologic surveillance and quality management procedures.

OBJECTIVES

Upon completion of this chapter, the student will be able to:

1. Demonstrate effective handwashing and hand sanitation technique.
2. Demonstrate a 3-minute surgical scrub.
3. Apply standard precautions and transmission-based isolation procedures according to Centers for Disease Control and Prevention (CDC) guidelines.
4. Distinguish between various types of isolation procedures and apply applicable precautions for each.
5. Practice procedures mandated by the Occupational Safety and Health Administration (OSHA) for the handling and disposal of infectious waste or equipment.

KEY TERMS

aerobe	endotoxin	immunosuppression	prokaryotic
anaerobe	enteric	infection	proliferation
bacteremia	epidemic	inhibition	prophylactic
bactericidal	eukaryotic	morphology	prophylaxis
bacteriostatic	exotoxin	mutualism	pus
cell-mediated	facilitate	mycology	sepsis
colonization	facultative	necrosis	septicemia
commensalism	fastidious	obligate	symbiosis
condensate	fomite	opportunistic	synergism
debilitated	hemolytic	optimum	vector
desiccation	homogeneous	parasitism	virology
endemic	humoral	pathogen	virulence
endocytosis	immunology	phagocytosis	virulent

Exercises

EQUIPMENT REQUIRED

- ☐ Antimicrobial liquid soap in dispenser
- ☐ Bar soap
- ☐ Disposable high-efficiency particulate aerosol (HEPA) filter masks
- ☐ Disposable isolation gowns
- ☐ Disposable nitrile and vinyl gloves in various sizes
- ☐ Hand sanitizing solution (liquid or foam) and dispenser
- ☐ Isolation head and foot coverings
- ☐ Paper towels
- ☐ Protective eyewear or face shields
- ☐ Sample isolation signs
- ☐ Sink with running water
- ☐ Sterile gloves in various sizes
- ☐ Stopwatch
- ☐ Surgical masks
- ☐ Surgical scrub brushes

EXERCISE 3.1 HANDWASHING

Proper handwashing before and after any patient contact is one of the single most important infection control procedures.

1. Remove jewelry and watch.
2. Adjust water flow and temperature using foot pedals, if available, as shown in Figure 3.1, or hand faucet controls.
3. Wet forearms and hands.
4. Apply disinfectant liquid soap liberally.
5. Wash with strong friction for as long as you feel appropriate. Have your partner use a stopwatch to time how long you wash. **Record the initial time on your laboratory report.**
6. You should scrub the following as shown in Figure 3.2:
   A. Palms
   B. Between digits
   C. Under fingernails and around cuticles with a brush
   D. Wrists and forearms

NOTE: Make sure you do not touch the sink with your hands or body.

7. Handwashing should be done for a minimum of 15 seconds.[3] If you did not achieve this time initially, repeat step 5. Sing a chorus of *Yankee Doodle* or *My Country 'Tis of Thee* to get the timing down.
8. Rinse from the forearm to the fingertips, ensuring that all soap solution has been removed.
9. Obtain paper towels aseptically.
10. Dry hands individually, using separate towels.
11. Turn off water faucets using a dry, clean towel if foot pedals are not available.
12. Discard paper towels in an appropriate waste container.

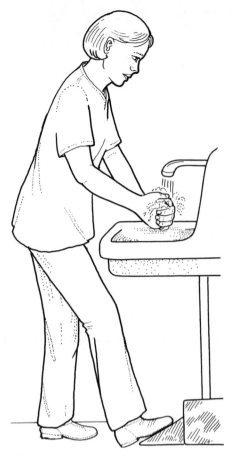

Figure 3.1. Adjusting water flow using foot pedals.

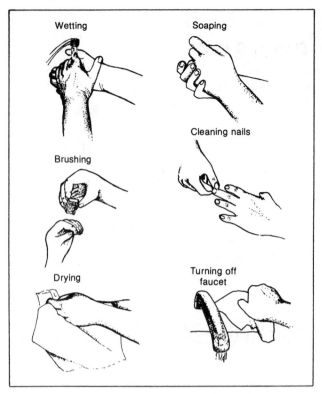

Figure 3.2. Handwashing technique. (From McLaughlin, AJ Jr: Manual of Infection Control in Respiratory Care. Little, Brown & Co., Boston, MA, p. 85, with permission.)

EXERCISE 3.2 HAND SANITATION

1. Remove jewelry and watch.
2. Fill your palm with liquid or foam sanitizing hand solution.
3. Rub into your hands, between fingers, and into palms and wrists for at least 10 seconds until dry.
4. Look up the recommendations for how often hand sanitizing lotion can be applied before handwashing is required. **Record this information on your laboratory report.**

EXERCISE 3.3 SURGICAL SCRUB

1. Obtain a package of surgical scrub brush with soap.
2. Remove jewelry and watch.
3. Adjust water flow and temperature using foot pedals. Wet forearms and hands.
4. Open scrub package and begin scrubbing hands and arms up to your elbow for at least 3 minutes.
5. Rinse from elbows toward fingertips, ensuring that all soap solution has been removed.
6. Obtain paper towels aseptically.
7. Dry hands individually, using separate towels.
8. Turn off water faucets using a dry, clean towel if foot pedals are not available.
9. Discard paper towels in an appropriate waste container.

EXERCISE 3.4 BARRIER PRECAUTIONS/PERSONAL PROTECTIVE EQUIPMENT

EXERCISE 3.4.1 STANDARD PRECAUTIONS/TRANSMISSION-BASED ISOLATION PROCEDURES

Protecting our patients and ourselves against infection requires strict adherence to current infection control procedures.[1,4] To create barriers to transmission, one must be aware of the routes of transmission of infectious disease (Fig. 3.3).

1. Review all signs and posters for standard precautions and transmission-based isolation procedures as illustrated in Figures 3.4 and 3.5.

2. Review all category-specific isolation precautions[4] as shown in Table 3.1. The CDC classifies four categories for isolation procedures: standard, airborne, droplet, and contact precautions. Standard precautions synthesized the major features of universal (blood and body fluid precautions) and body substance isolation.[5] Transmission-based precautions are designed for patients documented or suspected to be infected with highly transmissible or epidemiologically important pathogens for which additional precautions are needed to interrupt transmission.[5] Airborne precautions are designed to reduce the risk of transmission of infectious agents by droplet nuclei or dust particles. Droplet precautions reduce the transmission of infectious agents through large droplet contact (greater than 5 μ) such as occurs with coughing, sneezing, or talking. Immunocompromised patients, such as those with cancer, leukemia, severe burns, or organ transplants, are generally at increased risk for bacterial, fungal, parasitic, and viral infections from both endogenous and exogenous sources.[6] The use of standard precautions for all patients and transmission-based precautions for specified patients should reduce the acquisition by these patients of nosocomial infections.

3. Obtain all personal protective equipment (PPE) required for standard transmission based isolation procedures. Hands should be washed before this procedure. Apply the equipment in the following order[3] (Fig. 3.6):

    A. Hair and foot coverings. Make sure all of your hair is covered.

    B. Gown.
        i.   Open gown fully.
        ii. With the opening in the back, insert your arms into the sleeves.
        iii. Fasten ties at the neck and waist.

    C. Mask. Make sure that both your nose and mouth are completely covered and the mask is tied to the back of the head or straps are adjusted. A surgical mask should be changed frequently because it is ineffective once it becomes wet.

    D. Goggles or face shield. Although not part of required strict isolation equipment, goggles or face shield may be necessary if splashing of blood or body fluids is anticipated.

    E. Gloves. Gloves should fit well. Examine for any tears or holes and replace if necessary. Nitrile powder-free or vinyl gloves may be substituted if latex sensitivity or powdered gloves are a problem.

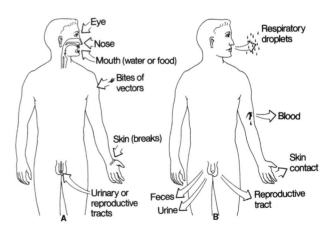

Figure 3.3. Routes of transmission of infectious diseases. (From Scanlon, VC and Sanders, T: Essentials of Anatomy and Physiology, ed 2. FA Davis, Philadelphia, 1991, p. 510, with permission.)

STANDARD PRECAUTIONS

FOR INFECTION CONTROL

Hand Hygiene

Wash after touching **body fluids**, after **removing gloves**, and between **patient contacts.** If hands are not visibly soiled, use an alcohol-based hand rub for routinely decontaminating hands.

Gloves

Wear **Gloves** before touching **body fluids**, **mucous membranes**, and **nonintact skin**.

Mask & Eye Protection or Face Shield

Protect eyes, nose, mouth during procedures that cause **splashes** or **sprays** of **body fluids**.

Gown

Wear **Gown** during procedures that may cause **splashes** or **sprays** of **body fluids**.

Patient-Care Equipment

Handle soiled equipment so as to prevent personal contamination and transfer to other patients.

Environmental Control

Follow hospital procedures for cleaning beds, equipment, and frequently touched surfaces.

Linen

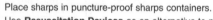
Handle linen soiled with **body fluids** so as to prevent personal contamination and transfer to other patients.

Occupational Health & Bloodborne Pathogens

Prevent injuries from needles, scalpels, and other sharp devices.
Never recap needles using both hands.
Place sharps in puncture-proof sharps containers.
Use **Resuscitation Devices** as an alternative to mouth-to-mouth resuscitation.

Patient Placement

Use a Private Room for a patient who contaminates the environment.

"Body Fluids" include **blood**, **secretions**, and **excretions**.

Condensed Version

Figure 3.4. Standard precautions. (Courtesy of Brevis Corp., Salt Lake City, Utah.)

CONTACT PRECAUTIONS

(in addition to Standard Precautions)

 VISITORS: Report to nurse before entering.

Gloves
Don gloves upon entry into the room or cubicle.
Wear gloves whenever touching the patient's intact skin or surfaces and articles in close proximity to the patient.
Remove gloves before leaving patient room.

Hand Hygiene
Hand Hygiene according to Standard Precautions.

Gowns
Don gown upon entry into the room or cubicle.
Remove gown and observe hand hygiene before leaving the patient-care environment.

Patient Transport
Limit transport of patients to medically necessary purposes.
Ensure that infected or colonized areas of the patient's body are contained and covered.
Remove and dispose of contaminated PPE and perform hand hygiene prior to transporting patients on Contact Precautions.
Don clean PPE to handle the patient at the transport destination.

Patient–Care Equipment
Use disposable noncritical patient-care equipment or implement patient-dedicated use of such equipment.

A

Figure 3.5. Transmission-based precautions. **(A)** Contact precautions, **(B)** Droplet precautions, **(C)** Airborne precautions. (Courtesy of Brevis Corp., Salt Lake City, UT.) *(continued)*

DROPLET PRECAUTIONS

(in addition to Standard Precautions)

VISITORS: Report to nurse before entering.

Use Droplet Precautions as recommended for patients known or suspected to be infected with pathogens transmitted by respiratory droplets that are generated by a patient who is coughing, sneezing or talking.

Personal Protective Equipment (PPE)

Don a mask upon entry into the patient room or cubicle.

Hand Hygiene

Hand Hygiene according to Standard Precautions.

Patient Placement

Private room, if possible. Cohort or maintain spatial separation of 3 feet from other patients or visitors if private room is not available.

Patient transport

Limit transport and movement of patients to **medically-necessary purposes.**

If transport or movement in any healthcare setting is necessary, instruct patient to **wear a mask** and follow Respiratory Hygiene/Cough Etiquette.

No mask is required for persons transporting patients on Droplet Precautions.

B

Figure 3.5. *(continued)*

AIRBORNE PRECAUTIONS
(in addition to Standard Precautions)

VISITORS: Report to nurse before entering.

Use Airborne Precautions as recommended for patients known or suspected to be infected with infectious agents transmitted person-to-person by the airborne route (e.g., M. tuberculosis, measles, chickenpox, disseminated herpes zoster).

Patient placement

Place patients in an **AIIR** (Airborne Infection Isolation Room).
Monitor air pressure daily with visual indicators (e.g., flutter strips).

Keep door closed when not required for entry and exit.

In ambulatory settings instruct patients with a known or suspected airborne infection to wear a surgical mask and observe Respiratory Hygiene/Cough Etiquette. Once in an AIIR, the mask may be removed.

Patient transport

Limit transport and movement of patients to **medically-necessary purposes.**

If transport or movement outside an AIIR is necessary, instruct patients to **wear a surgical mask**, if possible, and observe Respiratory Hygiene/Cough Etiquette.

Hand Hygiene

Hand Hygiene according to Standard Precautions.

Personal Protective Equipment (PPE)

Wear a fit-tested NIOSH-approved **N95** or higher level respirator for respiratory protection when entering the room of a patient when the following diseases are suspected or confirmed: Listed on back.

C

Figure 3.5. *(continued)*

Table 3.1 Isolation Precautions

CATEGORY	REQUIREMENTS	SELECTED INDICATIONS
Standard	Handwashing with nonantimicrobial soap	Routine; before and after all patient contact
	Handwashing with antimicrobial soap	For specific outbreaks as defined by infection control program
	Gloves	When touching blood, body fluids, secretions, mucous membranes, nonintact skin
	Mask, eye protections, face shield	For procedures likely to generate splashes or sprays of blood, body fluids, secretions, and excretions
	Gown	For procedures and activities that are likely to generate sprays or splashes or cause soiling
	Patient-care equipment	To prevent skin and mucous membrane exposures and contamination of clothing; clean and reprocess reusable equipment between patients; discard single-use items
	Environmental control	Routine care: cleaning and disinfection of environmental surfaces, beds, bedrails, bedside equipment; blood spills should be cleaned up promptly with 5.25% solution sodium hypochlorite diluted 1:10 with water
	Linen	Handle, transport, and process used linen soiled with blood, body fluids, secretions, and excretions to prevent skin and mucous membrane exposures, contamination of clothing and avoid transfer of microorganisms to other patients and environments
	Occupational health and blood-borne pathogens	Prevent injuries when using, cleaning, or disposing of needles, scalpels, and other sharps; do not bend, break, or otherwise manipulate by hand; never recap using any technique involving point of sharp toward any part of the body
	Private room	For patient who contaminates the environment or who cannot assist in maintaining hygiene or environmental control
Airborne	*In addition to standard precautions:* Private room with door closed and monitored negative air pressure; 6 to 12 air changes per hour; discharge of air outdoors or monitored HEPA filtration of room air Respiratory protection Limit patient transport, mask patient	Patients known or suspected to be infected with organisms transmitted by airborne droplet nuclei; measles (rubeola); chicken pox varicella; tuberculosis
Droplet	*In addition to standard precautions:* Private room Mask when working within 3 feet of patient Limit patient transport, mask patient	Known or suspected to be infected with microorganisms transmitted by large particle droplet (>5 µ) that can be generated during coughing, sneezing, talking, or performance of procedures Invasive *Haemophilus influenzae* type disease including meningitis, pneumonia, epiglottitis, and sepsis; invasive *Neisseria meningitidis* disease including meningitis, pneumonia and sepsis; diphtheria, *Mycoplasma* pneumonia, pertussis, pneumonic plague, streptococcal pharyngitis, pneumonia, or scarlet fever in infants and young children; adenovirus, influenza, mumps rubella

(continued)

Table 3.1 Isolation Precautions
(continued)

CATEGORY	REQUIREMENTS	SELECTED INDICATIONS
Contact	In addition to standard precautions: Private room Masks Gloves when entering room; change when soiled and before leaving room Gowns when entering room if soiling likely; change after contact with infective material	Gastrointestinal, respiratory, skin and wound, or colonization by multidrug-resistant bacterial infections such as methicillin-resistant *Staphylococcus aureus* (MRSA) Enteric infections with low infectious dose including *Clostridium difficile*; infectious diarrhea from *Escherichia coli*, *Shigella*, hepatitis A or rotovirus Respiratory syncytial virus, parainfluenza virus or enteroviral infections in infants and young children Skin infections that are highly contagious including diphtheria (cutaneous), herpes simplex virus, impetigo, major abscesses, cellulitis or decubiti, pediculosis, scabies; zoster; viral hemorrhagic conjunctivitis; viral hemorrhagic infections including Ebola, Lassa, and Marburg virus

Note: Hands must be washed after touching patient or potentially contaminated articles for all categories. Contaminated articles should be discarded or bagged and labeled.

4. Remove all PPE in the following sequence:
    A. Head and foot coverings.
    B. Mask and goggles.
    C. Gloves. Gloves should be removed by pulling down from the wrist and turning them inside out.
    D. Gown. After untying neck and waist, remove gown inside out.
5. Discard disposable items in infectious waste container. (For purposes of laboratory practice, PPE may be saved to reuse in later exercises.)
6. Wash hands.

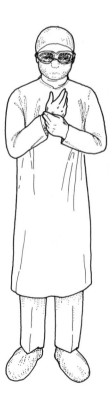

Figure 3.6. Personal protective equipment (PPE).

EXERCISE 3.4.2 APPLICATION OF STERILE GLOVES

When applying sterile gloves, it is important to follow the proper sequence of steps to prevent contamination, as shown in Figure 3.7.

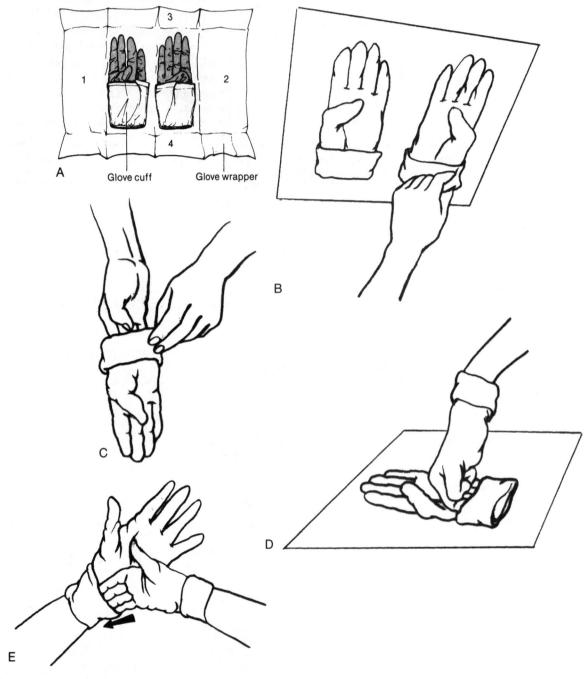

Figure 3.7. Application of sterile gloves. (From Frew, MA, Lane, K and Frew, DR: Comprehensive Medical Assisting, ed 3. FA Davis, Philadelphia, 1995, pp. 615–617, with permission.)

During this exercise you will be placing a glove on your dominant hand first, using the opposite (nondominant) hand to handle the glove. If you are right handed, your right hand is your dominant hand and your left hand is your nondominant hand. If you are left handed, the opposite is true.

1. Obtain proper size package of sterile gloves.
2. Wash hands.
3. Open package aseptically and unfold it completely, making sure both gloves are accessible. Do not touch the inside of the package (Fig. 3.7A).
4. Using your nondominant hand, pick up the cuffed (folded) portion of the glove that will be pulled onto your dominant hand. Make sure not to touch any part of the glove other than the outside of the folded portion of the cuff (Fig. 3.7B).
5. Slide your dominant hand into the glove as far as possible. Now raise your hand and apply the glove completely. Use your nondominant hand to pull the glove on while touching only the inside of the glove (Fig. 3.7C).
6. Using your gloved dominant hand, pick up the other glove, using two or three fingers inserted into the cuffed portion (Fig. 3.7D).
7. Slide your ungloved nondominant hand into the glove as far as possible. Now raise your hand and apply the glove completely. Do not touch your skin with the sterile gloved hand. Pull the glove on by the cuff while touching only the outside of the glove (Fig. 3.7E).
8. Remove gloves. Gloves should be removed by pulling them down from the wrist and turning them inside out.
9. Discard gloves in infectious waste container.

EXERCISE 3.4.3 AIRBORNE/DROPLET PRECAUTIONS

OSHA regulations for tuberculosis precautions now require the use of a high-efficiency particulate aerosol (HEPA) mask as part of personal protective equipment, or other similar devices recommended by the National Institute for Occupational Safety and Health (NIOSH).[5,6] NIOSH certifies three types of masks as acceptable: HEPA 100, with a 99.97% efficiency rate; HEPA 99, with a 99% efficiency rate; and HEPA 95, with a 95% efficiency rate. OSHA relies on NIOSH certification for its recommendations. Review the current CDC recommendations for respiratory/tuberculosis isolation precautions.

1. Obtain disposable HEPA filter mask. Read the directions on the manufacturer's label.
2. Apply the mask according to the manufacturer's directions, as shown in Figure 3.8. Make sure the mask fits well.

NOTE: Facial hair may interfere with the effective functioning of this mask. Also, healthcare providers may need medical clearance to wear these types of masks for any length of time. Pre-existing pulmonary disease or reduced flow rates may cause difficulty in breathing through these masks. Your medical director should be consulted regarding guidelines.

3. Leave the mask on for 5 minutes, as tolerated. Record your observations on your laboratory report.

• **Fitting instructions to be followed each time respirator is worn**

Prestretch top and bottom straps before placing respirator on the face.

Cup the respirator in your hand, with the nosepiece at your fingertips, allowing the headbands to hang freely below your hand.

Position the respirator under your chin with the nosepiece up. Pull the top strap over your head resting it high at the top back of your head. Pull the bottom strap over your head and position it around the neck below the ears.

Place your fingertips from both hands at the top of the metal nosepiece. Using two hands, mold the nose area to the shape of your nose by pushing inward while moving your fingertips down both sides of the nosepiece. Pinching the nosepiece using one hand may cause a bad fit and result in less effective respirator performance. Use two hands.

The seal of the respirator on the face should be fit checked prior to each wearing. To check fit, place both hands completely over the respirator and exhale. Be careful not to disturb the position of the respirator. If air leaks around nose, readjust the nosepiece as described in step 4.

If air leaks at the respirator edges, work the straps back along the sides of your head.

Figure 3.8. Application of high-efficiency particulate aerosol (HEPA) filter mask. (Courtesy of 3M Occupational Health and Environmental Safety Division, St. Paul, MN.)

REFERENCES

1. Occupational Safety and Health Administration: Regulations for bloodborne pathogens. Federal Register, 29 CFR Section 1910.103, January 29, 1992, pp. 41–47.
2. Scanlan, C et al (eds): Egan's Fundamentals of Respiratory Care, ed 6. Mosby, St. Louis, 1995, p. 52.
3. Guideline for Hand Hygiene in Health-Care Settings: Recommendations of the Healthcare Infection Control Practices Advisory Committee and the HICPAC/SHEA/APIC/IDSA Hand Hygiene Task Force. MMWR, October 25, 2002, 51(RR16); pp. 1–44.
4. Centers for Disease Control and Prevention: Guideline for isolation precautions in hospitals. Part II: Recommendations for isolation precautions in hospitals. AJIC 24:32–52, 1996.
5. Centers for Disease Control and Prevention: Guideline for isolation precautions in hospitals. Part II: Recommendations for isolation precautions in hospitals. AJIC 24:36–37, 1996.
6. Centers for Disease Control and Prevention: Guidelines for preventing the transmission of *Mycobacterium tuberculosis* in health care settings, 2005. MMWR, December 30, 2005, 54(RR17), pp. 1–141.

Laboratory Report

CHAPTER 3: INFECTION CONTROL

Name _____ Date _____

Course/Section _____ Instructor _____

Data Collection

EXERCISE 3.1 Handwashing

Time of initial handwashing in seconds: _____

EXERCISE 3.2 Hand Sanitation

Application of hand sanitizing lotion information: _____
_____

EXERCISE 3.4 Barrier Precautions/Personal Protective Equipment

EXERCISE 3.4.3 AIRBORNE/DROPLET PRECAUTIONS

Observations wearing HEPA filter mask: _____
_____
_____
_____

Critical Thinking Questions

1. Mr. Abraham is a 40-year-old man being mechanically ventilated with an oral endotracheal tube in place. You note on his chart that a methicillin-resistant form of *Staphylococcus aureus* (MRSA) has been cultured from his sputum.

    A. What types of transmission-based isolation precautions should be taken before entering the room?

    B. List the PPE required.

    C. What type of antimicrobial therapy would be recommended to treat this patient's infection?

2. Ms. Holland is a 27-year-old woman who is HIV positive. She was admitted with respiratory difficulty. Sputum analysis has proved positive for acid-fast bacillus.

    A. What type of transmission-based isolation precautions are indicated in this patient?

    B. Describe what infection control precautions (relating to the equipment, the patient, and yourself) should be taken when performing an arterial blood gas on this patient.

    C. You inadvertently spill some blood on the floor while performing the arterial blood gas on this patient. What action or actions should be taken to clean up the spill? Specify the solution used.

Procedural Competency Evaluation

STUDENT: **DATE:**

HAND HYGIENE

	PERFORMANCE RATING	PERFORMANCE LEVEL
Evaluator: ☐ Peer ☐ Instructor **Setting:** ☐ Lab ☐ Clinical Simulation		
Equipment Utilized: **Conditions (Describe):**		

Performance Level:

S or ✓ = Satisfactory, no errors of omission or commission
U = Unsatisfactory Error of Omission or Commission
NA = Not applicable

Performance Rating:

5   **Independent:** Near flawless performance; minimal errors; able to perform without supervision; seeks out new learning; shows initiative; A = 4.7–5.0 average

4   **Minimally Supervised:** Few errors, able to self-correct; seeks guidance when appropriate; B = 3.7–4.65

3   **Competent:** Minimal required level; no critical errors; able to correct with coaching; meets expectations; safe; C = 3.0–3.65

2   **Marginal:** Below average; critical errors or problem areas noted; would benefit from remediation; D = 2.0–2.99

1   **Dependent:** Poor; unacceptable performance; unsafe; gross inaccuracies; potentially harmful; F = < 2.0

Two or more errors of commission or omission of mandatory or essential performance elements will terminate the procedure, and require additional practice and/or remediation and reevaluation. Student is responsible for obtaining additional evaluation forms as needed from the Director of Clinical Education (DCE).

	Performance Rating	Performance Level
HANDWASHING WITH SOAP AND WATER		
1. Removes personal articles		
2. Adjusts water flow and temperature; avoids contact with sink		
3. Wets forearms and hands thoroughly		
4. Applies disinfectant soap liberally		
5. Washes hands with appropriate friction for a minimum of 15 seconds		
A. Palms		
B. Wrists		
C. Between Fingers		
D. Nails/Cuticles		
E. Forearms		
6. Washes appropriate length of time (repeats when indicated)		
7. Avoids hand/finger contact with fixtures		
8. Rinses thoroughly from the forearm to the fingertips		
9. Obtains paper towels without contamination		
10. Dries areas thoroughly		
11. Turns off water avoiding re-contamination		
12. Maintains processes equipment; disposes of infectious waste		
HAND DISINFECTION WITH ALCOHOL-BASED DISINFECTANT		
13. Removes personal articles		
14. Inspects hands to ensure that they are not soiled		
15. Applies gel to the palm of one hand		
16. Rubs hands together, covering all surfaces of the hands and fingers		
17. Continues to rub until all surfaces are dry		

SIGNATURES   Student: Evaluator: Date:

Clinical Performance Evaluation

PERFORMANCE RATING:

5 **Independent:** Near flawless performance; minimal errors; able to perform without supervision; seeks out new learning; shows initiative; A = 4.7–5.0 average

4 **Minimally Supervised:** Few errors, able to self-correct; seeks guidance when appropriate; B = 3.7–4.65

3 **Competent:** Minimal required level; no critical errors; able to correct with coaching; meets expectations; safe; C = 3.0–3.65

2 **Marginal:** Below average; critical errors or problem areas noted; would benefit from remediation; D = 2.0–2.99

1 **Dependent:** Poor; unacceptable performance; unsafe; gross inaccuracies; potentially harmful; F = < 2.0

Circle the appropriate response below. Please be consistent, objective, and honest in your assessment of the student's clinical performance and ability.

PERFORMANCE CRITERIA	SCORE				
COGNITIVE DOMAIN					
1. Consistently displays knowledge, comprehension, and command of essential concepts	5	4	3	2	1
2. Demonstrates the relationship between theory and clinical practice	5	4	3	2	1
3. Able to select, review, apply, analyze, synthesize, interpret, and evaluate information; makes recommendations to modify care plan	5	4	3	2	1
PSYCHOMOTOR DOMAIN					
4. Minimal errors, no critical errors; able to self-correct; performs all steps safely and accurately	5	4	3	2	1
5. Selects, assembles, and verifies proper function and cleanliness of equipment; assures operation and corrects malfunctions; provides adequate care and maintenance	5	4	3	2	1
6. Exhibits the required manual dexterity	5	4	3	2	1
7. Performs procedure in a reasonable time frame for clinical level	5	4	3	2	1
8. Applies and maintains aseptic technique and PPE as required	5	4	3	2	1
9. Maintains concise and accurate patient and clinical records	5	4	3	2	1
10. Reports promptly on patient status/needs to appropriate personnel	5	4	3	2	1
AFFECTIVE DOMAIN					
11. Exhibits courteous and pleasant demeanor; shows consideration and respect, honesty, and integrity	5	4	3	2	1
12. Communicates verbally and in writing clearly and concisely	5	4	3	2	1
13. Preserves confidentiality and adheres to all policies	5	4	3	2	1
14. Follows directions, exhibits sound judgment, and seeks help when required	5	4	3	2	1
15. Demonstrates initiative, self-direction, responsibility, and accountability	5	4	3	2	1

TOTAL POINTS = _____ /15 = AVERAGE GRADE = _____

ADDITIONAL COMMENTS: IDENTIFY AREAS OF EXCELLENCE; LIST ERRORS OF OMISSION OR COMMISSION, CRITICAL ERRORS

SUMMARY PERFORMANCE EVALUATION AND RECOMMENDATIONS

☐ PASS: Satisfactory Performance

  ☐ Minimal supervision needed, may progress to next level provided specific skills, clinical time completed

  ☐ Minimal supervision needed, able to progress to next level without remediation

☐ FAIL: Unsatisfactory Performance (check all that apply)

  ☐ Minor reevaluation only

  ☐ Needs additional clinical practice before reevaluation

  ☐ Needs additional laboratory practice before skills performed in clinical area

  ☐ Recommend clinical probation

SIGNATURES

Evaluator (print name): _____   Evaluator signature: _____   Date: _____

Student Signature: _____   Date: _____

Student Comments:

Procedural Competency Evaluation

STUDENT: **DATE:**

STANDARD PRECAUTIONS/TRANSMISSION-BASED ISOLATION PROCEDURES

	PERFORMANCE RATING	PERFORMANCE LEVEL
Evaluator: ☐ Peer ☐ Instructor **Setting:** ☐ Lab ☐ Clinical Simulation		
Equipment Utilized: **Conditions (Describe):**		
Performance Level: S or ✓ = Satisfactory, no errors of omission or commission U = Unsatisfactory Error of Omission or Commission NA = Not applicable		
Performance Rating: **5** **Independent:** Near flawless performance; minimal errors; able to perform without supervision; seeks out new learning; shows initiative; A = 4.7–5.0 average **4** **Minimally Supervised:** Few errors, able to self-correct; seeks guidance when appropriate; B = 3.7–4.65 **3** **Competent:** Minimal required level; no critical errors; able to correct with coaching; meets expectations; safe; C = 3.0–3.65 **2** **Marginal:** Below average; critical errors or problem areas noted; would benefit from remediation; D = 2.0–2.99 **1** **Dependent:** Poor; unacceptable performance; unsafe; gross inaccuracies; potentially harmful; F = < 2.0 *Two or more errors of commission or omission of mandatory or essential performance elements will terminate the procedure, and require additional practice and/or remediation and reevaluation. Student is responsible for obtaining additional evaluation forms as needed from the Director of Clinical Education (DCE).*		
EQUIPMENT AND PATIENT PREPARATION		
1. Common Performance Elements Steps 1–8		
ASSESSMENT AND IMPLEMENTATION		
2. Removes jewelry and watch		
3. Adjusts water flow and temperature		
4. Wets forearms and hands; applies disinfectant soap liberally		
5. Washes hands for a minimum of 15 seconds with strong friction; palms, between the digits, under fingernails, and around cuticles		
A. Never touches sink with hands		
6. Rinses from forearm to fingertips		
7. Obtains towels aseptically and dries hands using individual towels		
8. Turns off water using dry, clean towel		
9. Reviews patient chart and surveys room for any posted transmission-based precautions		
10. Obtains and applies appropriate PPE in the proper sequence: hair and foot coverings, gown, mask, goggles and/or face shield, and gloves		
11. Performs procedure		
FOLLOW-UP		
12. Bags, seals, and labels any contaminated equipment		
13. Removes PPE in proper sequence		
14. Disposes of any infectious waste		
15. Washes hands		
16. Transports contaminated equipment in low-traffic areas		

SIGNATURES   Student: Evaluator: Date:

Clinical Performance Evaluation

PERFORMANCE RATING:

5 **Independent:** Near flawless performance; minimal errors; able to perform without supervision; seeks out new learning; shows initiative; A = 4.7–5.0 average

4 **Minimally Supervised:** Few errors, able to self-correct; seeks guidance when appropriate; B = 3.7–4.65

3 **Competent:** Minimal required level; no critical errors; able to correct with coaching; meets expectations; safe; C = 3.0–3.65

2 **Marginal:** Below average; critical errors or problem areas noted; would benefit from remediation; D = 2.0–2.99

1 **Dependent:** Poor; unacceptable performance; unsafe; gross inaccuracies; potentially harmful; F = < 2.0

Circle the appropriate response below. Please be consistent, objective, and honest in your assessment of the student's clinical performance and ability.

PERFORMANCE CRITERIA	SCORE				
COGNITIVE DOMAIN					
1. Consistently displays knowledge, comprehension, and command of essential concepts	5	4	3	2	1
2. Demonstrates the relationship between theory and clinical practice	5	4	3	2	1
3. Able to select, review, apply, analyze, synthesize, interpret, and evaluate information; makes recommendations to modify care plan	5	4	3	2	1
PSYCHOMOTOR DOMAIN					
4. Minimal errors, no critical errors; able to self-correct; performs all steps safely and accurately	5	4	3	2	1
5. Selects, assembles, and verifies proper function and cleanliness of equipment; assures operation and corrects malfunctions; provides adequate care and maintenance	5	4	3	2	1
6. Exhibits the required manual dexterity	5	4	3	2	1
7. Performs procedure in a reasonable time frame for clinical level	5	4	3	2	1
8. Applies and maintains aseptic technique and PPE as required	5	4	3	2	1
9. Maintains concise and accurate patient and clinical records	5	4	3	2	1
10. Reports promptly on patient status/needs to appropriate personnel	5	4	3	2	1
AFFECTIVE DOMAIN					
11. Exhibits courteous and pleasant demeanor; shows consideration and respect, honesty, and integrity	5	4	3	2	1
12. Communicates verbally and in writing clearly and concisely	5	4	3	2	1
13. Preserves confidentiality and adheres to all policies	5	4	3	2	1
14. Follows directions, exhibits sound judgment, and seeks help when required	5	4	3	2	1
15. Demonstrates initiative, self-direction, responsibility, and accountability	5	4	3	2	1

TOTAL POINTS = _____ /15 = AVERAGE GRADE = _____

ADDITIONAL COMMENTS: IDENTIFY AREAS OF EXCELLENCE; LIST ERRORS OF OMISSION OR COMMISSION, CRITICAL ERRORS

SUMMARY PERFORMANCE EVALUATION AND RECOMMENDATIONS

☐ PASS: Satisfactory Performance

    ☐ Minimal supervision needed, may progress to next level provided specific skills, clinical time completed

    ☐ Minimal supervision needed, able to progress to next level without remediation

☐ FAIL: Unsatisfactory Performance (check all that apply)

    ☐ Minor reevaluation only

    ☐ Needs additional clinical practice before reevaluation

    ☐ Needs additional laboratory practice before skills performed in clinical area

    ☐ Recommend clinical probation

SIGNATURES

Evaluator (print name): _____ Evaluator signature: _____ Date: _____

Student Signature: _____ Date: _____

Student Comments:

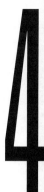
Sterilization and Disinfection

INTRODUCTION

As discussed in the previous chapter, the second component of good infection control is the prevention of nosocomial infections. An essential component is the disinfection and sterilization of equipment. While the majority of today's respiratory care equipment is single-patient use and disposable, rising costs of equipment and its disposal are making respiratory care departments rethink the use of permanent, nondisposable equipment.

There are several methods used for the **sterilization** and **disinfection** of respiratory care equipment. The first step is decontamination, which removes the infectious, organic residues from the equipment. Sterilization is the killing of all microorganisms. The process of sterilization may be physical (steam **autoclave**) or chemical (ethylene oxide). Disinfection, which usually is not effective against spores, can be achieved by pasteurization. Batch pasteurization has been instituted by many respiratory care departments as a way of holding down the rising costs of disposable supplies such as tubing. "Cold sterilization" with activated **glutaraldehyde** is a high-level disinfection method, rather than sterilization, due to the impossibility of preventing exposure during the rinse phase prior to packaging.

Respiratory care practitioners, as part of the healthcare team, should be intimately familiar with issues concerning the **etiology** and **epidemiology** of infectious disorders. Each practitioner must adhere to established guidelines. Knowledgeable respiratory care practitioners can serve as positive role models and educators to reinforce the importance of every healthcare provider's responsibility in preventing and controlling infection.

OBJECTIVES

Upon completion of this chapter, the student will be able to:

1. Differentiate between the methods for **decontamination**, **disinfection**, and **sterilization**.
2. Prepare equipment for the most commonly used methods of decontamination, disinfection, and sterilization.
3. Practice monitoring techniques for evaluating the effectiveness of infection control procedures.
4. Practice communication skills needed to explain infection control procedures to patients.
5. Practice documentation of infection control procedures.

KEY TERMS

antiseptic	decontamination	epidemiology	nosocomial
asepsis	disinfectant	etiology	pasteurization
aseptic	disinfection	glutaraldehyde	sterilization
autoclave			

Exercises

EQUIPMENT REQUIRED

- ☐ Agar plates
- ☐ Antimicrobial liquid soap in dispenser
- ☐ **Aseptic** area/field for drying equipment
- ☐ Bar soap
- ☐ Biological indicator vials
- ☐ Chemical indicator tape
- ☐ Culture swabs
- ☐ Detergent solution
- ☐ Disposable high-efficiency particulate aerosol (HEPA) filter masks
- ☐ Disposable isolation gowns
- ☐ Disposable latex and vinyl gloves in various sizes

- ☐ Infectious waste bags with biohazard labels
- ☐ Isolation head and foot coverings
- ☐ Paper towels
- ☐ Protective eyewear or face shields
- ☐ Sample syringes, "contaminated" equipment, and waste
- ☐ Sharps containers
- ☐ Sink with running water
- ☐ Surgical masks
- ☐ Various bags and wraps for equipment packaging
- ☐ Various size equipment brushes

EXERCISE 4.1 HANDLING AND DISPOSAL OF INFECTIOUS EQUIPMENT AND WASTE

In this exercise, you are simulating entering the room of a patient in contact isolation to discard disposable infectious waste and safely remove a piece of reusable respiratory equipment for transport to the disinfection area. The instructor will have the "room" prepared with equipment to be discarded and to be transported.

1. Wash your hands as previously instructed.
2. Apply the required PPE for contact isolation.
3. Enter the "patient's room."
4. Carefully dispose of any sharps (needles, syringes, lancets) into the puncture-proof sharps container (Fig. 4.1). If the container is full, replace it with a new one.
5. Obtain infectious waste bags labeled with a biohazard indicator.
6. Place the reusable equipment into the infectious waste bag, secure it, and label it as in Figure 4.2. Be careful not to contaminate the outside of the bag.
7. Leave the "room." Remove your PPE in the sequence previously described, and discard it in an infectious waste container.

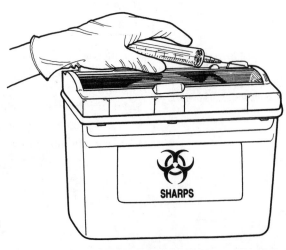

Figure 4.1. Puncture-proof sharps container with biohazard symbol.

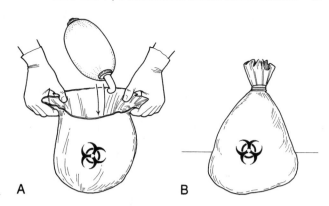

Figure 4.2. Bagging of contaminated equipment. **A** **B**

EXERCISE 4.2 PREPARATION OF EQUIPMENT FOR DISINFECTION/STERILIZATION BY AUTOCLAVE, ETHYLENE OXIDE, ACTIVATED GLUTARALDEHYDE, OR PASTEURIZATION

The instructor will provide nondisposable equipment for this exercise. Although specific requirements vary with the method of disinfection or sterilization to be used, there are steps in equipment preparation common to all modalities.

Not all schools have the facilities to conduct all parts of this exercise. If access to disinfection/sterilization equipment and areas is available, students should perform all elements. If not, students should perform steps 1 through 8 and then examine the materials necessary for the remaining steps. In the absence of such equipment, an alternative to this exercise is a tour or rotation through the sterilization/disinfection department at a clinical agency.

1. Put on PPE, including gloves and gown.

2. Completely disassemble the equipment into its smallest parts.

3. Examine the equipment for any tears, cracks, or pitting. Equipment should be discarded if defective because these defects can provide a safe hiding place for microorganisms.

4. Soak the equipment for at least 10 minutes in a warm solution of disinfecting detergent agent.

5. Scrub the equipment parts thoroughly, making sure to get into any crevices (Fig. 4.3).

6. Rinse the equipment thoroughly with tap water.

7. Set the equipment out to dry on aseptic absorbent disposable towels provided for this purpose.

8. Reassemble the equipment. Loosely secure any parts so that the disinfection/sterilization method can penetrate.

9. Once the equipment is reassembled, it is ready for the appropriate sterilization method:

   A. For autoclave or "gas sterilization" with ethylene oxide, the equipment is first packaged in the appropriate materials; sealed; labeled with time, date, load, and technician signature; and marked with chemical indicator tape (Fig. 4.4). The equipment is then sterilized and aerated, if necessary. Any required paperwork should be completed according to institution policy.

   B. For "cold sterilization" with glutaraldehyde, protective eyewear should be worn. The equipment is next soaked in the disinfecting solution for 10 minutes to 10 hours, depending on whether disinfection or sterilization is to be achieved. The technician then puts on sterile gloves and prepares a sterile field. The equipment is then aseptically rinsed with sterile water, dried on the sterile field, and packaged for storage. The package should be labeled with the date, time, and technician signature. Any required paperwork should be completed according to institution policy.

   C. For pasteurization, the equipment is loaded into the machine and run through the cycle. The equipment is then dried and packaged for storage. The package should be labeled with the date, time, and technician signature. Any required paperwork should be completed according to institution policy.

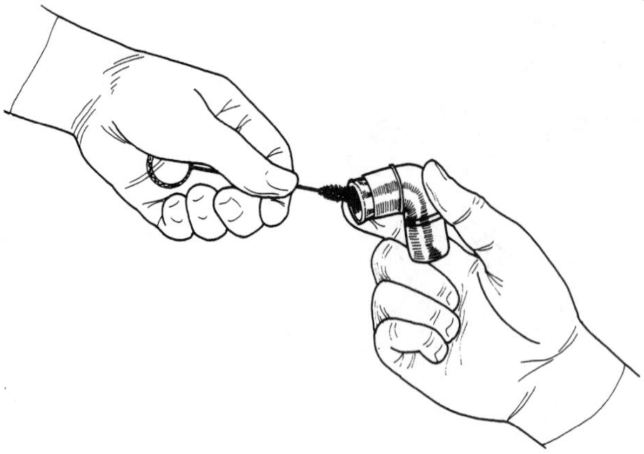

Figure 4.3. Scrubbing equipment.

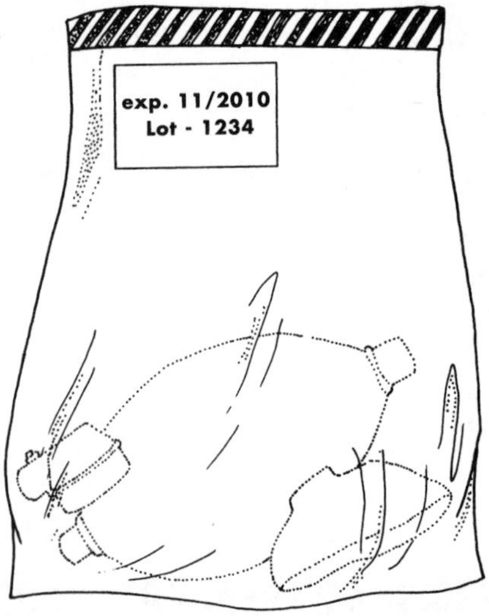

Figure 4.4. Packaging of equipment for sterilization.

exp. 11/2010
Lot - 1234

EXERCISE 4.3 MONITORING INFECTION CONTROL PROCEDURES

Monitoring of infection control techniques is essential in evaluating their effectiveness. This can be accomplished by a variety of microbial culture techniques, depending on the item to be cultured.

Not all schools have the facilities to conduct all parts of this exercise. If access to a microbiology laboratory is available, students should perform all elements.

EXERCISE 4.3.1 BIOLOGICAL MONITORS

Examine the biological monitor vials or strips used for autoclave and ethylene oxide sterilization (Fig. 4.5).

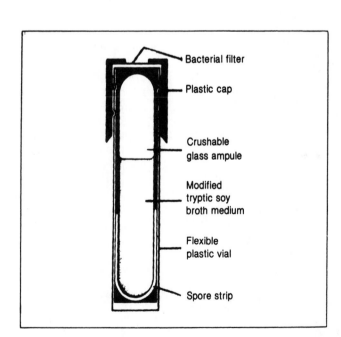

Figure 4.5. Biological indicator. (From McLaughlin, AJ Jr: Manual of Infection Control in Respiratory Care. Little, Brown & Co., Boston, MA, 1983, p. 72, with permission.)

- Bacterial filter
- Plastic cap
- Crushable glass ampule
- Modified tryptic soy broth medium
- Flexible plastic vial
- Spore strip

EXERCISE 4.3.2 SWAB CULTURING

Swab culturing may be used to take spot cultures of various surfaces, such as tracheostomy stoma sites (Fig. 4.6).

1. Wash your hands thoroughly.
2. Obtain the sterile swabs and culture medium tubes.
3. Using separate culture swabs and tubes, culture each of the following:
    A. The palms of your hands
    B. The drain area of the sink
    C. Bar soap
4. Rub the swab back and forth over the area to be cultured. Aseptically replace the swab in the culture tube.
5. Seal the culture tube. Label it with the date, time, and area cultured.
6. Send the culture tube to the microbiology laboratory for culturing and identification.
7. When results are available, **record them on your laboratory report.**

EXERCISE 4.3.3 CULTURING AEROSOL AND GAS SOURCES

For this exercise, the instructor will have a large-volume aerosol delivery system available.

1. Wash your hands thoroughly and put on gloves.
2. Obtain an agar plate.
3. Expose the surface of the plate to the aerosol directly, as shown in Figure 4.7, without allowing the tube to touch the surface of the agar. A commercially available funnel device may be used to minimize contamination of the sample.
4. Seal the agar plate. Label with the date, time, source of sample, and technician signature.
5. Send the sample for culturing.
6. When results are available, **record them on your laboratory report.**

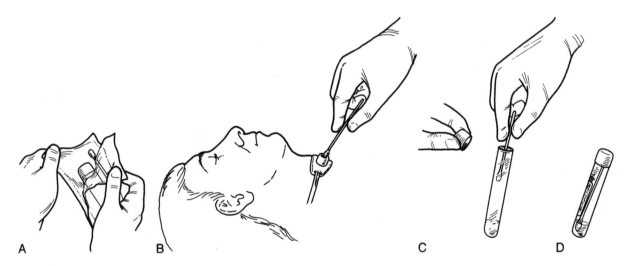

A   B   C   D

Figure 4.6. Swab culturing technique.

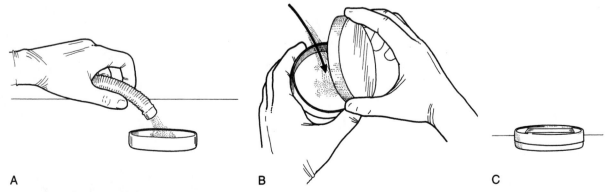

A   B   C

Figure 4.7. Technique for aerosol or gas source culturing.

Laboratory Report

CHAPTER 4: STERILIZATION AND DISINFECTION

Name _____   Date _____

Course/Section _____   Instructor _____

Data Collection

EXERCISE 4.3 Monitoring Infection Control Procedures

EXERCISE 4.3.2 SWAB CULTURING

Date	Time	Source	Results

EXERCISE 4.3.3 CULTURING AEROSOL AND GAS SOURCES

Date	Time	Source	Results

Critical Thinking Questions

1. Mrs. Pak is a 64-year-old female being mechanically ventilated for the last 10 days with an oral endotracheal tube in place. You note on her chart that *Pseudomonas aeruginosa* has been cultured from her sputum. Describe how intensive care unit and mechanical ventilation may have contributed to the development of this nosocomial infection.

2. Mr. Grand is a 47-year-old man who is positive for hepatitis B. He was admitted to the ICU and you are called to draw an arterial blood gas. Describe what infection control precautions (relating to the equipment, the patient, and yourself) should be taken when performing an arterial blood gas on this patient.

3. After an unsuccessful resuscitation, you are requested to remove the manual resuscitator bag from the patient's room. The nondisposable bag is made of a silicone material and is soiled heavily with bloody secretions. Describe how this equipment should be transported and disinfected.

Procedural Competency Evaluation

STUDENT: **DATE:**

DISINFECTION/STERILIZATION

					PERFORMANCE RATING	PERFORMANCE LEVEL
Evaluator: ☐ Peer ☐ Instructor		**Setting:** ☐ Lab		☐ Clinical Simulation		
Equipment Utilized:		**Conditions (Describe):**				

Performance Level:

S or ✓ = Satisfactory, no errors of omission or commission
U = Unsatisfactory Error of Omission or Commission
NA = Not applicable

Performance Rating:

5   **Independent:** Near flawless performance; minimal errors; able to perform without supervision; seeks out new learning; shows initiative; A = 4.7–5.0 average

4   **Minimally Supervised:** Few errors, able to self-correct; seeks guidance when appropriate; B = 3.7–4.65

3   **Competent:** Minimal required level; no critical errors; able to correct with coaching; meets expectations; safe; C = 3.0–3.65

2   **Marginal:** Below average; critical errors or problem areas noted; would benefit from remediation; D = 2.0–2.99

1   **Dependent:** Poor; unacceptable performance; unsafe; gross inaccuracies; potentially harmful; F = < 2.0

Two or more errors of commission or omission of mandatory or essential performance elements will terminate the procedure, and require additional practice and/or remediation and reevaluation. Student is responsible for obtaining additional evaluation forms as needed from the Director of Clinical Education (DCE).

EQUIPMENT AND PATIENT PREPARATION

	Rating	Level
1. Isolates, gathers, and transports equipment to processing site		
2. Applies PPE, including gloves and gown		
3. Disinfects sink (washer)		
4. Fills sink, adds detergent		
5. Sorts, disassembles equipment into smallest parts		
6. Examines equipment for any tears, cracks, or pitting; discards defective equipment		
7. Immerses equipment in solution and soaks for 20 minutes (institutes wash cycle)		
8. Scrubs parts thoroughly, including any crevices		
9. Rinses equipment thoroughly with tap water or sterile water, as appropriate (institutes rinse cycle)		
10. Removes and sets equipment out to dry on aseptic absorbent surface equipment; drains sink		
11. Prepares for appropriate sterilization method		
12. Reassembles equipment; loosely secures any parts so disinfection/sterilization method can penetrate		
13. Autoclave or gas sterilization: packages equipment in appropriate materials and marks with chemical or heat indicator tape		
14. Cold sterilization with glutaraldehyde: checks solution expiration date; immerses equipment into solution; soaks in disinfecting solution for 10 minutes to 10 hours, as specified; puts on sterile gloves and prepares sterile field; aseptically rinses equipment with sterile water; dries on sterile field, and packages for storage		
15. Pasteurization: loads equipment into machine and runs through cycle; dries and packages for storage		

FOLLOW-UP

	Rating	Level
16. Common Performance Elements Steps 11–16		
17. Verifies exposure to process and sterilization		
18. Aerates equipment as needed (for gas sterilization)		
19. Stores equipment; rotates stock		

SIGNATURES   Student: Evaluator: Date:

Clinical Performance Evaluation

PERFORMANCE RATING:

5 **Independent:** Near flawless performance; minimal errors; able to perform without supervision; seeks out new learning; shows initiative; A = 4.7–5.0 average

4 **Minimally Supervised:** Few errors, able to self-correct; seeks guidance when appropriate; B = 3.7–4.65

3 **Competent:** Minimal required level; no critical errors; able to correct with coaching; meets expectations; safe; C = 3.0–3.65

2 **Marginal:** Below average; critical errors or problem areas noted; would benefit from remediation; D = 2.0–2.99

1 **Dependent:** Poor; unacceptable performance; unsafe; gross inaccuracies; potentially harmful; F = < 2.0

Circle the appropriate response below. Please be consistent, objective, and honest in your assessment of the student's clinical performance and ability.

PERFORMANCE CRITERIA | SCORE

PERFORMANCE CRITERIA					
COGNITIVE DOMAIN					
1. Consistently displays knowledge, comprehension, and command of essential concepts	5	4	3	2	1
2. Demonstrates the relationship between theory and clinical practice	5	4	3	2	1
3. Able to select, review, apply, analyze, synthesize, interpret, and evaluate information; makes recommendations to modify care plan	5	4	3	2	1
PSYCHOMOTOR DOMAIN					
4. Minimal errors, no critical errors; able to self-correct; performs all steps safely and accurately	5	4	3	2	1
5. Selects, assembles, and verifies proper function and cleanliness of equipment; assures operation and corrects malfunctions; provides adequate care and maintenance	5	4	3	2	1
6. Exhibits the required manual dexterity	5	4	3	2	1
7. Performs procedure in a reasonable time frame for clinical level	5	4	3	2	1
8. Applies and maintains aseptic technique and PPE as required	5	4	3	2	1
9. Maintains concise and accurate patient and clinical records	5	4	3	2	1
10. Reports promptly on patient status/needs to appropriate personnel	5	4	3	2	1
AFFECTIVE DOMAIN					
11. Exhibits courteous and pleasant demeanor; shows consideration and respect, honesty, and integrity	5	4	3	2	1
12. Communicates verbally and in writing clearly and concisely	5	4	3	2	1
13. Preserves confidentiality and adheres to all policies	5	4	3	2	1
14. Follows directions, exhibits sound judgment, and seeks help when required	5	4	3	2	1
15. Demonstrates initiative, self-direction, responsibility, and accountability	5	4	3	2	1

TOTAL POINTS = _____ /15 = AVERAGE GRADE = _____

ADDITIONAL COMMENTS: IDENTIFY AREAS OF EXCELLENCE; LIST ERRORS OF OMISSION OR COMMISSION, CRITICAL ERRORS

SUMMARY PERFORMANCE EVALUATION AND RECOMMENDATIONS

☐ PASS: Satisfactory Performance

  ☐ Minimal supervision needed, may progress to next level provided specific skills, clinical time completed

  ☐ Minimal supervision needed, able to progress to next level without remediation

☐ FAIL: Unsatisfactory Performance (check all that apply)

  ☐ Minor reevaluation only

  ☐ Needs additional clinical practice before reevaluation

  ☐ Needs additional laboratory practice before skills performed in clinical area

  ☐ Recommend clinical probation

SIGNATURES

Evaluator (print name): _____ Evaluator signature: _____ Date: _____

Student Signature: _____ Date: _____

Student Comments:

5

Medical Record

INTRODUCTION

The medical record serves as the official document regarding the patient's medical history, illness, treatment, and response. It is a legal document and is the source document in any litigation. Therefore, it is extremely important that the information contained in the document be accurate and truly reflects the care rendered. Even in this day of computerized records, the old adage "If you didn't chart it, you didn't do it" still rings true. Several formats can be used to document respiratory care services. They are the narrative note, the SOAP method, check-list charting, and charting by exception (CBE). Charting by exception assumes that the response to an intervention was normal. Therefore, only abnormal findings are charted. While this may seem contradictory to our old adage, most computerized versions of CBE document and reflect the care rendered.

One of the most important sources for the information contained in the medical record is the patient. The physician, nurse, or respiratory therapist obtains very important information by interviewing the patient concerning the circumstances of the illness. The art of the patient interview is a skill that improves with practice. One of the key components of the process is to put the patient at ease and establish a rapport.

Another facet of the medical record is that it contains sensitive and personal information regarding the patient that is protected by federal law. The Health Insurance Portability and Accountability Act (HIPAA) of 1996 safeguards the confidential nature of that information. Violation of this act and the subsequent regulation known as the "Privacy Rule" issued by the Department of Health and Human Services may result in civil or criminal penalties.[1] Since the respiratory therapist has access to this confidential information, it must never be discussed outside of the scope of care.

OBJECTIVES

Upon completion of this chapter, the student will be able to:

1. Use therapeutic communication skills to establish patient rapport and elicit information during a patient interview.
2. Obtain specific patient information by reading the medical record.
3. Practice medical charting for the documentation of performance of patient assessment procedures utilizing SOAP and narrative charting techniques.
4. Edit and organize the information for an oral case presentation.

KEY TERMS

acute	diagnosis	ischemia	pleuritic (pain)
alleviating	dyspnea	lesions	pneumoconiosis
ambulatory	electrolyte	lethargic	pneumothorax
antecubital	epistaxis	malaise	polycythemia
asterixis	hematocrit	obtunded	sensorium
ataxia	homeostasis	orthopnea	somnolent
atrophy	hypertension	orthostatic	syncope
bilateral	hypertrophy	pallor	systemic
chronic	hypervolemia	palpation	tachycardia
contraindication	hypotension	paresthesia	tachypnea
debilitated	hypovolemia	paroxysmal (cough)	vascular

Exercises

EQUIPMENT REQUIRED

☐ Computerized medical documentation system if available

☐ Patient or student surrogate

☐ Sample medical records

☐ Sample respiratory care notes and flowsheets from clinical facilities

EXERCISE 5.1 CHART REVIEW, PATIENT INTERVIEW, AND HISTORY

Effective communication skills are necessary to establish a rapport with the patient and to elicit useful information to supplement the physical examination. Communication also provides the patient's perspective on the problem at hand.[1] In this exercise, the student will practice communication and questioning techniques, with a fellow student acting as the patient surrogate.

EXERCISE 5.1.1 REVIEW OF THE MEDICAL RECORD

Before entering the "patient's room," check the "chart" for all pertinent information. Your review of the chart should include the following priority areas:

1. Patient **demographics (age, height, gender, race, religion, insurance information)**
2. Chief complaint/**diagnosis**
3. History of present illness, including:
   A. Smoking history (pack/years)
   B. Allergies
   C. Current medications
4. Past medical history—major surgeries, **hypertension**, tuberculosis, diabetes, cardiac or pulmonary disease, and any other *major* illness
5. Social history—marital and family status, living arrangements, alcohol use, sexual activity
6. Occupational history
7. Family history
8. Results of recent diagnostic procedures (x-ray, laboratory, pulmonary function tests, electrocardiogram, etc.)

9. Recent progress notes

10. Physician orders

NOTE: This activity may be performed with actual patient charts if they are available in the lab, or by describing the information to your lab partner. It may also be performed in the clinical setting.

11. **Record your findings on your laboratory report.**

EXERCISE 5.1.2 PATIENT INTERVIEW AND HISTORY

Students should wash hands and apply standard precautions and transmission-based isolation procedures as appropriate. The exercise requires using a laboratory partner as a surrogate.

Approach your "patient" and perform the following, demonstrating effective listening as delineated in Table 5.1. Be sure to take notes so you can record the information at the end of the exercise.

1. Introduce yourself to the "patient" and explain why you are there.

2. Verify your "patient's" identification by asking his/her name and date of birth (DOB) and checking the name band.

3. The interview should be used to assess the following general information:

   A. Level of consciousness and **sensorium**—orientation to person, place, and time. Note any changes in mental status (since this is your lab partner, if he/she fall asleep, wake him/her up!)

   B. Ability to follow directions

   C. Emotional status

   D. Level of **dyspnea**

   E. Nutritional status

   F. Tolerance of activities of daily living (ADLs)

4. Ask the "patient" questions to verify the information obtained from the chart regarding the following:

   A. Demographics

   B. Chief complaint: onset, duration, frequency, severity (quantity), character (quality), location, radiation, aggravating factors, **alleviating** factors, associated manifestations

   C. Allergies

   D. Current medications

   E. History of present illness, including smoking history

   F. Past medical history

   G. Psychosocial assessment:

      i. Birthplace

      ii. Race

      iii. Religion

      iv. Culture

      v. Language(s) spoken

      vi. Highest education level

      vii. Sexual activity

      viii. Living arrangements (e.g., live alone?)

      ix. Alcohol intake

      x. Drug use

   H. Occupational history

      i. If retired or a full-time student, be sure to find out what jobs were held in the past that may have had risk of occupational exposure to environmental hazards.

5. Ask the "patient" questions to ascertain specific pulmonary symptoms:

   A. Dyspnea—on exertion or rest; **orthopnea**

   B. Cough

   C. Sputum production—amount, color, consistency, presence of blood

   D. Chest pain—quality, location, radiation, aggravating factors, alleviating factors, associated manifestations

6. Ask the "patient" questions to determine current comfort level or needs.

7. **Record your interview findings on your laboratory report.**

Table 5.1 Some Characteristics of an Effective Listener

1. Seek to understand the person who is speaking, not simply to respond to his or her statements.
2. Listen to a person's tone and inflection as well as his or her choice of words.
3. Look at the person speaking and pay attention to body language. Does the person's body give you the same message as his or her words?
4. Don't rush in with opinions and judgments. Give the person the freedom to express himself or herself.
5. When you speak, make it clear that you have understood what the person has said. You can even restate the person's point more clearly than he or she might have made it originally.

From Soreff, SM and Cadigan, RT: EMS Street Strategies, FA Davis, Philadelphia, 1992, p. 45, with permission.

EXERCISE 5.2 MEDICAL RECORD DOCUMENTATION (CHARTING)

The key elements of a respiratory care note are the date and time of the procedure, patient assessment before the intervention, assessment of the patient's response to the intervention, any adverse effects, and a signature. Some facilities use the SOAP methodology to construct a note.

S = Subjective findings: usually in the words of the patient, such as "I'm still coughing"
O = Objective findings: patient assessment and other data
A = Assessment: problem list (may include differential diagnosis)
P = Plan: are any modifications to the care plan necessary?

If a SOAP methodology is not used, the documentation may consist of a narrative note, a simple check-list, or charting by exception. Students should be familiar with the forms and types of charting required by the clinical agencies because it is the responsibility of the respiratory therapist to document according to facility policy.

EXERCISE 5.2.1 REVIEWING CLINICAL CHARTING FORMS

Review the types of forms used by the various clinical agencies that are affiliated with your respiratory care program. Compare the forms and note similarities and differences.

EXERCISE 5.2.2 WRITING A RESPIRATORY CARE NOTE

A respiratory care note may be written in the following forms: narrative, SOAP, PIP (problem, implementation, plan), APIE (assessment, problem, implementation, evaluation), check-list, and by exception.

Using the following information, construct a SOAP note, a narrative note, PIP, APIE, a check-list note, or documentation by exception. Your instructor may ask you to use all formats. **Record your notes on your laboratory report or a blank progress note form.**

Mrs. Puccini is a 65 year-old female admitted 2 days ago with chronic bronchitis. Prior to hospitalization, she was complaining of fever, cough, and producing large amounts of yellow-green mucus for 5 days. She had smoked 1½ packs of cigarettes per day since she was 18. Currently she is using a nasal cannula at 1 Lpm, her oxygen saturation is 92%, and her pretreatment heart rate is 88 beats per minute. She is still complaining of the cough and mucus production. You administer a nebulizer treatment with 0.5 mg ipratropium diluted in 3.0 ml of normal saline. There are bilateral coarse crackles present before and after the treatment. She expectorates a moderate amount of yellow mucus after the treatment. Her saturation is still 92% and her heart rate is 110/minute.

REFERENCES
1. Department of Health and Human Services: General overview of standsrds for privacy of individually identifiable health information. http://www.hhs.gov/ocr/hipaa/guidelines/overview.pdf.

Laboratory Report

CHAPTER 5: MEDICAL RECORD

Name _____ Date _____

Course/Section _____ Instructor _____

Data Collection

EXERCISE 5.1 Chart Review, Patient Interview, and History

EXERCISE 5.1.1 REVIEW OF THE MEDICAL RECORD

If an actual patient chart was used, **record your findings on the form below:**

Sex: M ❑ F ❑   Date of Birth: _____   Race: _____

Weight: _____   Height: _____   Ideal Body Wt (calculate): _____

Date of Admission: _____   LOS (if applicable): _____

CHIEF COMPLAINT: _____

Admitting Diagnosis: _____   Discharge Diagnoses: _____

HPI: _____

_____

Smoking History: Never smoked ❑ Smoker ❑ Former smoker ❑

Age started: _____   Age when quit: _____   Current age: _____   Packs/day: _____

Allergies: _____

Current Medications: _____

VS on Admission: _____

PMI *Do you have or have you ever had any of the following:*

HEENT: _____

Neuro: _____

Eyes: _____   Ears: _____   Nose: _____   Throat: _____

Lungs: _____

Dyspnea: _____   On exertion: _____   At rest: _____   Position: _____

Cough: _____   Sputum production: _____   Chest pain with cough: _____

Cor: _____

Liver Problems: _____   Hepatitis: A B C: _____

Endocrine: _____   Diabetes: _____   Thyroid: _____

Kidney Disease: _____

Gastrointestinal:

FEN(Feedings/Enteral/Nutritional status):

Genitourinary:

Bone/muscle: Osteoporosis: Other:

Skin:

Major Surgeries:

Psychosocial Assessment

Birthplace: Cultural or Ethnic Group:

Religion: Language(s) Spoken:

Highest Educational Level:

Sexual Activity:

Alcohol Intake:

Drug Use (illegal, prescription, etc.):

Ambulation:

Access/Lines (chest tubes, IV, a-line, central line, etc.):

Occupational History (If retired, what types of jobs did you have?):

Family History:

Results of Recent Diagnostic Procedures:

Recent Progress Notes:

Current Physician Orders:

Outcome:

EXERCISE 5.1.2 PATIENT INTERVIEW AND HISTORY

Sex: M ❑ F ❑   Date of Birth: Race:

Weight: Height: Ideal Body Wt (calculate):

CHIEF COMPLAINT:

Diagnosis:

HPI:

LOC:

Smoking History: Never smoked ❑ Smoker ❑ Former smoker ❑

Age started: Age when quit: Current age: Packs/day:

Allergies:

Current Medications:

Ambulation/Assess ADL:

PMI *Do you have or have you ever had any of the following:*

Major Surgeries:

HEENT:

Neurological Problems:

Seizure History:

Eyes: Ears: Nose: Throat:

Teeth: Dentures:

Lungs:

Asthma: since:

Emphysema: since:

Bronchitis: Pneumonia:

Tuberculosis: Other:

Dyspnea: On exertion: At rest: Position:

Cough: Sputum production: Chest pain with cough:

Heart: Chest pain:

Hypertension:

Heart attack: Pacemaker:

Liver problems: Hepatitis: A B C:

Endocrine: Diabetes: Thyroid:

Kidney disease:

Gastrointestinal:

GERD: Ulcers: Bowel problems:

FEN (Feedings/Enteral/Nutritional status):

Genitourinary:

Bone/muscle: Osteoporosis   Other:

Skin:

Psychosocial Assessment

Birthplace: Cultural or Ethnic Group:

Religion: Language(s) Spoken:

Highest Educational Level:

Sexual Activity:

Alcohol Intake:

Drug Use (illegal, prescription, etc.):

Occupational History (If retired, what types of jobs did you have?):

Family History:

Results of Recent Diagnostic Procedures:

Recent Progress Notes:

Current Physician Orders:

EXERCISE 5.2 Medical Record Documentation (Charting)

EXERCISE 5.2.2 WRITING A RESPIRATORY CARE NOTE

Note (or attach progress note form if instructed to do so) _____

S: _____

O: _____

_____

A: _____

_____

P: _____

_____

_____

_____

_____

Critical Thinking Questions

1. The staff respiratory therapist tells you that sometimes she is just too busy to chart all her treatments. Discuss the implications of not charting.

2. Puff Mommy, a famous recording star, is admitted to your hospital. That night, your best friend calls after hearing about the hospitalization on the evening news. She wants to know why she was admitted. How do you respond?

Procedural Competency Evaluation

STUDENT: DATE:

MEDICAL RECORDS REVIEW

		PERFORMANCE RATING	PERFORMANCE LEVEL
Evaluator: ☐ Peer ☐ Instructor **Setting:** ☐ Lab ☐ Clinical Simulation			
Equipment Utilized: **Conditions (Describe):**			

Performance Level:

     S or ✓ = Satisfactory, no errors of omission or commission
     U = Unsatisfactory Error of Omission or Commission
     NA = Not applicable

Performance Rating:

     5   **Independent:** Near flawless performance; minimal errors; able to perform without supervision; seeks out new learning; shows initiative; A = 4.7–5.0 average

     4   **Minimally Supervised:** Few errors, able to self-correct; seeks guidance when appropriate; B = 3.7–4.65

     3   **Competent:** Minimal required level; no critical errors; able to correct with coaching; meets expectations; safe; C = 3.0–3.65

     2   **Marginal:** Below average; critical errors or problem areas noted; would benefit from remediation; D = 2.0–2.99

     1   **Dependent:** Poor; unacceptable performance; unsafe; gross inaccuracies; potentially harmful; F = < 2.0

     Two or more errors of commission or omission of mandatory or essential performance elements will terminate the procedure, and require additional practice and/or remediation and reevaluation. Student is responsible for obtaining additional evaluation forms as needed from the Director of Clinical Education (DCE).

EQUIPMENT AND PATIENT PREPARATION

1. Obtains and verifies correct chart or electronic medical record		
2. Informs nurse or unit secretary if removing chart from the nurses' station		
3. Ensures compliance with HIPAA regulations regarding personal health information		

ASSESSMENT AND IMPLEMENTATION

4. Locates and evaluates:		
A. Patient demographics		
B. Chief complaint/diagnosis		
C. History of present illness		
D. Smoking history (pack years)		
E. Past medical history		
F. Allergies		
G. Current medications		
H. Psycho/social history		
I. Occupational history and exposures		
J. Family history		
5. Locates and evaluates the physician's orders or protocols		
6. Reviews physical examination results		
7. Reviews results of current diagnostic procedures including CXR, EKG, PFT, ABGs, labs		
8. Reads and evaluates most recent progress notes		
9. Charts procedure performed or shift note including all pertinent data		
10. Signs note with appropriate credential and has preceptor/instructor countersign		

FOLLOW-UP

11. Develops and documents SOAP, APIE, and care plan		
12. Returns chart to proper location and/or closes electronic record		

SIGNATURES   Student: Evaluator: Date:

Clinical Performance Evaluation

PERFORMANCE RATING:

5 **Independent:** Near flawless performance; minimal errors; able to perform without supervision; seeks out new learning; shows initiative; A = 4.7–5.0 average

4 **Minimally Supervised:** Few errors, able to self-correct; seeks guidance when appropriate; B = 3.7–4.65

3 **Competent:** Minimal required level; no critical errors; able to correct with coaching; meets expectations; safe; C = 3.0–3.65

2 **Marginal:** Below average; critical errors or problem areas noted; would benefit from remediation; D = 2.0–2.99

1 **Dependent:** Poor; unacceptable performance; unsafe; gross inaccuracies; potentially harmful; F = < 2.0

Circle the appropriate response below. Please be consistent, objective, and honest in your assessment of the student's clinical performance and ability.

PERFORMANCE CRITERIA	SCORE				
COGNITIVE DOMAIN					
1. Consistently displays knowledge, comprehension, and command of essential concepts	5	4	3	2	1
2. Demonstrates the relationship between theory and clinical practice	5	4	3	2	1
3. Able to select, review, apply, analyze, synthesize, interpret, and evaluate information; makes recommendations to modify care plan	5	4	3	2	1
PSYCHOMOTOR DOMAIN					
4. Minimal errors, no critical errors; able to self-correct; performs all steps safely and accurately	5	4	3	2	1
5. Selects, assembles, and verifies proper function and cleanliness of equipment; assures operation and corrects malfunctions; provides adequate care and maintenance	5	4	3	2	1
6. Exhibits the required manual dexterity	5	4	3	2	1
7. Performs procedure in a reasonable time frame for clinical level	5	4	3	2	1
8. Applies and maintains aseptic technique and PPE as required	5	4	3	2	1
9. Maintains concise and accurate patient and clinical records	5	4	3	2	1
10. Reports promptly on patient status/needs to appropriate personnel	5	4	3	2	1
AFFECTIVE DOMAIN					
11. Exhibits courteous and pleasant demeanor; shows consideration and respect, honesty, and integrity	5	4	3	2	1
12. Communicates verbally and in writing clearly and concisely	5	4	3	2	1
13. Preserves confidentiality and adheres to all policies	5	4	3	2	1
14. Follows directions, exhibits sound judgment, and seeks help when required	5	4	3	2	1
15. Demonstrates initiative, self-direction, responsibility, and accountability	5	4	3	2	1

TOTAL POINTS = _____ /15 = AVERAGE GRADE = _____

ADDITIONAL COMMENTS: IDENTIFY AREAS OF EXCELLENCE; LIST ERRORS OF OMISSION OR COMMISSION, CRITICAL ERRORS

SUMMARY PERFORMANCE EVALUATION AND RECOMMENDATIONS

☐ PASS: Satisfactory Performance

☐ Minimal supervision needed, may progress to next level provided specific skills, clinical time completed

☐ Minimal supervision needed, able to progress to next level without remediation

☐ FAIL: Unsatisfactory Performance (check all that apply)

☐ Minor reevaluation only

☐ Needs additional clinical practice before reevaluation

☐ Needs additional laboratory practice before skills performed in clinical area

☐ Recommend clinical probation

SIGNATURES

Evaluator (print name): _____   Evaluator signature: _____   Date: _____

Student Signature: _____   Date: _____

Student Comments:

Procedural Competency Evaluation

STUDENT: **DATE:**

MEDICAL RECORD DOCUMENTATION

		PERFORMANCE RATING	PERFORMANCE LEVEL
Evaluator: ☐ Peer ☐ Instructor **Setting:** ☐ Lab ☐ Clinical Simulation			

Equipment Utilized: **Conditions (Describe):**

Performance Level:

S or ✓ = Satisfactory, no errors of omission or commission
U = Unsatisfactory Error of Omission or Commission
NA = Not applicable

Performance Rating:

5   **Independent:** Near flawless performance; minimal errors; able to perform without supervision; seeks out new learning; shows initiative; A = 4.7–5.0 average

4   **Minimally Supervised:** Few errors, able to self-correct; seeks guidance when appropriate; B = 3.7–4.65

3   **Competent:** Minimal required level; no critical errors; able to correct with coaching; meets expectations; safe; C = 3.0–3.65

2   **Marginal:** Below average; critical errors or problem areas noted; would benefit from remediation; D = 2.0–2.99

1   **Dependent:** Poor; unacceptable performance; unsafe; gross inaccuracies; potentially harmful; F = < 2.0

Two or more errors of commission or omission of mandatory or essential performance elements will terminate the procedure, and require additional practice and/or remediation and reevaluation. Student is responsible for obtaining additional evaluation forms as needed from the Director of Clinical Education (DCE).

	Performance Rating	Performance Level
1. Identifies and selects the proper medical record		
2. Identifies the proper section of the chart for documenting respiratory care services		
3. Dates and times the entry		
4. Charts the respiratory care procedure according to facility policy		
5. Includes all patient assessment data		
6. Includes medication dosage and mode of delivery, if indicated		
7. Charts patient response to therapy		
8. Signs the note (including credential) according to facility policy		
9. If a paper record is used, returns the chart to the proper location		
10. If electronic record is used, closes the record and logs off the computer		

SIGNATURES   Student: Evaluator: Date:

Clinical Performance Evaluation

PERFORMANCE RATING:

5 **Independent:** Near flawless performance; minimal errors; able to perform without supervision; seeks out new learning; shows initiative; A = 4.7–5.0 average

4 **Minimally Supervised:** Few errors, able to self-correct; seeks guidance when appropriate; B = 3.7–4.65

3 **Competent:** Minimal required level; no critical errors; able to correct with coaching; meets expectations; safe; C = 3.0–3.65

2 **Marginal:** Below average; critical errors or problem areas noted; would benefit from remediation; D = 2.0–2.99

1 **Dependent:** Poor; unacceptable performance; unsafe; gross inaccuracies; potentially harmful; F = < 2.0

Circle the appropriate response below. Please be consistent, objective, and honest in your assessment of the student's clinical performance and ability.

PERFORMANCE CRITERIA / SCORE

PERFORMANCE CRITERIA					
COGNITIVE DOMAIN					
1. Consistently displays knowledge, comprehension, and command of essential concepts	5	4	3	2	1
2. Demonstrates the relationship between theory and clinical practice	5	4	3	2	1
3. Able to select, review, apply, analyze, synthesize, interpret, and evaluate information; makes recommendations to modify care plan	5	4	3	2	1
PSYCHOMOTOR DOMAIN					
4. Minimal errors, no critical errors; able to self-correct; performs all steps safely and accurately	5	4	3	2	1
5. Selects, assembles, and verifies proper function and cleanliness of equipment; assures operation and corrects malfunctions; provides adequate care and maintenance	5	4	3	2	1
6. Exhibits the required manual dexterity	5	4	3	2	1
7. Performs procedure in a reasonable time frame for clinical level	5	4	3	2	1
8. Applies and maintains aseptic technique and PPE as required	5	4	3	2	1
9. Maintains concise and accurate patient and clinical records	5	4	3	2	1
10. Reports promptly on patient status/needs to appropriate personnel	5	4	3	2	1
AFFECTIVE DOMAIN					
11. Exhibits courteous and pleasant demeanor; shows consideration and respect, honesty, and integrity	5	4	3	2	1
12. Communicates verbally and in writing clearly and concisely	5	4	3	2	1
13. Preserves confidentiality and adheres to all policies	5	4	3	2	1
14. Follows directions, exhibits sound judgment, and seeks help when required	5	4	3	2	1
15. Demonstrates initiative, self-direction, responsibility, and accountability	5	4	3	2	1

TOTAL POINTS = _____ /15 = AVERAGE GRADE = _____

ADDITIONAL COMMENTS: IDENTIFY AREAS OF EXCELLENCE; LIST ERRORS OF OMISSION OR COMMISSION, CRITICAL ERRORS

SUMMARY PERFORMANCE EVALUATION AND RECOMMENDATIONS

☐ PASS: Satisfactory Performance

    ☐ Minimal supervision needed, may progress to next level provided specific skills, clinical time completed

    ☐ Minimal supervision needed, able to progress to next level without remediation

☐ FAIL: Unsatisfactory Performance (check all that apply)

    ☐ Minor reevaluation only

    ☐ Needs additional clinical practice before reevaluation

    ☐ Needs additional laboratory practice before skills performed in clinical area

    ☐ Recommend clinical probation

SIGNATURES

Evaluator (print name): _____ Evaluator signature: _____ Date: _____

Student Signature: _____ Date: _____

Student Comments:

Procedural Competency Evaluation

STUDENT: _____ DATE: _____

PATIENT INTERVIEW AND HISTORY

					PERFORMANCE RATING	PERFORMANCE LEVEL
Evaluator: ☐ Peer ☐ Instructor			**Setting:** ☐ Lab	☐ Clinical Simulation		
Equipment Utilized:			**Conditions (Describe):**			

Performance Level:

    S or ✓ = Satisfactory, no errors of omission or commission
    U = Unsatisfactory Error of Omission or Commission
    NA = Not applicable

Performance Rating:

    5   **Independent:** Near flawless performance; minimal errors; able to perform without supervision; seeks out new learning; shows initiative; A = 4.7–5.0 average

    4   **Minimally Supervised:** Few errors, able to self-correct; seeks guidance when appropriate; B = 3.7–4.65

    3   **Competent:** Minimal required level; no critical errors; able to correct with coaching; meets expectations; safe; C = 3.0–3.65

    2   **Marginal:** Below average; critical errors or problem areas noted; would benefit from remediation; D = 2.0–2.99

    1   **Dependent:** Poor; unacceptable performance; unsafe; gross inaccuracies; potentially harmful; F = < 2.0

    Two or more errors of commission or omission of mandatory or essential performance elements will terminate the procedure, and require additional practice and/or remediation and reevaluation. Student is responsible for obtaining additional evaluation forms as needed from the Director of Clinical Education (DCE).

EQUIPMENT AND PATIENT PREPARATION

1. Common Performance Elements Steps 1–8

2. Limits distractions; performs in quiet location

ASSESSMENT AND IMPLEMENTATION

3. Common Performance Elements Steps 9 and 10

4. Utilizes therapeutic communication skills to determine level of consciousness and sensorium, orientation to person, place, time

5. Assesses ability to follow directions and level of cooperation

6. Evaluates emotional status, level of dyspnea, nutritional status, and tolerance of activities of daily living (ADL)

7. Asks patient chief complaint: onset, duration, frequency, severity (quantity), character (quality), location, radiation, aggravating factors, alleviating factors, associated manifestations

8. Asks about history of present illness

9. Determines smoking history (pack years)

10. Inquires about allergies and current medications

11. Asks the patient questions to ascertain specific pulmonary symptoms: dyspnea on exertion or rest, orthopnea, platypnea, pleurodynia

12. Asks about nature of cough

13. Inquires about sputum production: amount, color, consistency, odor, taste, presence of blood

14. Inquires about chest pain: quality, location, radiation, aggravating factors, alleviating factors, and associated manifestations

15. Inquires about past medical history, major illnesses, injuries, and surgeries

16. Performs psychosocial assessment as applicable:

    A. Birthplace   F. Highest education level
    B. Race   G. Alcohol intake
    C. Religion   H. Sexual activity
    D. Culture   I. Drug use
    E. Language(s) spoken   J. Home situation

17. Asks questions about occupational history and exposures

18. Performs review of systems (ROS) to ensure all pertinent information has been obtained

19. Asks the patient questions to determine current comfort level or needs

FOLLOW-UP

20. Common Performance Elements Steps 11–16

SIGNATURES   Student: _____   Evaluator: _____   Date: _____

Clinical Performance Evaluation

PERFORMANCE RATING:

5   **Independent:** Near flawless performance; minimal errors; able to perform without supervision; seeks out new learning; shows initiative; A = 4.7–5.0 average

4   **Minimally Supervised:** Few errors, able to self-correct; seeks guidance when appropriate; B = 3.7–4.65

3   **Competent:** Minimal required level; no critical errors; able to correct with coaching; meets expectations; safe; C = 3.0–3.65

2   **Marginal:** Below average; critical errors or problem areas noted; would benefit from remediation; D = 2.0–2.99

1   **Dependent:** Poor; unacceptable performance; unsafe; gross inaccuracies; potentially harmful; F = < 2.0

Circle the appropriate response below. Please be consistent, objective, and honest in your assessment of the student's clinical performance and ability.

PERFORMANCE CRITERIA	SCORE				
COGNITIVE DOMAIN					
1. Consistently displays knowledge, comprehension, and command of essential concepts	5	4	3	2	1
2. Demonstrates the relationship between theory and clinical practice	5	4	3	2	1
3. Able to select, review, apply, analyze, synthesize, interpret, and evaluate information; makes recommendations to modify care plan	5	4	3	2	1
PSYCHOMOTOR DOMAIN					
4. Minimal errors, no critical errors; able to self-correct; performs all steps safely and accurately	5	4	3	2	1
5. Selects, assembles, and verifies proper function and cleanliness of equipment; assures operation and corrects malfunctions; provides adequate care and maintenance	5	4	3	2	1
6. Exhibits the required manual dexterity	5	4	3	2	1
7. Performs procedure in a reasonable time frame for clinical level	5	4	3	2	1
8. Applies and maintains aseptic technique and PPE as required	5	4	3	2	1
9. Maintains concise and accurate patient and clinical records	5	4	3	2	1
10. Reports promptly on patient status/needs to appropriate personnel	5	4	3	2	1
AFFECTIVE DOMAIN					
11. Exhibits courteous and pleasant demeanor; shows consideration and respect, honesty, and integrity	5	4	3	2	1
12. Communicates verbally and in writing clearly and concisely	5	4	3	2	1
13. Preserves confidentiality and adheres to all policies	5	4	3	2	1
14. Follows directions, exhibits sound judgment, and seeks help when required	5	4	3	2	1
15. Demonstrates initiative, self-direction, responsibility, and accountability	5	4	3	2	1

TOTAL POINTS = _____ /15 = AVERAGE GRADE = _____

ADDITIONAL COMMENTS: IDENTIFY AREAS OF EXCELLENCE; LIST ERRORS OF OMISSION OR COMMISSION, CRITICAL ERRORS

SUMMARY PERFORMANCE EVALUATION AND RECOMMENDATIONS

☐ PASS: Satisfactory Performance

    ☐ Minimal supervision needed, may progress to next level provided specific skills, clinical time completed

    ☐ Minimal supervision needed, able to progress to next level without remediation

☐ FAIL: Unsatisfactory Performance (check all that apply)

    ☐ Minor reevaluation only

    ☐ Needs additional clinical practice before reevaluation

    ☐ Needs additional laboratory practice before skills performed in clinical area

    ☐ Recommend clinical probation

SIGNATURES

Evaluator (print name): _____   Evaluator signature: _____   Date: _____

Student Signature: _____   Date: _____

Student Comments:

Procedural Competency Evaluation

STUDENT: **DATE:**

CASE STUDY PRESENTATION

	PERFORMANCE RATING	PERFORMANCE LEVEL

Evaluator: ☐ Peer ☐ Instructor   **Setting:** ☐ Lab   ☐ Clinical Simulation

Equipment Utilized: **Conditions (Describe):**

Performance Level:

S or ✓ = Satisfactory, no errors of omission or commission
U = Unsatisfactory Error of Omission or Commission
NA = Not applicable

Performance Rating:

5 **Independent:** Near flawless performance; minimal errors; able to perform without supervision; seeks out new learning; shows initiative; A = 4.7–5.0 average

4 **Minimally Supervised:** Few errors, able to self-correct; seeks guidance when appropriate; B = 3.7–4.65

3 **Competent:** Minimal required level; no critical errors; able to correct with coaching; meets expectations; safe; C = 3.0–3.65

2 **Marginal:** Below average; critical errors or problem areas noted; would benefit from remediation; D = 2.0–2.99

1 **Dependent:** Poor; unacceptable performance; unsafe; gross inaccuracies; potentially harmful; F = < 2.0

Two or more errors of commission or omission of mandatory or essential performance elements will terminate the procedure, and require additional practice and/or remediation and reevaluation. Student is responsible for obtaining additional evaluation forms as needed from the Director of Clinical Education (DCE).

EQUIPMENT AND PATIENT PREPARATION

1. Common Performance Elements Steps 1–8		

ASSESSMENT AND IMPLEMENTATION

2. Common Performance Elements Steps 9 and 10		
3. Interviews patient and collects history		
4. Performs physical examination		
5. Ensures patient comfort and safety		

ORAL CASE PRESENTATION

6. Identifies self to audience		
7. Maintains patient confidentiality		
8. Relates patient information including: age, gender, race, height, and weight		
9. Relates advances directive status (full code, DNR)		
10. States chief complaint concisely		
11. States history of present illness (tells the story)		
12. States past medical history including major illnesses, injuries, and surgeries		
13. States psychosocial history		
14. Identifies employment history including present and past employment		
15. Identifies family history		
16. Identifies result of review of systems (ROS)		
17. Identifies results of physical examination including date and time performed		
18. Presents case in chronological order (tells the story)		
19. Presents discussion and summary		
20. Presents complete care plan		
21. Maintains poise and composure throughout presentation		
22. Communicates verbally clearly and loudly enough so audience can hear and comprehend		
23. Answers questions of audience and instructors in reasonable time frame		
24. Correlates theory to case presentation		
25. Completes presentation in reasonable time frame (15 to 30 minutes)		
26. Prepares and submits written case according to instructions		

SIGNATURES   Student: Evaluator: Date:

Clinical Performance Evaluation

PERFORMANCE RATING:

5 **Independent:** Near flawless performance; minimal errors; able to perform without supervision; seeks out new learning; shows initiative; A = 4.7–5.0 average

4 **Minimally Supervised:** Few errors, able to self-correct; seeks guidance when appropriate; B = 3.7–4.65

3 **Competent:** Minimal required level; no critical errors; able to correct with coaching; meets expectations; safe; C = 3.0–3.65

2 **Marginal:** Below average; critical errors or problem areas noted; would benefit from remediation; D = 2.0–2.99

1 **Dependent:** Poor; unacceptable performance; unsafe; gross inaccuracies; potentially harmful; F = < 2.0

Circle the appropriate response below. Please be consistent, objective, and honest in your assessment of the student's clinical performance and ability.

PERFORMANCE CRITERIA	SCORE				
COGNITIVE DOMAIN					
1. Consistently displays knowledge, comprehension, and command of essential concepts	5	4	3	2	1
2. Demonstrates the relationship between theory and clinical practice	5	4	3	2	1
3. Able to select, review, apply, analyze, synthesize, interpret, and evaluate information; makes recommendations to modify care plan	5	4	3	2	1
PSYCHOMOTOR DOMAIN					
4. Minimal errors, no critical errors; able to self-correct; performs all steps safely and accurately	5	4	3	2	1
5. Selects, assembles, and verifies proper function and cleanliness of equipment; assures operation and corrects malfunctions; provides adequate care and maintenance	5	4	3	2	1
6. Exhibits the required manual dexterity	5	4	3	2	1
7. Performs procedure in a reasonable time frame for clinical level	5	4	3	2	1
8. Applies and maintains aseptic technique and PPE as required	5	4	3	2	1
9. Maintains concise and accurate patient and clinical records	5	4	3	2	1
10. Reports promptly on patient status/needs to appropriate personnel	5	4	3	2	1
AFFECTIVE DOMAIN					
11. Exhibits courteous and pleasant demeanor; shows consideration and respect, honesty, and integrity	5	4	3	2	1
12. Communicates verbally and in writing clearly and concisely	5	4	3	2	1
13. Preserves confidentiality and adheres to all policies	5	4	3	2	1
14. Follows directions, exhibits sound judgment, and seeks help when required	5	4	3	2	1
15. Demonstrates initiative, self-direction, responsibility, and accountability	5	4	3	2	1

TOTAL POINTS =   /15 = AVERAGE GRADE =

ADDITIONAL COMMENTS: IDENTIFY AREAS OF EXCELLENCE; LIST ERRORS OF OMISSION OR COMMISSION, CRITICAL ERRORS

SUMMARY PERFORMANCE EVALUATION AND RECOMMENDATIONS

☐ PASS: Satisfactory Performance

☐ Minimal supervision needed, may progress to next level provided specific skills, clinical time completed

☐ Minimal supervision needed, able to progress to next level without remediation

☐ FAIL: Unsatisfactory Performance (check all that apply)

☐ Minor reevaluation only

☐ Needs additional clinical practice before reevaluation

☐ Needs additional laboratory practice before skills performed in clinical area

☐ Recommend clinical probation

SIGNATURES

Evaluator (print name):   Evaluator signature: Date:

Student Signature: Date:

Student Comments:

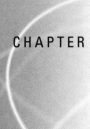

6 Patient Assessment: Basic Skills Vital Signs

INTRODUCTION

Effective patient assessment is the single most important component in providing competent respiratory care. Initiation, modification, and discontinuance of all respiratory care procedures depend on adequately assessing the patient's changing condition.[1] Incorporation of assessment data with the information gathered by the patient interview gives the respiratory care practitioner a clearer understanding of the patient's clinical picture. Therefore, to effectively participate in the decision-making process or to successfully implement respiratory care, therapist-driven protocols (TDPs), the respiratory care practitioner must be proficient in patient assessment techniques.

The basic elements of patient assessment include the following:

1. Scene survey
2. Primary survey
3. Secondary survey
4. Vital signs
5. Pulse oximetry

This chapter will focus on the basic techniques of vital sign assessment, including pulse oximetry. We will explore pulse oximetry and other noninvasive blood gas monitoring techniques more comprehensively in Chapter 25. The more advanced skills of physical assessment of the chest and auscultation will be discussed in the next chapter.

OBJECTIVES

Upon completion of this chapter, the student will be able to:

1. Conduct a primary survey.
2. Perform a secondary survey (head-to-toe assessment).
3. Practice the techniques of simple vital sign measurements:
   A. Temperature
   B. Pulse
   C. Breathing
   D. Blood pressure
4. Perform pulse oximetry.
5. Practice medical charting for the documentation of performance of patient assessment procedures.
6. Apply infection control guidelines and standards associated with equipment and procedures, according to OSHA regulations and CDC guidelines.

KEY TERMS

While many of these key terms are not in the body of the text, they may be used to discuss patient status during assessment

acute	chronic	hypopnea	prone
ambulatory	clubbing	hypotension	proximal
aneroid	collateral	hypothermia	sensorium
antecubital	contraindication	hypovolemia	somnolent
anterior	cyanosis	inferior	stoma
apical	debilitated	invasive	sphygmomanometer
apnea	decubitus	ischemia	subcutaneous
aspiration	diaphoresis	jaundice	emphysema
asterixis	distal	Kussmaul's respiration	superior
auscultation	dyspnea	lateral	supine
asymmetrical	ecchymosis	lethargic	syncope
ataxia	edema	malaise	systemic
atelectasis	electrolyte	medial	systolic pressure
atrophy	epistaxis	obtunded	tachycardia
bilateral	epithelium	orthopnea	tachypnea
binaural	erythema	orthostatic	torr
Biot's respiration	eupnea	pallor	turgor
blanching	febrile	palpation	unilateral
bradycardia	flaring	paradoxical	vascular
cachectic	hematocrit	paresthesia	vasoconstriction
catheter	hyperpnea	percussion	vasodilation
caudad	hypertension	perfusion	ventilation
cephalad	hyperthermia	phalanges	
Cheyne Stokes	hypertrophy	polycythemia	
respiration	hypervolemia	posterior	

Exercises

EQUIPMENT REQUIRED

- ☐ Alcohol prep pads
- ☐ **Binaural** stethoscopes (teaching models, if available)
- ☐ Disposable (nonlatex) gloves, various sizes
- ☐ Electronic digital oral or ear thermometers and sheaths
- ☐ Hospital bed or equivalent
- ☐ Human patient simulator mannequin (if available)

- ☐ Patient mannequin (or student)
- ☐ Pulse oximeter and probes (disposable and permanent)
- ☐ **Sphygmomanometer**
- ☐ Stopwatch
- ☐ Various pulse oximeter probes
- ☐ Various size blood pressure cuffs
- ☐ Watch with second hand

EXERCISE 6.1 PRIMARY SURVEY

The primary survey includes the initial impression of the patient, observing for any immediate life-threatening conditions only. The primary survey consists of checking airway, breathing, and circulation (the ABCs): Airway—is the airway open? Breathing—is breathing present? Circulation—is pulse present? Is there any severe bleeding? Immediate action must be taken for any life-threatening condition before proceeding to the next step. Remember to check the scene for safety (see Chapter 1) before approaching the patient. **Record your findings on your laboratory report.**

It is expected that the student will have already had instruction in basic life support for healthcare providers before this laboratory exercise.

In this exercise the instructor will set up one or more of the following scenarios. Refer to current American Heart Association (AHA) or American Red Cross (ARC) cardiopulmonary resuscitation (CPR) guidelines for specific details.

Students should apply standard precautions and transmission-based isolation procedures as appropriate. Approach the "patient" and assess the ABCs. Perform any necessary steps as determined by your findings.

1. A conscious and alert patient who is breathing and has a pulse
    A. Determine responsiveness.
    B. Quickly observe the patient for chest rise and fall.
    C. Ask the patient a question that requires a response to determine whether the subject has a patent airway and is able to move air.
    D. Quickly observe for any severe bleeding by scanning the patient from head to toe.
2. An unconscious patient who is breathing and has a pulse
    A. Determine unresponsiveness.
    B. Activate the emergency medical services (EMS) system.
    C. Use the head tilt/chin lift maneuver (Fig. 6.1) to open the airway. Look, listen, and feel for breathing (Fig. 6.2). If spinal injury is suspected, use a modified jaw thrust (Fig. 6.3) to open the airway.
        i. If the patient is breathing, maintain head tilt/chin lift position with one hand. Continue to monitor for breathing and carotid pulse.
3. An unconscious patient who is not breathing but who has a pulse
    A. Determine unresponsiveness.
    B. Activate the EMS system.
    C. Use the head tilt/chin lift maneuver to open the airway, and maintain it with one hand. Look, listen, and feel for breathing.
    D. If breathing is absent, begin rescue breathing. Various methods of ventilation are shown in Figure 6.4.
    E. Practice mouth-to-mask ventilation, as shown in Figure 6.5.

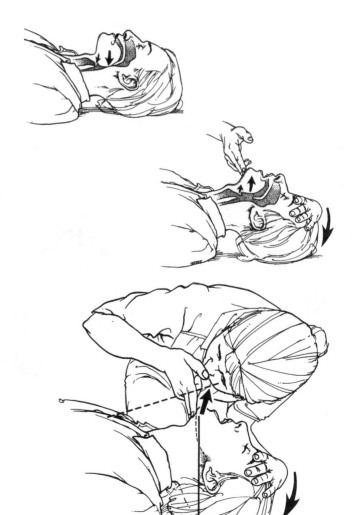

Figure 6.1. Opening the airway. (Reproduced with permission from Chandra, NC and Hazinski, MF: *Textbook of Basic Life Support for Healthcare Providers.* American Heart Association, Dallas, 1994.)

Figure 6.2. Determining breathlessness. (Reproduced with permission from Chandra, NC and Hazinski, MF: *Textbook of Basic Life Support for Healthcare Providers.* American Heart Association, Dallas, 1994.)

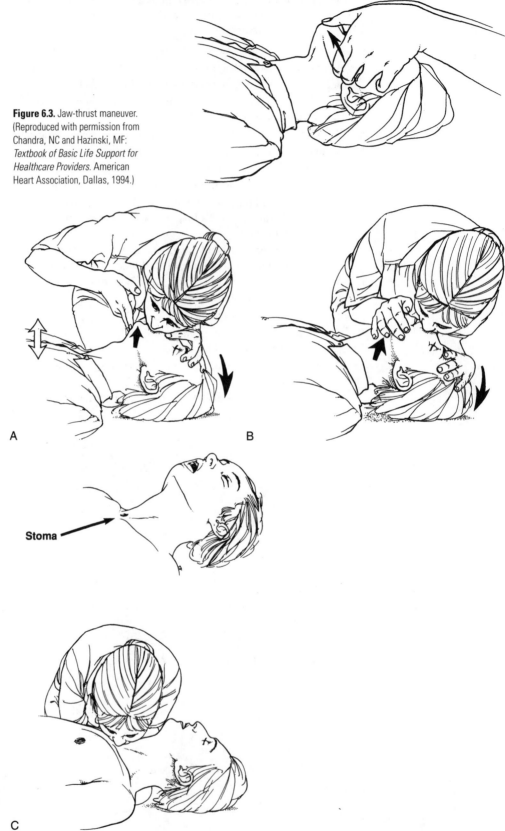

Figure 6.3. Jaw-thrust maneuver. (Reproduced with permission from Chandra, NC and Hazinski, MF: *Textbook of Basic Life Support for Healthcare Providers*. American Heart Association, Dallas, 1994.)

A

B

Stoma

Figure 6.4. Methods of rescue breathing: **(A)** Mouth-to-mouth breathing, **(B)** Mouth-to-nose breathing, **(C)** Mouth-to-stoma breathing. (Reproduced with permission from Chandra, NC and Hazinski, MF: *Textbook of Basic Life Support for Healthcare Providers*. American Heart Association, Dallas, 1994.)

C

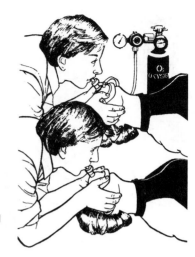

Figure 6.5. Mouth-to-mask ventilation with a one-way valve and supplemental oxygen. (Courtesy of Laerdal Medical Corporation, Wappingers Falls, NY.)

NOTE: Ventilations should be simulated if a student is acting as the surrogate patient.

    F.   Check the carotid pulse for 5 to 10 seconds (Fig. 6.6). If the pulse is present, continue rescue breathing. Monitor the pulse periodically.

4.   An unconscious patient who is not breathing and has no pulse

    A.   Determine unresponsiveness.

    B.   Activate the EMS system.

    C.   Position the patient.

    D.   Use the head tilt/chin lift maneuver to open the airway, and maintain it with one hand. Look, listen, and feel for breathing.

        i.   If breathing is absent, give ventilations.

    E.   Check the carotid pulse for 5 to 10 seconds.

        i.   If pulse is absent, begin chest compressions (Fig. 6.7) and continue CPR according to current AHA or ARC guidelines.

    NOTE: Compressions should be simulated if a student is acting as the surrogate patient.

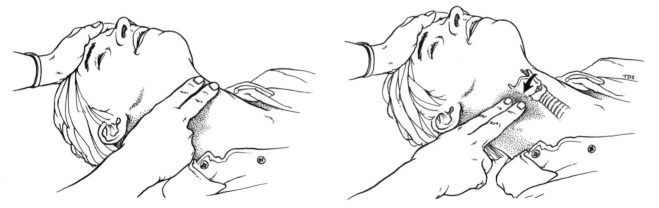

Figure 6.6. Checking the carotid pulse. (Reproduced with permission from Chandra, NC and Hazinski, MF: *Textbook of Basic Life Support for Healthcare Providers.* American Heart Association, Dallas, 1994.)

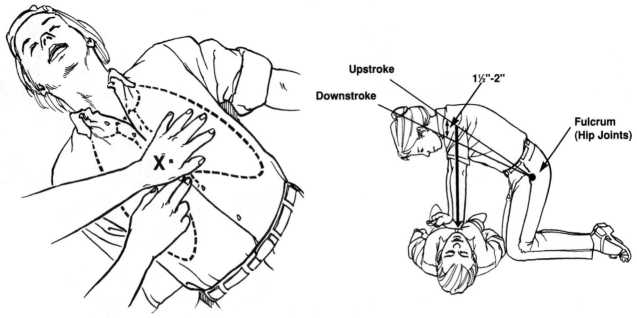

Figure 6.7. Proper positioning for chest compressions. (Reproduced with permission from Chandra, NC and Hazinski, MF: *Textbook of Basic Life Support for Healthcare Providers.* American Heart Association, Dallas, 1994.)

EXERCISE 6.2 SECONDARY SURVEY

The secondary survey is a brief head-to-toe observation of your patient to ascertain any injuries or problems other than the chief complaint that may require attention.

Perform a brief head-to-toe survey of your lab partner or human patient simulator, as shown in Figure 6.8. Wash your hands and apply standard precautions and transmission-based isolation procedures as appropriate.

1. *Head.* Examine the head as follows:
   A. Observe and palpate for the presence of any cuts or bruises.
   B. Inspect the nose and ears for fluid or blood.
   C. Inspect the mouth for blood, broken teeth, or loose teeth.
   D. Check the breath odor.
   E. Check skin temperature and texture.
   F. Check mucous membranes for color.

2. *Neck.* Inspect and palpate the neck for the following:
   A. Any masses
   B. Jugular vein distention (JVD)
   C. Medic Alert pendant
   D. Presence of stoma
   E. Subcutaneous emphysema
   F. Tracheal deviation
   G. Transtracheal oxygen catheter
   H. Use of accessory muscles
   I. Any other invasive catheters

3. *Chest.* This area will be covered in the next exercise.

4. *Abdomen.* Palpate the four quadrants and observe for the following:
   A. Pain
   B. Distention
   C. Rigidity
   D. Bruising

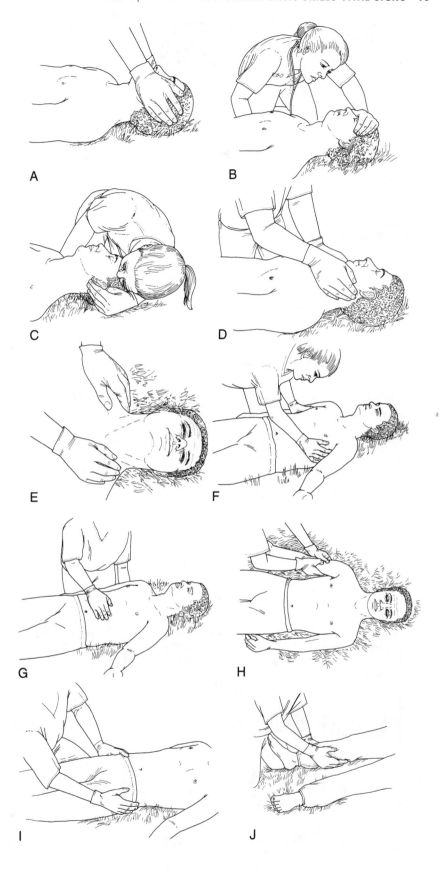

A

B

C

D

E

F

G

H

I

J

Figure 6.8. Head-to-toe survey.

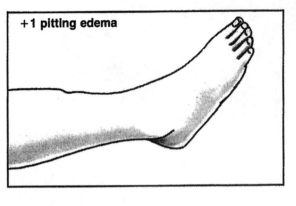

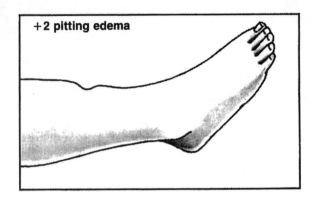

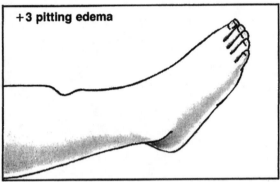

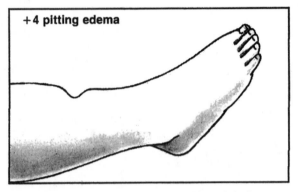

Figure 6.9. Evaluating pitting edema. (From Morton, PG: Health Assessment in Nursing, ed 2. FA Davis, Philadelphia, 1993, p. 399, with permission.)

5. *Extremities.* Observe and palpate for the following:
   A. Deformities
   B. Edema (Fig. 6.9)
   C. Peripheral pulses
   D. Temperature and color
   E. Capillary refill
   F. Clubbing of the distal phalanges (Fig. 6.10)
   G. Tobacco stains on the fingers
   H. Medic Alert bracelet
6. Record your findings on your laboratory report.

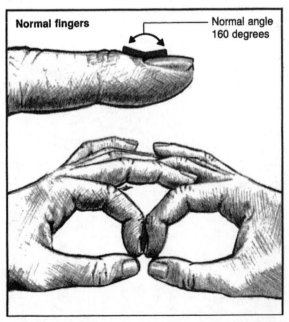

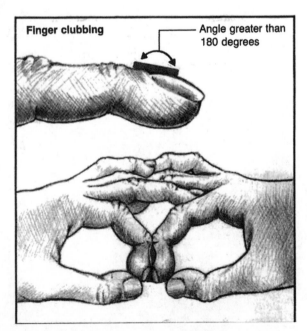

Figure 6.10. Clubbing. (From Morton, PG: Health Assessment in Nursing, ed 2. FA Davis, Philadelphia, 1993, p. 261, with permission.)

EXERCISE 6.3 VITAL SIGNS

EXERCISE 6.3.1 TAKING ORAL/AXILLARY/EAR TEMPERATURES

*Each student will measure the axillary, oral, and ear temperature of a laboratory partner. Various thermometers are shown in Figure 6.11. The causes of **hyperthermia** and **hypothermia** are shown in Table 6.1. Wash your hands and apply standard precautions and transmission-based isolation procedures as appropriate.*

1. Place the thermometer probe in a disposable sheath.
2. Press the "Start" button.
3. Place the probe of the thermometer under your lab partner's tongue and leave it in place until the thermometer indicates a final reading (several seconds).
4. Remove the thermometer, discard the sheath, **and record the temperature on your laboratory report.**
5. Repeat for axillary temperature with a nondisposable thermometer. Keep under the arm for at least 10 minutes and **record the temperature on your laboratory report.**
6. Repeat for tympanic temperature (ear temperature as available) and **record the temperature on your laboratory report.**

Chemical dot thermometer

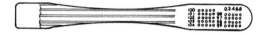

Digital thermometer

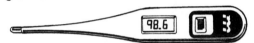

Electronic digital thermometer

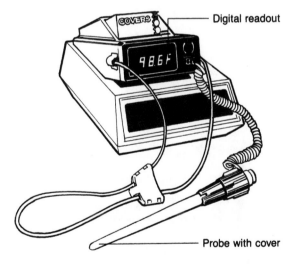

Digital readout

Probe with cover

Figure 6.11. Several types of thermometers measure body temperature: chemical dot, digital, and electronic digital. Each type provides accurate readings when used properly. (From Morton, PG: Health Assessment in Nursing, ed 2. FA Davis, Philadelphia, 1993, p. 74, with permission.)

Table 6.1 Causes of Hypothermia and Hyperthermia

Causes of Hypothermia	Causes of Hyperthermia
Cold exposure	Fever
Shock, blood loss	Heat exposure
Drugs	Drugs
Brain injuries	Dehydration
	Anesthesia
	Atelectasis
	Surgery
	Brain injuries

EXERCISE 6.3.2 LOCATION AND MEASUREMENT OF PULSE

1. **Location of Common Pulse Points** Wash your hands and apply standard precautions and transmission-based isolation procedures as appropriate. Identify the following pulse points as shown in Figure 6.12 on your laboratory partner or yourself:

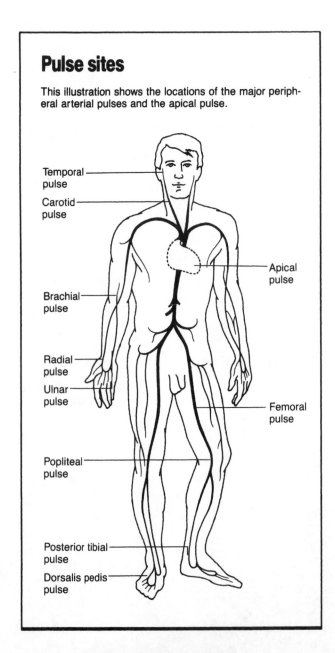

Figure 6.12. Location of pulses. (From Morton, PG: Health Assessment in Nursing, ed 2. FA Davis, Philadelphia, 1993, p. 96, with permission.)

Radial

Ulnar

Brachial

Carotid

Femoral

Temporal

Popliteal

Dorsalis pedis

Posterior tibial

NOTE: To properly palpate pulses, use the index and middle fingers as shown in Figure 6.13. Press firmly but gently. *The thumb should not be used.* Excessive pressure can obliterate the pulse. Ideally, the pulse should be measured for a full minute, particularly in subjects with an irregular heart rate or rhythm.

2. **Measurement of Pulse Rate** Wash your hands and apply standard precautions and transmission based isolation procedures as appropriate.

  A. Using a watch with a second hand, measure your partner's radial pulse for 15 and 60 seconds. **Record the results on your laboratory report.**

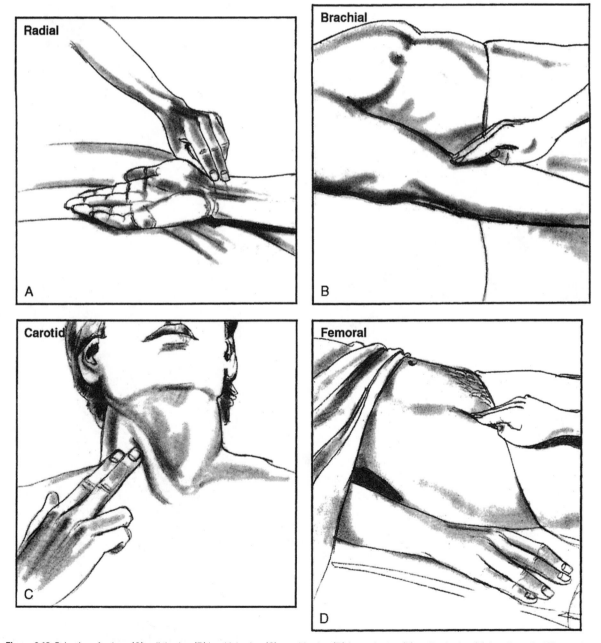

Figure 6.13. Palpation of pulses: **(A)** radial pulse, **(B)** brachial pulse, **(C)** carotid pulse, **(D)** femoral pulse, **(E)** popliteal pulse, **(F)** dorsalis pedis, **(G)** posterior tibial. (From Morton, PG: Health Assessment in Nursing, ed 2. FA Davis, Philadelphia, 1993, pp. 312–313, with permission.) *(continued)*

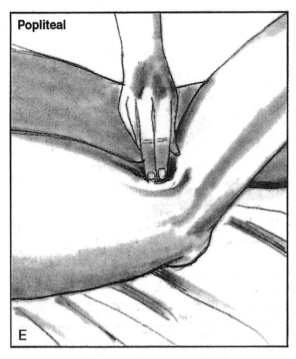

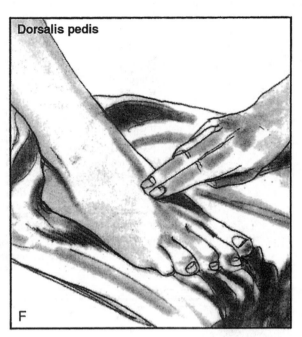

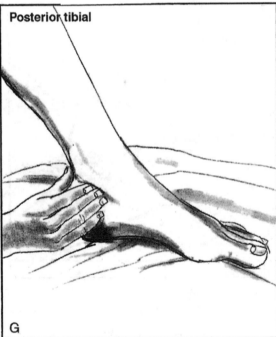

Figure 6.13. *(continued)*

    B.   Describe the quality of the pulses you felt. Include assessment of pulse strength and regularity. **Record this on your laboratory report.**

    C.   Have your partner run or up and down a flight of stairs or run in place for 1 minute. Remeasure the radial pulse. **Record the result on your laboratory report.**

3.   **Measurement of Apical Radial Pulse** The apex of the heart is located on the left side of the chest. You can hear the heart beating with a stethoscope. The causes of bradycardia and tachycardia are shown in Table 6.2.

    A.   Measure the apical pulse rate on your laboratory partner and compare it with the result from step 2.

    B.   **Record the pulse rate on your laboratory report.**

4.   **Capillary Refill** Capillary refill helps one to assess local perfusion.

    A.   Gently squeeze the tip of each finger (one at a time) until a blanching is noticed (nail bed turns white), as shown in Figure 6.14.

Table 6.2 Causes of Bradycardia and Tachycardia

Causes of Bradycardia	Causes of Tachycardia
Heart block	Hypoxia
Athletic conditioning	Fever
Hypothermia	Anxiety/stress
Severe trauma	Pain
Adrenergic blocking agents	Drugs
Vagal stimulation	Hyperthyroidism
Increased intracranial pressure	Shock
Drugs	Hypercapnia
	Heart dysrhythmias

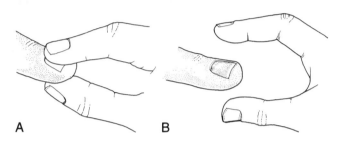

Figure 6.14. Assessing capillary refill.

A   B

B. Using a stopwatch, record the time it takes for the fingertip to turn pink. A slow refill (longer than 3 seconds) indicates poor perfusion.

EXERCISE 6.3.3 ASSESSMENT OF BREATHING (RESPIRATION)

1. Measuring Respiratory Frequency
   A. Wash your hands and apply standard precautions and transmission-based isolation procedures as appropriate.
   B. Observe your partner's chest for movement. The chest rises during inspiration. Count one full respiration as a cycle from the beginning of one inspiration to the beginning of the next.

   NOTE: Many patients unintentionally alter their respiratory rate or pattern if they become aware that you are counting their respirations. This can be avoided if you appear to be taking the pulse while you are actually counting the respiratory rate.

   C. Using a watch with a second hand, count your partner's respirations (f) for 15 and 60 seconds. **Record the results on your laboratory report.**
   D. Describe the quality of the respirations you observed. Assessment should include evaluation of the rate and depth, whether there is labored breathing, and the pattern of respiration.

2. Inspiration:Expiration (I:E) Ratio

   Expiration is normally twice as long as inspiration. The ratio of inspiratory time (I) to expiratory time (E) should be approximately 1:2. It is extremely difficult to manually measure the I:E ratio. In a clinical setting (e.g., a patient on mechanical ventilation) the I:E ratio is measured by computerized technology. However, it is clinically important to be able to assess and compare the length of inspiratory and expiratory cycles with "normal."

   Formulas:

   f = respiratory rate
   T (total time) $= 60/f$
   $E = T - I$
   $I = T - E$
   $I{:}E = 1{:}E/I$
   $I = T/I + E$

A. Using a watch with a second hand, measure the time it takes for one full respiration from the beginning of inspiration to the beginning of the next inspiration.

B. Watch your laboratory partner closely. Measure your partner's inspiratory time (from beginning of inspiration to beginning of expiration) in seconds. **Record the results on your laboratory report.**

C. Measure your partner's expiratory time (from beginning of expiration to beginning of inspiration) in seconds. **Record the results on your laboratory report.**

NOTE: The inspiratory time and expiratory time should equal the total time. Because of the difficulty of manual measurement, times may not be exact.

EXERCISE 6.3.4 ARTERIAL BLOOD PRESSURE

Most healthcare facilities have aneroid sphygmomanometers mounted on a wheeled cart or on the wall, as shown in Figure 6.15. Some facilities may be using various types of electronic devices.

To measure blood pressure with an aneroid sphygmomanometer, take your laboratory partner's blood pressure while he or she is sitting. **Record the results on your laboratory report.**

1. Wash or sanitize your hands and apply standard precautions and transmission-based isolation procedures as appropriate.

2. Wrap the sphygmomanometer cuff snugly around your partner's arm approximately 1 inch above the inner aspect of the elbow (the antecubital area), as shown in Figure 6.16. Proper cuff size is essential. The cuff should be about 1.5 times the size of the limb. Ensure that the cuff bladder is centered over the brachial artery. Most cuffs have arrows to indicate artery and cuff alignment. The gauge should be kept at the level of your partner's arm. Your partner's arm should be kept at heart level. The arm must remain relaxed. Any muscle tension used to keep the arm straight will alter the reading.

3. Palpate the brachial pulse and then rapidly inflate the cuff to approximately 30 mm Hg above the level at which the pulse disappears.

4. Deflate the cuff *slowly* until the pulse reappears. Make a mental note of that number. Deflate the cuff completely.

5. Place the stethoscope in your ears and place the bell of the stethoscope over the brachial pulse, slightly distal to or partially under the cuff, as shown in Figure 6.17.

6. Watching the manometer, pump up the cuff until the level is about 30 mm Hg above the point at which the pulse disappeared (from step 4).

7. Slowly open the air valve to deflate the cuff and watch carefully as the needle drops. The speed should be approximately 2 to 4 mm Hg per second.

8. While watching the manometer, listen for the sound of blood pulsating through the brachial artery. The point at which this occurs is the systolic pressure. Make a mental note of this number. This is the systolic pressure.

9. Continue to deflate the cuff at the same rate until all sound disappears. Note this number. This is the diastolic pressure.

10. Remove the cuff and **record the blood pressure on your laboratory report as systolic/diastolic.**

11. Repeat the blood pressure measurement while your partner is standing and then lying down. **Record these measurements on your laboratory report.**

Figure 6.15. Aneroid sphygmomanometer. (From Morton, PG: Health Assessment in Nursing, ed 2. FA Davis, Philadelphia, 1993, p. 75, with permission.)

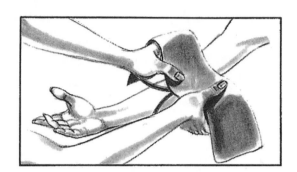

Figure 6.16. Blood pressure cuff application. (From Morton, PG: Health Assessment in Nursing, ed 2. FA Davis, Philadelphia, 1993, p. 99, with permission.)

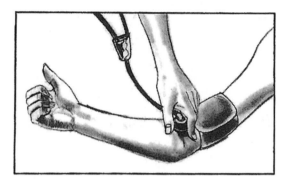

Figure 6.17. Measuring blood pressure. (From Morton, PG: Health Assessment in Nursing, ed 2. FA Davis, Philadelphia, 1993, p. 99, with permission.)

12. Have your partner run in place for 1 minute and then repeat the standing blood pressure measurement. **Record the measurement on your laboratory report.**

EXERCISE 6.4 BASIC PULSE OXIMETRY

Pulse oximetry has literally become the fifth vital sign. This noninvasive technique of quickly assessing oxygenation status is simple and should be done during initial patient assessment and as often as necessary. It is important to report the results in conjunction with any oxygen therapy. If the reading was obtained on room air, then that should be included in the findings. Pulse oximetry will be explored in more depth in Chapter 25.

Obtain a pulse oximetry reading on your partner and **record the results on your laboratory report.**

1. Wash or sanitize your hands and apply standard precautions and transmission-based isolation procedures as appropriate.
2. Select a pulse oximeter and finger probe.
3. Turn the unit on and ensure that it is functioning.
4. Select a finger and ensure that there is adequate circulation to the digit.
5. Apply the probe as shown in Figure 6.18.
6. Wait about 30 seconds for the reading to stabilize.
7. Observe both the oximetry and pulse reading. Does the pulse correlate with your findings in Exercise 6.3.2?
8. Note whether the "patient" is breathing room air or supplemental oxygen.
9. **Record the pulse, oximetry, and oxygen percentage on your laboratory report.**

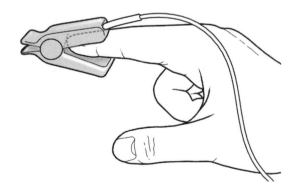

Figure 6.18. Proper orientation of oximeter finger probe.

REFERENCES

1. Wilkins, RL and Stoller, JK: Egan's Fundamentals of Respiratory Care, ed 8. Mosby, St. Louis, 2003, p. 309.

Laboratory Report

CHAPTER 6: PATIENT ASSESSMENT: BASIC SKILLS VITAL SIGNS

Name _____   Date _____

Course/Section _____   Instructor _____

Data Collection

EXERCISE 6.1 Primary Survey

Findings: _____

_____

EXERCISE 6.2 Secondary Survey

1. Head _____

2. Neck _____

3. Chest _____

4. Abdomen _____

5. Extremities _____

EXERCISE 6.3 Vital Signs

EXERCISE 6.3.1 TAKING ORAL/AXILLARY/EAR TEMPERATURES

Temperature = _____ °F

Convert temperature to Celsius. **Show your work!**

°C = 5(°F − 32)/9   Temperature = _____ °C

Temperature = 35 °C

Convert temperature to Fahrenheit. **Show your work!**

°F = °C × 9/5 + 32   Temperature = _____°F

EXERCISE 6.3.2 LOCATION AND MEASUREMENT OF PULSE

60-second pulse = _____/minute

15-second pulse = _____ × 4 = _____/minute

Compare the two measurement methods: _____

_____

Quality of pulse: _____

Pulse after exercise = _____/minute

Apical pulse rate (resting) = _____/minute

Pulse deficit = Apical − Radial = _____/minute

Capillary refill time = _____seconds

EXERCISE 6.3.3 ASSESSMENT OF BREATHING (RESPIRATION)

1. Measuring respiratory frequency

    A. f: 15 seconds = _____ × 4 = _____/minute

    B. f: 30 seconds = _____ /minute

    C. Quality of respirations: _____

2. Inspiration:Expiration ratio

    A. Measured respiratory total time = _____ seconds

    B. Measured inspiratory time : = _____ seconds

3. Calculating expiratory time. Using steps 2.A and 2.B, calculate the following. **Show your work!**

    A. Expiratory time $T − I = E$ _____ (seconds)

    B. I:E ratio = 1: _____

    C. Measured expiratory time = _____ seconds

4. Calculating inspiratory time. (Do not use your measured value of I time for this calculation!) Using steps 2. A and 2.C, calculate the following. **Show your work!**

    A. $T − E$ (measured) = I _____ seconds

    B. I:E ratio = 1: _____

EXERCISE 6.3.4 ARTERIAL BLOOD PRESSURE

1. Blood pressure (BP) sitting = _____ mm Hg

2. Pulse pressure = Systolic − Diastolic = _____

3. BP standing = _____ mm Hg

4. BP supine = _____ mm Hg

5. BP after exercise = _____ mm Hg

EXERCISE 6.4 Basic Pulse Oximetry

1. Pulse: _____

2. Oximetry reading:_____

3. Pulse correlation:_____

4. Oxygen or room air:_____

Critical Thinking Questions

1. When would it be recommended to count the pulse for 30 to 60 seconds rather than 15 seconds?

2. What conditions or circumstances may cause the apical and radial pulse to be different from each other?

3. A patient is noted to be tachycardic with a pulse rate of 140/minute. What other signs and symptoms would you expect to find on physical examination if the tachycardia is caused by hypoxia?

4. Name two respiratory care procedures or modalities that can interfere with the accurate measurement of an oral temperature.

5. Convert the following Fahrenheit temperatures to Celsius. **Show your work!**

   A.   95 °F = _____°C

   B.   105 °F = _____°C

6. If the patient's total respiratory time and respiratory rate stayed the same but expiratory time was increased, would inspiratory time increase or decrease?

7. If the patient's total respiratory time was 6 seconds, what would this person's respiratory rate per minute be? **Show your work!**

8. If a patient's I:E ratio was 1:2 and expiration was 4 seconds long, what would the inspiratory time be? **Show your work!**

9. If a patient's I:E ratio was 1:3 and respiratory rate was 30/minute, calculate the following. **Show your work!**

   T = _____ Inspiratory time = _____ Expiratory time = _____

10. Explain how and why pulsus paradoxus occurs.

11. Differentiate between pulsus paradoxus and pulsus alternans.

12. How will the blood pressure measurement be affected if excessive pressure is used in cuff inflation or if pressure is held in the cuff too long?

13. What happens if a blood pressure cuff is too small?

14. **Scenario 1:** You have entered the patient's room to administer a respiratory treatment. You find the patient lying face-down on the bathroom floor.

    A. What are the first three steps you would take under these circumstances?

    B. You have determined that the victim is not breathing. You attempt manual ventilation and do not see the chest rise and fall or feel air entering the victim. What are the first three steps you would take under these circumstances?

15. **Scenario 2:** A patient with diabetes enters the emergency department (ED) in a coma. You perform a basic assessment on this patient.

    A. What would you expect to find when assessing the patient's breath?

    B. The patient's capillary refill time is noted to be 10 seconds. What would this indicate? Why?

    C. What type of respiratory rate and pattern would you expect to find?

16. **Scenario 3:** You are called to the ED to evaluate Mr. C.O. Tu. Mr. Tu has a long-standing history of chronic obstructive pulmonary disease (COPD). He has been brought to the ED by ambulance. He complains of increasing shortness of breath and productive cough with thick, green sputum.

    A. Identify five clinical findings you could detect by direct observation that would indicate to you that Mr. Tu has an increased work of breathing.

    B. What values would you expect to find when measuring vital signs (pulse, respirations, blood pressure, and temperature) and pulse oximetry?

Procedural Competency Evaluation

STUDENT: DATE:

VITAL SIGNS: PULSE AND RESPIRATION

Evaluator: ☐ Peer ☐ Instructor   **Setting:** ☐ Lab ☐ Clinical Simulation

Equipment Utilized: **Conditions (Describe):**

Performance Level:

S or ✓ = Satisfactory, no errors of omission or commission
U = Unsatisfactory Error of Omission or Commission
NA = Not applicable

Performance Rating:

5   **Independent:** Near flawless performance; minimal errors; able to perform without supervision; seeks out new learning; shows initiative; A = 4.7–5.0 average

4   **Minimally Supervised:** Few errors, able to self-correct; seeks guidance when appropriate; B = 3.7–4.65

3   **Competent:** Minimal required level; no critical errors; able to correct with coaching; meets expectations; safe; C = 3.0–3.65

2   **Marginal:** Below average; critical errors or problem areas noted; would benefit from remediation; D = 2.0–2.99

1   **Dependent:** Poor; unacceptable performance; unsafe; gross inaccuracies; potentially harmful; F = < 2.0

Two or more errors of commission or omission of mandatory or essential performance elements will terminate the procedure, and require additional practice and/or remediation and reevaluation. Student is responsible for obtaining additional evaluation forms as needed from the Director of Clinical Education (DCE).

Columns: PERFORMANCE RATING | PERFORMANCE LEVEL

EQUIPMENT AND PATIENT PREPARATION

1. Common Performance Elements Steps 1–8

ASSESSMENT AND IMPLEMENTATION

2. Common Performance Elements Steps 9 and 10
3. Locates pulse site
4. Measures pulse for at least 15 seconds, or a full minute if pulse is irregular
  A. Assesses rhythm and quality of the pulse
5. Measures respiration for at least 15 seconds
  A. Assesses depth of breathing and I:E ratio
  B. Assesses rhythm and quality of respirations
6. Assesses degree of labored breathing, orthopnea, platypnea, pleurodynia, accessory muscle use, pursed-lip breathing, retractions, nasal flaring, and abdominal paradox
7. Measures pulse oximeter saturation and pulse reading (see PCE for Pulse Oximetry)
8. Compares pulse reading to oximeter or cardiac monitor rate
9. Measures blood pressure (see PCE for Blood Pressure)
10. Looks up and notes patient's temperature on vital signs flowsheet or chart

FOLLOW-UP

11. Common Performance Elements Steps 11–16

SIGNATURES   Student: Evaluator: Date:

Clinical Performance Evaluation

PERFORMANCE RATING:

5 **Independent:** Near flawless performance; minimal errors; able to perform without supervision; seeks out new learning; shows initiative; A = 4.7–5.0 average

4 **Minimally Supervised:** Few errors, able to self-correct; seeks guidance when appropriate; B = 3.7–4.65

3 **Competent:** Minimal required level; no critical errors; able to correct with coaching; meets expectations; safe; C = 3.0–3.65

2 **Marginal:** Below average; critical errors or problem areas noted; would benefit from remediation; D = 2.0–2.99

1 **Dependent:** Poor; unacceptable performance; unsafe; gross inaccuracies; potentially harmful; F = < 2.0

Circle the appropriate response below. Please be consistent, objective, and honest in your assessment of the student's clinical performance and ability.

PERFORMANCE CRITERIA

	SCORE				
COGNITIVE DOMAIN					
1. Consistently displays knowledge, comprehension, and command of essential concepts	5	4	3	2	1
2. Demonstrates the relationship between theory and clinical practice	5	4	3	2	1
3. Able to select, review, apply, analyze, synthesize, interpret, and evaluate information; makes recommendations to modify care plan	5	4	3	2	1
PSYCHOMOTOR DOMAIN					
4. Minimal errors, no critical errors; able to self-correct; performs all steps safely and accurately	5	4	3	2	1
5. Selects, assembles, and verifies proper function and cleanliness of equipment; assures operation and corrects malfunctions; provides adequate care and maintenance	5	4	3	2	1
6. Exhibits the required manual dexterity	5	4	3	2	1
7. Performs procedure in a reasonable time frame for clinical level	5	4	3	2	1
8. Applies and maintains aseptic technique and PPE as required	5	4	3	2	1
9. Maintains concise and accurate patient and clinical records	5	4	3	2	1
10. Reports promptly on patient status/needs to appropriate personnel	5	4	3	2	1
AFFECTIVE DOMAIN					
11. Exhibits courteous and pleasant demeanor; shows consideration and respect, honesty, and integrity	5	4	3	2	1
12. Communicates verbally and in writing clearly and concisely	5	4	3	2	1
13. Preserves confidentiality and adheres to all policies	5	4	3	2	1
14. Follows directions, exhibits sound judgment, and seeks help when required	5	4	3	2	1
15. Demonstrates initiative, self-direction, responsibility, and accountability	5	4	3	2	1

TOTAL POINTS =   /15 = AVERAGE GRADE =

ADDITIONAL COMMENTS: IDENTIFY AREAS OF EXCELLENCE; LIST ERRORS OF OMISSION OR COMMISSION, CRITICAL ERRORS

SUMMARY PERFORMANCE EVALUATION AND RECOMMENDATIONS

☐ PASS: Satisfactory Performance

    ☐ Minimal supervision needed, may progress to next level provided specific skills, clinical time completed

    ☐ Minimal supervision needed, able to progress to next level without remediation

☐ FAIL: Unsatisfactory Performance (check all that apply)

    ☐ Minor reevaluation only

    ☐ Needs additional clinical practice before reevaluation

    ☐ Needs additional laboratory practice before skills performed in clinical area

    ☐ Recommend clinical probation

SIGNATURES

Evaluator (print name):   Evaluator signature: Date:

Student Signature: Date:

Student Comments:

Procedural Competency Evaluation

STUDENT: **DATE:**

BLOOD PRESSURE

	PERFORMANCE RATING	**PERFORMANCE LEVEL**

Evaluator: ☐ Peer ☐ Instructor   **Setting:** ☐ Lab   ☐ Clinical Simulation

Equipment Utilized: **Conditions (Describe):**

Performance Level:

S or ✓ = Satisfactory, no errors of omission or commission
U = Unsatisfactory Error of Omission or Commission
NA = Not applicable

Performance Rating:

5   **Independent:** Near flawless performance; minimal errors; able to perform without supervision; seeks out new learning; shows initiative; A = 4.7–5.0 average

4   **Minimally Supervised:** Few errors, able to self-correct; seeks guidance when appropriate; B = 3.7–4.65

3   **Competent:** Minimal required level; no critical errors; able to correct with coaching; meets expectations; safe; C = 3.0–3.65

2   **Marginal:** Below average; critical errors or problem areas noted; would benefit from remediation; D = 2.0–2.99

1   **Dependent:** Poor; unacceptable performance; unsafe; gross inaccuracies; potentially harmful; F = < 2.0

Two or more errors of commission or omission of mandatory or essential performance elements will terminate the procedure, and require additional practice and/or remediation and reevaluation. Student is responsible for obtaining additional evaluation forms as needed from the Director of Clinical Education (DCE).

	PERFORMANCE RATING	PERFORMANCE LEVEL
EQUIPMENT AND PATIENT PREPARATION		
1. Common Performance Elements Steps 1–8		
ASSESSMENT AND IMPLEMENTATION		
2. Common Performance Elements Steps 9 and 10		
3. Determines patient's usual blood pressure readings, if able		
4. Selects correct size sphygmomanometer cuff for patient's age and weight		
5. Wraps cuff snugly around patient's arm (should wrap 1 1/2 times)		
6. Positions aneroid gauge level with arm at heart level		
7. Has patient relax arm while supporting it		
8. Palpates brachial pulse and inflates cuff approximately 30 mm Hg above level until pulse disappears		
A. Notes pressure at point when pulse disappears		
9. Deflates cuff slowly until pulse reappears		
A. Notes pressure at that point		
10. Places stethoscope in ears and places bell of stethoscope over the brachial pulse, slightly distal to or partially under cuff		
11. Reinflates cuff 30 mm Hg above expected systolic pressure determined in steps 8 and 9		
12. Deflates cuff slowly, observing manometer; notes systolic and diastolic pressures		
13. Completely deflates and removes cuff		
14. Records the blood pressure		
FOLLOW-UP		
15. Common Performance Elements Steps 11–16		

SIGNATURES   Student: Evaluator: Date:

Clinical Performance Evaluation

PERFORMANCE RATING:

5 **Independent:** Near flawless performance; minimal errors; able to perform without supervision; seeks out new learning; shows initiative; A = 4.7–5.0 average

4 **Minimally Supervised:** Few errors, able to self-correct; seeks guidance when appropriate; B = 3.7–4.65

3 **Competent:** Minimal required level; no critical errors; able to correct with coaching; meets expectations; safe; C = 3.0–3.65

2 **Marginal:** Below average; critical errors or problem areas noted; would benefit from remediation; D = 2.0–2.99

1 **Dependent:** Poor; unacceptable performance; unsafe; gross inaccuracies; potentially harmful; F = < 2.0

Circle the appropriate response below. Please be consistent, objective, and honest in your assessment of the student's clinical performance and ability.

PERFORMANCE CRITERIA

PERFORMANCE CRITERIA	SCORE				
COGNITIVE DOMAIN					
1. Consistently displays knowledge, comprehension, and command of essential concepts	5	4	3	2	1
2. Demonstrates the relationship between theory and clinical practice	5	4	3	2	1
3. Able to select, review, apply, analyze, synthesize, interpret, and evaluate information; makes recommendations to modify care plan	5	4	3	2	1
PSYCHOMOTOR DOMAIN					
4. Minimal errors, no critical errors; able to self-correct; performs all steps safely and accurately	5	4	3	2	1
5. Selects, assembles, and verifies proper function and cleanliness of equipment; assures operation and corrects malfunctions; provides adequate care and maintenance	5	4	3	2	1
6. Exhibits the required manual dexterity	5	4	3	2	1
7. Performs procedure in a reasonable time frame for clinical level	5	4	3	2	1
8. Applies and maintains aseptic technique and PPE as required	5	4	3	2	1
9. Maintains concise and accurate patient and clinical records	5	4	3	2	1
10. Reports promptly on patient status/needs to appropriate personnel	5	4	3	2	1
AFFECTIVE DOMAIN					
11. Exhibits courteous and pleasant demeanor; shows consideration and respect, honesty, and integrity	5	4	3	2	1
12. Communicates verbally and in writing clearly and concisely	5	4	3	2	1
13. Preserves confidentiality and adheres to all policies	5	4	3	2	1
14. Follows directions, exhibits sound judgment, and seeks help when required	5	4	3	2	1
15. Demonstrates initiative, self-direction, responsibility, and accountability	5	4	3	2	1

TOTAL POINTS = _____ /15 = AVERAGE GRADE = _____

ADDITIONAL COMMENTS: IDENTIFY AREAS OF EXCELLENCE; LIST ERRORS OF OMISSION OR COMMISSION, CRITICAL ERRORS

SUMMARY PERFORMANCE EVALUATION AND RECOMMENDATIONS

☐ PASS: Satisfactory Performance

    ☐ Minimal supervision needed, may progress to next level provided specific skills, clinical time completed

    ☐ Minimal supervision needed, able to progress to next level without remediation

☐ FAIL: Unsatisfactory Performance (check all that apply)

    ☐ Minor reevaluation only

    ☐ Needs additional clinical practice before reevaluation

    ☐ Needs additional laboratory practice before skills performed in clinical area

    ☐ Recommend clinical probation

SIGNATURES

Evaluator (print name): _____ Evaluator signature: _____ Date: _____

Student Signature: _____ Date: _____

Student Comments:

Procedural Competency Evaluation

STUDENT: **DATE:**

PULSE OXIMETRY

		PERFORMANCE RATING	PERFORMANCE LEVEL

Evaluator: ☐ Peer ☐ Instructor   **Setting:** ☐ Lab   ☐ Clinical Simulation

Equipment Utilized: **Conditions (Describe):**

Performance Level:

  S or ✓ = Satisfactory, no errors of omission or commission
  U = Unsatisfactory Error of Omission or Commission
  NA = Not applicable

Performance Rating:

  5 **Independent:** Near flawless performance; minimal errors; able to perform without supervision; seeks out new learning; shows initiative; A = 4.7–5.0 average

  4 **Minimally Supervised:** Few errors, able to self-correct; seeks guidance when appropriate; B = 3.7–4.65

  3 **Competent:** Minimal required level; no critical errors; able to correct with coaching; meets expectations; safe; C = 3.0–3.65

  2 **Marginal:** Below average; critical errors or problem areas noted; would benefit from remediation; D = 2.0–2.99

  1 **Dependent:** Poor; unacceptable performance; unsafe; gross inaccuracies; potentially harmful; F = < 2.0

  Two or more errors of commission or omission of mandatory or essential performance elements will terminate the procedure, and require additional practice and/or remediation and reevaluation. Student is responsible for obtaining additional evaluation forms as needed from the Director of Clinical Education (DCE).

	PERFORMANCE RATING	PERFORMANCE LEVEL
EQUIPMENT AND PATIENT PREPARATION		
1. Common Performance Elements Steps 1–8		
2. Determines F_iO_2 and/or ventilator settings		
3. Visually inspects the power cord (if applicable) and probes cable for any frayed or exposed wires		
ASSESSMENT AND IMPLEMENTATION		
4. Common Performance Elements Steps 9 and 10		
5. Assesses patient by measuring the patient's pulse rate manually and/or verifying the heart rate displayed on ECG monitor (if applicable)		
6. Confirms the F_iO_2 and/or ventilator settings in the patient's room		
7. Turns on the oximeter and allows for appropriate warm-up		
8. Selects a site for the probe application and checks for adequate perfusion; removes nail polish or artificial nails if necessary		
9. Cleans site and nondisposable probe with alcohol prep pad		
10. Attaches probe to the selected site and secures		
11. Allows for proper stabilization		
12. Observes the pulse rate on the oximeter and correlates it with the manually measured rate and/or ECG rate		
13. Records the pulse rate, saturation, respiratory rate, and pattern		
FOLLOW-UP		
14. Common Performance Elements Steps 11–16		
15. Disconnects and turns unit off if not a continuous monitoring situation		
16. Disinfects probe if nondisposable		

SIGNATURES   Student: Evaluator: Date:

Clinical Performance Evaluation

PERFORMANCE RATING:

5 **Independent:** Near flawless performance; minimal errors; able to perform without supervision; seeks out new learning; shows initiative; A = 4.7–5.0 average

4 **Minimally Supervised:** Few errors, able to self-correct; seeks guidance when appropriate; B = 3.7–4.65

3 **Competent:** Minimal required level; no critical errors; able to correct with coaching; meets expectations; safe; C = 3.0–3.65

2 **Marginal:** Below average; critical errors or problem areas noted; would benefit from remediation; D = 2.0–2.99

1 **Dependent:** Poor; unacceptable performance; unsafe; gross inaccuracies; potentially harmful; F = < 2.0

Circle the appropriate response below. Please be consistent, objective, and honest in your assessment of the student's clinical performance and ability.

PERFORMANCE CRITERIA	SCORE				
COGNITIVE DOMAIN					
1. Consistently displays knowledge, comprehension, and command of essential concepts	5	4	3	2	1
2. Demonstrates the relationship between theory and clinical practice	5	4	3	2	1
3. Able to select, review, apply, analyze, synthesize, interpret, and evaluate information; makes recommendations to modify care plan	5	4	3	2	1
PSYCHOMOTOR DOMAIN					
4. Minimal errors, no critical errors; able to self-correct; performs all steps safely and accurately	5	4	3	2	1
5. Selects, assembles, and verifies proper function and cleanliness of equipment; assures operation and corrects malfunctions; provides adequate care and maintenance	5	4	3	2	1
6. Exhibits the required manual dexterity	5	4	3	2	1
7. Performs procedure in a reasonable time frame for clinical level	5	4	3	2	1
8. Applies and maintains aseptic technique and PPE as required	5	4	3	2	1
9. Maintains concise and accurate patient and clinical records	5	4	3	2	1
10. Reports promptly on patient status/needs to appropriate personnel	5	4	3	2	1
AFFECTIVE DOMAIN					
11. Exhibits courteous and pleasant demeanor; shows consideration and respect, honesty, and integrity	5	4	3	2	1
12. Communicates verbally and in writing clearly and concisely	5	4	3	2	1
13. Preserves confidentiality and adheres to all policies	5	4	3	2	1
14. Follows directions, exhibits sound judgment, and seeks help when required	5	4	3	2	1
15. Demonstrates initiative, self-direction, responsibility, and accountability	5	4	3	2	1

TOTAL POINTS = _____ /15 = AVERAGE GRADE = _____

ADDITIONAL COMMENTS: IDENTIFY AREAS OF EXCELLENCE; LIST ERRORS OF OMISSION OR COMMISSION, CRITICAL ERRORS

SUMMARY PERFORMANCE EVALUATION AND RECOMMENDATIONS

☐ PASS: Satisfactory Performance

    ☐ Minimal supervision needed, may progress to next level provided specific skills, clinical time completed

    ☐ Minimal supervision needed, able to progress to next level without remediation

☐ FAIL: Unsatisfactory Performance (check all that apply)

    ☐ Minor reevaluation only

    ☐ Needs additional clinical practice before reevaluation

    ☐ Needs additional laboratory practice before skills performed in clinical area

    ☐ Recommend clinical probation

SIGNATURES

Evaluator (print name): _____ Evaluator signature: _____ Date: _____

Student Signature: _____ Date: _____

Student Comments:

Patient Assessment: Advanced Skills

7

INTRODUCTION

The next steps in the assessment of the client by the respiratory care practitioner are the physical examination of the chest and **auscultation** of breath sounds. To achieve proficiency, these skills require practice and exposure to many different types of patients in varying clinical scenarios. The data obtained from physical examination of the chest and auscultation, combined with the primary and secondary scene survey and vital signs, can be used to begin to formulate or amend a respiratory care plan. In this chapter the following skills will be practiced:

1. Physical assessment of the chest

    A. Inspection

    B. Palpation

    C. Diagnostic chest percussion

2. Auscultation

OBJECTIVES

Upon completion of this chapter, the student will be able to:

1. Practice the physical assessment techniques of inspection, palpation, and percussion of the chest.
2. Practice auscultation.
3. Differentiate the various breath sounds heard during auscultation.
4. Practice medical charting for the documentation of performance of patient assessment procedures.
5. Apply infection control guidelines and standards associated with equipment and procedures, according to OSHA regulations and CDC guidelines.

KEY TERMS

adventitious
anterior
auscultation
basilar
bifurcation
binaural
bronchoconstriction
bronchodilation
bronchophony
bronchorrhea
bronchospasm
consolidation
contralateral
copious
crackles (fine)
crackles (coarse)

crepitus
decubitus
density
egophony
empyema
eupnea
fetid
flail
fremitus
hyperinflation
hyperresonant
inspissated
kyphosis
lesions
lethargic
lordosis

mucoid
mucopurulent
nodules
paroxysmal (cough)
patency
pectoriloquy
pectus carinatum
pectus excavatum
phonation
pleural effusion
pleural friction rub
pleuritic (pain)
pneumoconiosis
pneumothorax
purulent
rales

resonance
retractions
rhonchi
scoliosis
serous
stridor
tenacious
tetany
Trendelenburg position
turbulent
tympanitic
wheezing
whispered pectoriloquy

Exercises

EQUIPMENT REQUIRED

- [ ] Alcohol prep pads
- [ ] **Binaural** stethoscopes (teaching models, if available)
- [ ] DVD or video player and monitor
- [ ] Human patient simulator
- [ ] MP3, CD, or cassette player
- [ ] Patient mannequin (or student)
- [ ] Recording of breath sounds
- [ ] Video of physical assessment of the chest

EXERCISE 7.1 PHYSICAL ASSESSMENT OF THE CHEST

EXERCISE 7.1.1 INSPECTION

For a practitioner to perform a complete physical assessment, the room should be well lit and the patient should ideally be naked to the waist. However, for female patients the patient's modesty must be considered and safeguarded. The patient should be in the Fowler's position and the practitioner should explain the process and reassure the patient before performing the assessment.

This section is best completed using a male volunteer with shirt removed. A video demonstration may be substituted. Wash your hands and apply standard precautions and transmission-based isolation procedures as appropriate. Have the subject sit upright.

1. Observe the "patient" for overall appearance, age, sex, and weight.
2. Stand directly in front of the "patient" and observe the chest for the following:
   A. General shape and appearance (Fig. 7.1)
3. **Anterior** to posterior diameter
4. Sternal deformities
   A. Surgical or other scars
   B. **Symmetrical** expansion (Fig. 7.2): observe for any paradoxical or unequal expansion
   C. Presence of chest tubes
5. From the back of the "patient," observe spinal curvature.
6. Observe skin for cyanosis, pallor, mottling, diaphoresis, swelling, bruises, and **erythema**.
7. Observe skin for any obvious masses, **lesions**, or **nodules**.
8. Assess the respiratory pattern. Look for regularity, accessory muscle use, rate and depth, and patient positioning for breathing (Fig. 7.3).
9. Observe for retractions, pursed lip breathing, and nasal flaring.
10. **Record your findings on your laboratory report.**

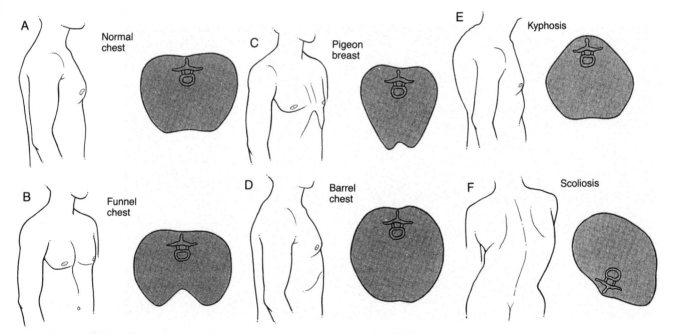

Figure 7.1. Common abnormalities of the chest. (From Monahan, FD, Drake, T and Neighbors, M: Nursing Care of Adults. WB Saunders, Philadelphia, 1994, p. 419, with permission.)

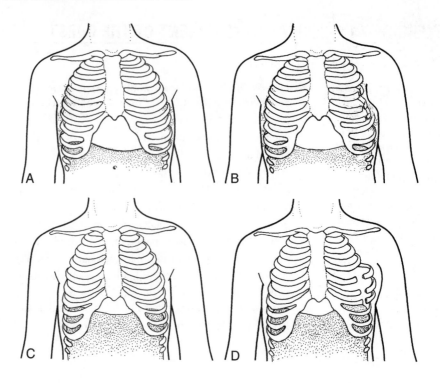

Figure 7.2. Normal and paradoxical motion. **(A)** Normal inspiration, **(B)** paradoxical inspiration, **(C)** normal expiration, and **(D)** paradoxical expiration.

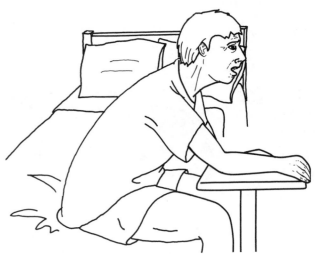

Figure 7.3. The tripod position.

EXERCISE 7.1.2 PALPATION

1. Palpate the position of the trachea by inserting two fingers from the same hand on either side of the trachea and moving your fingers downward (Fig. 7.4).
2. Palpate the skin for the presence of subcutaneous emphysema, which may be felt as **crepitus** crackling under the skin ("Rice Krispies").
3. Place your hands in the "butterfly" position with your thumbs on the spine and your hands on the posterior rib margins. Palpate for equal **bilateral** expansion using the steps in Figure 7.5.
4. Tactile **fremitus**. Palpate the chest wall over each of the lung lobes as shown in Figure 7.6 while the "patient" says "ninety-nine." Feel for any vibrations with the palms of your hands. Avoid bony prominences.
5. Palpate for spinal curvature. Place two fingers from the same hand along either side of the spine and move them downward, using sufficient pressure to cause skin blanching. Note any deviations.
6. Assess peripheral perfusion by palpating pulses and capillary refill.
7. **Record your findings on your laboratory report.**

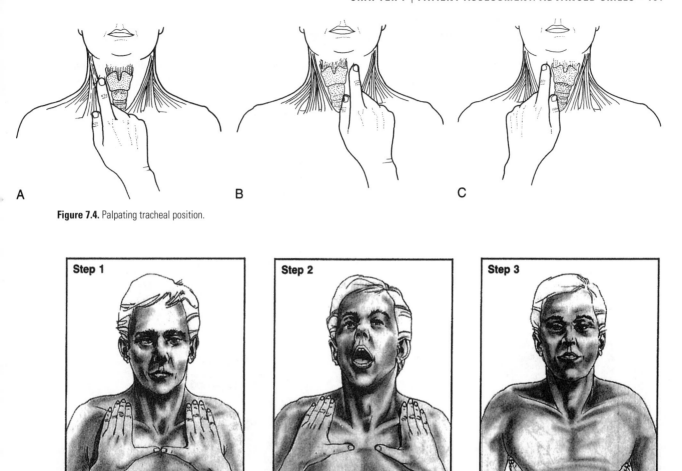

Figure 7.4. Palpating tracheal position.

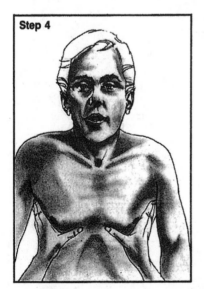
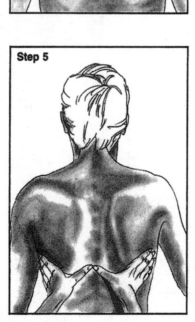
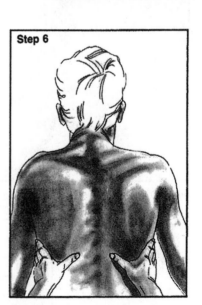

Figure 7.5. Palpation for chest excursion. (From Morton, PG: Health Assessment in Nursing, ed 2. FA Davis, Philadelphia, 1993, pp. 266–267, with permission.)

EXERCISE 7.1.3 DIAGNOSTIC CHEST PERCUSSION

Diagnostic chest percussion may be performed by directly striking the chest wall with a finger between the ribs. It may be performed indirectly by placing one hand on the chest wall and striking the middle or index finger with your other hand, as shown in Figure 7.7. Comparison of bilateral percussion notes for quality and intensity should be made. Table 7.1 shows the important percussion notes, location, and common causes. Diaphragmatic excursion can also be estimated by percussion of the posterior chest wall.[1]

1. Percuss over a solid structure such as the liver, thigh, or heart to create a dull percussion note.
2. Percuss over normal lung tissue to hear a resonant percussion note. Compare the sounds bilaterally.
3. Percuss over the stomach to hear a **hyperresonant** or **tympanitic** percussion note.
4. Estimate diaphragmatic excursion by first instructing the patient to take a full, deep breath. Determine the lowest margin of **resonance** by percussing over the lower lung field and moving downward in small increments until a definite change in the percussion note is detected. Then instruct the "patient" to exhale maximally and hold this position while percussion is repeated.
5. **Record your findings on your laboratory report.**

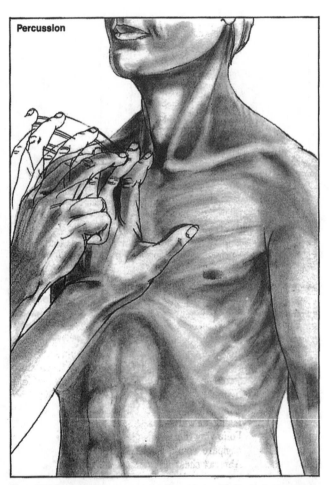

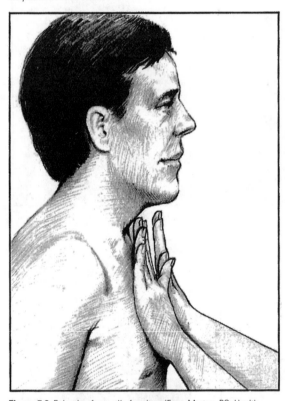

Figure 7.6. Palpating for tactile fremitus. (From Morton, PG: Health Assessment in Nursing, ed 2. FA Davis, Philadelphia, 1993, p. 275, with permission.)

Figure 7.7. Diagnostic chest percussion. (From Morton, PG: Health Assessment in Nursing, ed 2. FA Davis, Philadelphia, 1993, p. 268, with permission.)

Table 7.1 Percussion Sounds

SOUND	QUALITY	SOURCE
Resonant	Hollow	Normal lung
Dull	Thud-like	Liver, consolidated lung, pleural effusion
Hyperresonant/tympanitic	Drum-like	Hyperinflated lung (as in emphysema), gastric air bubble, pneumothorax
Flat	Flat	Muscle, bone

EXERCISE 7.2 AUSCULTATION

The stethoscope (Fig. 7.8) is a valuable and essential assessment tool for the respiratory care practitioner. It consists of four basic parts: (a) a bell for low-frequency sounds, such as heart sounds; (b) a diaphragm for higher pitched lung sounds; (c) tubing, which is ideally 11 to 16 inches in length and thick enough to exclude external noise; and (d) binaural earpieces, which should be pointed in toward the ear canals.[2] Students should apply standard precautions and transmission-based isolation procedures as appropriate.

1. Listen to the breath sound tape (if available).
2. **Auscultate** your laboratory partner.
    A. Check your stethoscope for function. Wipe the earpieces and diaphragm with an alcohol swab. Place the earpieces securely in your ears. Turn the head of the stethoscope to the diaphragm side and gently tap on it. If you do not hear anything, turn the chest piece 180 degrees and repeat. Examine the chest piece and tubing regularly for cracks and other defects. Clean the earpieces of wax and dirt with an alcohol prep pad.
    B. Warm the diaphragm piece with your hands.
    C. Instruct your "patient" to sit up, lean forward, and breathe through the mouth with the head turned away from you. Place the diaphragm firmly against the chest wall.
    D. Identify the location of normal breath sounds, as shown in Figure 7.9.
    E. Auscultate the posterior chest wall in at least six places, comparing sounds bilaterally, as shown in Figure 7.10. You may proceed from apices to bases or from bases to apices as long as you make bilateral comparisons.
    F. Auscultate the anterior chest wall, with the "patient" leaning slightly back, in at least six places. Compare sounds bilaterally.
3. **Record your findings on your laboratory report.**

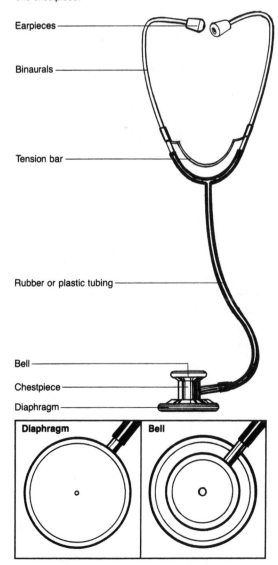

Stethoscope
All stethoscopes have earpieces, binaurals, tubing, and a chestpiece (head). However, some have several removable chestpieces suitable for adult and pediatric clients. Others, designed specifically for use on an adult or a child, have only one chestpiece.

Earpieces

Binaurals

Tension bar

Rubber or plastic tubing

Bell

Chestpiece

Diaphragm

Diaphragm	Bell

Figure 7.8. Components of a stethoscope. (From Morton, PG: Health Assessment in Nursing, ed 2. FA Davis, Philadelphia, 1993, p. 99, with permission.)

Anterior chest

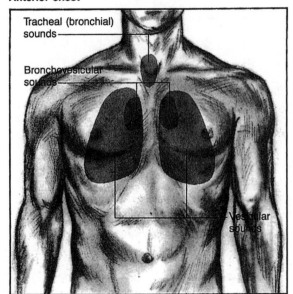

Posterior chest

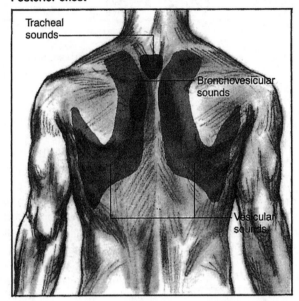

Figure 7.9. Location of normal breath sounds. (From Morton, PG: Health Assessment in Nursing, ed 2. FA Davis, Philadelphia, 1993, p. 270, with permission.)

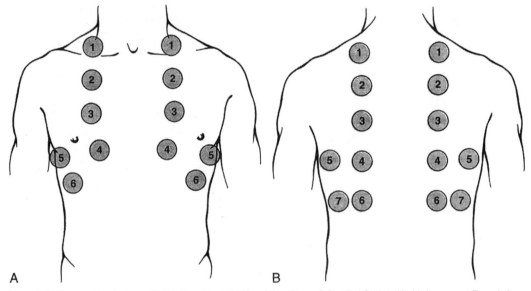

Figure 7.10. Sequence for chest auscultation. (From Hogstel, MO and Keen-Payne, R: Practical Guide to Health Assessment Through the Lifespan. FA Davis, Philadelphia, 1993, pp. 94–95, with permission.)

REFERENCES

1. Wilkins, RL and Krider, SJ: Clinical Assessment in Respiratory Care, ed 5. Mosby, St. Louis, 2005, p. 63.
2. Wilkins, RL, Krider, SJ and Sheldon, RL: Clinical Assessment in Respiratory Care, ed 3. Mosby, St. Louis, 1990, p. 62.

Laboratory Report

CHAPTER 7: PATIENT ASSESSMENT: ADVANCED SKILLS

Name _____ Date _____

Course/Section _____ Instructor _____

Data Collection

EXERCISE 7.1 Physical Examination of the Chest

EXERCISE 7.1.1 INSPECTION

Findings: _____

_____

_____

EXERCISE 7.1.2 PALPATION

Findings: _____

_____

_____

EXERCISE 7.1.3 PERCUSSION

Findings: _____

_____

_____

EXERCISE 7.2 Physical Examination of the Chest: Auscultation

Auscultate lab partner. Findings:_____

_____

_____

_____

Critical Thinking Questions

Scenario 1: You continue to evaluate Mr. C.O. Tu, who has a long-standing history of chronic obstructive pulmonary disease (COPD). Recall that he has been brought to the ED by ambulance. He complains of increasing shortness of breath and productive cough with thick, green sputum.

During physical examination of the chest, you notice a hyperresonant percussion note with decreased fremitus over most of the lung fields except for the right lower lobe (RLL), which has a dull percussion note and increased fremitus.

1. Identify a possible explanation for these differences in your findings.

2. Based on your findings, describe what you would expect to hear on auscultation over the RLL.

Scenario 2: Bill Long, a 34-year-old man, presents to the ED with left-sided chest pain and shortness of breath. It is suspected that he has a left-sided pneumothorax.

1. What findings on physical examination would help establish the diagnosis?

2. What diagnostic tests should be performed to confirm the diagnosis?

Procedural Competency Evaluation

STUDENT: **DATE:**

PHYSICAL ASSESSMENT OF THE CHEST

Evaluator: ☐ Peer ☐ Instructor	**Setting:** ☐ Lab ☐ Clinical Simulation
Equipment Utilized:	**Conditions (Describe):**

PERFORMANCE RATING / *PERFORMANCE LEVEL*

Performance Level:

S or ✓ = Satisfactory, no errors of omission or commission
U = Unsatisfactory Error of Omission or Commission
NA = Not applicable

Performance Rating:

5   **Independent:** Near flawless performance; minimal errors; able to perform without supervision; seeks out new learning; shows initiative; A = 4.7–5.0 average

4   **Minimally Supervised:** Few errors, able to self-correct; seeks guidance when appropriate; B = 3.7–4.65

3   **Competent:** Minimal required level; no critical errors; able to correct with coaching; meets expectations; safe; C = 3.0–3.65

2   **Marginal:** Below average; critical errors or problem areas noted; would benefit from remediation; D = 2.0–2.99

1   **Dependent:** Poor; unacceptable performance; unsafe; gross inaccuracies; potentially harmful; F = < 2.0

Two or more errors of commission or omission of mandatory or essential performance elements will terminate the procedure, and require additional practice and/or remediation and reevaluation. Student is responsible for obtaining additional evaluation forms as needed from the Director of Clinical Education (DCE).

EQUIPMENT AND PATIENT PREPARATION

1. Common Performance Elements Steps 1–8

ASSESSMENT AND IMPLEMENTATION

2. Common Performance Elements Steps 9 and 10
3. Observes patient for overall appearance, age, sex, and weight
4. Notes patient positioning (tripod, high Fowler's, etc.)
5. Stands directly in front of the patient and observes chest for shape and appearance, anterior-posterior diameter, sternal deformities, surgical or other scars, and symmetrical expansion
6. Observes for normal or abnormal spinal curvatures
7. Observes for any paradoxical or unequal expansion
8. Observes for retractions, pursed-lip breathing, nasal flaring, and abdominal paradox
9. Observes for presence of chest tubes
10. Observes the skin for cyanosis, pallor, mottling, diaphoresis, swelling, pitting edema, turgor, dryness, bruises, erythema, or petechiae
11. Observes skin for any masses, lesions, or nodules
12. Assesses respiratory pattern: regularity, rate and depth of breathing, and accessory muscle use
13. Evaluates for orthopnea, platypnea, pleurodynia
14. Palpates position of the trachea
15. Palpates skin for presence of subcutaneous emphysema
16. Palpates for bilateral chest expansion
17. Palpates chest wall for tactile fremitus
18. Palpates for spinal curvature
19. Palpates pulses and assesses capillary refill
20. Performs diagnostic chest percussion
21. Auscultates chest for normal, abnormal, and adventitious breath sounds (See PCE for Auscultation)

FOLLOW-UP

22. Common Performance Elements Steps 11–16

SIGNATURES   Student: Evaluator: Date:

Clinical Performance Evaluation

PERFORMANCE RATING:

5   **Independent:** Near flawless performance; minimal errors; able to perform without supervision; seeks out new learning; shows initiative; A = 4.7–5.0 average

4   **Minimally Supervised:** Few errors, able to self-correct; seeks guidance when appropriate; B = 3.7–4.65

3   **Competent:** Minimal required level; no critical errors; able to correct with coaching; meets expectations; safe; C = 3.0–3.65

2   **Marginal:** Below average; critical errors or problem areas noted; would benefit from remediation; D = 2.0–2.99

1   **Dependent:** Poor; unacceptable performance; unsafe; gross inaccuracies; potentially harmful; F = < 2.0

Circle the appropriate response below. Please be consistent, objective, and honest in your assessment of the student's clinical performance and ability.

PERFORMANCE CRITERIA	SCORE				
COGNITIVE DOMAIN					
1. Consistently displays knowledge, comprehension, and command of essential concepts	5	4	3	2	1
2. Demonstrates the relationship between theory and clinical practice	5	4	3	2	1
3. Able to select, review, apply, analyze, synthesize, interpret, and evaluate information; makes recommendations to modify care plan	5	4	3	2	1
PSYCHOMOTOR DOMAIN					
4. Minimal errors, no critical errors; able to self-correct; performs all steps safely and accurately	5	4	3	2	1
5. Selects, assembles, and verifies proper function and cleanliness of equipment; assures operation and corrects malfunctions; provides adequate care and maintenance	5	4	3	2	1
6. Exhibits the required manual dexterity	5	4	3	2	1
7. Performs procedure in a reasonable time frame for clinical level	5	4	3	2	1
8. Applies and maintains aseptic technique and PPE as required	5	4	3	2	1
9. Maintains concise and accurate patient and clinical records	5	4	3	2	1
10. Reports promptly on patient status/needs to appropriate personnel	5	4	3	2	1
AFFECTIVE DOMAIN					
11. Exhibits courteous and pleasant demeanor; shows consideration and respect, honesty, and integrity	5	4	3	2	1
12. Communicates verbally and in writing clearly and concisely	5	4	3	2	1
13. Preserves confidentiality and adheres to all policies	5	4	3	2	1
14. Follows directions, exhibits sound judgment, and seeks help when required	5	4	3	2	1
15. Demonstrates initiative, self-direction, responsibility, and accountability	5	4	3	2	1

TOTAL POINTS =   /15 = AVERAGE GRADE =

ADDITIONAL COMMENTS: IDENTIFY AREAS OF EXCELLENCE; LIST ERRORS OF OMISSION OR COMMISSION, CRITICAL ERRORS

SUMMARY PERFORMANCE EVALUATION AND RECOMMENDATIONS

☐ PASS: Satisfactory Performance

     ☐ Minimal supervision needed, may progress to next level provided specific skills, clinical time completed

     ☐ Minimal supervision needed, able to progress to next level without remediation

☐ FAIL: Unsatisfactory Performance (check all that apply)

     ☐ Minor reevaluation only

     ☐ Needs additional clinical practice before reevaluation

     ☐ Needs additional laboratory practice before skills performed in clinical area

     ☐ Recommend clinical probation

SIGNATURES

Evaluator (print name):   Evaluator signature: Date:

Student Signature: Date:

Student Comments:

Procedural Competency Evaluation

STUDENT: **DATE:**

AUSCULTATION		PERFORMANCE RATING	PERFORMANCE LEVEL
Evaluator: ☐ Peer ☐ Instructor **Setting:** ☐ Lab ☐ Clinical Simulation			
Equipment Utilized: **Conditions (Describe):**			

Performance Level:
 	
    S or ✓ = Satisfactory, no errors of omission or commission
    U = Unsatisfactory Error of Omission or Commission
    NA = Not applicable			

Performance Rating:
 	
  5   **Independent:** Near flawless performance; minimal errors; able to perform without supervision; seeks out new learning; shows initiative; A = 4.7–5.0 average
  4   **Minimally Supervised:** Few errors, able to self-correct; seeks guidance when appropriate; B = 3.7–4.65
  3   **Competent:** Minimal required level; no critical errors; able to correct with coaching; meets expectations; safe; C = 3.0–3.65
  2   **Marginal:** Below average; critical errors or problem areas noted; would benefit from remediation; D = 2.0–2.99
  1   **Dependent:** Poor; unacceptable performance; unsafe; gross inaccuracies; potentially harmful; F = < 2.0
 	
    Two or more errors of commission or omission of mandatory or essential performance elements will terminate the procedure, and require additional practice and/or remediation and reevaluation. Student is responsible for obtaining additional evaluation forms as needed from the Director of Clinical Education (DCE).			

EQUIPMENT AND PATIENT PREPARATION			
1. Common Performance Elements Steps 1–8			
ASSESSMENT AND IMPLEMENTATION			
2. Common Performance Elements Steps 9 and 10			
3. Clean earpieces, bell, and diaphragm of stethoscope with alcohol swab			
4. Warms stethoscope diaphragm with hand			
5. Places stethoscope in ears with earpieces facing forward into the ear canal			
A. Verifies function by gently tapping on diaphragm with earpieces in place			
6. Positions patient:			
A. Has patient sit upright leaning forward (if possible), facing away			
B. If not able to sit up, gets assistance to turn patient to side to auscultate posterior chest			
7. Auscultates the anterior chest in at least six positions, comparing sounds bilaterally			
8. Auscultates the lateral chest bilaterally			
9. Auscultates the posterior chest in at least six positions, comparing sounds bilaterally			
10. Correctly interprets breath sounds			
FOLLOW-UP			
11. Properly identifies normal, abnormal, and adventitious breath sounds and their possible causes			
12. Common Performance Elements Steps 11–16			

SIGNATURES   Student: Evaluator: Date:

Clinical Performance Evaluation

PERFORMANCE RATING:

5 **Independent:** Near flawless performance; minimal errors; able to perform without supervision; seeks out new learning; shows initiative; A = 4.7–5.0 average

4 **Minimally Supervised:** Few errors, able to self-correct; seeks guidance when appropriate; B = 3.7–4.65

3 **Competent:** Minimal required level; no critical errors; able to correct with coaching; meets expectations; safe; C = 3.0–3.65

2 **Marginal:** Below average; critical errors or problem areas noted; would benefit from remediation; D = 2.0–2.99

1 **Dependent:** Poor; unacceptable performance; unsafe; gross inaccuracies; potentially harmful; F = < 2.0

Circle the appropriate response below. Please be consistent, objective, and honest in your assessment of the student's clinical performance and ability.

PERFORMANCE CRITERIA	SCORE				
COGNITIVE DOMAIN					
1. Consistently displays knowledge, comprehension, and command of essential concepts	5	4	3	2	1
2. Demonstrates the relationship between theory and clinical practice	5	4	3	2	1
3. Able to select, review, apply, analyze, synthesize, interpret, and evaluate information; makes recommendations to modify care plan	5	4	3	2	1
PSYCHOMOTOR DOMAIN					
4. Minimal errors, no critical errors; able to self-correct; performs all steps safely and accurately	5	4	3	2	1
5. Selects, assembles, and verifies proper function and cleanliness of equipment; assures operation and corrects malfunctions; provides adequate care and maintenance	5	4	3	2	1
6. Exhibits the required manual dexterity	5	4	3	2	1
7. Performs procedure in a reasonable time frame for clinical level	5	4	3	2	1
8. Applies and maintains aseptic technique and PPE as required	5	4	3	2	1
9. Maintains concise and accurate patient and clinical records	5	4	3	2	1
10. Reports promptly on patient status/needs to appropriate personnel	5	4	3	2	1
AFFECTIVE DOMAIN					
11. Exhibits courteous and pleasant demeanor; shows consideration and respect, honesty, and integrity	5	4	3	2	1
12. Communicates verbally and in writing clearly and concisely	5	4	3	2	1
13. Preserves confidentiality and adheres to all policies	5	4	3	2	1
14. Follows directions, exhibits sound judgment, and seeks help when required	5	4	3	2	1
15. Demonstrates initiative, self-direction, responsibility, and accountability	5	4	3	2	1

TOTAL POINTS = _____ /15 = AVERAGE GRADE = _____

ADDITIONAL COMMENTS: IDENTIFY AREAS OF EXCELLENCE; LIST ERRORS OF OMISSION OR COMMISSION, CRITICAL ERRORS

SUMMARY PERFORMANCE EVALUATION AND RECOMMENDATIONS

☐ PASS: Satisfactory Performance

　　☐ Minimal supervision needed, may progress to next level provided specific skills, clinical time completed

　　☐ Minimal supervision needed, able to progress to next level without remediation

☐ FAIL: Unsatisfactory Performance (check all that apply)

　　☐ Minor reevaluation only

　　☐ Needs additional clinical practice before reevaluation

　　☐ Needs additional laboratory practice before skills performed in clinical area

　　☐ Recommend clinical probation

SIGNATURES

Evaluator (print name): _____ Evaluator signature: _____ Date: _____

Student Signature: _____ Date: _____

Student Comments: _____

Procedural Competency Evaluation

STUDENT: **DATE:**

COMMON PERFORMANCE ELEMENTS

Evaluator: ☐ Peer ☐ Instructor		**Setting:** ☐ Lab		☐ Clinical Simulation	
Equipment Utilized:		**Conditions (Describe):**			

Performance Level:

S or ✓ = Satisfactory, no errors of omission or commission
U = Unsatisfactory Error of Omission or Commission
NA = Not applicable

Performance Rating:

5   **Independent:** Near flawless performance; minimal errors; able to perform without supervision; seeks out new learning; shows initiative; A = 4.7–5.0 average

4   **Minimally Supervised:** Few errors, able to self-correct; seeks guidance when appropriate; B = 3.7–4.65

3   **Competent:** Minimal required level; no critical errors; able to correct with coaching; meets expectations; safe; C = 3.0–3.65

2   **Marginal:** Below average; critical errors or problem areas noted; would benefit from remediation; D = 2.0–2.99

1   **Dependent:** Poor; unacceptable performance; unsafe; gross inaccuracies; potentially harmful; F = < 2.0

Two or more errors of commission or omission of mandatory or essential performance elements will terminate the procedure, and require additional practice and/or remediation and reevaluation. Student is responsible for obtaining additional evaluation forms as needed from the Director of Clinical Education (DCE).

	PERFORMANCE RATING	PERFORMANCE LEVEL
PATIENT AND EQUIPMENT PREPARATION		
1. Verifies, interprets, and evaluates physician's order or protocol		
2. Scans chart for any other pertinent data and notes, including diagnosis, medications, therapies, radiographic and other laboratory results		
3. Washes hands or applies disinfectant		
4. Selects, obtains, assembles equipment correctly, verifies function		
5. Trouble shoots equipment and corrects malfunctions if indicated		
6. Applies personal protective equipment (PPE); observes standard precautions and transmission-based isolation procedures as appropriate		
7. Identifies patient, introduces self and department		
8. Explains purpose of the procedure and confirms patient understanding		
ASSESSMENT AND IMPLEMENTATION		
9. Positions patient for procedure		
10. Assesses patient including, where applicable, vital signs, SpO$_2$, breath sounds, and ventilatory status		
FOLLOW-UP		
11. Reassesses and reinstructs patient as needed		
12. Ensures patient comfort and safety		
13. Maintains/processes equipment		
14. Disposes of infectious waste and washes hands or applies disinfectant		
15. Records pertinent data in chart and departmental records		
16. Notifies appropriate personnel and makes any necessary recommendations or modifications to the patient care plan		

SIGNATURES   Student: Evaluator: Date:

Clinical Performance Evaluation

PERFORMANCE RATING:

5 Independent: Near flawless performance; minimal errors; able to perform without supervision; seeks out new learning; shows initiative; A = 4.7–5.0 average

4 Minimally Supervised: Few errors, able to self-correct; seeks guidance when appropriate; B = 3.7–4.65

3 Competent: Minimal required level; no critical errors; able to correct with coaching; meets expectations; safe; C = 3.0–3.65

2 Marginal: Below average; critical errors or problem areas noted; would benefit from remediation; D = 2.0–2.99

1 Dependent: Poor; unacceptable performance; unsafe; gross inaccuracies; potentially harmful; F = < 2.0

Circle the appropriate response below. Please be consistent, objective, and honest in your assessment of the student's clinical performance and ability.

PERFORMANCE CRITERIA	SCORE				
COGNITIVE DOMAIN					
1. Consistently displays knowledge, comprehension, and command of essential concepts	5	4	3	2	1
2. Demonstrates the relationship between theory and clinical practice	5	4	3	2	1
3. Able to select, review, apply, analyze, synthesize, interpret, and evaluate information; makes recommendations to modify care plan	5	4	3	2	1
PSYCHOMOTOR DOMAIN					
4. Minimal errors, no critical errors; able to self-correct; performs all steps safely and accurately	5	4	3	2	1
5. Selects, assembles, and verifies proper function and cleanliness of equipment; assures operation and corrects malfunctions; provides adequate care and maintenance	5	4	3	2	1
6. Exhibits the required manual dexterity	5	4	3	2	1
7. Performs procedure in a reasonable time frame for clinical level	5	4	3	2	1
8. Applies and maintains aseptic technique and PPE as required	5	4	3	2	1
9. Maintains concise and accurate patient and clinical records	5	4	3	2	1
10. Reports promptly on patient status/needs to appropriate personnel	5	4	3	2	1
AFFECTIVE DOMAIN					
11. Exhibits courteous and pleasant demeanor; shows consideration and respect, honesty, and integrity	5	4	3	2	1
12. Communicates verbally and in writing clearly and concisely	5	4	3	2	1
13. Preserves confidentiality and adheres to all policies	5	4	3	2	1
14. Follows directions, exhibits sound judgment, and seeks help when required	5	4	3	2	1
15. Demonstrates initiative, self-direction, responsibility, and accountability	5	4	3	2	1

TOTAL POINTS = _____ /15 = AVERAGE GRADE = _____

ADDITIONAL COMMENTS: IDENTIFY AREAS OF EXCELLENCE; LIST ERRORS OF OMISSION OR COMMISSION, CRITICAL ERRORS

_____

_____

SUMMARY PERFORMANCE EVALUATION AND RECOMMENDATIONS

☐ PASS: Satisfactory Performance

    ☐ Minimal supervision needed, may progress to next level provided specific skills, clinical time completed

    ☐ Minimal supervision needed, able to progress to next level without remediation

☐ FAIL: Unsatisfactory Performance (check all that apply)

    ☐ Minor reevaluation only

    ☐ Needs additional clinical practice before reevaluation

    ☐ Needs additional laboratory practice before skills performed in clinical area

    ☐ Recommend clinical probation

SIGNATURES

Evaluator (print name): _____ Evaluator signature: _____ Date: _____

Student Signature: _____ Date: _____

Student Comments: _____

8 Bedside Assessment of Pulmonary Mechanics

INTRODUCTION

Often the respiratory care practitioner is called to the bedside to obtain data relevant to the state of the patient's ability to breathe. Simple bedside measurements can be performed. These data are essential, in conjunction with clinical assessment, when making decisions regarding initiation, modification, or discontinuance of respiratory modalities and procedures, especially mechanical ventilation.

These studies include, but are not limited to, the following parameters:

1. Tidal volume (V_T), minute ventilation (V_E), and alveolar ventilation (V_A)

2. Maximum inspiratory pressure (MIP)

3. Maximum expiratory pressure (MEP)

4. Slow vital capacity (SVC)

5. Peak expiratory flow rate (PEFR)

OBJECTIVES

Upon completion of this chapter, the student will be able to:

1. Perform bedside assessment of pulmonary mechanics in the laboratory and clinical settings.
2. Select, use, and maintain the equipment necessary to perform bedside assessment of pulmonary mechanics, including **vane** and electronic respirometers.
3. Apply infection control guidelines and standards associated with each piece of equipment, according to OSHA regulations, CDC guidelines, and American Thoracic Society (ATS) standards.
4. Given a patient scenario, select the appropriate tests and relate the clinical significance of the measured parameters to treatment decisions.
5. Explain alternative ways of obtaining data when dealing with patients with limited mental or functional capacity or language barriers.
6. Practice communication skills needed to instruct patients in the performance of pulmonary mechanics testing.
7. Practice medical charting for the documentation of performance of bedside pulmonary mechanics procedures.

KEY TERMS

atmospheric temperature and pressure, saturated (ATPS)	compliance	lumen
	deadspace	resistance
	elastance	spirometer
body temperature and pressure, saturated (BTPS)	facilitate	transducer
	flow rate	turbulent
	laminar	vane

Exercises

EQUIPMENT REQUIRED

- ☐ Briggs adaptors
- ☐ BTPS conversion chart
- ☐ Corrugated tubing
- ☐ Disposable gloves
- ☐ Disposable mouthpieces
- ☐ Electronic and vane respirometers
- ☐ Human patient simulator mannequin (if available)
- ☐ Inspiratory force adaptors (disposable)
- ☐ Intubated or tracheostomized airway management trainer
- ☐ Masks
- ☐ Noseclips
- ☐ One-way valves
- ☐ Peak flowmeters (disposable or permanent)
- ☐ Predicted values nomograms
- ☐ Pressure manometer with positive and negative ranges
- ☐ Watch with a second hand

These exercises require students to work in groups of two. The students may carry out all the exercises with the same partner, or the instructor may want to change pairs to enhance the ability of each student to communicate and explain the procedure to a different person.

In an actual clinical situation, the patient may be receiving supplemental oxygen via mask or may be on a ventilator. To obtain bedside pulmonary mechanics, the patient would have to be removed from these devices and an alternative mode of oxygen delivery instituted. In these circumstances, the practitioner should monitor the patient carefully for signs of hypoxia while the parameters are being obtained. This includes observation of the patient, use of pulse oximetry, and cardiac monitors. Placing the patient on a nasal cannula may be one alternative. The therapist should consult with the physician or follow departmental policies under these circumstances. If the patient is on a ventilator, the practitioner must ensure that the ventilator connector is handled aseptically. The ventilator alarms may need to be temporarily bypassed, but the practitioner must ensure they are reset and functional once the procedure is concluded. The patient must be immediately returned to the ventilator if there is any indication that the patient is not tolerating the testing. Results of the testing may be interpreted based on normal and critical values, shown in Table 8.1

Table 8.1 Normal and Critical Values for Bedside Spirometry

PARAMETER	NORMAL VALUE	MINIMAL ACCEPTABLE VALUE
Tidal volume	5–8 mL/kg	—
Vital capacity	50–70 mL/kg	10–15 mL/kg
Minute ventilation	6–10 Lpm	—
Peak flow	300–600 Lpm	80–100 Lpm
Negative inspiratory force	–60 to –100 cm H_2O	–20 cm H_2O
Maximum expiratory pressure	+60 to +100 cm H_2O	+20 cm H_2O

EXERCISE 8.1 OBTAINING V_T, V_E, AND V_A

*This exercise requires data to be obtained using a device called a respirometer. The two major types of respirometers are a rotating **vane spirometer**, as shown in Figure 8.1, and electronic respirometers, as shown in Figure 8.2.*

1. Gather the necessary equipment: watch with a second hand, spirometer, disposable noseclips, mouthpieces, one way valves, and tubing to prevent cross contamination with the spirometer.
2. A one-way valve should be used each time this procedure is performed. The one-way valve is for single patient use only.
3. Wash hands and apply standard precautions and transmission based isolation procedures as appropriate.
4. Assemble the equipment as shown in Figure 8.3.
   A. Attach a single length of large-bore corrugated tubing to the T-piece opening. Attach the mouthpiece to the opposite end of the corrugated tubing.
   B. Attach a single length of corrugated tubing to the expiratory side of the T-piece one way valve assembly. Place a 22-mm outer diameter (OD)/15-mm inner diameter (ID) adaptor to the opposite end of the corrugated tubing.
   C. Attach the respirometer to the expiratory side of the 22-mm OD/15-mm ID adaptor.
   D. Verify the appropriate direction of flow by ensuring that one-way valves allow for inspiration from the room and expiration into the respirometer.
5. Introduce yourself. **Record your partner's age, sex, height, and weight on your laboratory report.**
6. Explain the procedure and the purpose of the testing to your partner. Demonstrate if necessary.
7. Instruct your partner to put the mouthpiece into his or her mouth. Emphasize the importance of maintaining a tight seal around the mouthpiece. Explain the purpose of using the noseclips.
8. Allow your partner to stabilize, or "get used to," breathing through the mouthpiece and spirometer.
9. Turn the spirometer on. Activate the spirometer by pressing the "Reset" button to zero the dial, and begin recording your partner's exhaled volumes.
10. Simultaneously, count your partner's breath rate.
11. Measure these parameters for *one full minute*. At the end of precisely one minute, press the "Stop" or "Off" button to stop the recording and preserve the data.
12. **Record the data on your laboratory report. Record the room temperature. Look up conversion factor for that room temperature. Convert to BTPS.**
13. Disassemble and properly clean the equipment.
    A. In the event that multiple measurements are required on an individual patient, the one-way valve assembly may be aseptically stored in the patient's room. Otherwise the assembly should be discarded after use.
    B. The respirometer should be wiped down with a 70% isopropyl alcohol solution between patients.
    C. For patients with active tuberculosis or any other disorder requiring airborne or droplet isolation precautions, the respirometer should be sterilized between patients.

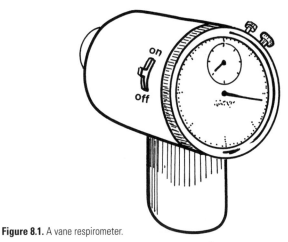

Figure 8.1. A vane respirometer.

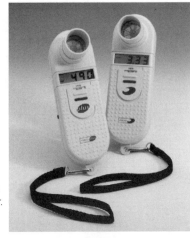

Figure 8.2. Electronic ultrasonic vortex flow-sensing respirometer. (Courtesy of Cardinal Health, Dublin, OH.)

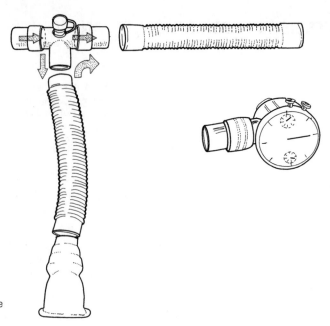

Figure 8.3. Assembly of one-way valve monitoring circuit.

EXERCISE 8.2 OBTAINING NEGATIVE INSPIRATORY FORCE AND MAXIMUM EXPIRATORY PRESSURE

1. Gather the necessary equipment: mask or mouthpiece and noseclips, disposable inspiratory force adaptor with one-way valve, and pressure manometer.
2. Wash your hands and apply standard precautions and transmission based isolation procedures as appropriate.
3. Assemble the equipment as shown in Figure 8.4.
   A. Attach the small-bore tubing to the nipple on the inspiratory force meter.
   B. Attach the opposite end of the small-bore tubing to the inspiratory force adaptor or the port on the one-way valve setup.
   C. The inspiratory force adaptor will fit directly onto an endotracheal or tracheostomy tube. For nonintubated patients, attach the adaptor to a mask or mouthpiece.
   D. Explain the procedure to your partner. Demonstrate if necessary.

Figure 8.4. Assembled equipment for inspiratory force measurement. (From Black, LF and Hyatt, RE: Am Rev Respir Dis 103:641–650, 1971, with permission.)

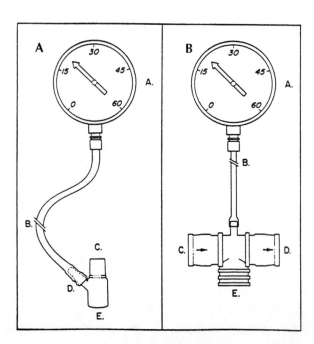

E. Completely occlude the opening on the inspiratory force adaptor with your finger and instruct your partner to inhale as hard as possible from the normal resting exhalation position. If the one-way valve is used, no occlusion is needed. Note the maximum negative pressure achieved.

F. Repeat the procedure two more times.

G. **Record the data from the three trials on your laboratory report.**

4. Using the same equipment, completely occlude the opening of the adaptor and instruct your partner to take a deep breath and then to exhale as hard as possible.

A. Repeat the procedure two more times.

B. **Record the data from the three trials on your laboratory report.**

EXERCISE 8.3 OBTAINING A SLOW VITAL CAPACITY

*NOTE: If a vane type spirometer, such as a Wright respirometer, is used, high **flow rates** will warp the vanes. Do not perform a forced vital capacity (FVC) with this device!*

1. Gather and assemble the necessary equipment: respirometer, one-way valves, mouthpiece or mask, and noseclips as in Exercise 8.1.

2. Wash hands and apply standard precautions and transmission-based isolation procedures as appropriate.

3. Turn the spirometer on and reset to zero.

4. Explain the procedure by instructing your partner to take in the deepest breath possible and then exhale *slowly* and completely into the spirometer. Demonstrate if necessary.

5. Ensure a tight seal by making sure that the mouthpiece is secure, that noseclips are in place, or, if using a mask, that there are no leaks.

6. Coach the "patient" throughout the procedure. Turn off the respirometer or press the "Stop" button when exhalation is complete.

7. Repeat the procedure two more times and **record the data on your laboratory report. Convert values to BTPS.**

EXERCISE 8.4 OBTAINING PEAK EXPIRATORY FLOW RATE MEASUREMENTS

1. Obtain a peak flowmeter and a mouthpiece (Fig. 8.5). The use of noseclips is recommended.

2. Wash hands and apply standard precautions and transmission-based isolation procedures as appropriate.

3. Instruct your partner to take in a deep breath and then to blow as hard as possible into the peak flowmeter. Ensure a tight seal. Exhalation down to residual volume is not necessary. Demonstrate if necessary.

4. Repeat the procedure two more times and **record the data on your laboratory report. Convert values to BTPS.**

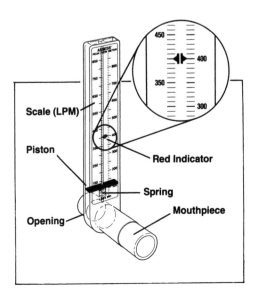

Figure 8.5. Peak flowmeter. (Courtesy of HealthScan Products, Inc., Cedar Grove, NJ.)

EXERCISE 8.5 OBTAINING DATA ON PATIENTS WITH ARTIFICIAL AIRWAYS

1. Obtain one-way valves, corrugated tubing, and Briggs adaptors.
2. Assemble the equipment as previously described.
3. Wash your hands and apply standard precautions and transmission-based isolation procedures as appropriate.
4. Attach equipment to the adaptor of the artificial airway as shown in Figure 8.6.
5. If a human patient simulator mannequin is used, measure the V_E and f and calculate the V_T. **Record this information on your laboratory report.**

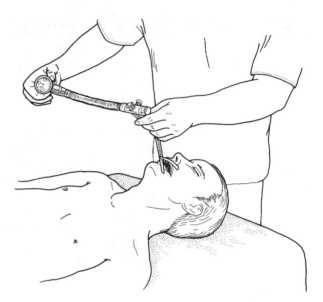

Figure 8.6. Attaching monitoring equipment to an artificial airway.

Laboratory Report

CHAPTER 8: BEDSIDE ASSESSMENT OF PULMONARY MECHANICS

Name _____ Date _____

Course/Section _____ Instructor _____

Data Collection

Laboratory partner(s): _____

Age:	Sex:	Height:	Weight:	Race:

Calculate Ideal Body Wt (show work)

_____

EXERCISE 8.1 Obtaining V_T, V_E, and V_A

V_E: _____ Breath rate: _____ Room Temperature: _____ °F

Calculate your partner's average tidal volume using the following formula: $V_T = V_E/f$. *Don't forget the proper units!*

$V_T =$ _____

Calculate your partner's alveolar ventilation using the formula: $V_A = (V_T - V_D) f$. *Don't forget the proper units!*

$V_D =$ _____

$V_A =$ _____

Conversion factor for room temperature = _____

Convert V_E to BTPS (show your work) = _____

Convert V_T to BTPS (show your work) = _____

EXERCISE 8.2 Obtaining Negative Inspiratory Force and Maximum Expiratory Pressure

	Trial 1	Trial 2	Trial 3
MIP			
MEP			

Circle the value to be reported.

EXERCISE 8.3 Obtaining a Slow Vital Capacity

	Trial 1	Trial 2	Trial 3
SVC (ATPS)			
SVC (BTPS)			

Convert to BTPS = _____ (show your work).
Circle the value to be reported.

EXERCISE 8.4 Obtaining Peak Expiratory Flow Rate Measurements

	Trial 1	Trial 2	Trial 3
PEFR			

Circle the value to be reported.

EXERCISE 8.5 Obtaining Data on Patients with Artificial Airways

V_E: _____ Breath rate: _____ Room Temperature: _____ °F

Calculate average V_T

$V_T =$

Convert to BTPS correction factor

V_E (BTPS) =

V_T (BTPS) =

Critical Thinking Questions

1. Calculate the missing values. Show your work!

Weight	200 lb	60 kg	140 lb
V_r	400 mL		
f	14	20	15
V_E		12.6 L	
V_D			
V_A			6.0 L

2. Why is it necessary to obtain at least three trials? Which trial(s) would you report to the physician?

3. Which measurement(s) required the most cooperation from your partner to obtain results?

4. Dr. Shah asks you to perform a bedside evaluation on Mrs. Hernandez, a 29-year-old, 150-lb. woman admitted with a diagnosis of myasthenia gravis. As you begin to explain the procedure, you realize that she speaks and understands only Spanish.

   A. How would you alter your instructions or actions to the patient in order to obtain the data under these circumstances?

   B. What is the clinical significance of monitoring these parameters in a patient with Mrs. Hernandez's condition?

5. You are able to obtain the following parameters:

V_T:	300 mL
f:	25/min
V_E:	7.7 Lpm
MIP:	−40 cm H_2O
SVC:	1.5 Lpm
PEFR:	200 Lpm

   A. For each of these parameters, indicate whether it is within normal limits, abnormal, or a critical value.

   B. What is your overall impression and interpretation of these results?

   C. What would be your recommendations to the physician regarding evaluation and treatment of this patient?

   D. Which of these parameters is indicative of the patient's ability to cough and deep breathe?

   E. Which of these parameters is most indicative of respiratory muscle strength?

6. Dr. Shah now tells you that she suspects that Mrs. Hernandez has diplococcal pneumonia. What infection control procedures related to the patient, the equipment, and yourself did you practice to ensure that the infection will not be spread to you or to other patients? What, if any, additional procedures would you follow if Mrs. Hernandez was suspected of having tuberculosis?

7. Two hours later, the bedside evaluation is repeated and the following data are obtained: V_T 200 mL; f 40/minute. Based on these data, which of the following would most likely be increased above normal? Circle as many as are appropriate.

A. V_E

B. V_A

C. V_D

D. $PaCO_2$

8. In a patient with an artificial airway, which test(s), if any, could not be performed?

9. Which parameters *can* be obtained in a comatose patient?

Procedural Competency Evaluation

STUDENT: **DATE:**

BEDSIDE PULMONARY MECHANICS

	PERFORMANCE RATING	PERFORMANCE LEVEL
Evaluator: ☐ Peer ☐ Instructor **Setting:** ☐ Lab ☐ Clinical Simulation		
Equipment Utilized: **Conditions (Describe):**		

Performance Level:

    S or ✓ = Satisfactory, no errors of omission or commission

    U = Unsatisfactory Error of Omission or Commission

    NA = Not applicable

Performance Rating:

    5   **Independent:** Near flawless performance; minimal errors; able to perform without supervision; seeks out new learning; shows initiative; A = 4.7–5.0 average

    4   **Minimally Supervised:** Few errors, able to self-correct; seeks guidance when appropriate; B = 3.7–4.65

    3   **Competent:** Minimal required level; no critical errors; able to correct with coaching; meets expectations; safe; C = 3.0–3.65

    2   **Marginal:** Below average; critical errors or problem areas noted; would benefit from remediation; D = 2.0–2.99

    1   **Dependent:** Poor; unacceptable performance; unsafe; gross inaccuracies; potentially harmful; F = < 2.0

    Two or more errors of commission or omission of mandatory or essential performance elements will terminate the procedure, and require additional practice and/or remediation and reevaluation. Student is responsible for obtaining additional evaluation forms as needed from the Director of Clinical Education (DCE).

EQUIPMENT AND PATIENT PREPARATION		
1. Common Performance Elements Steps 1–8		
2. Obtains all mouthpieces, one-way valve, and disposable adapters for equipment		
ASSESSMENT AND IMPLEMENTATION		
3. Common Performance Elements Steps 9 and 10		
4. Uses nose clips or mask if needed		
A. Obtains required parameters:		
B. Minute Volume, *f*		
C. V_T (computed)		
D. RSBI (computed)		
E. SVC or FVC (forced expiration should not be performed with handheld vane-type respirometer)		
5. Repeats the following at least 3 times for best result:		
A. SVC		
B. NIF/MIP		
C. PEFR		
6. Performs MVV for 12–15 seconds and extrapolates for lpm; ensures the patient is sitting upright		
FOLLOW-UP		
7. Common Performance Elements Steps 11–16		
8. Records best effort for each value		

SIGNATURES   Student: Evaluator: Date:

Clinical Performance Evaluation

PERFORMANCE RATING:

5 **Independent:** Near flawless performance; minimal errors; able to perform without supervision; seeks out new learning; shows initiative; A = 4.7–5.0 average

4 **Minimally Supervised:** Few errors, able to self-correct; seeks guidance when appropriate; B = 3.7–4.65

3 **Competent:** Minimal required level; no critical errors; able to correct with coaching; meets expectations; safe; C = 3.0–3.65

2 **Marginal:** Below average; critical errors or problem areas noted; would benefit from remediation; D = 2.0–2.99

1 **Dependent:** Poor; unacceptable performance; unsafe; gross inaccuracies; potentially harmful; F = < 2.0

Circle the appropriate response below. Please be consistent, objective, and honest in your assessment of the student's clinical performance and ability.

PERFORMANCE CRITERIA	SCORE				
COGNITIVE DOMAIN					
1. Consistently displays knowledge, comprehension, and command of essential concepts	5	4	3	2	1
2. Demonstrates the relationship between theory and clinical practice	5	4	3	2	1
3. Able to select, review, apply, analyze, synthesize, interpret, and evaluate information; makes recommendations to modify care plan	5	4	3	2	1
PSYCHOMOTOR DOMAIN					
4. Minimal errors, no critical errors; able to self-correct; performs all steps safely and accurately	5	4	3	2	1
5. Selects, assembles, and verifies proper function and cleanliness of equipment; assures operation and corrects malfunctions; provides adequate care and maintenance	5	4	3	2	1
6. Exhibits the required manual dexterity	5	4	3	2	1
7. Performs procedure in a reasonable time frame for clinical level	5	4	3	2	1
8. Applies and maintains aseptic technique and PPE as required	5	4	3	2	1
9. Maintains concise and accurate patient and clinical records	5	4	3	2	1
10. Reports promptly on patient status/needs to appropriate personnel	5	4	3	2	1
AFFECTIVE DOMAIN					
11. Exhibits courteous and pleasant demeanor; shows consideration and respect, honesty, and integrity	5	4	3	2	1
12. Communicates verbally and in writing clearly and concisely	5	4	3	2	1
13. Preserves confidentiality and adheres to all policies	5	4	3	2	1
14. Follows directions, exhibits sound judgment, and seeks help when required	5	4	3	2	1
15. Demonstrates initiative, self-direction, responsibility, and accountability	5	4	3	2	1

TOTAL POINTS = _____ /15 = AVERAGE GRADE = _____

ADDITIONAL COMMENTS: IDENTIFY AREAS OF EXCELLENCE; LIST ERRORS OF OMISSION OR COMMISSION, CRITICAL ERRORS

SUMMARY PERFORMANCE EVALUATION AND RECOMMENDATIONS

☐ PASS: Satisfactory Performance

    ☐ Minimal supervision needed, may progress to next level provided specific skills, clinical time completed

    ☐ Minimal supervision needed, able to progress to next level without remediation

☐ FAIL: Unsatisfactory Performance (check all that apply)

    ☐ Minor reevaluation only

    ☐ Needs additional clinical practice before reevaluation

    ☐ Needs additional laboratory practice before skills performed in clinical area

    ☐ Recommend clinical probation

SIGNATURES

Evaluator (print name): _____ Evaluator signature: _____ Date: _____

Student Signature: _____ Date: _____

Student Comments:

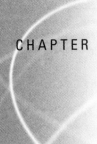

Oxygen Supply Systems

INTRODUCTION

Most respiratory therapy devices require some type of pressurized gas source. The gas source and its system are considered *primary equipment*, and the delivery devices (such as oxygen masks) are *secondary equipment*.[1] Primary systems include cylinders, piped systems, and bulk gas and liquid systems. Primary systems are too often overlooked by respiratory care practitioners, but a thorough understanding of them is necessary for safe patient care. To illustrate this point, in an issue of *Respiratory Care Manager*, a critical incident was reported in which oxygen was contaminated with trichloroethylene, a toxic substance; this may have contributed to the deaths of five patients.[2] Although the practitioner may have an advanced comprehension of pathophysiology and the goals of medical gas therapy, he or she must also have a sound working knowledge of the capabilities and safe handling of the related equipment. If these systems fail, thorough knowledge would enable a quick and effective response by the respiratory care practitioner.[1]

OBJECTIVES

Upon completion of this chapter, the student will be able to:

1. Identify the contents of medical gas cylinders.
2. Identify the markings on a medical gas cylinder as defined by the Department of Transportation (DOT).
3. Differentiate between the **American Standard Safety System (ASSS)** index for large cylinders, the **Diameter Index Safety System (DISS)**, and the **Pin Index Safety System (PISS)** for small cylinders.
4. Demonstrate the safe handling, transport, and storage of medical gas cylinders.
5. Identify the components of a bulk liquid system.
6. Identify the components of a reserve system.
7. Operate and troubleshoot an air compressor.
8. Identify the components of a single-stage and a multistage **regulator**.
9. Identify the components of a Bourdon gauge regulator.
10. Identify the components of a Thorpe tube flowmeter.
11. Differentiate between a pressure-compensated and a nonpressure-compensated flowmeter.
12. Calculate the duration of flow of a cylinder.
13. Set up and safely operate a blender.
14. Locate and identify zone valves in a healthcare facility.
15. Identify and safely use wall outlet quick-connect systems.

KEY TERMS

ambient
American Standard Safety
    System (ASSS)
boiling point
combustible
compensation
critical pressure
critical temperature
density
Diameter Index Safety System
    (DISS)

evaporation
flammable
fractional distillation
frangible
fusible
Joint Commission on
    Accreditation of Healthcare
    Organizations (JCAHO)
melting point
Pin Index Safety System
    (PISS)

pounds per square inch
    (psi)
pounds per square inch gauge
    (psig)
reducing valve
regulator
reservoir
specific gravity
sublimation
volatile

Exercises

EQUIPMENT REQUIRED

- ☐ Adjustable wrenches
- ☐ Air compressor
- ☐ Blender
- ☐ Bourdon gauge regulators
- ☐ Cylinder trucks and circle stands
- ☐ E cylinder keys
- ☐ Gasloc® seals (PISS cylinder washers)
- ☐ High-pressure air and oxygen hoses with DISS connectors and quick-connect types
- ☐ H- and E-sized oxygen and other types of medical gas cylinders

- ☐ Liter metering devices
- ☐ Samples of quick-connect adaptors and wall plates
- ☐ Sample of wall outlet box and components
- ☐ Single-stage and multistage regulators
- ☐ Screwdrivers: flathead and Phillips, Allen wrenches
- ☐ Stopwatch
- ☐ Thorpe tube flowmeters, with and without regulators
- ☐ Torx wrench

EXERCISE 9.1 MEDICAL GAS CYLINDERS

EXERCISE 9.1.1 SAFE STORAGE OF CYLINDERS—DIAGRAM

Carefully observe the diagram shown in Figure 9.1 and identify at least four cylinder storage safety violations. **Record your list on your laboratory report.**

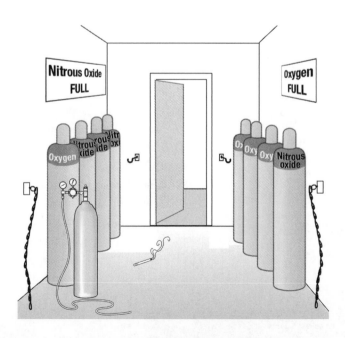

Figure 9.1. Scene survey.

EXERCISE 9.1.2 SAFE STORAGE OF CYLINDERS

In this exercise, the instructor has prepared a scenario in which medical gas cylinders are being stored improperly. Carefully observe the area. Identify and correct the safety violations (at least four are present). **Record each safety violation observed and corrective actions taken on your laboratory report.**

EXERCISE 9.1.3 SAFE HANDLING AND TRANSPORT OF CYLINDERS

1. Wheel an H cylinder on its truck (Fig. 9.2) from one side of the laboratory to the other. Be sure to push, not pull.
2. Take the H cylinder off of its truck. Carefully walk it across the room and safely secure it in a circle stand (donut) or other type of cylinder stand (see Fig. 9.2).
3. Repeat steps 1 and 2 for an E cylinder.

EXERCISE 9.1.4 CYLINDER MARKINGS

Your instructor will supply you with two different types and sizes of medical gas cylinders. Observe the cylinder markings, as shown in Figure 9.3. **Record the following data on your laboratory report:**

Size of each cylinder
Contents of each cylinder
Safety system of each cylinder outlet
Date of manufacture of each cylinder
Retest date of each cylinder
Ownership of each cylinder
Serial number
Filling pressure

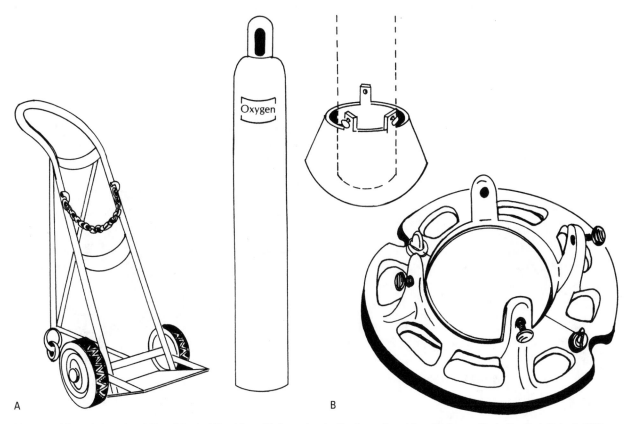

A   B

Figure 9.2. (A) H cylinder and truck (From Eubanks, DH and Bone, RC: Comprehensive Respiratory Care: A Learning System. Mosby-Year Book, St. Louis, 1990, p. 136, with permission); **(B)** Circle stand (From Eubanks, DH and Bone, RC: Comprehensive Respiratory Care: A Learning System. Mosby-Year Book, St. Louis, 1990, p. 136, with permission).

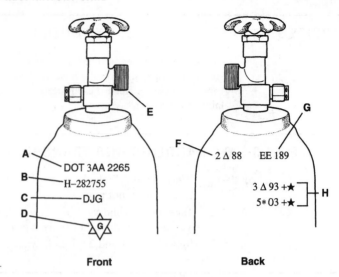

Figure 9.3. Location of cylinder markings.   **Front**   **Back**

EXERCISE 9.1.5 SAFETY SYSTEM CONNECTIONS

1. Obtain an H cylinder with a regulator and an E cylinder with a regulator. Observe the gas outlets and points of regulator attachments. Differentiate between the Compressed Gas Association–American Standard Safety System (ASSS), the Diameter Index Safety System (DISS), and the Pin Index Safety System (PISS). Identify the safety systems shown in Figure 9.4. **Record the corresponding letter from the diagram on your laboratory report.**

   Post

   Threaded ASSS outlet

   Valve stem

   DISS

   Frangible disk or fusible plug

   PISS

2. Using the H cylinder, identify the location of the frangible disk or fusible plug pressure relief valves on the valve stem. **Record the corresponding letter from Figure 9.4 on your laboratory report.**

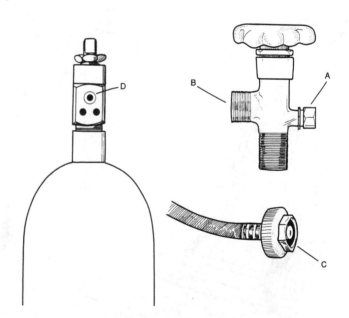

Figure 9.4. Identification of safety systems.

EXERCISE 9.2 REDUCING VALVES, REGULATORS, AND FLOWMETERS

EXERCISE 9.2.1 REDUCING VALVES

1. Identify the components of the reducing valve shown in Figure 9.5 and **record the labeled parts on your laboratory report:**
    ASSS high-pressure inlet
    DISS gas outlet
    Bourdon gauge pressure manometer
    Bourdon gauge flowmeter
    Bourdon gauge flow control
    Pressure relief valve(s)

2. Determine whether the reducing valve is adjustable or preset. **Record your observation on your laboratory report.**

3. Announce out loud that you are about to "crack" a cylinder. Make sure no one is facing the gas outlet while this is being done. "Crack" the cylinder by quickly opening and closing the main valve so that a brief blast of gas is released. Then attach the regulator to the cylinder. Turn on the cylinder and **record the pressure on your laboratory report.**

EXERCISE 9.2.2 BOURDON GAUGE REGULATOR

1. Identify the components of a Bourdon gauge regulator, as shown in Figure 9.6 and **record the labeled parts on your laboratory report.**
    High-pressure inlet
    Gas outlet (oxygen nipple adapter)
    Bourdon gauge pressure manometer
    Bourdon gauge flowmeter
    Pressure relief valve(s)
    Bourdon gauge flow control
    T-valve
    PISS yoke
    PISS pins
    Gasloc® seal (O-ring or washer)

A. Attach the Bourdon gauge regulator to an H or E cylinder, as available.

B. Turn on the cylinder completely. **Record the pressure on your laboratory report.**

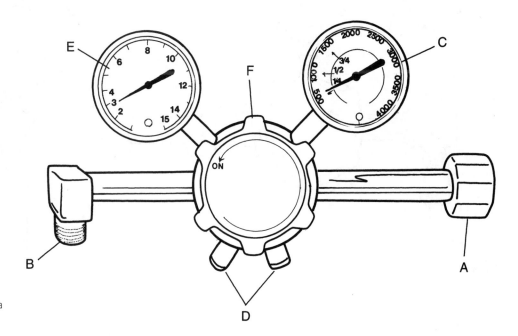

Figure 9.5. Components of a reducing valve.

C. Turn the flow to 5 Lpm. Occlude the orifice with your finger. **Record your observations on your laboratory report.**

2. Obtain an E cylinder with a Bordon gauge regulator. Turn the flowmeter on to 3 Lpm. Lay the cylinder on its side and observe the flowmeter gauge reading. **Record this on your laboratory report.**

3. Obtain an E cylinder. Replace the Gasloc® seal (washer) on the regulator and reattach it. If an H cylinder was used for step 2, set the Bourdon gauge flowmeter on this E cylinder to 5 Lpm. **Record the pressure on your laboratory report.**

4. Turn the flowmeter off. Turn the regulator off. "Bleed" the pressure from the regulator by turning the flowmeter on until the pressure gauge returns to zero. Turn the flowmeter off.

EXERCISE 9.2.3 THORPE TUBE FLOWMETERS

1. Identify the components of a Thorpe tube flowmeter, as shown in Figure 9.7 and **record the labeled parts on your laboratory report.**

    DISS or quick-connect high-pressure gas inlet

    DISS gas outlet

    Thorpe tube

    Flowmeter needle valve control knob

    PTO (pressure take-off) 50-psi outlet

    Flow indicator ball

2. Attach a Thorpe tube flowmeter with a regulator to an H cylinder. Turn the cylinder on. **Record the pressure and your observations on your laboratory report.**

3. Turn the flow up to 8 Lpm. Completely occlude the orifice with your finger. **Record your observations on your laboratory report.**

4. Obtain an E cylinder with a regulator with a Thorpe tube flowmeter. Turn the flowmeter on to 3 Lpm. Lay the cylinder on its side and observe the flowmeter gauge reading. **Record this on your laboratory report and contrast this with what happened with the Bourdon gauge regulator in the previous Exercise 9.2.2.**

5. Turn the flowmeter off. Turn the regulator off. "Bleed" the pressure from the regulator by turning the flowmeter on until the pressure gauge returns to zero. Turn the flowmeter off.

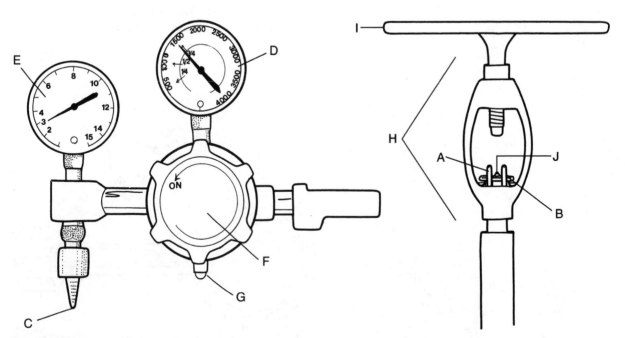

Figure 9.6. Components of a Bourdon gauge regulator.

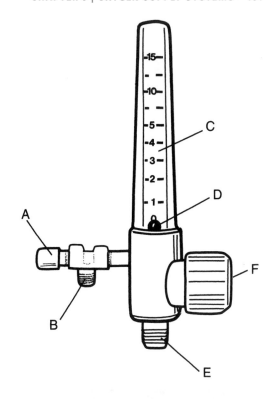

Figure 9.7. Components of a Thorpe tube flowmeter.

EXERCISE 9.2.4 CALCULATION OF CYLINDER DURATION

For the pressures and flows recorded in Exercises 9.2.2 and 9.2.3, calculate the duration of flow for the E and H cylinders using the following formula and the appropriate conversion factor from Table 9.1.

Duration of flow = Pressure in cylinder × Cylinder factor / Flow rate

Remember, this will give you the duration of flow in minutes. You must divide by 60 to obtain duration in hours. **Show your work!**

Table 9.1 Cylinder Conversion Factors

CYLINDER SIZE	CONVERSION FACTOR
D	0.16
E	0.28
G	2.41
H or K	3.14

EXERCISE 9.3 AIR COMPRESSORS

1. Identify the following components of an air compressor, as shown in Figure 9.8. **Record the labeled parts on your laboratory report.**
    Electrical cord
    Pressure outlets
    Pressure manometer
    Pressure adjustment
    Filter
    On/off switch
2. Turn on the compressor and start timing with the stopwatch. What is the operating pressure of the device? How long did it take the compressor to achieve the operating pressure? **Record the pressure and time on your laboratory report.**

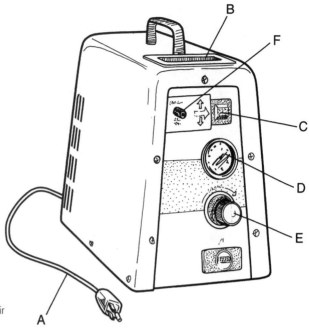

Figure 9.8. Components of an air compressor.

EXERCISE 9.4 BLENDERS

1. Identify the components of an air/oxygen blender as shown in Figure 9.9.
   Air inlet
   Oxygen inlet
   Gas outlet
   Alarm
   F_IO_2 adjustment control
2. Connect the pressure hoses to the appropriate connections. Identify the safety system. Turn on the gas supplies. Adjust the F_IO_2 to 0.40. **Record your observations, if any, on your laboratory report.**
3. Disconnect the air pressure hose. **Record your observations on your laboratory report.**
4. Reattach the air. Disconnect the oxygen hose. **Record your observations on your laboratory report.**
5. Reattach the oxygen hose
6. Attach a flowmeter to the blender outlet. Adjust blender to 60%. Turn flow to 8 Lpm. Analyze the blender output. **Record measured F_IO_2 on your laboratory report.**

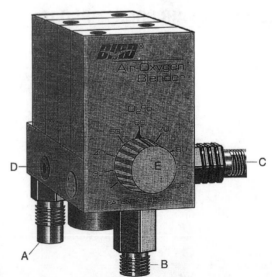

Figure 9.9. Components of an air/oxygen blender. (Courtesy of Bird Products Corporation, Palm Springs, CA.)

EXERCISE 9.5 BULK STORAGE SYSTEMS

EXERCISE 9.5.1 LIQUID STORAGE SYSTEM

1. Identify the components of a liquid bulk storage system, as shown in Figure 9.10, and **record the labeled parts on your laboratory report.**
   Liquid container: carbon steel-protected outer shell
   Gas vent valve
   Vaporizer panels
   Control panel
   Main line to hospital

EXERCISE 9.5.2 BANK AND RESERVE SYSTEMS

1. Identify the components of a bank system, as shown in Figure 9.11, and **record the labeled parts on your laboratory report.**
   Gas cylinders
   Connecting pipes
   Main-line pressure alarm
   Bank manometers
   Main supply line
   Switch-over
   Check valves
   Main supply manometer

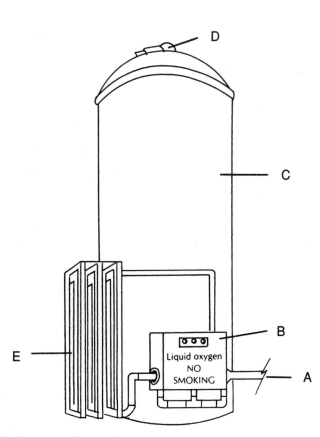

Figure 9.10. Components of a bulk liquid oxygen system. (Adapted from Eubanks, DH and Bone, RC: Principles and Applications of Cardiorespiratory Care Equipment, Mosby-Year Book, St. Louis, 1994, p. 9.)

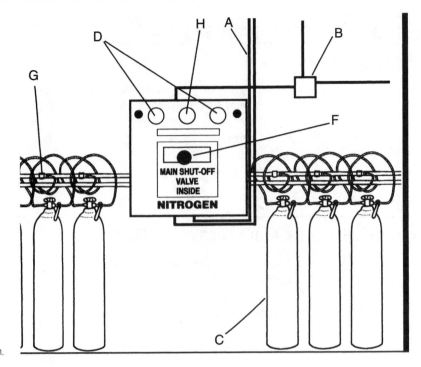

Figure 9.11. Components of a bank system.

EXERCISE 9.6 ZONE VALVES AND WALL OUTLETS

This exercise may need to be performed in the clinical setting because of the lack of availability of the necessary equipment in the laboratory.

1. Locate the two zone valves (Fig. 9.12) (in the healthcare facility, if not available in the lab). Determine which rooms or units would be affected by shutting off these valves. Observe the line pressures for air, oxygen, and vacuum. **Record the pressures for each on your laboratory report.**

2. Identify the types of wall outlet quick-connect systems, as shown in Figure 9.13.

3. Locate a wall outlet (Fig. 9.14) at your institution. Identify the type of quick-connect used and **record this on your laboratory report.**

4. Unscrew the face plate of a sample wall outlet (make sure the compressed gas system is turned off if a functional outlet is used). Take notice of the locking mechanism that holds the flowmeter in place. Take the mechanism apart. Examine the O-rings that prevent leakage for cracks or pitting. Replace if needed. Reassemble and replace when finished.

5. Locate and identify the types of wall outlet quick-connects used in the lab or at clinical sites. Obtain a flowmeter with the same type of connection. Practice engaging and disengaging the flowmeter. **Record the type of wall outlet quick-connects and your observations on your laboratory report.** If different types are used, compare and contrast the ease of use.

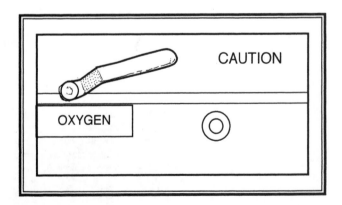

Figure 9.12. Zone valve.

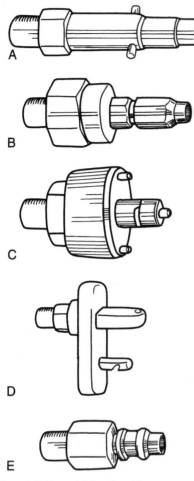

Figure 9.13. Types of wall outlet quick-connect systems. **(A)** Oxyquip '07 O.E.S.; **(B)** Schrader; **(C)** Ohmeda; **(D)** Chemetron; **(E)** Puritan Bennett.

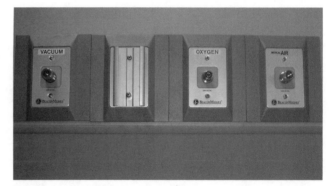

Figure 9.14. Wall outlets.

REFERENCES
1. McPherson, S: Respiratory Care Equipment, ed 5. Mosby, St Louis, 1995, p 24.
2. Tainted O_2 linked to ICU deaths. Respiratory Care Manager 5:4, 1996.

Laboratory Report

CHAPTER 9: OXYGEN SUPPLY SYSTEMS

Name _____ Date _____

Course/Section _____ Instructor _____

Data Collection

EXERCISE 9.1 Medical Gas Cylinders

EXERCISE 9.1.1 SAFE STORAGE OF CYLINDERS—DIAGRAM

1. _____

2. _____

3. _____

4. _____

5. _____

EXERCISE 9.1.2 SAFE STORAGE OF CYLINDERS

Identify the safety violations and corrective actions taken:

1. _____

2. _____

3. _____

4. _____

5. _____

EXERCISE 9.1.4 CYLINDER MARKINGS

	Cylinder A	Cylinder B
Size		
Contents		
Safety system		
Date of manufacture		
Retest date		
Ownership		
Serial number		
Filling pressure		

EXERCISE 9.1.5 SAFETY SYSTEM CONNECTIONS

Identify the corresponding letter from Figure 9.4:

Threaded ASSS outlet

DISS

PISS

Frangible disk or fusible plug

Post

Valve stem

EXERCISE 9.2 Reducing Valves, Regulators, and Flowmeters

EXERCISE 9.2.1 REDUCING VALVES

A. _____

B. _____

C. _____

D. _____

E. _____

F. _____

Adjustable or preset? _____

Pressure recorded: _____

EXERCISE 9.2.2 BOURDON GAUGE REGULATOR

A. _____

B. _____

C. _____

D. _____

E. _____

F. _____

G. _____

H. _____

I. _____

J. _____

Pressure in the cylinder: _____

What occurred when the orifice of the Bourdon gauge was occluded? _____

_____

What occurred to the readings when the tank was laid on its side? _____

_____

EXERCISE 9.2.3 THORPE TUBE FLOWMETERS

A. _____

B. _____

C. _____

D. _____

E. _____

F. _____

What occurred immediately when the cylinder was turned on? _____

_____

Pressure in the cylinder: _____

What happened when you occluded the outlet of the Thorpe tube flowmeter? _____

_____

What happened to the readings when the tank was laid on its side? _____

EXERCISE 9.2.4 CALCULATION OF CYLINDER DURATION

Duration of E cylinder: _____

Duration of H cylinder: _____

Show your work! _____

EXERCISE 9.3 Air Compressors

A. _____

B. _____

C. _____

D. _____

E. _____

F. _____

Operating pressure reading from the compressor: _____

Time until operating pressure was achieved: _____

EXERCISE 9.4 Blenders

A. _____

B. _____

C. _____

D. _____

E. _____

Observations: _____

_____

_____

_____

Analyzed F_IO_2:_____

_____

EXERCISE 9.5 Bulk Storage Systems

EXERCISE 9.5.1 LIQUID STORAGE SYSTEMS

A. _____

B. _____

C. _____

D. _____

E. _____

EXERCISE 9.5.2 BANK AND RESERVE SYSTEMS

A. _____

B. _____

C. _____

D. _____

E. _____

F. _____

G. _____

H. _____

EXERCISE 9.6 Zone Valves and Wall Outlets

Location of zone valves and areas controlled by each: _____

Oxygen line pressure: _____

Air line pressure: _____

Vacuum line pressure: _____

Type of wall outlet quick-connects: _____

Type of wall outlet(s): _____

Critical Thinking Questions

1. Why is it necessary to "crack" a cylinder before attaching a regulator?

2. Identify at least three ways to determine whether a flowmeter is compensated.

3. Which would be preferred to transport a patient on a stretcher, a Bourdon gauge flowmeter or a Thorpe tube flowmeter? Explain why.

4. Which would be preferred to transport a patient in a wheelchair with a tank carrier attached? Why?

5. Identify the following [flammability must be categorized as "flammable" (F), "nonflammable" (NF), or "supports combustion" (SC)]:

Symbol	Gas	Color Code	Combustion
O_2			
$O_2 + N_2$			
CO_2			
CO_2/O_2			
N_2			
He			
He/O_2			
N_2O			
NO			
$(CH_2)_3$			
ETO			

6. Mr. Butinsky is using a nasal cannula at 3 Lpm. The nurse calls you and tells you that the patient must go to x-ray in a wheel chair. Describe the specific equipment required to transport this patient to x-ray.

Procedural Competency Evaluation

STUDENT: DATE:

BULK MEDICAL GAS SUPPLY SYSTEM

		PERFORMANCE RATING	PERFORMANCE LEVEL
Evaluator: ☐ Peer ☐ Instructor **Setting:** ☐ Lab ☐ Clinical Simulation			
Equipment Utilized: **Conditions (Describe):**			

Performance Level:
    S or ✓ = Satisfactory, no errors of omission or commission
    U = Unsatisfactory Error of Omission or Commission
    NA = Not applicable			

Performance Rating:			
5 **Independent:** Near flawless performance; minimal errors; able to perform without supervision; seeks out new learning; shows initiative; A = 4.7–5.0 average			
4 **Minimally Supervised:** Few errors, able to self-correct; seeks guidance when appropriate; B = 3.7–4.65			
3 **Competent:** Minimal required level; no critical errors; able to correct with coaching; meets expectations; safe; C = 3.0–3.65			
2 **Marginal:** Below average; critical errors or problem areas noted; would benefit from remediation; D = 2.0–2.99			
1 **Dependent:** Poor; unacceptable performance; unsafe; gross inaccuracies; potentially harmful; F = < 2.0			
Two or more errors of commission or omission of mandatory or essential performance elements will terminate the procedure, and require additional practice and/or remediation and reevaluation. Student is responsible for obtaining additional evaluation forms as needed from the Director of Clinical Education (DCE).			

LIQUID BULK SYSTEM

1. Identifies the liquid gas container		
2. Identifies gas vent valve		
3. Identifies vaporizer panels		
4. Identifies control and alarm panels		
5. Identifies main delivery line and emergency shut off valve		

BANK AND RESERVE SYSTEMS

6. Identifies gas cylinders and contents		
7. Identifies connecting piping		
8. Identifies main line pressure alarm		
9. Identifies manometers for each side of the bank		
10. Identifies main supply line		
11. Identifies main supply manometer and reads the service pressure		
12. Identifies the manual or automatic switch-over mechanism		
13. Switches service from one side to the other		
14. Disconnects cylinders to be replaced		
15. Connects full cylinders to the pipe connectors		
16. Opens valves on all cylinders and checks for leaks		
17. Ensures adequate service pressure is maintained		

SIGNATURES   Student: Evaluator: Date:

Clinical Performance Evaluation

PERFORMANCE RATING:

5 **Independent:** Near flawless performance; minimal errors; able to perform without supervision; seeks out new learning; shows initiative; A = 4.7–5.0 average

4 **Minimally Supervised:** Few errors, able to self-correct; seeks guidance when appropriate; B = 3.7–4.65

3 **Competent:** Minimal required level; no critical errors; able to correct with coaching; meets expectations; safe; C = 3.0–3.65

2 **Marginal:** Below average; critical errors or problem areas noted; would benefit from remediation; D = 2.0–2.99

1 **Dependent:** Poor; unacceptable performance; unsafe; gross inaccuracies; potentially harmful; F = < 2.0

Circle the appropriate response below. Please be consistent, objective, and honest in your assessment of the student's clinical performance and ability.

PERFORMANCE CRITERIA	SCORE				
COGNITIVE DOMAIN					
1. Consistently displays knowledge, comprehension, and command of essential concepts	5	4	3	2	1
2. Demonstrates the relationship between theory and clinical practice	5	4	3	2	1
3. Able to select, review, apply, analyze, synthesize, interpret, and evaluate information; makes recommendations to modify care plan	5	4	3	2	1
PSYCHOMOTOR DOMAIN					
4. Minimal errors, no critical errors; able to self-correct; performs all steps safely and accurately	5	4	3	2	1
5. Selects, assembles, and verifies proper function and cleanliness of equipment; assures operation and corrects malfunctions; provides adequate care and maintenance	5	4	3	2	1
6. Exhibits the required manual dexterity	5	4	3	2	1
7. Performs procedure in a reasonable time frame for clinical level	5	4	3	2	1
8. Applies and maintains aseptic technique and PPE as required	5	4	3	2	1
9. Maintains concise and accurate patient and clinical records	5	4	3	2	1
10. Reports promptly on patient status/needs to appropriate personnel	5	4	3	2	1
AFFECTIVE DOMAIN					
11. Exhibits courteous and pleasant demeanor; shows consideration and respect, honesty, and integrity	5	4	3	2	1
12. Communicates verbally and in writing clearly and concisely	5	4	3	2	1
13. Preserves confidentiality and adheres to all policies	5	4	3	2	1
14. Follows directions, exhibits sound judgment, and seeks help when required	5	4	3	2	1
15. Demonstrates initiative, self-direction, responsibility, and accountability	5	4	3	2	1

TOTAL POINTS = _____ /15 = AVERAGE GRADE = _____

ADDITIONAL COMMENTS: IDENTIFY AREAS OF EXCELLENCE; LIST ERRORS OF OMISSION OR COMMISSION, CRITICAL ERRORS

SUMMARY PERFORMANCE EVALUATION AND RECOMMENDATIONS

☐ PASS: Satisfactory Performance

    ☐ Minimal supervision needed, may progress to next level provided specific skills, clinical time completed

    ☐ Minimal supervision needed, able to progress to next level without remediation

☐ FAIL: Unsatisfactory Performance (check all that apply)

    ☐ Minor reevaluation only

    ☐ Needs additional clinical practice before reevaluation

    ☐ Needs additional laboratory practice before skills performed in clinical area

    ☐ Recommend clinical probation

SIGNATURES

Evaluator (print name): _____ Evaluator signature: _____ Date: _____

Student Signature: _____ Date: _____

Student Comments: _____

Procedural Competency Evaluation

STUDENT: **DATE:**

GAS PRESSURE AND FLOW REGULATION

	PERFORMANCE RATING	PERFORMANCE LEVEL
Evaluator: ☐ Peer ☐ Instructor **Setting:** ☐ Lab ☐ Clinical Simulation		
Equipment Utilized: **Conditions (Describe):**		

Performance Level:

    S or ✓ = Satisfactory, no errors of omission or commission
    U = Unsatisfactory Error of Omission or Commission
    NA = Not applicable

Performance Rating:

  5   **Independent:** Near flawless performance; minimal errors; able to perform without supervision; seeks out new learning; shows initiative; A = 4.7–5.0 average

  4   **Minimally Supervised:** Few errors, able to self-correct; seeks guidance when appropriate; B = 3.7–4.65

  3   **Competent:** Minimal required level; no critical errors; able to correct with coaching; meets expectations; safe; C = 3.0–3.65

  2   **Marginal:** Below average; critical errors or problem areas noted; would benefit from remediation; D = 2.0–2.99

  1   **Dependent:** Poor; unacceptable performance; unsafe; gross inaccuracies; potentially harmful; F = < 2.0

    Two or more errors of commission or omission of mandatory or essential performance elements will terminate the procedure, and require additional practice and/or remediation and reevaluation. Student is responsible for obtaining additional evaluation forms as needed from the Director of Clinical Education (DCE).

GAS PRESSURE AND FLOW REGULATION

1. Identifies and verifies contents of cylinder by label and color		
2. Identifies and interprets marking on cylinder		
3. Identifies the safety systems on large and small cylinders, wall outlets, regulators, and flowmeters		
4. Selects the proper regulator and flowmeter for large and small cylinders and wall outlets		
5. Observes proper handling, transportation, and storage of cylinder		
6. Demonstrates proper "cracking" of cylinder; alerts any bystanders		
7. Verifies presence of gas-loc (O-ring, washer, gasket) seal on E cylinder		
8. Properly connects regulator to cylinder		
A. Detects and corrects any leaks		
9. Properly opens cylinder valve for gas delivery		
A. Reads cylinder pressure correctly		
10. Identifies type of flowmeter and determines if it is compensated or non-compensated		
11. Connects flowmeter correctly to wall outlet		
A. Detects and corrects any leaks		
12. Adjusts liter flow		
13. Occludes outlet of flowmeter and explains observations		

FOLLOW-UP

14. Determines length of duration of cylinder		
15. Closes cylinder valve and bleeds pressure from regulator		
16. Removes regulator from cylinder		
17. Stores cylinder properly		
18. Discusses hazards associated with cylinder		
19. Discusses hazards associated with regulator		

SIGNATURES   Student: Evaluator: Date:

Clinical Performance Evaluation

PERFORMANCE RATING:

5 **Independent:** Near flawless performance; minimal errors; able to perform without supervision; seeks out new learning; shows initiative; A = 4.7–5.0 average

4 **Minimally Supervised:** Few errors, able to self-correct; seeks guidance when appropriate; B = 3.7–4.65

3 **Competent:** Minimal required level; no critical errors; able to correct with coaching; meets expectations; safe; C = 3.0–3.65

2 **Marginal:** Below average; critical errors or problem areas noted; would benefit from remediation; D = 2.0–2.99

1 **Dependent:** Poor; unacceptable performance; unsafe; gross inaccuracies; potentially harmful; F = < 2.0

Circle the appropriate response below. Please be consistent, objective, and honest in your assessment of the student's clinical performance and ability.

PERFORMANCE CRITERIA	SCORE				
COGNITIVE DOMAIN					
1. Consistently displays knowledge, comprehension, and command of essential concepts	5	4	3	2	1
2. Demonstrates the relationship between theory and clinical practice	5	4	3	2	1
3. Able to select, review, apply, analyze, synthesize, interpret, and evaluate information; makes recommendations to modify care plan	5	4	3	2	1
PSYCHOMOTOR DOMAIN					
4. Minimal errors, no critical errors; able to self-correct; performs all steps safely and accurately	5	4	3	2	1
5. Selects, assembles, and verifies proper function and cleanliness of equipment; assures operation and corrects malfunctions; provides adequate care and maintenance	5	4	3	2	1
6. Exhibits the required manual dexterity	5	4	3	2	1
7. Performs procedure in a reasonable time frame for clinical level	5	4	3	2	1
8. Applies and maintains aseptic technique and PPE as required	5	4	3	2	1
9. Maintains concise and accurate patient and clinical records	5	4	3	2	1
10. Reports promptly on patient status/needs to appropriate personnel	5	4	3	2	1
AFFECTIVE DOMAIN					
11. Exhibits courteous and pleasant demeanor; shows consideration and respect, honesty, and integrity	5	4	3	2	1
12. Communicates verbally and in writing clearly and concisely	5	4	3	2	1
13. Preserves confidentiality and adheres to all policies	5	4	3	2	1
14. Follows directions, exhibits sound judgment, and seeks help when required	5	4	3	2	1
15. Demonstrates initiative, self-direction, responsibility, and accountability	5	4	3	2	1

TOTAL POINTS =   /15 = AVERAGE GRADE =

ADDITIONAL COMMENTS: IDENTIFY AREAS OF EXCELLENCE; LIST ERRORS OF OMISSION OR COMMISSION, CRITICAL ERRORS

SUMMARY PERFORMANCE EVALUATION AND RECOMMENDATIONS

☐ PASS: Satisfactory Performance

    ☐ Minimal supervision needed, may progress to next level provided specific skills, clinical time completed

    ☐ Minimal supervision needed, able to progress to next level without remediation

☐ FAIL: Unsatisfactory Performance (check all that apply)

    ☐ Minor reevaluation only

    ☐ Needs additional clinical practice before reevaluation

    ☐ Needs additional laboratory practice before skills performed in clinical area

    ☐ Recommend clinical probation

SIGNATURES

Evaluator (print name):   Evaluator signature: Date:

Student Signature: Date:

Student Comments:

Procedural Competency Evaluation

STUDENT: **DATE:**

OXYGEN BLENDER

				PERFORMANCE RATING	PERFORMANCE LEVEL
Evaluator: ☐ Peer ☐ Instructor	**Setting:** ☐ Lab ☐ Clinical Simulation				
Equipment Utilized:	**Conditions (Describe):**				

Performance Level:

    S or ✓ = Satisfactory, no errors of omission or commission
    U = Unsatisfactory Error of Omission or Commission
    NA = Not applicable

Performance Rating:

  5   **Independent:** Near flawless performance; minimal errors; able to perform without supervision; seeks out new learning; shows initiative; A = 4.7–5.0 average

  4   **Minimally Supervised:** Few errors, able to self-correct; seeks guidance when appropriate; B = 3.7–4.65

  3   **Competent:** Minimal required level; no critical errors; able to correct with coaching; meets expectations; safe; C = 3.0–3.65

  2   **Marginal:** Below average; critical errors or problem areas noted; would benefit from remediation; D = 2.0–2.99

  1   **Dependent:** Poor; unacceptable performance; unsafe; gross inaccuracies; potentially harmful; F = < 2.0

Two or more errors of commission or omission of mandatory or essential performance elements will terminate the procedure, and require additional practice and/or remediation and reevaluation. Student is responsible for obtaining additional evaluation forms as needed from the Director of Clinical Education (DCE).

EQUIPMENT AND PATIENT PREPARATION

1. Common Performance Elements Steps 1–8		
2. Selects appropriate blender and gas sources		
3. Attaches high-pressure hoses to appropriate gas source		
4. Adjusts blender to the appropriate F_IO_2		
5. Attaches the prescribed oxygen delivery device		
6. Analyzes the set F_IO_2 to assure blender accuracy		

FOLLOW-UP

7. Common Performance Elements Steps 11–16		

SIGNATURES   Student: Evaluator: Date:

Clinical Performance Evaluation

PERFORMANCE RATING:

5   **Independent:** Near flawless performance; minimal errors; able to perform without supervision; seeks out new learning; shows initiative; A = 4.7–5.0 average

4   **Minimally Supervised:** Few errors, able to self-correct; seeks guidance when appropriate; B = 3.7–4.65

3   **Competent:** Minimal required level; no critical errors; able to correct with coaching; meets expectations; safe; C = 3.0–3.65

2   **Marginal:** Below average; critical errors or problem areas noted; would benefit from remediation; D = 2.0–2.99

1   **Dependent:** Poor; unacceptable performance; unsafe; gross inaccuracies; potentially harmful; F = < 2.0

Circle the appropriate response below. Please be consistent, objective, and honest in your assessment of the student's clinical performance and ability.

PERFORMANCE CRITERIA	SCORE				
COGNITIVE DOMAIN					
1. Consistently displays knowledge, comprehension, and command of essential concepts	5	4	3	2	1
2. Demonstrates the relationship between theory and clinical practice	5	4	3	2	1
3. Able to select, review, apply, analyze, synthesize, interpret, and evaluate information; makes recommendations to modify care plan	5	4	3	2	1
PSYCHOMOTOR DOMAIN					
4. Minimal errors, no critical errors; able to self-correct; performs all steps safely and accurately	5	4	3	2	1
5. Selects, assembles, and verifies proper function and cleanliness of equipment; assures operation and corrects malfunctions; provides adequate care and maintenance	5	4	3	2	1
6. Exhibits the required manual dexterity	5	4	3	2	1
7. Performs procedure in a reasonable time frame for clinical level	5	4	3	2	1
8. Applies and maintains aseptic technique and PPE as required	5	4	3	2	1
9. Maintains concise and accurate patient and clinical records	5	4	3	2	1
10. Reports promptly on patient status/needs to appropriate personnel	5	4	3	2	1
AFFECTIVE DOMAIN					
11. Exhibits courteous and pleasant demeanor; shows consideration and respect, honesty, and integrity	5	4	3	2	1
12. Communicates verbally and in writing clearly and concisely	5	4	3	2	1
13. Preserves confidentiality and adheres to all policies	5	4	3	2	1
14. Follows directions, exhibits sound judgment, and seeks help when required	5	4	3	2	1
15. Demonstrates initiative, self-direction, responsibility, and accountability	5	4	3	2	1

TOTAL POINTS =   /15 = AVERAGE GRADE =

ADDITIONAL COMMENTS: IDENTIFY AREAS OF EXCELLENCE; LIST ERRORS OF OMISSION OR COMMISSION, CRITICAL ERRORS

SUMMARY PERFORMANCE EVALUATION AND RECOMMENDATIONS

☐ PASS: Satisfactory Performance

    ☐ Minimal supervision needed, may progress to next level provided specific skills, clinical time completed

    ☐ Minimal supervision needed, able to progress to next level without remediation

☐ FAIL: Unsatisfactory Performance (check all that apply)

    ☐ Minor reevaluation only

    ☐ Needs additional clinical practice before reevaluation

    ☐ Needs additional laboratory practice before skills performed in clinical area

    ☐ Recommend clinical probation

SIGNATURES

Evaluator (print name):   Evaluator signature: Date:

Student Signature: Date:

Student Comments:

10 Oxygen Analysis

INTRODUCTION

Determining the **accuracy** of the delivered F_IO_2 is an important part of oxygen administration. The only way to verify the concentration being delivered is by oxygen analysis. The concentration of oxygen can be measured by three different physical principles (**paramagnetic**, electromechanical, and electrochemical). The most commonly used type works by the electrochemical principle and that is the **galvanic** fuel cell analyzer.

OBJECTIVES

Upon completion of this chapter, the student will be able to:

1. Given a specific oxygen analyzer, identify its component parts.
2. Calibrate an oxygen analyzer on room air and 100% oxygen.
3. Given an oxygen delivery system, analyze the F_IO_2.
4. Describe the effects of moisture buildup and pressure on the measured F_IO_2.

KEY TERMS

accuracy
calibration
diffusion
efficacy

gain
galvanic
paramagnetic

permeability
polarographic
sensor

Exercises

EQUIPMENT REQUIRED

- [ ] Oxygen analyzers
- [ ] In-line adaptors
- [ ] Fuel cell cap
- [ ] Oxygen gas source—H or E cylinders
- [ ] Large wrench
- [ ] Cylinder stands
- [ ] Regulator with flowmeter
- [ ] Oxygen nipple adaptors
- [ ] Oxygen connection tubing

- [ ] Large-bore corrugated tubing
- [ ] Large-volume jet nebulizer
- [ ] Sterile water
- [ ] Plastic bag
- [ ] Small screwdriver
- [ ] Scissors
- [ ] Spare batteries (see manufacturer's specifications)

EXERCISE 10.1 IDENTIFICATION OF OXYGEN ANALYZERS

1. Examine the device and identify the component parts, as shown in Figure 10.1. Depending on the style of analyzer and its manufacturer, the component parts may vary. Refer to the individual operating manual for specifics.

    A. Analog scale or LED readout
    B. Calibration knob
    C. Sensor plug
    D. Sensor
    E. Batteries (not shown)
    F. Alarms (if applicable)
    G. In-line adaptor

2. Identify the brand and type of analyzer you are using. Identify the components. **Record the information on your laboratory report.**

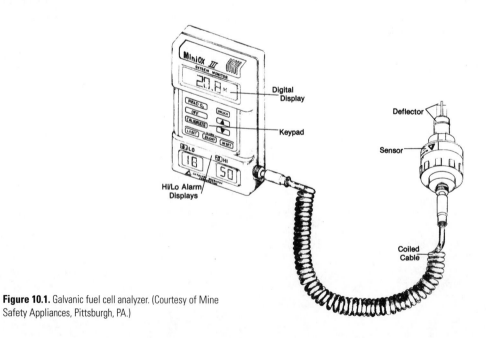

Figure 10.1. Galvanic fuel cell analyzer. (Courtesy of Mine Safety Appliances, Pittsburgh, PA.)

EXERCISE 10.2 CALIBRATION OF OXYGEN ANALYZERS

Regular calibration of oxygen analyzers is required to ensure the accuracy of measured F_iO_2. All oxygen delivery systems should be checked at least once daily. More frequent checks by calibrated analyzers may be necessary in specific types of systems. The AARC clinical practice guidelines (CPGs) should be utilized. The frequency of analysis, whether continuous or intermittent, determines how often calibration is needed.

1. Obtain the analyzer.
2. Set up the oxygen source by attaching a regulator with a Thorpe tube flowmeter to an H cylinder.
3. Attach an oxygen nipple adaptor to the DISS connection of the flowmeter outlet.
4. Secure the oxygen connecting tubing to the oxygen nipple adaptor.
5. Check that the analyzer is in good operating condition. Make sure that the analog scale/LED, sensor cable, and electrode or fuel cell are intact.
6. Prepare analyzer for use.
7. Attach the sensor cable to the analyzer. Some types of fuel cell analyzers may also have on/off switches for the alarms and LED readings.
8. With the sensor exposed to room air, adjust the calibration knob to read 21% oxygen.
9. Place the sensor inside a plastic bag, as shown in Figure 10.2. Place the oxygen connecting tubing inside the bag with the sensor. Turn on the flowmeter to 10 Lpm (flow needed may vary depending on the size of the bag used). Loosely hold the bag closed.
10. Allow the analyzer reading to stabilize. This may take 20 to 30 seconds depending on the type of analyzer. Excessively long stabilization time or failure to reach greater than 80% oxygen may indicate that the sensor must be replaced.
11. While the sensor is exposed to 100% oxygen, adjust the calibration knob (gain) to read 100%.
12. Shut off the oxygen. Remove the sensor from the bag. Relocate the analyzer to a different part of the room and recheck at 21% calibration. Adjust if necessary.
13. After the calibration procedure is performed, the analyzer is now ready for use.
14. Turn off the analyzer when not in use.

EXERCISE 10.3 OXYGEN ANALYSIS

For this exercise, assembly of the oxygen delivery system to be analyzed is required. See Figure 10.3 for the placement of the analyzer in line in a setup of a large-volume jet nebulizer.

1. Cut a single length of large-bore tubing (6 inches) from a roll, if it is not already available.
2. Place the analyzer sensor into an in-line adaptor. Make sure it fits tightly.
3. Attach a single length of large-bore tubing to one end of the in-line adaptor.
4. Fill the nebulizer with sterile water. Adjust the nebulizer to an F_iO_2 of 0.40. Turn the flowmeter on to 10 Lpm.
5. Attach the in-line adaptor with sensor at the end of the aerosol tubing as close to the delivery device (mask or T-piece) as possible.
6. Position the sensor so that moisture cannot collect on the surface of the membrane. The sensor should be facing down, as shown in Figure 10.4. Make sure the sensor and adaptor are secured tightly in the circuit.

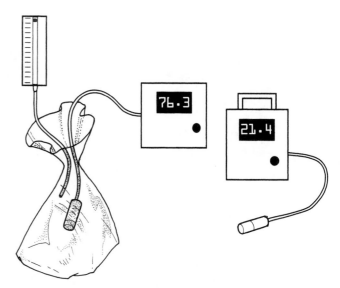

Figure 10.2. Calibration of an oxygen analyzer.

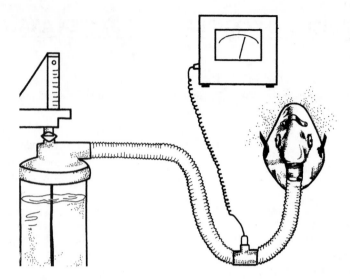

Figure 10.3. Oxygen analysis.

7. Allow the reading to stabilize. **Record the results on your laboratory report.**

8. If a disposable nebulizer is used, the F_IO_2 setting may not be accurate. If the reading on the analyzer does not match the set F_IO_2, adjust the nebulizer setting to the prescribed F_IO_2. Note any necessary adjustment. **Record the actual nebulizer setting on your laboratory report.**

9. Repeat the procedure for an F_IO_2 of 0.60. **Record the results on your laboratory report.**

10. Turn off the analyzer when not in use.

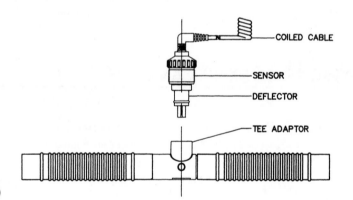

Figure 10.4. In-line placement of analyzer sensor. (Courtesy of Mine Safety Appliances, Pittsburgh, PA.)

Laboratory Report

CHAPTER 10: OXYGEN ANALYSIS

Name _____ Date _____

Course/Section _____ Instructor _____

Data Collection

EXERCISE 10.1 Identification of Oxygen Analyzer

Brand and type analyzer: _____

List component parts: _____

_____

_____

_____

_____

_____

EXERCISE 10.3 Oxygen Analysis

1. Analysis of 40% _____

  A. Initial reading: _____

  B. Adjusted nebulizer setting: _____

2. Analysis of 60% _____

  A. Initial reading: _____

  B. Adjusted nebulizer setting: _____

Critical Thinking Questions

1. Which type of analyzing method directly measures the concentration of oxygen?

   A. Which method directly measures partial pressure?

2. How would decreased barometric pressure or increased altitude affect the reading of an oxygen analyzer?

   A. Why?

3. How would moisture or condensation buildup on the sensor membrane affect the measured F_IO_2?

   A. What measures can be taken to prevent this?

4. How would positive pressure ventilation affect the measured F_IO_2?

5. Explain why routine oxygen analysis is important in:

   A. Monitoring a newborn on supplemental oxygen.

   B. Using an oxygen system that is comprised of compressed air and oxygen bleed-in.

   C. Monitoring a home care patient using an oxygen concentrator.

Procedural Competency Evaluation

STUDENT: **DATE:**

OXYGEN ANALYSIS

Evaluator: ☐ Peer ☐ Instructor **Setting:** ☐ Lab ☐ Clinical Simulation	**PERFORMANCE RATING**	**PERFORMANCE LEVEL**

Equipment Utilized: **Conditions (Describe):**

Performance Level:

    S or ✓ = Satisfactory, no errors of omission or commission
    U = Unsatisfactory Error of Omission or Commission
    NA = Not applicable

Performance Rating:

    5   **Independent:** Near flawless performance; minimal errors; able to perform without supervision; seeks out new learning; shows initiative; A = 4.7–5.0 average

    4   **Minimally Supervised:** Few errors, able to self-correct; seeks guidance when appropriate; B = 3.7–4.65

    3   **Competent:** Minimal required level; no critical errors; able to correct with coaching; meets expectations; safe; C = 3.0–3.65

    2   **Marginal:** Below average; critical errors or problem areas noted; would benefit from remediation; D = 2.0–2.99

    1   **Dependent:** Poor; unacceptable performance; unsafe; gross inaccuracies; potentially harmful; F = < 2.0

    Two or more errors of commission or omission of mandatory or essential performance elements will terminate the procedure, and require additional practice and/or remediation and reevaluation. Student is responsible for obtaining additional evaluation forms as needed from the Director of Clinical Education (DCE).

	Performance Rating	Performance Level
EQUIPMENT AND PATIENT PREPARATION		
1. Common Performance Elements Steps 1–8		
2. Identifies the type of oxygen analyzers: electrochemical, polarographic, and galvanic		
ASSESSMENT AND IMPLEMENTATION		
3. Common Performance Elements Steps 9 and 10		
4. Assembles oxygen delivery device to be analyzed		
5. Assembles additional oxygen flowmeter and attaches nipple adaptor		
6. Secures oxygen connecting tubing to the adaptor		
7. With the sensor exposed to room air, calibrates analyzer to room air and adjusts display if needed		
8. Places sensor in 100% oxygen source gas (in bag, loosely held closed) and calibrates analyzer; adjusts reading if needed		
9. Analyzes desired oxygen source; allows analyzer reading to stabilize		
10. Adjusts F_IO_2 if necessary		
FOLLOW-UP		
11. Adjusts high and low F_IO_2 alarms for continuous monitoring		
12. Caps sensor; unplugs analyzer when not in use		
13. Common Performance Elements Steps 11–16		

SIGNATURES   Student: Evaluator: Date:

Clinical Performance Evaluation

PERFORMANCE RATING:

5   **Independent:** Near flawless performance; minimal errors; able to perform without supervision; seeks out new learning; shows initiative; A = 4.7–5.0 average

4   **Minimally Supervised:** Few errors, able to self-correct; seeks guidance when appropriate; B = 3.7–4.65

3   **Competent:** Minimal required level; no critical errors; able to correct with coaching; meets expectations; safe; C = 3.0–3.65

2   **Marginal:** Below average; critical errors or problem areas noted; would benefit from remediation; D = 2.0–2.99

1   **Dependent:** Poor; unacceptable performance; unsafe; gross inaccuracies; potentially harmful; F = < 2.0

Circle the appropriate response below. Please be consistent, objective, and honest in your assessment of the student's clinical performance and ability.

PERFORMANCE CRITERIA | SCORE

PERFORMANCE CRITERIA					
COGNITIVE DOMAIN					
1. Consistently displays knowledge, comprehension, and command of essential concepts	5	4	3	2	1
2. Demonstrates the relationship between theory and clinical practice	5	4	3	2	1
3. Able to select, review, apply, analyze, synthesize, interpret, and evaluate information; makes recommendations to modify care plan	5	4	3	2	1
PSYCHOMOTOR DOMAIN					
4. Minimal errors, no critical errors; able to self-correct; performs all steps safely and accurately	5	4	3	2	1
5. Selects, assembles, and verifies proper function and cleanliness of equipment; assures operation and corrects malfunctions; provides adequate care and maintenance	5	4	3	2	1
6. Exhibits the required manual dexterity	5	4	3	2	1
7. Performs procedure in a reasonable time frame for clinical level	5	4	3	2	1
8. Applies and maintains aseptic technique and PPE as required	5	4	3	2	1
9. Maintains concise and accurate patient and clinical records	5	4	3	2	1
10. Reports promptly on patient status/needs to appropriate personnel	5	4	3	2	1
AFFECTIVE DOMAIN					
11. Exhibits courteous and pleasant demeanor; shows consideration and respect, honesty, and integrity	5	4	3	2	1
12. Communicates verbally and in writing clearly and concisely	5	4	3	2	1
13. Preserves confidentiality and adheres to all policies	5	4	3	2	1
14. Follows directions, exhibits sound judgment, and seeks help when required	5	4	3	2	1
15. Demonstrates initiative, self-direction, responsibility, and accountability	5	4	3	2	1

TOTAL POINTS =   /15 = AVERAGE GRADE =

ADDITIONAL COMMENTS: IDENTIFY AREAS OF EXCELLENCE; LIST ERRORS OF OMISSION OR COMMISSION, CRITICAL ERRORS

SUMMARY PERFORMANCE EVALUATION AND RECOMMENDATIONS

☐ PASS: Satisfactory Performance

    ☐ Minimal supervision needed, may progress to next level provided specific skills, clinical time completed

    ☐ Minimal supervision needed, able to progress to next level without remediation

☐ FAIL: Unsatisfactory Performance (check all that apply)

    ☐ Minor reevaluation only

    ☐ Needs additional clinical practice before reevaluation

    ☐ Needs additional laboratory practice before skills performed in clinical area

    ☐ Recommend clinical probation

SIGNATURES

Evaluator (print name):   Evaluator signature: Date:

Student Signature: Date:

Student Comments:

11 Oxygen Therapy Administration

INTRODUCTION

Oxygen is one of the most commonly administered respiratory drugs. Although administration of oxygen requires relatively simple skills, it is often misused or abused. There are a variety of devices that can be used to deliver oxygen. The respiratory care practitioner must have a complete knowledge and understanding of the uses and limitations of these devices, as well as the indications and hazards of oxygen therapy. The primary **goal** of oxygen therapy is to reduce **morbidity** and **mortality** associated with **hypoxia**. Proper administration, using the correct device and assessing the adequacy of the delivered F_IO_2, can have significant positive impact on patient outcomes. Recently designed high-flow cannula and mask devices have helped make F_IO_2 delivery more efficient without having to resort to more invasive methods.

OBJECTIVES

Upon completion of this chapter, the student will be able to:

1. Identify and assemble various oxygen delivery devices, such as the nasal cannula, high-flow nasal cannula, simple mask, partial rebreathing mask, nonrebreathing mask, high-flow nonrebreathing mask, and air entrainment (Venturi) masks.
2. Classify each oxygen delivery device as high-flow or low-flow.
3. Estimate the F_IO_2 for an oxygen delivery device, given the operating flow rate.
4. Given a patient scenario, select and administer the appropriate oxygen device.
5. Demonstrate effective communication skills needed for patient–practitioner interaction.
6. Calculate inspiratory flow demands and total flows delivered for a given F_IO_2, using air-to-oxygen mixing ratios.
7. Assess a patient for response to oxygen therapy.
8. Identify and correct common problems associated with oxygen delivery devices.

KEY TERMS

entrainment	hypoxia	jet	mortality
goal	indication	morbidity	Venturi

Exercises

EQUIPMENT REQUIRED

- Alcohol swabs
- Cylinder stands
- Gloves
- High-flow nasal cannula and humidifier system
- High-flow nonrebreathing mask
- In-line adaptor
- Nasal cannulas
- Nonrebreathing masks
- "No Smoking" signs
- One-way valves
- Oxygen analyzer
- Oxygen connection tubing
- Oxygen gas source: H, E cylinders with

- regulators or piped in wall
- Oxygen nipple adaptors
- Partial rebreathing masks
- Plastic bags
- Prefilled bubble humidifiers
- Pulse oximeter with probes
- Simple masks
- Sterile water
- Vane respirometer
- Venturi masks, various brands and styles
- Watch with a second hand
- Wrenches

Students should perform these exercises in groups of two. Students may carry out all the exercises with the same partner, or the instructor may want to change pairs to enhance the ability of each student to communicate and explain the procedure to a different person. Additionally, a human patient simulator may be used to demonstrate a realistic clinical response to oxygen therapy.

EXERCISE 11.1 OXYGEN DEVICE IDENTIFICATION

Examine each of the following devices, identify all component parts, and **record the corresponding letters *(if shown)* on your laboratory report.**

EXERCISE 11.1.1 NASAL CANNULA (FIG. 11.1)

- Nasal prongs
- Elastic strap or lariat ear tubes
- Oxygen connecting tube

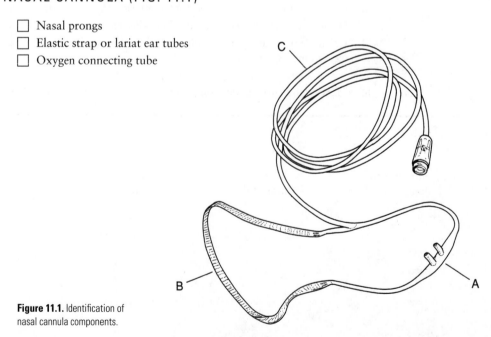

Figure 11.1. Identification of nasal cannula components.

EXERCISE 11.1.2 HIGH-FLOW NASAL CANNULA (FIG. 11.2)

☐ Wide-bore nasal prongs
☐ Elastic strap or lariat ear tubes
☐ Oxygen connecting tube
☐ Specialized nondisposable humidifier

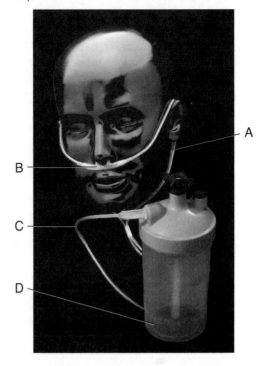

Figure 11.2. High flow nasal cannula. (Courtesy of Salter Labs, Arvin, CA.)

EXERCISE 11.1.3 SIMPLE MASK (FIG. 11.3)

☐ Transparent plastic mask
☐ Oxygen inlet
☐ Exhalation ports
☐ Malleable metal nosepiece

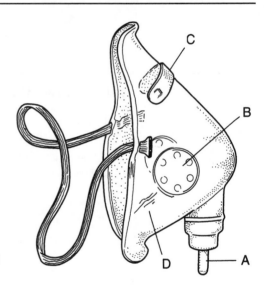

Figure 11.3. Identification of simple mask components.

EXERCISE 11.1.4 PARTIAL REBREATHING MASK (FIG. 11.4)

- ☐ Gas inlet
- ☐ Exhalation ports
- ☐ Reservoir bag
- ☐ Malleable metal nosepiece

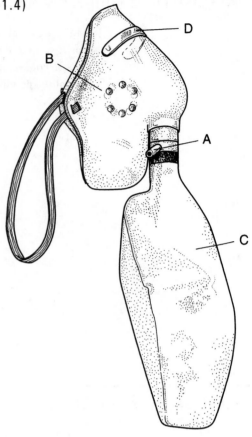

Figure 11.4. Identification of partial rebreathing mask components.

EXERCISE 11.1.5 NONREBREATHING MASK (FIG. 11.5)

- ☐ Gas inlet
- ☐ Nonrebreathing one-way valve
- ☐ Exhalation ports and valve
- ☐ Reservoir bag

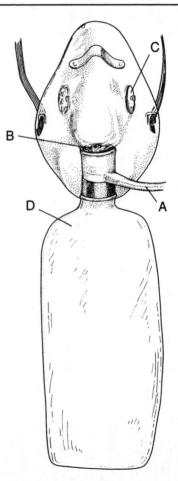

Figure 11.5. Identification of nonrebreathing mask components.

EXERCISE 11.1.6 HIGH-FLOW NONREBREATHING MASK

Obtain a high-flow nonrebreathing mask (if available), compare it to the nonrebreathing mask (Fig. 11.5), and **note and record the differences on your lab report.**

EXERCISE 11.1.7 AIR ENTRAINMENT (VENTURI) MASK (FIG. 11.6)

☐ Oxygen inlet
☐ Jet
☐ Air entrainment port
☐ Exhalation valve
☐ Venturi tube

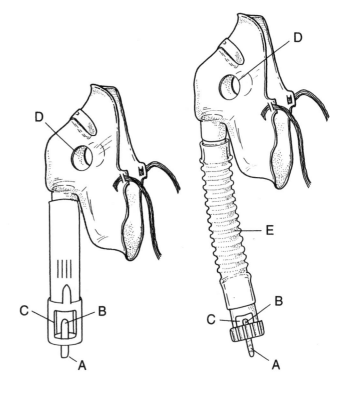

Figure 11.6. Identification of air entrainment mask components.

EXERCISE 11.2 OXYGEN THERAPY ADMINISTRATION

EXERCISE 11.2.1 NASAL CANNULA

Nasal cannulas deliver a varying F_IO_2. Refer to Table 11.1 for the approximate F_IO_2 that can be delivered using this oxygen administration method.

1. Verify "physician's" order or protocol.
2. Obtain the following equipment:
    Nasal cannula
    H cylinder or piped-in oxygen gas source
    Regulator and/or flowmeter
    Bubble humidifier
    Oxygen nipple adaptor
    "No Smoking" signs
3. Wash or sanitize your hands and apply PPE as appropriate.
4. With your laboratory partner acting as your patient, or using a human patient simulator, perform the following:

Table 11.1 Approximate F_IO_2 for Nasal Cannula (NC)

O_2 Flow	Approximate F_IO_2
1 Lpm	0.24
2 Lpm	0.28
3 Lpm	0.32
4 Lpm	0.36
5 Lpm	0.40
6 Lpm	0.44
High-flow NC at 15 Lpm	1.0

A. Introduce yourself, verify your "patient's identification," explain the procedure, and confirm "patient" understanding.

B. Assess your "patient" before beginning oxygen therapy by measuring pulse, respiratory rate, quality of respirations, color, and SpO_2. Interview the "patient" to determine whether dyspnea is present. **Record the results on your laboratory report.**

C. Explain safety considerations regarding smoking and electrical devices to your "patient." Verify "patient" understanding.

D. Post "No Smoking" signs.

5. Set up the equipment as shown in Figure 11.7:

A. Attach the regulator to the oxygen cylinder.

B. Attach the bubble humidifier to the DISS outlet of the flowmeter.

NOTE: A humidifier may not be necessary with flow rates less than 4 Lpm, but according to the AARC clinical practice guidelines it should be used with flow rates of 4 Lpm or higher. Policy may vary at your clinical sites.

C. While aseptically keeping the nasal cannula in its wrapper, attach the oxygen connecting tubing from the nasal cannula to the outlet of the humidifier.

D. Adjust the flowmeter to the prescribed level. **Record the liter flow on your laboratory report.**

E. Pinch the oxygen connecting tubing to obstruct flow to verify function of the humidifier. If the humidifier fails to make a whistling sound, check all connections for leaks.

F. Place the cannula in the "patient's" nose and adjust the straps for fit. For lariat-style cannula, place the ear loops behind the "patient's" ears and adjust the fit. Verify "patient" comfort.

G. Reassess the "patient" after 5 minutes.

6. Repeat the exercise with a high-flow nasal cannula and special nondisposable humidifier.

A. **Record pulse, respiratory rate, and SpO_2 before and after application of the device.**

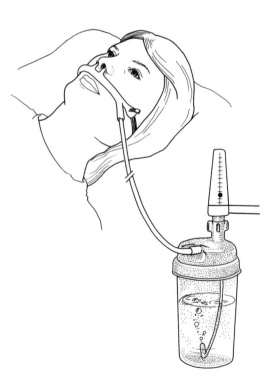

Figure 11.7. Nasal cannula equipment assembly.

EXERCISE 11.2.2 SIMPLE MASK

Simple oxygen masks also deliver a varying F_IO_2. Refer to Table 11.2 for the approximate F_IO_2 that can be delivered using the simple mask as well as by partial rebreathing and nonrebreathing masks.

Table 11.2 Approximate F_IO_2 for Oxygen Mask Devices

MASK	LITER FLOW	APPROXIMATE F_IO_2
Simple	6–10 Lpm	35–50%
Partial rebreathing	Enough to keep bag inflated (8–12 Lpm)	Up to 70%
Nonrebreathing	Enough to keep bag inflated (8–12 Lpm)	Up to 100%

1. Verify "physician's" order or protocol.
2. Obtain the following equipment:
   Simple mask
   H cylinder or piped-in oxygen gas source
   Regulator or flowmeter
   Bubble humidifier
   Oxygen nipple adaptor
   "No Smoking" signs
3. Wash or sanitize your hands and apply PPE as appropriate.
4. With your laboratory partner acting as your patient, perform the following:
   A. Introduce yourself, verify your "patient's" identification, explain the procedure, and verify "patient" understanding.
   B. Assess your "patient" before beginning oxygen therapy by measuring pulse, respiratory rate, quality of respirations, color, and SpO_2. Interview the "patient" to determine whether dyspnea is present.
5. Set up the equipment as shown in Figure 11.8:
   A. Attach the regulator to the oxygen cylinder.
   B. Attach the bubble humidifier to the DISS outlet of the flowmeter.
   C. While aseptically keeping the simple mask in its wrapper, attach the oxygen connecting tubing from the mask to the outlet of the humidifier. Attach the other end to the mask oxygen inlet connector.
   D. Adjust the flowmeter to the prescribed level.
   NOTE: All masks should be used with a minimum flow rate of 5 Lpm.[1]
   E. Pinch the oxygen connecting tubing to obstruct flow to verify function of the humidifier. If the humidifier fails to make a whistling sound, check all connections for leaks.
   F. Place the mask over the "patient's" nose and mouth. Adjust the straps and nose bridge for fit. Verify "patient" comfort.
   G. Reassess the "patient" after 5 minutes.

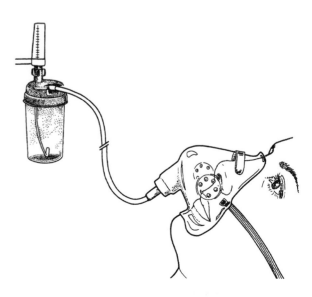

Figure 11.8. Simple mask equipment assembly.

EXERCISE 11.2.3 PARTIAL REBREATHING OR NONREBREATHING MASK

Refer to Table 11.2 for the approximate F_iO_2 delivered by partial rebreathing and nonrebreathing masks.

1. Verify "physician's" order or protocol.
2. Obtain the following equipment:
   Partial rebreathing or nonrebreathing mask
   H cylinder or piped-in oxygen gas source
   Regulator or flowmeter
   Bubble humidifier
   Oxygen nipple adaptor
   "No Smoking" signs
3. Wash or sanitize your hands and apply PPE.
4. With your laboratory partner acting as your patient, or using a human patient simulator, perform the following:
   A. Introduce yourself, verify your "patient's" identification, explain the procedure, and verify "patient" understanding.
   B. Assess your "patient" before beginning oxygen therapy by measuring pulse, respiratory rate, quality of respirations, and color. A pulse oximeter should also be used. Interview the "patient" to determine whether dyspnea is present.
5. Set up the equipment as shown in Figure 11.9:
   A. Attach the regulator to the oxygen cylinder.
   B. Attach the bubble humidifier to the DISS outlet of the flowmeter.
   C. While aseptically keeping the mask in its wrapper, attach the oxygen connecting tubing from the mask to the outlet of the humidifier. Attach the other end to the mask oxygen inlet connector.
   D. Adjust the flowmeter to between 8 and 12 Lpm.
   E. Pinch the oxygen connecting tubing to obstruct flow to verify function of the humidifier. If the humidifier fails to make a whistling sound, check all connections for leaks.
   F. Place the mask over the "patient's" nose and mouth. Adjust the straps and nose bridge for fit. Verify "patient" comfort.
   G. Readjust flow to ensure that the bag remains inflated during peak inspiration. **Record the liter flow on your laboratory report.**
   H. Reassess the "patient" after 5 minutes.
6. Repeat the exercise with a high-flow nonrebreathing mask.

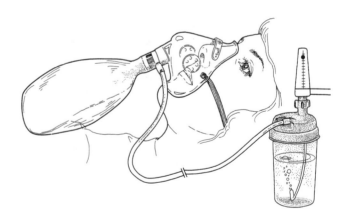

Figure 11.9. Partial or nonrebreathing mask equipment assembly.

EXERCISE 11.3 AIR ENTRAINMENT (VENTURI) MASK

The F_IO_2 delivered by these devices depends on the air entrainment ratios shown in Table 11.3.

Table 11.3 Air:Oxygen Entrainment Mixing Ratios

Air:Oxygen Ratio	F_IO_2
25:1	24%
10:1	28%
8:1	30%
7:1	32%
5:1	35%
3:1	40%
2:1	45%
1.7:1	50%
1:1	60%
0.6:1	70%

EXERCISE 11.3.1 ADMINISTRATION OF OXYGEN VIA AIR ENTRAINMENT DEVICE

1. Verify "physician's" order or protocol.
2. Obtain the following equipment:
   Air entrainment (Venturi) mask, jet, or entrainment port adaptors
   H cylinder or piped-in oxygen gas source
   Regulator or flowmeter
   Oxygen nipple adaptor
   "No Smoking" signs
3. Wash or sanitize your hands and apply PPE as appropriate.
4. With your laboratory partner acting as your patient, perform the following:
   A. Introduce yourself, verify your "patient's" identification, explain the procedure, and verify "patient" understanding.
   B. Assess your "patient" before beginning oxygen therapy by measuring pulse, respiratory rate, quality of respirations, and color. A pulse oximeter may be used. Interview the "patient" to determine whether dyspnea is present.
5. Set up the equipment as shown in Figure 11.10
   A. Attach the regulator to the oxygen cylinder.
   B. Attach the oxygen nipple to the DISS outlet of the flowmeter.
   NOTE: A bubble humidifier should not be used with this device.
   C. While aseptically keeping the mask in its wrapper, attach the oxygen connecting tubing from the mask to the oxygen nipple. Attach the other end to the mask oxygen inlet connector.
   D. Adjust the flowmeter to the recommended liter flow for the F_IO_2 being used.
   E. Place the mask over the "patient's" nose and mouth. Adjust the straps and nose bridge for fit. Verify "patient" comfort.
   F. Reassess the "patient" after 5 minutes.

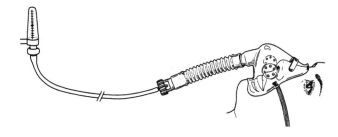

Figure 11.10. Air entrainment mask equipment assembly.

EXERCISE 11.3.2 ACCURACY OF F_IO_2 WITH AIR ENTRAINMENT DEVICES

1. Set the Venturi device on 40% and adjust the oxygen flow to the manufacturer's recommended setting. **Record the manufacturer brand of mask used on your laboratory report.**

2. Calibrate and set up an oxygen analyzer.

3. While the oxygen is on, remove the mask from the Venturi device. Attach an oxygen sensor to an in-line adaptor and connect the Venturi device to the adaptor. A single length of large-bore corrugated tubing may be required to make this connection.

4. Measure the F_IO_2, allowing time for the reading to stabilize. **Record the liter flow used and the F_IO_2 measured on your laboratory report.**

5. Decrease the oxygen flow rate to any liter flow of your choice below the manufacturer's recommended setting. Measure the F_IO_2, allowing time for the reading to stabilize. **Record the results on your laboratory report.**

6. Increase the oxygen flow rate to any liter flow of your choice above the manufacturer's recommended setting. Measure the F_IO_2, allowing time for the reading to stabilize. **Record the results on your laboratory report.**

7. Adjust the Venturi device to another F_IO_2 of your choice.

8. Repeat steps 4, 5, and 6 for this new F_IO_2. **Record the results on your laboratory report.**

9. Place the Venturi device in a plastic bag. Insert an oxygen analyzer sensor into the bag. Measure the F_IO_2 and **record the results on your laboratory report.**

10. Place the Venturi mask on a mannequin or human patient simulator. Cover the air entrainments ports with a sheet or blanket pulled up to the "patient's" chin. Analyze the F_IO_2 by placing a oxygen sensor with in-line adapter between the mask and Venturi device. **Record the F_IO_2 on your laboratory report.**

EXERCISE 11.3.3 ADEQUACY OF FLOW RATES FROM AN AIR ENTRAINMENT DEVICE

1. Measure your laboratory partner's minute ventilation. **Record the results on your laboratory report.**

2. Calculate your partner's estimated inspiratory flow demand. **Record the results on your laboratory report.**

   NOTE: The inspiratory flow demands can be estimated as three times the minute ventilation (V_E).

3. With the Venturi device set at 40%, calculate the total flow being delivered from the mask using the following formula:

   Total flow = (Sum of air:oxygen entrainment ratios) × Flow rate

4. Based on your calculations, adjust the flow rate to meet your laboratory partner's inspiratory flow demand. **Record this flow on your laboratory report.**

EXERCISE 11.4 TROUBLESHOOTING

EXERCISE 11.4.1 TROUBLESHOOTING COMMON PROBLEMS

1. The instructor or your laboratory partner will set up one of the following suggested problems related to oxygen delivery devices. The student will inspect the equipment, identify the problem, and correct it.

   A. Incorrect equipment setup

   B. Incorrect liter flow used for device

   C. Loose humidifier cap

   D. Kinked oxygen connecting tubing

   E. Tubing disconnection

2. **Record the problem and corrective action on your laboratory report.**

EXERCISE 11.4.2 TROUBLESHOOTING DIAGRAMS

Figures 11.11 and 11.12 illustrate one or more problems with the setup of the oxygen delivery systems. Identify the problem(s) and the corrective action to be taken. **Record these on your laboratory report.**

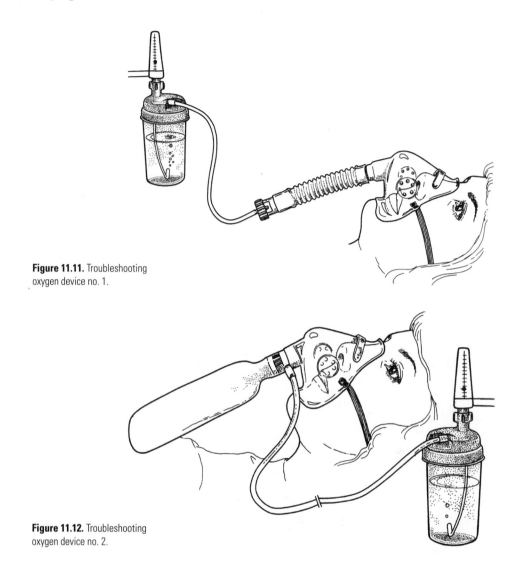

Figure 11.11. Troubleshooting oxygen device no. 1.

Figure 11.12. Troubleshooting oxygen device no. 2.

REFERENCES
1. Wilkins, R: Egan's Fundamentals of Respiratory Care, ed 8. Mosby, St. Louis, 2003.

Laboratory Report

CHAPTER 11: OXYGEN THERAPY ADMINISTRATION

Name _____ Date _____

Course/Section _____ Instructor _____

Data Collection

EXERCISE 11.1 Oxygen Device Identification

EXERCISE 11.1.1 NASAL CANNULA

A._____

B._____

C._____

EXERCISE 11.1.2 HIGH-FLOW NASAL CANNULA

A._____

B._____

C._____

D. _____

EXERCISE 11.1.3 SIMPLE MASK

A._____

B._____

C._____

D. _____

EXERCISE 11.1.4 PARTIAL REBREATHING MASK

A._____

B._____

C._____

D. _____

EXERCISE 11.1.5 NONREBREATHING MASK

A._____

B. _____

C._____

D. _____

EXERCISE 11.1.6 HIGH-FLOW NONREBREATHING MASK

Observations: _____

_____

EXERCISE 11.1.7 AIR ENTRAINMENT (VENTURI) MASK

A._____

B. _____

C._____

D. _____

E. _____

EXERCISE 11.2 Oxygen Therapy Administration

EXERCISE 11.2.1 NASAL CANNULA

Nasal Cannula	
Before Oxygen Administration	**After Oxygen Administration**
Pulse:	
Respiratory rate (f):	
SpO_2:	
Prescribed liter flow:	
Estimated F_IO_2:	
High-Flow Nasal Cannula	
Before Oxygen Administration	**After Oxygen Administration**
Pulse:	
Respiratory rate (f):	
SpO_2:	
Prescribed liter flow:	
Estimated F_IO_2:	

EXERCISE 11.2.2 SIMPLE MASK

Before Oxygen Administration	After Oxygen Administration
Pulse:	
Respiratory rate (*f*):	
SpO$_2$:	
Prescribed liter flow:	
Estimated F$_I$O$_2$:	

EXERCISE 11.2.3 PARTIAL REBREATHING AND NONREBREATHING MASKS

Partial Rebreather	
Before Oxygen Administration	**After Oxygen Administration**
Pulse:	
Respiratory rate (*f*):	
SpO$_2$:	
Prescribed liter flow:	
Estimated F$_I$O$_2$:	
Nonrebreather	
Before Oxygen Administration	**After Oxygen Administration**
Pulse:	
Respiratory rate (*f*):	
SpO$_2$:	
Prescribed liter flow:	
Estimated F$_I$O$_2$:	
High-Flow Nonrebreather	
Before Oxygen Administration	**After Oxygen Administration**
Pulse:	
Respiratory rate (*f*):	
SpO$_2$:	
Prescribed liter flow:	
Estimated F$_I$O$_2$:	

EXERCISE 11.3 Air Entrainment (Venturi) Mask

EXERCISE 11.3.2 ACCURACY OF F$_I$O$_2$ WITH AIR ENTRAINMENT DEVICES

F$_I$O$_2$ set: 40%	Manufacturer and brand:	Recommended liter flow:
Measured F$_I$O$_2$:		
Decreased liter flow to:		Measured F$_I$O$_2$:
Increased liter flow to:		Measured F$_I$O$_2$:
F$_I$O$_2$ set:	Manufacturer and brand:	Recommended liter flow:
Measured F$_I$O$_2$:		
Decreased liter flow to:		Measured F$_I$O$_2$:
Increased liter flow to:		Measured F$_I$O$_2$:
Measured F$_I$O$_2$ of Venturi device in bag:		
Explain why this result was obtained:		
Measured F$_I$O$_2$ of Venturi device covered with sheet:		
Explain why this result was obtained:		

EXERCISE 11.3.3. ADEQUACY OF FLOW RATES FROM AN AIR ENTRAINMENT DEVICE

Measured minute ventilation (V_E): _____

Estimated inspiratory flow demand: _____

Total flow delivered at 40%: _____

What adjustment to the liter flow, if any, would you have to make to meet your partner's flow demand? _____

_____

EXERCISE 11.4 Troubleshooting

EXERCISE 11.4.1 TROUBLESHOOTING COMMON PROBLEMS

EQUIPMENT USED: _____

Problem identified: _____

Corrective action: _____

EQUIPMENT USED: _____

Problem identified: _____

Corrective action: _____

EXERCISE 11.4.2 TROUBLESHOOTING DIAGRAMS

Identify problem—Figure 11.11: _____

Corrective action: _____

Identify problem—Figure 11.12: _____

Corrective action: _____

Critical Thinking Questions

Mrs. Plaskowitz is a 60-year-old woman with COPD who is admitted to the ER via ambulance wearing a nonrebreathing mask at 10 Lpm. Mrs. Plaskowitz, who was awake and alert when the ambulance arrived at her home, is now extremely lethargic and somnolent. The ER physician orders you change the oxygen delivery device to a nasal cannula.

1.   Briefly explain the cause of the patient's lethargy.

2.   If the patient were to remain on the nonrebreathing mask for at least 24 hours, what complications or hazards could result from (a) the delivery method, and (b) the resulting oxygen concentration?

3.   What liter flow would you recommend to the physician for the nasal cannula?

4.   The pulmonary physician, who has been called in on this case, requests that you change the delivery device to a Venturi mask at a comparable F_IO_2.

   A.   What F_IO_2 should be used?

   B.   The patient is noted to have a minute ventilation of 15 Lpm. What is the minimum liter flow, at this F_IO_2, required to meet the patient's inspiratory flow demand? **Show your work!**

5.   Why is a minimum flow rate of 5 Lpm recommended for oxygen delivery by mask?

6.   Explain the difference between a high-flow and a low-flow oxygen delivery system. Give an example of each.

7.   You observe a patient wearing a nonrebreathing mask and note that the bag completely deflates with each inspiration. What actions, if any, should be taken?

8.   What oxygen delivery device would you recommend for a patient who has just been successfully resuscitated and is spontaneously breathing?

9.   List at least three factors that will affect the F_IO_2 delivered by a low-flow oxygen system.

10. Complete the following table by calculating or providing the missing parameters. **Show your work!**

F_IO_2	O_2 Flow Rate	Entrainment Ratio	Total Flow
	14 Lpm		24 Lpm
0.28	8 Lpm		
0.40			40 Lpm
		5:1	36 Lpm
	3 Lpm	7:1	
0.45	5 Lpm		
0.50	14 Lpm		
0.32	5 Lpm		

Procedural Competency Evaluation

STUDENT: **DATE:**

OXYGEN THERAPY

Evaluator: ☐ Peer ☐ Instructor	**Setting:** ☐ Lab ☐ Clinical Simulation
Equipment Utilized:	**Conditions (Describe):**

Performance Level:

    S or ✓ = Satisfactory, no errors of omission or commission
    U = Unsatisfactory Error of Omission or Commission
    NA = Not applicable

Performance Rating:

5   **Independent:** Near flawless performance; minimal errors; able to perform without supervision; seeks out new learning; shows initiative; A = 4.7–5.0 average

4   **Minimally Supervised:** Few errors, able to self-correct; seeks guidance when appropriate; B = 3.7–4.65

3   **Competent:** Minimal required level; no critical errors; able to correct with coaching; meets expectations; safe; C = 3.0–3.65

2   **Marginal:** Below average; critical errors or problem areas noted; would benefit from remediation; D = 2.0–2.99

1   **Dependent:** Poor; unacceptable performance; unsafe; gross inaccuracies; potentially harmful; F = < 2.0

Two or more errors of commission or omission of mandatory or essential performance elements will terminate the procedure, and require additional practice and/or remediation and reevaluation. Student is responsible for obtaining additional evaluation forms as needed from the Director of Clinical Education (DCE).

	PERFORMANCE RATING	PERFORMANCE LEVEL
EQUIPMENT AND PATIENT PREPARATION		
1. Common Performance Elements Steps 1 and 8		
2. Educates patient on oxygen safety		
ASSESSMENT AND IMPLEMENTATION		
3. Common Performance Elements Steps 9–10		
4. Assesses vital signs, respirations, and SpO$_2$		
5. Attaches oxygen delivery device to nipple adaptor or humidifier if flow rate ≥4 Lpm		
6. Adjusts the flowmeter to prescribed or appropriate liter flow		
7. Verifies oxygen flow or concentration		
8. Places the administration device properly and comfortably on the patient's face		
9. Confirms fit and verifies patient comfort		
10. Assesses adequacy of the therapy		
11. Makes any necessary flow rate adjustments		
FOLLOW-UP		
12. Common Performance Elements Steps 11–16		

SIGNATURES   Student: Evaluator: Date:

Clinical Performance Evaluation

PERFORMANCE RATING:

5   **Independent:** Near flawless performance; minimal errors; able to perform without supervision; seeks out new learning; shows initiative; A = 4.7–5.0 average

4   **Minimally Supervised:** Few errors, able to self-correct; seeks guidance when appropriate; B = 3.7–4.65

3   **Competent:** Minimal required level; no critical errors; able to correct with coaching; meets expectations; safe; C = 3.0–3.65

2   **Marginal:** Below average; critical errors or problem areas noted; would benefit from remediation; D = 2.0–2.99

1   **Dependent:** Poor; unacceptable performance; unsafe; gross inaccuracies; potentially harmful; F = < 2.0

Circle the appropriate response below. Please be consistent, objective, and honest in your assessment of the student's clinical performance and ability.

PERFORMANCE CRITERIA	SCORE				
COGNITIVE DOMAIN					
1. Consistently displays knowledge, comprehension, and command of essential concepts	5	4	3	2	1
2. Demonstrates the relationship between theory and clinical practice	5	4	3	2	1
3. Able to select, review, apply, analyze, synthesize, interpret, and evaluate information; makes recommendations to modify care plan	5	4	3	2	1
PSYCHOMOTOR DOMAIN					
4. Minimal errors, no critical errors; able to self-correct; performs all steps safely and accurately	5	4	3	2	1
5. Selects, assembles, and verifies proper function and cleanliness of equipment; assures operation and corrects malfunctions; provides adequate care and maintenance	5	4	3	2	1
6. Exhibits the required manual dexterity	5	4	3	2	1
7. Performs procedure in a reasonable time frame for clinical level	5	4	3	2	1
8. Applies and maintains aseptic technique and PPE as required	5	4	3	2	1
9. Maintains concise and accurate patient and clinical records	5	4	3	2	1
10. Reports promptly on patient status/needs to appropriate personnel	5	4	3	2	1
AFFECTIVE DOMAIN					
11. Exhibits courteous and pleasant demeanor; shows consideration and respect, honesty, and integrity	5	4	3	2	1
12. Communicates verbally and in writing clearly and concisely	5	4	3	2	1
13. Preserves confidentiality and adheres to all policies	5	4	3	2	1
14. Follows directions, exhibits sound judgment, and seeks help when required	5	4	3	2	1
15. Demonstrates initiative, self-direction, responsibility, and accountability	5	4	3	2	1

TOTAL POINTS =   /15 = AVERAGE GRADE =

ADDITIONAL COMMENTS: IDENTIFY AREAS OF EXCELLENCE; LIST ERRORS OF OMISSION OR COMMISSION, CRITICAL ERRORS

SUMMARY PERFORMANCE EVALUATION AND RECOMMENDATIONS

☐ PASS: Satisfactory Performance

    ☐ Minimal supervision needed, may progress to next level provided specific skills, clinical time completed

    ☐ Minimal supervision needed, able to progress to next level without remediation

☐ FAIL: Unsatisfactory Performance (check all that apply)

    ☐ Minor reevaluation only

    ☐ Needs additional clinical practice before reevaluation

    ☐ Needs additional laboratory practice before skills performed in clinical area

    ☐ Recommend clinical probation

SIGNATURES

Evaluator (print name):   Evaluator signature: Date:

Student Signature: Date:

Student Comments:

12 Humidity Devices

INTRODUCTION

The major functions of the upper airway are to warm, filter, and humidify the air that is breathed. Many conditions, such as the presence of an artificial airway, **dehydration**, fever, and the breathing of **anhydrous** gases, alter the efficiency of the upper airway in performing these functions. The respiratory care practitioner, in these circumstances, may deliver adjunctive humidity therapy to patients to minimize mucosal drying and irritation and to prevent secretions from becoming **inspissated**. The safe operation and use of these devices requires an understanding of their capabilities and as well as their limitations.

OBJECTIVES

Upon completion of this chapter, the student will be able to:

1. Identify the components of the heat and moisture exchanger (HME) and bubble and wick humidifiers.
2. Differentiate between the types of humidifiers, including their clinical uses, advantages, and disadvantages.
3. Assemble and operate the various types of humidifiers.
4. Perform monitoring, maintenance, and troubleshooting techniques.
5. Relate, according to AARC clinical practice guidelines, the proper amount of humidification for patients with artificial airways.

KEY TERMS

adhesion
ambient
anhydrous
anion
calorie
cation
cold stress
colloid
condensate
crystalloid

dehydration
density
desiccation
epithelium
evaporation
facilitate
hydration
hygrometer
hygroscopic
hypertonic

hypotonic
inspissated
isotonic
neutral thermal environment
osmosis
relative humidity
solute
solution
solvent

Exercises

EQUIPMENT REQUIRED

- [ ] Beaker or graduated cylinder
- [ ] Bubble humidifier
- [ ] Clean towels
- [ ] Compressed gas source
- [ ] Continuous fill system
- [ ] Corrugated tubing
- [ ] Heat and moisture exchangers, various types and brands

- [ ] Lung simulator (optional)
- [ ] Manual resuscitator with mask
- [ ] Regulator with flowmeter
- [ ] Scissors
- [ ] Sterile water bags or bottles
- [ ] Temperature probe with adaptor
- [ ] Wick humidifier

EXERCISE 12.1 BUBBLE HUMIDIFIER

EXERCISE 12.1.1 IDENTIFICATION OF COMPONENTS

Identify the components of a bubble humidifier, as shown in Figure 12.1, and **record the following on your laboratory report:**

DISS connection
Outlet
Capillary inlet tube
Pop-off valve
Bubble diffuser

EXERCISE 12.1.2 SETUP OF A BUBBLE HUMIDIFIER

1. If a dry humidifier (not prefilled) is used, fill the humidifier to the fill line with sterile water.
2. Connect the bubble humidifier to the DISS outlet of a flowmeter.
3. Adjust the flow rate to 5 Lpm.
4. **Record your observations on your laboratory report.**
5. Shut the flowmeter off.
6. Remove the plastic protector from the outlet of the humidifier.
7. Readjust the flowmeter to 5 Lpm.
8. Obstruct the outlet of the humidifier.
9. **Record your observations on your laboratory report.**
10. Loosen the cap from the bottle.
11. **Record your observations on your laboratory report.**

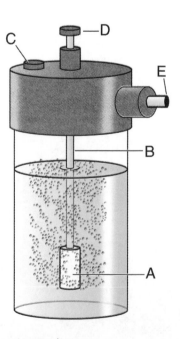

Figure 12.1. Identification of bubble humidifier components.

12. Tighten the cap. Attach a small-bore oxygen connecting tube to the humidifier outlet.

13. Kink the tubing by bending it in half.

14. **Record your observations on your laboratory report.**

15. Turn the flowmeter to flush.

16. **Record your observations on your laboratory report.**

EXERCISE 12.2 HEAT AND MOISTURE EXCHANGER (HME)

Examine a heat and moisture exchanger. Compare HMEs from several manufacturers, as shown in Figure 12.2. Perform the following:

1. Read the manufacturer's insert. **Record the brand used, expected H$_2$O content, and resistance specifications on your laboratory report.**

2. Ventilate through the HME with a handheld resuscitator. Alternatively, connect the HME to a lung simulator and attempt to bag through the HME. **Record your observations on your laboratory report.**

3. Fill the HME with water. Let it stand for 5 minutes, then drain the excess water.

4. Ventilate through the HME with a handheld resuscitator. Alternatively, connect the HME to a lung simulator and attempt to bag through the HME.

5. **Record your observations on your laboratory report.**

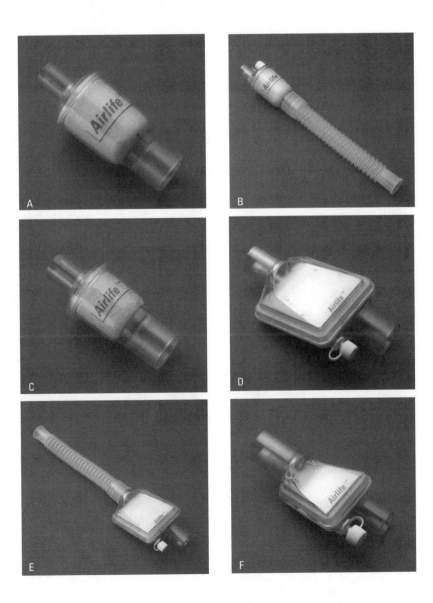

Figure 12.2. Heat and moisture exchangers.
(Courtesy of Cardinal Health, Dublin, OH.)

EXERCISE 12.3 WICK HUMIDIFIER

EXERCISE 12.3.1 COMPONENTS OF A WICK HUMIDIFIER

Identify the components of a wick humidifier (such as ConchaTherm® or Fisher & Paykel), as shown in Figure 12.3, and **record them on your laboratory report.**

Inlet

Outlet

Heating element

Wick element

On/off switch

Temperature probe

EXERCISE 12.3.2 ASSEMBLY OF A WICK HUMIDIFIER AND CONTINUOUS FEED SYSTEM

For this exercise, a compressor or high-flow gas generator may be used.

1. **Note the temperature in the room prior to the start of the exercise.**
2. Connect 12 6-inch lengths of corrugated tubing, cut in half with a T-drainage bag at the most dependent loop, to the outlet of the humidifier.
3. Connect the flowmeter to a compressed gas source (air or oxygen). Attach an adaptor that will connect the small-bore outlet of the flowmeter to large-bore corrugated tubing.
4. Attach three to six lengths of corrugated tubing from the flowmeter adaptor to the inlet of the humidifier.
5. Assemble the unit with a continuous feed system, as shown in Figure 12.4, and attach the water bag or bottle.
6. Open the clamp to the feed system, if applicable, and allow it to fill the humidifier to the fill line. If a continuous feed is not available, aseptically fill the humidifier with sterile water.
7. Ensure that the heating unit is plugged in.
8. Attach a temperature probe at the end of the tubing, using a monitoring adaptor.
9. Turn the flow to 15 Lpm and adjust the temperature setting to 37°C.
10. Place your hand by the end of the corrugated tubing and **record your observations on your laboratory report.**
11. Time how long it takes for the unit to reach 37°C.

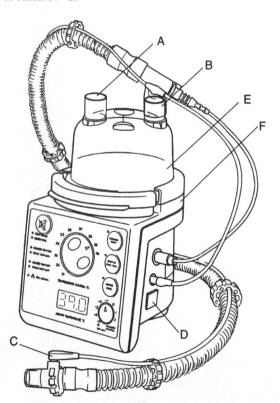

Figure 12.3. Components of a wick humidifier. (Courtesy of Fisher & Paykel Healthcare, Aukland, New Zealand.)

12. Once it has reached 37°C, wait another 15 minutes. Note the water level in the humidifier; drain the condensate away from the unit and measure.

13. Record the original room temperature, the time to reach set temperature, the highest temperature reached, the amount of condensate measured, and the ending water level on your laboratory report.

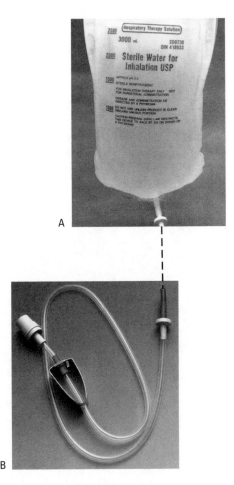

Figure 12.4. Setup of a continuous feed system. (Courtesy of Cardinal Health, Dublin, OH.)

Laboratory Report

CHAPTER 12: HUMIDITY DEVICES

Name _____ Date _____

Course/Section _____ Instructor _____

Data Collection

EXERCISE 12.1 Bubble Humidifier

EXERCISE 12.1.1 IDENTIFICATION OF COMPONENTS

A. _____

B. _____

C. _____

D. _____

E. _____

EXERCISE 12.1.2 SETUP OF A BUBBLE HUMIDIFIER

OBSERVATIONS

Plastic protector on, flow rate to 5 Lpm: _____

_____

Obstruct the outlet of the humidifier, flow rate to 5 Lpm: _____

_____

Loosen the cap from the bottle: _____

_____

Kinked tubing: _____

_____

Flowmeter to flush: _____

_____

EXERCISE 12.2 Heat and Moisture Exchanger (HME)

Brand used: _____

Expected H$_2$O content: _____

Resistance specifications: _____

_____

Ventilate through dry HME: _____

Resistance recorded on simulator: _____

HME wet: _____

Resistance recorded on simulator: _____

EXERCISE 12.3 Wick Humidifier

EXERCISE 12.3.1 COMPONENTS OF A WICK HUMIDIFIER

Brand used: _____

Components identified:

A. _____

B. _____

C. _____

D. _____

E. _____

F. _____

EXERCISE 12.3.2 ASSEMBLY OF A WICK HUMIDIFIER AND CONTINUOUS FEED SYSTEM

WICK HUMIDIFIER

Temperature: _____

Amount of condensate: _____

Observations: _____

_____

_____

_____

_____

_____

CONTINUOUS FEED

Temperature: _____

Amount of condensate: _____

Observations: _____

_____

_____

_____

_____

_____

Critical Thinking Questions

1. What are the limitations of a heat and moisture exchanger? What are the advantages? What effect does moisture have on HME function?

2. Which humidifiers are the most efficient? What effect does temperature have on the efficiency of the unit? According to AARC clinical practice guidelines, what is the minimum water vapor content (mg/L) that must be provided to patients with artificial airways?

3. What are the advantages and disadvantage of using a continuous feed system to fill a humidifier?

4. Define *humidity*. What is the purpose of using humidifiers in the clinical setting? What complications can result if inadequate humidification is provided?

5. According to AARC clinical practice guidelines, what are the recommended liter flows when using a bubble humidifier?

6. For each of the following scenarios, identify what type of humidifier you would use. Explain your rationale.

   A. Nasal cannula at 3 Lpm

   B. Nasal cannula at 6 Lpm

   C. Postoperative patient on short-term mechanical ventilation

   D. Long-term mechanically ventilated patient with inspissated secretions

Procedural Competency Evaluation

STUDENT: **DATE:**

HUMIDIFICATION THERAPY

Evaluator: ☐ Peer ☐ Instructor	**Setting:** ☐ Lab ☐ Clinical Simulation	
Equipment Utilized:	**Conditions (Describe):**	

Performance Level:

S or ✓ = Satisfactory, no errors of omission or commission
U = Unsatisfactory Error of Omission or Commission
NA = Not applicable

Performance Rating:

5   **Independent:** Near flawless performance; minimal errors; able to perform without supervision; seeks out new learning; shows initiative; A = 4.7–5.0 average

4   **Minimally Supervised:** Few errors, able to self-correct; seeks guidance when appropriate; B = 3.7–4.65

3   **Competent:** Minimal required level; no critical errors; able to correct with coaching; meets expectations; safe; C = 3.0–3.65

2   **Marginal:** Below average; critical errors or problem areas noted; would benefit from remediation; D = 2.0–2.99

1   **Dependent:** Poor; unacceptable performance; unsafe; gross inaccuracies; potentially harmful; F = < 2.0

Two or more errors of commission or omission of mandatory or essential performance elements will terminate the procedure, and require additional practice and/or remediation and reevaluation. Student is responsible for obtaining additional evaluation forms as needed from the Director of Clinical Education (DCE).

PERFORMANCE RATING | PERFORMANCE LEVEL

EQUIPMENT AND PATIENT PREPARATION

1. Common Performance Elements Steps 1–8

ASSESSMENT AND IMPLEMENTATION

2. Common Performance Elements Steps 9 and 10

3. Identifies the following types of humidifiers: bubble, wick, jet, HME

4. Bubble humidifier: uses when oxygen flow is 4 Lpm or higher with nasal cannula

5. For HME: assures no contraindications are present to its use according to AARC CPG.

   A. Places in circuit at proper location

6. Wick humidifier: obtains and sets up continuous feed system for sterile water and water traps.

7. Assembles servo heating system and verifies function. Sets temperature between 32–37°C as appropriate.

   A. Jet nebulizer (aerosol generator): Obtains pre-filled nebulizer and aerosol drainage bags

8. Adjusts liter flow to ensure patient inspiratory demands being met (minimum VE × 3)

   A. For wick: uses high-flow flowmeter if needed.

   B. For jet nebulizer: if F_iO_2 60% or higher, sets up tandem nebulizer or GIN nebulizer

9. Obtains and calibrates oxygen analyzer

10. Analyzes F_iO_2 delivered and adjusts device if needed

11. Applies device to the patient

12. Verifies gas temperature after appropriate time period

FOLLOW-UP

13. Common Performance Elements Steps 11–16

14. Replaces HME if visibly soiled or resistance to breathing has significantly increased

15. Replaces pre-filled sterile water reservoir on bubble humidifier and jet nebulizer as needed

16. Replaces sterile water bag on continuous feed system as needed

17. Empties drainage reservoir or water traps as needed

SIGNATURES   Student: Evaluator: Date:

Clinical Performance Evaluation

PERFORMANCE RATING:

5 **Independent:** Near flawless performance; minimal errors; able to perform without supervision; seeks out new learning; shows initiative; A = 4.7–5.0 average

4 **Minimally Supervised:** Few errors, able to self-correct; seeks guidance when appropriate; B = 3.7–4.65

3 **Competent:** Minimal required level; no critical errors; able to correct with coaching; meets expectations; safe; C = 3.0–3.65

2 **Marginal:** Below average; critical errors or problem areas noted; would benefit from remediation; D = 2.0–2.99

1 **Dependent:** Poor; unacceptable performance; unsafe; gross inaccuracies; potentially harmful; F = < 2.0

Circle the appropriate response below. Please be consistent, objective, and honest in your assessment of the student's clinical performance and ability.

PERFORMANCE CRITERIA	SCORE				
COGNITIVE DOMAIN					
1. Consistently displays knowledge, comprehension, and command of essential concepts	5	4	3	2	1
2. Demonstrates the relationship between theory and clinical practice	5	4	3	2	1
3. Able to select, review, apply, analyze, synthesize, interpret, and evaluate information; makes recommendations to modify care plan	5	4	3	2	1
PSYCHOMOTOR DOMAIN					
4. Minimal errors, no critical errors; able to self-correct; performs all steps safely and accurately	5	4	3	2	1
5. Selects, assembles, and verifies proper function and cleanliness of equipment; assures operation and corrects malfunctions; provides adequate care and maintenance	5	4	3	2	1
6. Exhibits the required manual dexterity	5	4	3	2	1
7. Performs procedure in a reasonable time frame for clinical level	5	4	3	2	1
8. Applies and maintains aseptic technique and PPE as required	5	4	3	2	1
9. Maintains concise and accurate patient and clinical records	5	4	3	2	1
10. Reports promptly on patient status/needs to appropriate personnel	5	4	3	2	1
AFFECTIVE DOMAIN					
11. Exhibits courteous and pleasant demeanor; shows consideration and respect, honesty, and integrity	5	4	3	2	1
12. Communicates verbally and in writing clearly and concisely	5	4	3	2	1
13. Preserves confidentiality and adheres to all policies	5	4	3	2	1
14. Follows directions, exhibits sound judgment, and seeks help when required	5	4	3	2	1
15. Demonstrates initiative, self-direction, responsibility, and accountability	5	4	3	2	1

TOTAL POINTS = /15 = AVERAGE GRADE =

ADDITIONAL COMMENTS: IDENTIFY AREAS OF EXCELLENCE; LIST ERRORS OF OMISSION OR COMMISSION, CRITICAL ERRORS

SUMMARY PERFORMANCE EVALUATION AND RECOMMENDATIONS

☐ PASS: Satisfactory Performance

    ☐ Minimal supervision needed, may progress to next level provided specific skills, clinical time completed

    ☐ Minimal supervision needed, able to progress to next level without remediation

☐ FAIL: Unsatisfactory Performance (check all that apply)

    ☐ Minor reevaluation only

    ☐ Needs additional clinical practice before reevaluation

    ☐ Needs additional laboratory practice before skills performed in clinical area

    ☐ Recommend clinical probation

SIGNATURES

Evaluator (print name):   Evaluator signature: Date:

Student Signature: Date:

Student Comments:

Procedural Competency Evaluation

STUDENT: **DATE:**

HUMIDIFICATION WITH ARTIFICIAL AIRWAY

Evaluator: ☐ Peer ☐ Instructor	**Setting:** ☐ Lab ☐ Clinical Simulation
Equipment Utilized:	**Conditions (Describe):**

Performance Level:

S or ✓ = Satisfactory, no errors of omission or commission
U = Unsatisfactory Error of Omission or Commission
NA = Not applicable

Performance Rating:

5   **Independent:** Near flawless performance; minimal errors; able to perform without supervision; seeks out new learning; shows initiative; A = 4.7–5.0 average

4   **Minimally Supervised:** Few errors, able to self-correct; seeks guidance when appropriate; B = 3.7–4.65

3   **Competent:** Minimal required level; no critical errors; able to correct with coaching; meets expectations; safe; C = 3.0–3.65

2   **Marginal:** Below average; critical errors or problem areas noted; would benefit from remediation; D = 2.0–2.99

1   **Dependent:** Poor; unacceptable performance; unsafe; gross inaccuracies; potentially harmful; F = < 2.0

Two or more errors of commission or omission of mandatory or essential performance elements will terminate the procedure, and require additional practice and/or remediation and reevaluation. Student is responsible for obtaining additional evaluation forms as needed from the Director of Clinical Education (DCE).

	PERFORMANCE RATING	PERFORMANCE LEVEL
EQUIPMENT AND PATIENT PREPARATION		
1. Common Performance Elements Steps 1–8		
ASSESSMENT AND IMPLEMENTATION		
2. Common Performance Elements Steps 9 and 10		
3. Identifies the proper heated humidifier to be used with an artificial airway		
4. Obtains and sets up continuous feed system for sterile water and water traps.		
5. Assembles servo heating system and verifies function. Sets temperature between 32–37°C as appropriate.		
6. Adjusts liter flow to ensure patient inspiratory demand		
7. Obtains and calibrates oxygen analyzer.		
8. Analyzes F_IO_2 delivered and adjusts device if needed		
9. Selects and applies trach collar or T-piece to the artificial airway		
10. Applies device to the patient		
11. Verifies gas temperature after appropriate time period		
FOLLOW-UP		
12. Common Performance Elements Steps 11–16		
13. Replaces sterile water bag on continuous feed system as needed.		
14. Empties drainage reservoir or water traps as needed		

SIGNATURES   Student: Evaluator: Date:

Clinical Performance Evaluation

PERFORMANCE RATING:

5 **Independent:** Near flawless performance; minimal errors; able to perform without supervision; seeks out new learning; shows initiative; A = 4.7–5.0 average

4 **Minimally Supervised:** Few errors, able to self-correct; seeks guidance when appropriate; B = 3.7–4.65

3 **Competent:** Minimal required level; no critical errors; able to correct with coaching; meets expectations; safe; C = 3.0–3.65

2 **Marginal:** Below average; critical errors or problem areas noted; would benefit from remediation; D = 2.0–2.99

1 **Dependent:** Poor; unacceptable performance; unsafe; gross inaccuracies; potentially harmful; F = < 2.0

Circle the appropriate response below. Please be consistent, objective, and honest in your assessment of the student's clinical performance and ability.

PERFORMANCE CRITERIA	SCORE				
COGNITIVE DOMAIN					
1. Consistently displays knowledge, comprehension, and command of essential concepts	5	4	3	2	1
2. Demonstrates the relationship between theory and clinical practice	5	4	3	2	1
3. Able to select, review, apply, analyze, synthesize, interpret, and evaluate information; makes recommendations to modify care plan	5	4	3	2	1
PSYCHOMOTOR DOMAIN					
4. Minimal errors, no critical errors; able to self-correct; performs all steps safely and accurately	5	4	3	2	1
5. Selects, assembles, and verifies proper function and cleanliness of equipment; assures operation and corrects malfunctions; provides adequate care and maintenance	5	4	3	2	1
6. Exhibits the required manual dexterity	5	4	3	2	1
7. Performs procedure in a reasonable time frame for clinical level	5	4	3	2	1
8. Applies and maintains aseptic technique and PPE as required	5	4	3	2	1
9. Maintains concise and accurate patient and clinical records	5	4	3	2	1
10. Reports promptly on patient status/needs to appropriate personnel	5	4	3	2	1
AFFECTIVE DOMAIN					
11. Exhibits courteous and pleasant demeanor; shows consideration and respect, honesty, and integrity	5	4	3	2	1
12. Communicates verbally and in writing clearly and concisely	5	4	3	2	1
13. Preserves confidentiality and adheres to all policies	5	4	3	2	1
14. Follows directions, exhibits sound judgment, and seeks help when required	5	4	3	2	1
15. Demonstrates initiative, self-direction, responsibility, and accountability	5	4	3	2	1

TOTAL POINTS = _____ /15 = AVERAGE GRADE = _____

ADDITIONAL COMMENTS: IDENTIFY AREAS OF EXCELLENCE; LIST ERRORS OF OMISSION OR COMMISSION, CRITICAL ERRORS

SUMMARY PERFORMANCE EVALUATION AND RECOMMENDATIONS

☐ PASS: Satisfactory Performance

☐ Minimal supervision needed, may progress to next level provided specific skills, clinical time completed

☐ Minimal supervision needed, able to progress to next level without remediation

☐ FAIL: Unsatisfactory Performance (check all that apply)

☐ Minor reevaluation only

☐ Needs additional clinical practice before reevaluation

☐ Needs additional laboratory practice before skills performed in clinical area

☐ Recommend clinical probation

SIGNATURES

Evaluator (print name): _____ Evaluator signature: _____ Date: _____

Student Signature: _____ Date: _____

Student Comments:

CHAPTER 13 Aerosol Generators

INTRODUCTION

An **aerosol** is defined as a suspension of solid or liquid particles in a gas. Aerosols may be administered to deliver medication or to deliver a **bland solution** for the purpose of sputum induction, treatment of upper airway edema, or humidification of a bypassed or compromised upper airway.[1]

There are many devices used by the respiratory care practitioner to generate aerosols for application to the upper or lower airway. These devices include small-volume nebulizers (SVNs), large-volume nebulizers (LVNs), gas injection nebulizers (GINs), nasal atomizers, metered dose inhalers (MDIs) and auxiliary spacing devices, dry powder inhalers (DPIs), and ultrasonic nebulizers (USNs).

The selection and utilization of the most appropriate device is based on the specific clinical application and the desired therapeutic goals. The respiratory care practitioner should consider several factors in this selection, including the intended target area of the respiratory tract to be treated; the proven efficacy of the technique being used; patient preference, coordination, and cooperation; availability of medications; convenience; and patient tolerance.[2] Before one can apply these devices in the clinical setting, the operating principles, advantages, and limitations of each device must be understood.

This chapter focuses on aerosol delivery devices used for continuous aerosol therapy. Chapter 14 emphasizes medication delivery devices and techniques.

OBJECTIVES

Upon completion of this chapter, the student will be able to:

1. Differentiate between the types of aerosol generators by operating principle.
2. Given a specific clinical situation, select and apply the appropriate aerosol delivery device.
3. Discuss the limitations of each type of aerosol delivery device.
4. List the hazards and complications associated with aerosol delivery.
5. Practice communication skills needed to explain the application of an aerosol device to a patient and confirm patient understanding.
6. Practice medical charting for the therapeutic application of an aerosol delivery device.
7. Apply infection control guidelines and standards associated with aerosol delivery equipment and procedures, according to OSHA regulations and CDC guidelines.

KEY TERMS

aerosol	baffle	density	solution
amplitude	bland	nebulizer	tandem
atomizer	couplant	piezoelectric	titrate

Exercises

EQUIPMENT REQUIRED

- ☐ Aerosol masks
- ☐ Briggs adaptors (T-pieces)
- ☐ Compressed gas sources (oxygen and air)
- ☐ Corrugated tubing
- ☐ Face tents
- ☐ Flowmeters
- ☐ Gas injection **nebulizer** (GIN)
- ☐ Heating elements
- ☐ Intubated and tracheostomized airway management trainer
- ☐ Large-volume nebulizers (LVNs)
- ☐ Normal saline vials (3 or 5 mL)

- ☐ Oxygen analyzer and in-line adaptor
- ☐ Oxygen nipple adaptors
- ☐ Oxygen supply tubing
- ☐ Scissors
- ☐ Sterile water
- ☐ Stethoscope
- ☐ Temperature probes and in-line adaptors
- ☐ Tracheostomy collars
- ☐ Ultrasonic nebulizer
- ☐ Watch with second hand
- ☐ Water traps or water drainage bags
- ☐ Y-connectors

EXERCISE 13.1 LARGE-VOLUME NEBULIZER (LVN)

EXERCISE 13.1.1 COMPONENTS OF AN LVN

Examine a large-volume nebulizer and identify the components shown in Figure 13.1. **Record the components in your laboratory report.**

DISS connection

Air entrainment ports

F_IO_2 adjustment (entrainment selector)

Jet

Baffle

Capillary tube

Pressure pop-off (not shown)

Filter

Outlet

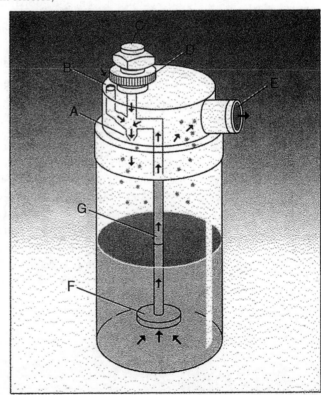

Figure 13.1. Components of a large-volume nebulizer. (From Persing, G: Entry-level Respiratory Care Review, ed 2. WB Saunders, Philadelphia, 1996, p. 41, with permission.)

EXERCISE 13.1.2 ASSEMBLY OF AN LVN

1. Assemble the nebulizer according to the manufacturer's instructions.
2. Aseptically fill the nebulizer with sterile water. If a prefilled nebulizer is used, be sure not to contaminate the internal surfaces.
3. Attach the heating element and adjust the settings, if possible, to achieve 37°C.
4. Attach the nebulizer to the DISS outlet of a flowmeter.
5. Adjust the F_IO_2 by turning the entrainment selector to the 100% setting.
6. Turn the flow to 10 Lpm and observe the mist density and output, the total flow, and the size of the entrainment port.
7. Turn the flowmeter to 15 Lpm or as high as it will go. **Record the highest flow achievable on your laboratory report.**
8. Return the flow to 10 Lpm.
9. Set the entrainment selector to 35% oxygen. Note any changes in the mist density and output, the total flow, and the size of the entrainment port. **Record your observations on your laboratory report.**
10. Set the entrainment selector in between any two oxygen settings.
11. Attach six lengths of corrugated tubing.
12. Place the temperature probe adaptor one tubing length from the patient interface. Insert the temperature probe.
13. Place another temperature probe adaptor about halfway between the nebulizer and the patient interface. Insert the temperature probe.
14. **Record the beginning temperature on both probes. Note the time.**
15. Measure the time it takes for the temperature to reach 37°C on each probe. **Record the times and final temperatures on your laboratory report.**
16. Analyze the F_IO_2 and **record it on your laboratory report.**
17. Adjust the F_IO_2 by turning the entrainment selector to 0.40. Analyze the F_IO_2 and readjust the entrainment selector if necessary to ensure that the nebulizer is delivering 40% oxygen.
18. Put water in the corrugated tubing so that the lumen of the tube is occluded in the loop, or "belly," of the tubing, as shown in Figure 13.2.
19. Analyze the F_IO_2 and **record it on your laboratory report.**
20. Drain the water from the tubing by "milking" the tubing away from the device and into a waste receptacle.
21. Attach a water trap by cutting the corrugated tubing in the belly of the tubing and attaching the trap to the ends of the tubing, as shown in Figure 13.3.
22. Turn the liter flow to 5 Lpm. Observe the mist output and **record your observations on your laboratory report.**

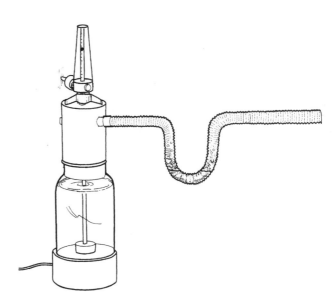

Figure 13.2. Water in the corrugated tubing.

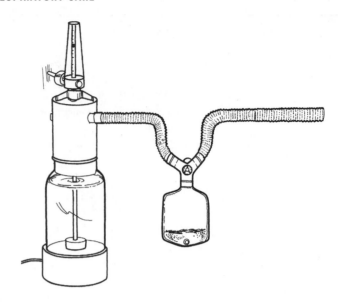

Figure 13.3. Insertion of a water trap in a nebulizer setup.

EXERCISE 13.2 AEROSOL DELIVERY DEVICES

EXERCISE 13.2.1 IDENTIFICATION OF AEROSOL DELIVERY DEVICES

Identify the following devices shown in Figure 13.4. **Record the letter corresponding to the device on your laboratory report.**

Face tent
Aerosol mask
Tracheostomy collar (mask)
Briggs adaptor (T-piece)

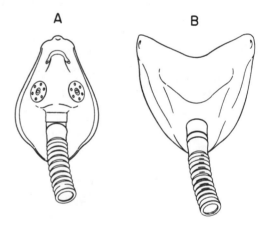

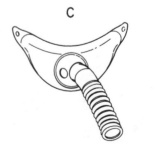

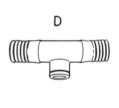

Figure 13.4. Aerosol delivery devices.

EXERCISE 13.2.2 APPLICATION OF AN AEROSOL GENERATING DEVICE

For these exercises, role-playing is required. The students are divided into groups of two. The students may do all the exercises with the same partner, or the instructor might want to change the pairs to enhance the ability of each student to communicate and explain the procedure to a different person. Using your laboratory partner as a patient, or a human patient simulator or mannequin, set up and deliver a heated aerosol at an F_IO_2 of 0.40 (unless otherwise specified by your instructor) for each of the following scenarios: a spontaneously breathing patient (Fig. 13.5); a spontaneously breathing patient with facial injuries (Fig. 13.6); a tracheostomized patient (Fig. 13.7); and an intubated patient (Fig. 13.8).

1. Check the "chart."
   Verify the physician's order or protocol for mode of delivery and F_IO_2.
   Check the patient's diagnosis.
2. Gather the necessary equipment:
   Large-volume nebulizer, prefilled if available
   Corrugated tubing
   Sterile water
   Heating element
   Temperature probe and in-line adaptor
   Oxygen flowmeter and gas source
   Water trap or aerosol T-drainage bag
   Scissors
   Appropriate aerosol delivery device (mask, T-piece, tracheostomy collar, or face tent)
3. Wash or sanitize your hands. Apply standard precautions and transmission-based isolation procedures as appropriate.
4. Introduce yourself and your department. Verify the "patient's" identification. Explain the procedure to the "patient" and confirm "patient" understanding.
5. Assemble the equipment.
6. Adjust the gas source to the appropriate flow rate for adequate flow to meet the "patient's" inspiratory demand. In most cases this is between 8 and 12 Lpm. For oxygen concentrations of 60% or above, a tandem or double setup or gas injection system should be used. This is demonstrated in Exercise 13.5. *REMEMBER: Never place "dead" equipment on a patient!*
7. Attach the delivery device to the "patient." Ensure "patient" comfort.
8. Analyze the F_IO_2 and adjust the entrainment selector if necessary.
9. Document the procedure appropriately. **"Chart" your therapy on your laboratory report.**

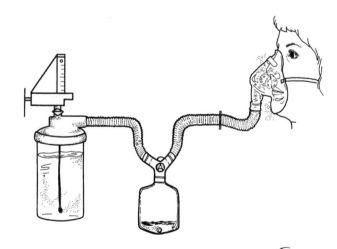

Figure 13.5. Aerosol setup with a face mask.

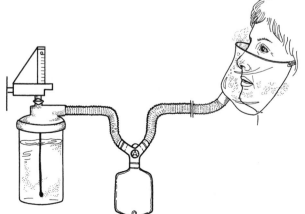

Figure 13.6. Aerosol setup with a face tent.

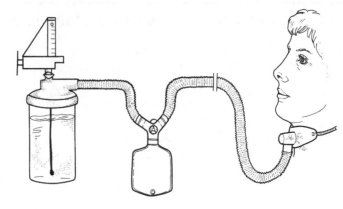

Figure 13.7. Aerosol setup with a tracheostomy collar.

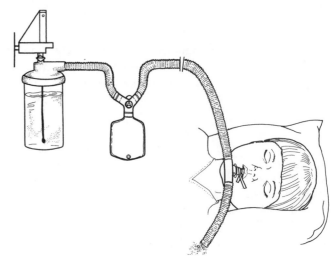

Figure 13.8. Aerosol setup with a Briggs adaptor.

EXERCISE 13.3 ULTRASONIC NEBULIZER (USN)

EXERCISE 13.3.1 LARGE-VOLUME USN

Identify the components of the large-volume ultrasonic nebulizer shown in Figure 13.9. **Record them on your laboratory report.**

On/off switch
Continuous feed inlet
Couplant chamber
Diaphragm
Medication chamber
Amplitude adjustor
Blower
Piezoelectric element

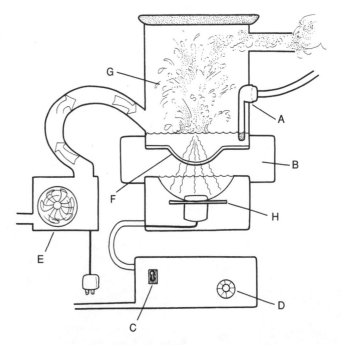

Figure 13.9. Components of an ultrasonic nebulizer.

1. Fill the couplant chamber with tap water.
2. Aseptically fill the medication chamber with 50 mL of sterile water.
3. Plug the unit into an electrical outlet.
4. Turn the unit on with the amplitude at its lowest setting. Note the time and gradually turn the amplitude to the maximum setting. **Record your observations on your laboratory report.**
5. Track the time required for the unit to go dry and **record it on your laboratory report.**
6. Refill the medication chamber.
7. Insert an in-line adaptor to **titrate** oxygen into the gas flow. Attach one end of a small-bore oxygen tube to the adaptor and the other end to a flowmeter. Adjust the flow to obtain an F_IO_2 of 0.30.
8. Drain the tap water from the couplant chamber. Fill it with sterile distilled water.
9. Reassemble the USN and turn it on. **Record your observations of USN function on your laboratory report.**

EXERCISE 13.3.2 MEDICATION SMALL-VOLUME USN

1. Obtain a small-volume medication USN. Identify the brand and model, components, and controls of your unit and **record them on your laboratory report.**
2. Insert disposable diaphragm.
3. Add 1 mL of normal saline solution (NSS) to medication chamber.
4. Turn unit on and note mist density. Adjust if possible.
5. Continue to add NSS to maximum capacity. **Note this amount on your laboratory report.**

EXERCISE 13.4 GAS TITRATION

1. Assemble the gas titration system as shown in Figure 13.10 with the nebulizer attached to a compressed gas source.
2. Turn the flow to 10 Lpm.
3. Adjust the oxygen flowmeter to achieve the following values of F_IO_2:
   0.24
   0.30
   0.45
4. **Record your observations and liter flows required on your laboratory report.**

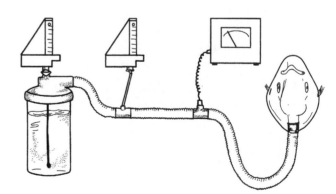

Figure 13.10. Setup for titrating to a specific F_IO_2.

EXERCISE 13.5 TANDEM NEBULIZER SETUP

1. Assemble two large-volume nebulizers in **tandem,** as shown in Figure 13.11.
2. Set the flowmeters on each device to 10 Lpm.
3. Turn the flow rate up to 15 Lpm. **Record your observations on your laboratory report.** Return the flow to 10 Lpm.
4. Set the entrainment selector on each nebulizer to the following: 0.50, 0.60, and 0.80. Observe the mist **density** and output and the total flow. **Record your observations for each setting on your laboratory report.**

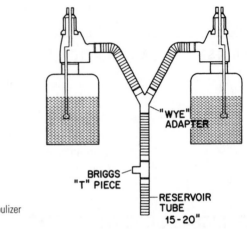

Figure 13.11. Tandem nebulizer setup.

REFERENCES

1. American Association for Respiratory Care: AARC clinical practice guideline: Bland aerosol administration: 2003 update. Respir Care 48(5):539–533, 2003.
2. American Association for Respiratory Care: AARC clinical practice for guideline: Selection of an aerosol delivery device. Respir Care 37:891–897, 1992.

Laboratory Report

CHAPTER 13: AEROSOL GENERATORS

Name _____ Date _____

Course/Section _____ Instructor _____

Data Collection

EXERCISE 13.1 Large-volume Nebulizer (LVN)

EXERCISE 13.1.1 COMPONENTS OF AN LVN

Components: _____

_____

_____

_____

_____

_____

EXERCISE 13.1.2 ASSEMBLY OF AN LVN

OBSERVATIONS

Type and brand of nebulizer used: _____

_____

Mist density at 100%: _____

Mist density at 35%: _____

Total flow at 100%: _____

Total flow at 35%: _____

Entrainment port at 100%: _____

Entrainment port at 35%: _____

F_IO_2 set between _____ and _____

Analyzed at: _____

Heating element setting: _____

INITIAL TEMPERATURES

Probe nearest humidifier: _____

Probe nearest patient interface: _____

TIME TO ACHIEVE 37 °C

Probe nearest humidifier: _____

Probe nearest patient interface: _____

FINAL TEMPERATURES

Probe nearest humidifier: _____

Probe nearest patient interface: _____

WATER IN THE TUBING

F_IO_2 analyzed at: _____

5 Lpm flow: _____

EXERCISE 13.2 Aerosol Delivery Devices

EXERCISE 13.2.1 IDENTIFICATION OF AEROSOL DELIVERY DEVICES

_____

_____

_____

_____

EXERCISE 13.2.2 APPLICATION OF AN AEROSOL GENERATING DEVICE

Chart the procedures for each of the following scenarios.

1. Spontaneously breathing patient: _____

_____

2. Spontaneously breathing patient with facial injuries: _____

_____

3. Intubated patient: _____

_____

4. Tracheostomized patient: _____

_____

EXERCISE 13.3 Ultrasonic Nebulizer (USN)

EXERCISE 13.3.1 LARGE-VOLUME USN

Components:

_____

_____

_____

_____

_____

_____

_____

OBSERVATIONS: Amplitude at maximum

_____

_____

_____

Time until unit is dry: _____

Liter flow to achieve F_IO_2 of 0.30: _____

OBSERVATIONS: Drained couplant chamber

_____

_____

OBSERVATIONS: Couplant filled with sterile water

_____

_____

EXERCISE 13.3.2 MEDICATION SMALL-VOLUME USN

Brand and model used: _____

_____

_____

Components and controls: _____

_____

Amount of saline solution added: _____

EXERCISE 13.4 Gas Titration Utilizing Aerosol Generators

Observations: _____

_____

_____

_____

Liter flow required to achieve

1. 0.24: _____

2. 0.30: _____

3. 0.45: _____

EXERCISE 13.5 Tandem Nebulizer Setup

Observations of mist density and total flow:

$F_IO_2 = 0.50$: _____

$F_IO_2 = 0.60$: _____

$F_IO_2 = 0.80$: _____

Critical Thinking Questions

1. What was the effect on the F_IO_2 of water in the corrugated tubing? Why did that effect occur?

2. What effect did increasing the amplitude of the USN have on the density of the aerosol? What determines the particle size of the USN?

3. The physician orders an ultrasonic treatment to be given to a patient who requires nasal oxygen at 5 Lpm. How would you adapt the equipment?

4. Under what circumstances would it be necessary to utilize tandem nebulizers?

Procedural Competency Evaluation

STUDENT: **DATE:**

AEROSOL GENERATORS: LARGE-VOLUME NEBULIZERS (LVNS)

	PERFORMANCE RATING	PERFORMANCE LEVEL
Evaluator: ☐ Peer ☐ Instructor **Setting:** ☐ Lab ☐ Clinical Simulation		
Equipment Utilized: **Conditions (Describe):**		
Performance Level: S or ✓ = Satisfactory, no errors of omission or commission U = Unsatisfactory Error of Omission or Commission NA = Not applicable		
Performance Rating: 5 **Independent:** Near flawless performance; minimal errors; able to perform without supervision; seeks out new learning; shows initiative; A = 4.7–5.0 average 4 **Minimally Supervised:** Few errors, able to self-correct; seeks guidance when appropriate; B = 3.7–4.65 3 **Competent:** Minimal required level; no critical errors; able to correct with coaching; meets expectations; safe; C = 3.0–3.65 2 **Marginal:** Below average; critical errors or problem areas noted; would benefit from remediation; D = 2.0–2.99 1 **Dependent:** Poor; unacceptable performance; unsafe; gross inaccuracies; potentially harmful; F = < 2.0 *Two or more errors of commission or omission of mandatory or essential performance elements will terminate the procedure, and require additional practice and/or remediation and reevaluation. Student is responsible for obtaining additional evaluation forms as needed from the Director of Clinical Education (DCE).*		

EQUIPMENT AND PATIENT PREPARATION		
1. Common Performance Elements Steps 1–8		
2. Selects appropriate aerosol generator and delivery device to achieve therapeutic objectives		
A. LVN, tandem set-up, gas injection nebulizer (GIN)		
ASSESSMENT AND IMPLEMENTATION		
3. Common Performance Elements Steps 9 and 10		
4. Sets flow rate to appropriate level (8–12 Lpm or GIN recommendation) to achieve adequate mist and total flow		
5. Determines pt total flow demand		
A. Determines total flow being generated by device		
B. Adjusts gas source and/or mist density to the appropriate flow rate for adequate flow to meet the patient's inspiratory demand.		
C. For oxygen concentrations 60% or higher, uses a tandem or double nebulizer setup, or GIN		
6. Attaches the delivery device to the patient and ensures patient comfort		
7. Analyzes the F_IO_2 and adjusts the entrainment selector or mist density if applicable		
8. Reassesses the patient after application of the aerosol device		
9. Collects sputum, labels, and sends to lab if indicated		
FOLLOW-UP		
10. Common Performance Elements Steps 11–16		

SIGNATURES   Student: Evaluator: Date:

Clinical Performance Evaluation

PERFORMANCE RATING:

5   **Independent:** Near flawless performance; minimal errors; able to perform without supervision; seeks out new learning; shows initiative; A = 4.7–5.0 average

4   **Minimally Supervised:** Few errors, able to self-correct; seeks guidance when appropriate; B = 3.7–4.65

3   **Competent:** Minimal required level; no critical errors; able to correct with coaching; meets expectations; safe; C = 3.0–3.65

2   **Marginal:** Below average; critical errors or problem areas noted; would benefit from remediation; D = 2.0–2.99

1   **Dependent:** Poor; unacceptable performance; unsafe; gross inaccuracies; potentially harmful; F = < 2.0

Circle the appropriate response below. Please be consistent, objective, and honest in your assessment of the student's clinical performance and ability.

PERFORMANCE CRITERIA	SCORE				
COGNITIVE DOMAIN					
1. Consistently displays knowledge, comprehension, and command of essential concepts	5	4	3	2	1
2. Demonstrates the relationship between theory and clinical practice	5	4	3	2	1
3. Able to select, review, apply, analyze, synthesize, interpret, and evaluate information; makes recommendations to modify care plan	5	4	3	2	1
PSYCHOMOTOR DOMAIN					
4. Minimal errors, no critical errors; able to self-correct; performs all steps safely and accurately	5	4	3	2	1
5. Selects, assembles, and verifies proper function and cleanliness of equipment; assures operation and corrects malfunctions; provides adequate care and maintenance	5	4	3	2	1
6. Exhibits the required manual dexterity	5	4	3	2	1
7. Performs procedure in a reasonable time frame for clinical level	5	4	3	2	1
8. Applies and maintains aseptic technique and PPE as required	5	4	3	2	1
9. Maintains concise and accurate patient and clinical records	5	4	3	2	1
10. Reports promptly on patient status/needs to appropriate personnel	5	4	3	2	1
AFFECTIVE DOMAIN					
11. Exhibits courteous and pleasant demeanor; shows consideration and respect, honesty, and integrity	5	4	3	2	1
12. Communicates verbally and in writing clearly and concisely	5	4	3	2	1
13. Preserves confidentiality and adheres to all policies	5	4	3	2	1
14. Follows directions, exhibits sound judgment, and seeks help when required	5	4	3	2	1
15. Demonstrates initiative, self-direction, responsibility, and accountability	5	4	3	2	1

TOTAL POINTS =   /15 = AVERAGE GRADE =

ADDITIONAL COMMENTS: IDENTIFY AREAS OF EXCELLENCE; LIST ERRORS OF OMISSION OR COMMISSION, CRITICAL ERRORS

SUMMARY PERFORMANCE EVALUATION AND RECOMMENDATIONS

☐ PASS: Satisfactory Performance

    ☐ Minimal supervision needed, may progress to next level provided specific skills, clinical time completed

    ☐ Minimal supervision needed, able to progress to next level without remediation

☐ FAIL: Unsatisfactory Performance (check all that apply)

    ☐ Minor reevaluation only

    ☐ Needs additional clinical practice before reevaluation

    ☐ Needs additional laboratory practice before skills performed in clinical area

    ☐ Recommend clinical probation

SIGNATURES

Evaluator (print name):   Evaluator signature: Date:

Student Signature: Date:

Student Comments:

14 Cardiopulmonary Pharmacology Review

INTRODUCTION

A primary responsibility of the respiratory care practitioner (RCP) is the delivery of pharmacological agents to the upper and lower airways. The respiratory tract is an ideal route of administration for these agents because they are rapidly absorbed, reduced dosages can be used, and the side effects are minimized. There are a variety of indications for the use of these drugs, including **bronchodilation**, sputum **induction**, mobilization of secretions, and delivery of anti-inflammatory and anti-infective agents. As a result, there are many drugs that can be delivered. New drugs and delivery devices are frequently being approved by the FDA and marketed. It is imperative that the RCP keep up with the rapid changes in drugs and delivery methods. The therapist must have a complete understanding of the classification, indications, contraindications, mechanism of action, and modes of delivery. In addition, the RCP must also know the sequence of administration, which drugs can or cannot be combined, and how to use any special administration equipment. The therapist needs to be able to explain the use of new devices to patients for home care use.

OBJECTIVES

Upon completion of this chapter, the student will be able to:

1. State the dosage, action, and route and mode of delivery for the following respiratory medications.
2. Identify any specialized delivery devices [e.g., DPI (dry powder inhaler)] and proprietary names used.
3. Identify the generic names for each:
   A. Accolate
   B. Advair
   C. Aerobid
   D. Alupent
   E. Asmanex, Nasonex
   F. Atrovent
   G. Coly-Mycin
   H. Combivent
   I. Cromolyn
   J. Curosurf
   K. DuoNeb
   L. Foradil
   M. Flovent, Flonase

    N.   Infasurf

    O.   Maxair Autohaler

    P.   Mucomyst

    Q.   NebuPent

    R.   Proventil, Ventolin

    S.   Pulmicort, Rhinocort

    T.   Pulmicort Respules

    U.   Pulmozyme

    V.   Serevent

    W.   Singulair

    X.   Spiriva

    Y.   Symbicort

    Z.   TOBI

    AA. Vanceril

    BB. VapoNefrin, Micronefrin

    CC. Xopenex

    DD. Other as specified by instructor

4. Practice calculation of drug dosages.

KEY TERMS

adrenergic	drugs	muscarinic	receptor
affinity	dyskinesia	nicotonic	sedation
agonist	enzyme	osteoporosis	solubility
anaphylaxis	excretion	parasympatholytic	surfactant
antagonist	hormone	parasympathomimetic	sympatholytic
anticholinergic	hypersensitivity	parenteral	sympathomimetic
antihistamine	hypoglycemia	pharmaceutical	synergism
antitussive	idiosyncrasy	pharmacodynamics	systemic
atopic	inotropic	pharmacognosy	tachyphylaxis
β agonist	interaction	pharmacokinetics	thrush
bronchoactive	ionization	pharmacology	tolerance
bronchodilation	leukotriene	potency	topical
catecholamines	metabolism	potentiation	toxicology
cholinergic	metabolite	prophylactic	vascular
chronotropic	mucokinetic	protein binding	vasoconstriction
decongestant	mucolytic	racemic	vasodilation

Exercises

EQUIPMENT REQUIRED

- [ ] *Physicians' Desk Reference* (PDR)
- [ ] Drug package inserts or manufacturer's information
- [ ] Internet access
- [ ] Internet drug database sites

EXERCISE 14.1 REVIEW OF RESPIRATORY MEDICATIONS

EXERCISE 14.1.1 PHARMACOLOGIC TERMINOLOGY

For the following definitions, provide the correct term and **record the terms on your laboratory report.**

1. Hand-bulb device to produce large-particle spray
2. Absorbing moisture
3. Applied to skin or mucous membranes for systemic effect
4. Having attraction to
5. Usefulness
6. Bringing harm
7. Complex protein catalyst
8. Containing small blood vessels
9. Decreased response or sensitivity to subsequent repeated doses of same substance or need for increasing doses to maintain constant response
10. Device to initiate an action or process
11. Effects = algebraic sum
12. Prevention
13. Specialized area in a cell that recognizes and bonds with specific substances producing some effect on the cell
14. Relief of pain
15. Route of administration other than GI tract
16. Strength
17. Sudden tolerance
18. Injected into the skin
19. Applied to certain area (i.e., skin or mucous membrane) for localized effect
20. Washing out of organ or cavity
21. Study of natural drugs and their constituents, sources
22. Study of harmful effects of drugs in an organism
23. Study or phase of drugs including dosage, preparation, dispensation, and routes of administration
24. Under the tongue
25. Injected under the skin
26. Sympathetic blood vessel receptors
27. Severe allergic reaction
28. Cough suppressant
29. Adrenergic receptors in heart
30. Natural or synthetic chemicals similar in structure to epinephrine
31. Produces effect of acetylcholine
32. Affecting time or rate
33. Increasing urination
34. Difficulty performing movement
35. Process of elimination as in waste matter or normal discharge
36. Coughing up and spitting out of sputum
37. Allergic asthma
38. Substance originating in an organ or gland and transported by bloodstream to other areas where it has a regulatory effect
39. Abnormally increased susceptibility to stimulus of any kind
40. Peculiar or individual reaction
41. Affecting the force of muscle contraction
42. Inflammatory mediator, product of arachidonic acid metabolism
43. Product of chemical reaction
44. Breaking down of mucus
45. Stimulation of parasympathetic neuroeffector sites, includes increased mucous and salivary gland discharge, decreased heart rate, vasodilation, and hypotension

46. "Pins and needles"
47. Combination of left and right image stereoisomer
48. Collection receptacle for medication of nebulizer
49. Administration of a drug to allay irritability or excitement, calming effect
50. Auxiliary device for MDI (metered-dose inhaler)
51. Stimulating epinephrine receptors
52. Narrowing or spasm of blood vessels

EXERCISE 14.1.2 CLASSIFICATION, GENERIC NAMES, AND SUPPLY OF COMMON RESPIRATORY DRUGS

1. Using the PDR and other reference materials, complete Table 14.1 and answer the questions. Your instructor may add or delete from the medication list.
2. Classify as follows using the abbreviations as shown:
   A. Sympathomimetic Bronchodilator = SPM
   B. Parasympatholytic Bronchodilator = PSPM
   C. Anti-infective = AI
   D. Antiasthmatic Mast Cell Stabilizer = AM
   E. Antiasthmatic Leukotriene Modifier = AL
   F. Mucolytic = ML
   G. Steroid = ST
   H. Surface Active = SA
3. **Record your answers on your laboratory report and answer the following questions:**
   A. Which medication(s) contain(s) fluticasone?
   B. DuoNeb and Combivent contain which two drugs?
   C. What is the generic name of Proventil and Ventolin?
   D. Which bronchodilator should *not* be a first-line drug for acute bronchospasm?
   E. TOBI and Pulmozyme are commonly used to treat the respiratory complications associated with what disease?

Table 14.1 Respiratory Medication Summary

Brand Name	Generic Name	Class	Forms	Dose	Hazards
Advair					
Atrovent					
Azmacort					
Beclovent					
Intal					
Curosurf					
Flovent					
Maxair					
Mucomyst					
Pentamidine					
Pulmozyme					
Spiriva					
Serevent					
Singulair					
Symbicort					
Tilade					

(continued)

Brand Name	Generic Name	Class	Forms	Dose	Hazards
TOBI					
Ventolin					
Xopenex					

EXERCISE 14.2 CALCULATION OF DRUG DOSAGES

To calculate percent solutions and dosages, the following formula is most often used:

$$\frac{\text{Original amount, mg}}{\text{Original amount, mL}} = \frac{\text{Desired amount, mg}}{\text{Desired amount, mL}}$$

Original mg $\times$ desired mL = desired mg $\times$ original mL

The components are cross-multiplied and solved for missing value.

Table 14.2 identifies frequently used conversion factors required for **pharmacology** calculations.

Calculate the following dosages of commonly used respiratory care medications:

1. A physician orders a 2.5-mL/kg dose of Curosurf surfactant replacement therapy for a 4.4-lb neonate. You are to administer it one-half dosage at a time. How many milliliters would be required for the initial application? **Show your work and answer on your laboratory report.**

2. A standard dose of 0.3 mL of a 5% solution of metaproterenol is given. How many milligrams are being administered? **Show your work and answer on your laboratory report.**

3. A 2.5-mg dose of a 0.5% solution of albuterol sulfate is being administered four times daily from a 20-mL multidose vial. How many patients could be treated in one day at this dose from this vial? **Show your work and answer on your laboratory report.**

4. 300 mg of pentamidine are mixed in 6 mL of sterile water. What is the percent solution being administered? How much would need to be administered if a 60-mg dose was ordered? **Show your work and answer on your laboratory report.**

5. 5 mL of 20% Mucomyst are ordered. How many milligrams are being administered? **Show your work and answer on your laboratory report.**

6. Ipratropium bromide unit-dose solution comes in a 0.02% solution. If the active ingredient is 500 μg, what is the equivalent amount of active ingredient in milliliters? **Show your work and answer on your laboratory report.**

7. The unit-dose Atrovent has been back-ordered. What drug could you recommend to the physician to substitute for the Atrovent? If this drug came in a 0.4-mg/mL solution and the physician ordered a 1-mg dose, how many milliliters would need to be drawn up to nebulize this dose? **Show your work and answers on your laboratory report.**

8. Dornase alfa has been ordered for a patient with cystic fibrosis. A single 2.5-mL ampule contains a 2.5-mg dose. What is the percent solution of this medication? **Show your work and answer on your laboratory report.**

Table 14.2 Frequently Used Pharmacology Conversion Factors

2.2 lb = 1 kg (body weight)
1,000 μg = 1 mg
1,000 mg = 1 g
1,000 mL = 1 L
5 mL = 1 tsp
1:00 solution = 1% = 10 mg/mL

Laboratory Report

CHAPTER 14: CARDIOPULMONARY PHARMACOLOGY REVIEW

Name   Date

Course/Section   Instructor

Data Collection

EXERCISE 14.1 Review of Respiratory Medications

EXERCISE 14.1.1 PHARMACOLOGIC TERMINOLOGY

1.	14.	27.	40.
2.	15.	28.	41.
3.	16.	29.	42.
4.	17.	30.	43.
5.	18.	31.	44.
6.	19.	32.	45.
7.	20.	33.	46.
8.	21.	34.	47.
9.	22.	35.	48.
10.	23.	36.	49.
11.	24.	37.	50.
12.	25.	38.	51.
13.	26.	39.	52.

EXERCISE 14.1.2 CLASSIFICATION, GENERIC NAMES, AND SUPPLY OF COMMON RESPIRATORY DRUGS

Brand Name	Generic Name	Class	Forms	Dose	Hazards
Advair					
Atrovent					
Azmacort					
Beclovent					
Intal					
Curosurf					
Flovent					
Maxair					
Mucomyst					
Pentamidine					
Pulmozyme					
Spiriva					
Serevent					
Singulair					
Symbicort					
Tilade					
TOBI					
Ventolin					
Xopenex					

A._____

B._____

C._____

D._____

E._____

EXERCISE 14.2 Calculation of Drug Dosages

1. _____

2. _____

3. _____

4. _____

5. _____

6. _____

7. Drug: _____

   Dosage: _____

8. _____

Critical Thinking Questions

1. List two hazards or complications of each of the following and explain how each could be assessed and prevented or treated:

   A. An aerosolized sympathomimetic

   B. A parasympatholytic bronchodilator

   C. A mucolytic agent

   D. 3% hypertonic saline

   E. Aerosolized anti-infective agent

Procedural Competency Evaluation

STUDENT: **DATE:**

CALCULATION OF DRUG DOSAGES

	PERFORMANCE RATING	PERFORMANCE LEVEL

Evaluator: ☐ Peer ☐ Instructor   **Setting:** ☐ Lab   ☐ Clinical Simulation

Equipment Utilized: **Conditions (Describe):**

Performance Level:

S or ✓ = Satisfactory, no errors of omission or commission
U = Unsatisfactory Error of Omission or Commission
NA = Not applicable

Performance Rating:

5   **Independent:** Near flawless performance; minimal errors; able to perform without supervision; seeks out new learning; shows initiative; A = 4.7–5.0 average

4   **Minimally Supervised:** Few errors, able to self-correct; seeks guidance when appropriate; B = 3.7–4.65

3   **Competent:** Minimal required level; no critical errors; able to correct with coaching; meets expectations; safe; C = 3.0–3.65

2   **Marginal:** Below average; critical errors or problem areas noted; would benefit from remediation; D = 2.0–2.99

1   **Dependent:** Poor; unacceptable performance; unsafe; gross inaccuracies; potentially harmful; F = < 2.0

Two or more errors of commission or omission of mandatory or essential performance elements will terminate the procedure, and require additional practice and/or remediation and reevaluation. Student is responsible for obtaining additional evaluation forms as needed from the Director of Clinical Education (DCE).

1. Converts body weight in pounds to body weight in kilograms		
2. Converts the amount of active drug from micrograms to milligrams		
3. Calculates the amount of drug to be administered if given a drug strength in mg/kg		
4. Calculates the amount of drug in milligrams to be administered given the percent solution and milliliters		
5. Calculates the percent solution of a drug given the amount of drug in mg/ml		
6. Calculates the amount of drug to be administered in milliliters given the drug in percent solution and micrograms		

SIGNATURES   Student: Evaluator: Date:

Clinical Performance Evaluation

PERFORMANCE RATING:

5   **Independent:** Near flawless performance; minimal errors; able to perform without supervision; seeks out new learning; shows initiative; A = 4.7–5.0 average

4   **Minimally Supervised:** Few errors, able to self-correct; seeks guidance when appropriate; B = 3.7–4.65

3   **Competent:** Minimal required level; no critical errors; able to correct with coaching; meets expectations; safe; C = 3.0–3.65

2   **Marginal:** Below average; critical errors or problem areas noted; would benefit from remediation; D = 2.0–2.99

1   **Dependent:** Poor; unacceptable performance; unsafe; gross inaccuracies; potentially harmful; F = < 2.0

Circle the appropriate response below. Please be consistent, objective, and honest in your assessment of the student's clinical performance and ability.

PERFORMANCE CRITERIA

		SCORE			
COGNITIVE DOMAIN					
1. Consistently displays knowledge, comprehension, and command of essential concepts	5	4	3	2	1
2. Demonstrates the relationship between theory and clinical practice	5	4	3	2	1
3. Able to select, review, apply, analyze, synthesize, interpret, and evaluate information; makes recommendations to modify care plan	5	4	3	2	1
PSYCHOMOTOR DOMAIN					
4. Minimal errors, no critical errors; able to self-correct; performs all steps safely and accurately	5	4	3	2	1
5. Selects, assembles, and verifies proper function and cleanliness of equipment; assures operation and corrects malfunctions; provides adequate care and maintenance	5	4	3	2	1
6. Exhibits the required manual dexterity	5	4	3	2	1
7. Performs procedure in a reasonable time frame for clinical level	5	4	3	2	1
8. Applies and maintains aseptic technique and PPE as required	5	4	3	2	1
9. Maintains concise and accurate patient and clinical records	5	4	3	2	1
10. Reports promptly on patient status/needs to appropriate personnel	5	4	3	2	1
AFFECTIVE DOMAIN					
11. Exhibits courteous and pleasant demeanor; shows consideration and respect, honesty, and integrity	5	4	3	2	1
12. Communicates verbally and in writing clearly and concisely	5	4	3	2	1
13. Preserves confidentiality and adheres to all policies	5	4	3	2	1
14. Follows directions, exhibits sound judgment, and seeks help when required	5	4	3	2	1
15. Demonstrates initiative, self-direction, responsibility, and accountability	5	4	3	2	1

TOTAL POINTS =   /15 = AVERAGE GRADE =

ADDITIONAL COMMENTS: IDENTIFY AREAS OF EXCELLENCE; LIST ERRORS OF OMISSION OR COMMISSION, CRITICAL ERRORS

SUMMARY PERFORMANCE EVALUATION AND RECOMMENDATIONS

☐ PASS: Satisfactory Performance

    ☐ Minimal supervision needed, may progress to next level provided specific skills, clinical time completed

    ☐ Minimal supervision needed, able to progress to next level without remediation

☐ FAIL: Unsatisfactory Performance (check all that apply)

    ☐ Minor reevaluation only

    ☐ Needs additional clinical practice before reevaluation

    ☐ Needs additional laboratory practice before skills performed in clinical area

    ☐ Recommend clinical probation

SIGNATURES

Evaluator (print name):   Evaluator signature: Date:

Student Signature: Date:

Student Comments:

15

Aerosol and Medication Therapy

INTRODUCTION

As discussed in the previous chapter, there are many different types of bronchoactive drugs that can be administered. These medications can be delivered using several different devices, such as dry powder inhalers, metered dose inhalers, small-volume nebulizers, continuous nebulizers, and ultrasonic nebulizing devices. Some medications such as pentamidine or surfactants may require specialized delivery devices. Techniques for delivery of aerosol medications include short-term intermittent treatments and long-term or continuous nebulization. To effectively deliver medications, the practitioner must be able to recommend and select the appropriate medication and delivery device, and then prepare the medication for administration. In addition, monitoring and evaluation of therapeutic effectiveness and adverse reactions must be performed and appropriately documented with each procedure.

The practitioner should always be cognizant of potential limitations to these procedures caused by such factors as device design, use of accessory devices, use of artificial airways, mechanical ventilation, condition or irritation of the airways, medication dosage, inadequate instruction or technique, and patient compliance.

OBJECTIVES

Upon completion of this chapter, the student will be able to:

1. Select and use various aerosol delivery devices and adjunctive equipment given specific clinical situations.
2. Discuss the indications, advantages, disadvantages, limitations, contraindications, and hazards of each type of aerosol delivery device and method used for medication delivery.
3. Perform patient assessment and monitor and evaluate patient response to aerosolized medication administration.
4. Obtain a sputum specimen for analysis using sputum induction techniques.
5. Chart an aerosol medication treatment.
6. Practice communication skills needed for the administration of an aerosol medication treatment.
7. Apply infection control guidelines and standards associated with equipment and procedures used for aerosol medication delivery, according to OSHA regulations and CDC guidelines.

KEY TERMS

actuator	holding chamber	propellant
dispersal agent	induction	spacer

Exercises

EQUIPMENT REQUIRED

- [ ] Aeroneb-Pro™ nebulizer
- [ ] Aerosol masks
- [ ] Auxiliary spacing devices (spacers or holding chambers)
- [ ] Circulaire™ nebulizer
- [ ] Compressed gas source, air or oxygen
- [ ] Continuous bronchodilator medication nebulizers (Heart™, Miniheart™, Uniheart™, Flowmist™, or Hope™)
- [ ] Demonstration discus
- [ ] Dry powder inhalers and demo units
- [ ] In-line MDI adaptors for ventilator circuits
- [ ] Intubated and trached airway training mannequin
- [ ] Large-bore aerosol tubing
- [ ] Metered dose inhalers, placebo and sample medications
- [ ] Multidose normal saline solution
- [ ] Multidose vials, Mucomyst (acetylcysteine)
- [ ] Multidose vials, sympathomimetic bronchodilators, variety

- [ ] Oxygen connecting tubing
- [ ] Oxygen nipple adaptors
- [ ] Peak flowmeters with disposable mouthpieces
- [ ] Respirgard™ or Iso-neb™ nebulizers
- [ ] Scissors
- [ ] Small-volume nebulizers, mouthpieces
- [ ] Sputum specimen cup
- [ ] Sterile water
- [ ] Stethoscopes
- [ ] 3% hypertonic saline solution (optional)
- [ ] Tissues
- [ ] T-piece or Briggs adaptor
- [ ] Tracheostomy collars
- [ ] Ultrasonic nebulizer
- [ ] Unit-dose normal saline solutions
- [ ] Unit-dose parasympatholytic bronchodilator
- [ ] Unit-dose Pulmicort Respules®
- [ ] Unit-dose racemic epinephrine
- [ ] Unit-dose sympathomimetic bronchodilators, variety
- [ ] Watch with second hand

EXERCISE 15.1 SMALL-VOLUME NEBULIZERS

EXERCISE 15.1.1 IDENTIFICATION OF COMPONENT PARTS

Examine the small-volume nebulizer and identify the components shown in Figure 15.1. **Record the corresponding letters on your laboratory report.**

Capillary tube
Baffle
Jet
Gas source inlet
Outlet
Reservoir tubing
Mouthpiece

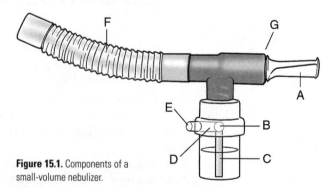

Figure 15.1. Components of a small-volume nebulizer.

EXERCISE 15.1.2 OPERATION OF A SMALL-VOLUME NEBULIZER

1. Assemble a small-volume nebulizer, as shown in Figure 15.2.
2. Attach the connecting tubing of the nebulizer to the nipple adaptor of a flowmeter or compressor outlet.
3. Aseptically instill 1 mL of normal saline into the medication cup. Do not allow the tip of the saline vial to touch any inside surface of the nebulizer.

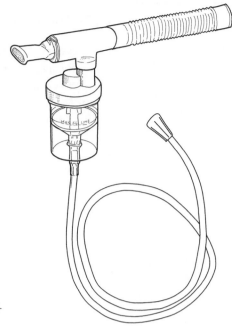

Figure 15.2. Assembly of a small-volume nebulizer.

4. Turn the flow to 6 Lpm. **Record your observations regarding mist density on your laboratory report.**
5. Now instill an additional 2 mL of saline into the medication cup. **Record your observations regarding mist density on your laboratory report.**
6. Turn the flow to 10 Lpm. **Record your observations on your laboratory report.**
7. Turn the flow down to 2 Lpm. **Record your observations regarding mist density on your laboratory report.**
8. Add an additional 3 mL to the nebulizer and turn the flow to 6 Lpm. **Record your observations regarding mist density on your laboratory report.**

EXERCISE 15.2 IDENTIFICATION OF COMPONENT PARTS OF ADDITIONAL DELIVERY DEVICES

EXERCISE 15.2.1 DRY POWDERED INHALER (DPI) DEVICES AND MEDICATIONS

1. Examine the two dry powder inhalers in Figure 15.3. Identify the medication associated with each DPI listed and **record on your laboratory report.** Practice using each device. Practice explaining how to use the device to your "patient."
2. Practice using each device. Practice explaining how to use the device to your "patient."
3. Identify the specific medication associated with each of the DPI devices.
4. Identify the nonactive ingredients and dispersal agents for one of the medications and **record this information on your laboratory report.**

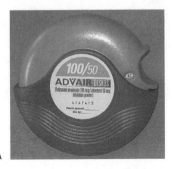
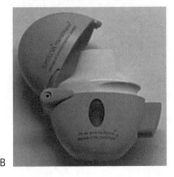

Figure 15.3. Dry powder inhalers:
(A) Advair Diskus® and **(B)**
Spiriva.   A   B

EXERCISE 15.2.2 METERED DOSE INHALERS (MDIS) AND MEDICATIONS

1. Examine a metered dose inhaler and identify the component parts shown in Figure 15.4.
2. Examine the auxiliary spacing devices (spacers) shown in Figure 15.5.
3. Examine the in-line adaptors for MDI delivery to ventilated patients, as shown in Figure 15.6.
4. Practice using the Maxair Autohaler™ MDI device (Fig. 15.7).

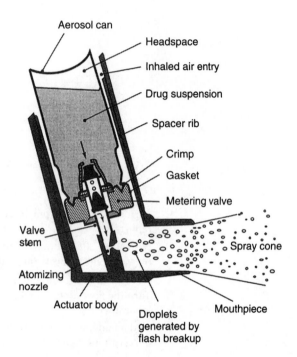

Figure 15.4. Components of a metered dose inhaler. (From Witek, TJ Jr and Schachter, EN: Pharmacology and Therapeutics in Respiratory Care. WB Saunders, Philadelphia, 1994, p. 40, with permission.)

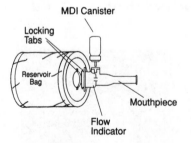

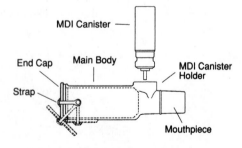

Figure 15.5. Spacing devices. (From Rau, JL Jr: Respiratory Care Pharmacology, ed 4. Mosby-Year Book, St. Louis, 1994, p. 53, with permission.)

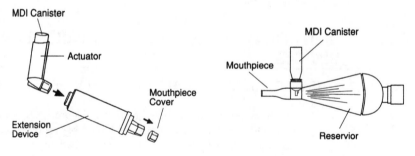

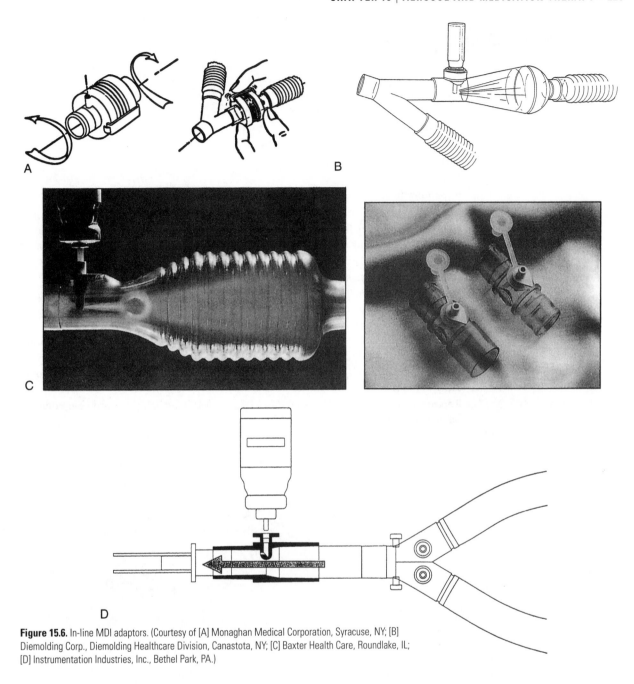

Figure 15.6. In-line MDI adaptors. (Courtesy of [A] Monaghan Medical Corporation, Syracuse, NY; [B] Diemolding Corp., Diemolding Healthcare Division, Canastota, NY; [C] Baxter Health Care, Roundlake, IL; [D] Instrumentation Industries, Inc., Bethel Park, PA.)

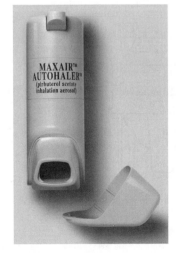

Figure 15.7. Maxair Autohaler™ MDI (Courtesy of Graceway Pharmaceuticals, Exton PA.)

EXERCISE 15.3 SPECIALTY NEBULIZERS

1. Examine filtered nebulizer systems such as the IsoPro™ or Respirgard™ nebulizers and identify the component parts shown in Figures 15.8.

   Mouthpiece

   One-way valve

   Medication reservoir

   Nebulizer

   Expiratory filter

   Connecting tubing

2. Compare a filtered nebulizer system such as the Respirgard™ or Iso-neb™ with a small-volume nebulizer and a large-volume nebulizer. **Record your comparisons on your laboratory report.**

3. Examine the Heart nebulizer and identify the component parts shown in Figure 15.9.

4. Do the same for the Circulaire™ nebulizer shown in Figure 15.10. Compare these devices with a small-volume nebulizer and a large-volume nebulizer. **Record your comparisons on your laboratory report.**

5. Repeat for AeronebPro™ (Fig. 15.11) system if available. **Record your comparisons on your laboratory report.**

6. Repeat for Pari™ nebulizer if available (Fig. 15.12). **Record your comparisons on your laboratory report.**

7. Repeat for AeroEclipse™ BAN nebulizer (Fig. 15.13) if available. **Record your comparisons on your laboratory report.**

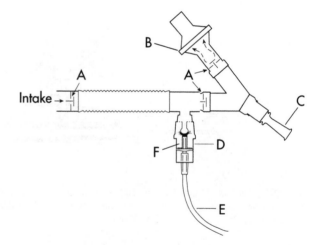

Figure 15.8. Respirgard™ nebulizer. (From Rau, JL Jr: Respiratory Care Pharmacology, ed 4. Mosby-Year Book, St. Louis, 1994, p. 291, with permission.)

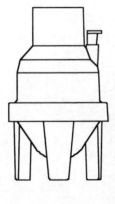

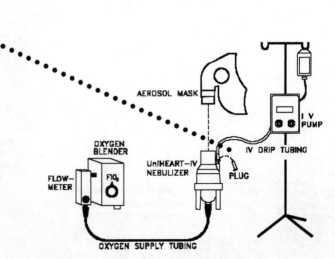

Figure 15.9. Heart nebulizer. (Courtesy of VORTRAN Medical Technology, Inc., Sacramento, CA.)

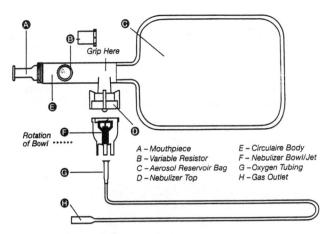

A – Mouthpiece   E – Circulaire Body
B – Variable Resistor   F – Nebulizer Bowl/Jet
C – Aerosol Reservoir Bag   G – Oxygen Tubing
D – Nebulizer Top   H – Gas Outlet

Figure 15.10. Circulaire™ nebulizer. (Courtesy of Westmed, Inc., Tucson, AZ.)

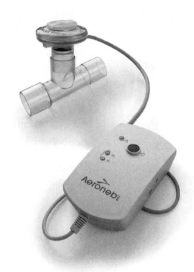

Figure 15.11. AeronebPro™ nebulizer. (Courtesy of Cardinal Health, Dublin, OH.)

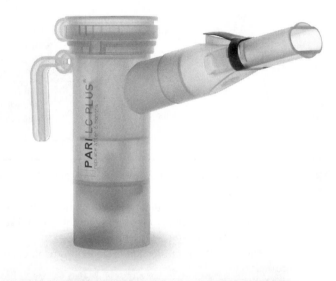

Figure 15.12. PARI LC® PLUS nebulizer. (PARI LC(R) PLUS is a registered trademark of PARI GmbH.)

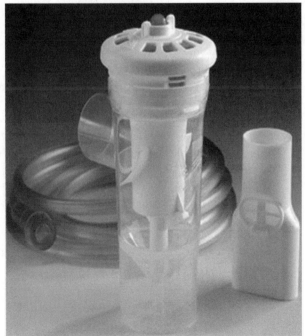

Figure 15.13. AeroEclipse™ nebulizer. (Courtesy of Monaghan Medical Corporation, Plattsburgh, NY.)

EXERCISE 15.4 AEROSOL MEDICATION ADMINISTRATION

There are many factors to consider when selecting an aerosol delivery device. Some are patient-related, others are related to the drug selected. These factors are summarized in Table 15.1.

NOTE: For the following exercises, placebo medications may be used. However, for any student with asthma or reactive airways disease, an actual bronchodilator may be administered with a prescription if the student is agreeable.

Table 15.1 Factors Influencing the Selection of an Aerosol Delivery Device

General Considerations	Disease state and severity Ease of use Power source Cost Drug availability Contamination Practitioner safety Patient age and cooperation
SVN	Patient unable to follow directions Poor vital capacity (<1.0 L) Unable to perform inspiratory hold maneuver Tachypnea (>25 bpm) Medication only available as a solution
MDI	Oriented, cooperative, coordinated patient Adequate vital capacity Respiratory rate <25 bpm Drug only available in MDI form
DPI	Poor MDI coordination Sensitivity to propellants (CFC) Drug availability Inspiratory flow >60 Lpm

EXERCISE 15.4.1 DRY POWDERED INHALER (DPI) ADMINISTRATION

1. Gather the necessary equipment for DPI administration of a sympathomimetic bronchodilator, parasympatholytic bronchodilator, and steroid. **Note which medications and devices were used on your laboratory report.**
2. Check the "chart" for medication order or protocol, diagnosis, history, and other pertinent information.
3. Wash or sanitize your hands. Apply standard precautions and transmission-based isolation procedures as appropriate.
4. Introduce yourself and your department to your "patient." Verify "patient" identification. Explain the purpose of the procedure and verify "patient" understanding.
5. Position the "patient" in an upright position.
6. Assess the "patient" before therapy for heart rate and pattern, respiratory rate and pattern, auscultation, and peak flow measurement.
7. Instruct your "patient" on DPI administration as follows:
   A. Explain which medications are being used and what they do.
   B. Demonstrate how to place the medication capsule or blister pack in the device, if applicable.
   C. Explain and demonstrate how to puncture the DPI capsule with the device.
   D. Instruct the "patient" to hold the device upright and not to turn or tip the device.
   E. Instruct the "patient" to inhale quickly (flow >60 Lpm), maintain breath hold for 5 to 10 seconds, and exhale normally.
   F. Assess the "patient," including V_E, peak flow, and breath sounds.
   G. Administer the DPI in the appropriate sequence.
   H. Reassess the "patient" when finished.
   I. Have the "patient" rinse mouth and gargle after administration of the steroid.
   J. Reinstruct if necessary.
   K. **"Chart" your therapy on your laboratory report.**

EXERCISE 15.4.2 METERED DOSE INHALER (MDI) ADMINISTRATION

1. Gather the necessary equipment for MDI administration: metered dose inhaler, spacer, peak flowmeter, disposable mouthpiece, and watch with second hand.
2. Note the type of propellant and nonactive ingredients contained in the MDI medication and **record on your laboratory report.**
3. Check the "chart" for medication order or protocol, diagnosis, history, and other pertinent information.
4. Wash or sanitize your hands. Apply standard precautions and transmission-based isolation procedures as appropriate.
5. Introduce yourself and your department to your "patient." Verify "patient" identification. Explain the purpose of the procedure and verify "patient" understanding.
6. Position the "patient" in an upright position.
7. Assess the "patient" before therapy for heart rate and pattern, respiratory rate and pattern, auscultation, and peak flow measurement.
8. Instruct your "patient" on MDI administration as follows:
    A. Remove the dustcap and inspect the actuator mouthpiece for any foreign objects.
    B. Shake the MDI. Actuate one puff into the air while holding the canister upside-down if more than 24 hours have elapsed since the last use.
    C. Place the spacer onto the end of the actuator adaptor.
    D. Place the spacer mouthpiece into the mouth. Keep the tongue relaxed and the teeth out of the way of the opening. Exhale normally, not to residual volume (RV).
    E. Begin a slow inspiration through the mouth and activate the MDI as inhalation continues.
    F. Inhale maximally. Maintain inspiratory hold for 5 to 10 seconds if possible.
    G. Wait at least 1 to 2 minutes between puffs.
9. Recap the mouthpiece.
10. If an inhaled corticosteroid is being used, have the "patient" rinse mouth and gargle throat with water when finished.
11. Reassess your "patient's" pulse, respiratory rate, breath sounds, and peak flow.
12. Instruct the "patient" to rinse the mouthpiece and spacer with warm water at least daily.
13. Instruct the "patient" on how to determine MDI contents remaining:
    A. Two hundred puffs per MDI.
    B. Floating canister in water. A full canister will sink, an empty canister will float.
    C. Commercial dose counter (Fig. 15.14).
14. Once a week, disinfect the mouthpiece assembly in a solution of one-half white vinegar and one-half water for 20 to 30 minutes. Rinse thoroughly and air dry.
15. **Chart the therapy on your laboratory report.**

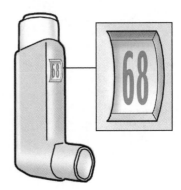

Figure 15.14. Dose counter.

EXERCISE 15.4.3 SMALL-VOLUME NEBULIZER (SVN) ADMINISTRATION

NOTE: For the following exercises, normal saline may be used. However, for any student with asthma or reactive airways disease, an actual bronchodilator may be administered with a prescription if the student is agreeable.

1. Gather the necessary equipment to deliver a medication via small-volume nebulizer by mouthpiece: small-volume nebulizer, connecting tubing, nipple adaptor, compressed gas source (air or oxygen), mouthpiece, one 6-inch length of large-bore corrugated aerosol tubing, unit-dose normal saline, unit-dose or multidose vial of an aerosolized bronchodilator, watch with second hand, stethoscope, and peak flowmeter.

2. Check the "chart" for order or protocol, diagnosis, history, and other pertinent information.

3. Wash or sanitize your hands and apply standard precautions and transmission-based isolation procedures as applicable.

4. Assemble the SVN.

5. Introduce yourself and your department. Verify "patient" identification, explain the procedure, and verify "patient" understanding.

6. Position the "patient" in an upright seated position, if possible.

7. Perform pretreatment assessment of heart rate and pattern, respiratory rate and pattern, auscultation, and peak flow measurement.

8. Aseptically fill the nebulizer with the ordered medication and diluent.

9. Set the compressed gas source to 6 to 8 Lpm.

10. Place the mouthpiece in the "patient's" mouth and instruct the "patient" to take slow, deep breaths with occasional inspiratory hold as tolerated.

11. Periodically reassess pulse throughout the treatment.

12. Modify the "patient's" technique as needed based on response, and reinstruct as necessary.

13. Terminate the treatment when complete medication dosage is nebulized or significant adverse reactions occur.

14. Reassess vital signs, breath sounds, and peak flow.

15. Encourage "patient" to cough and expectorate sputum. Observe for volume, color, consistency, odor, and presence or absence of blood.

16. Rinse the nebulizer with sterile water and air dry. Place it aseptically in a patient treatment bag.
    NOTE: The nebulizer should not be rinsed with tap water because of the possible contamination with *Legionella*.[1]

17. **Chart the therapy on your laboratory report.**

18. Notify appropriate personnel of any adverse reactions or other concerns.

EXERCISE 15.4.4 AEROSOL DELIVERY BY MASK

Repeat Exercise 15.4.3 using an aerosol mask in place of the mouthpiece for administration, as shown in Figure 15.15.

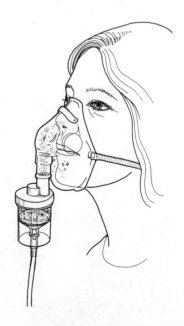

Figure 15.15. Aerosol delivery by mask.

EXERCISE 15.4.5 AEROSOL DELIVERY BY TRACHEOSTOMY COLLAR

Repeat Exercise 15.4.3 using a tracheostomy collar, as shown in Figure 15.16.

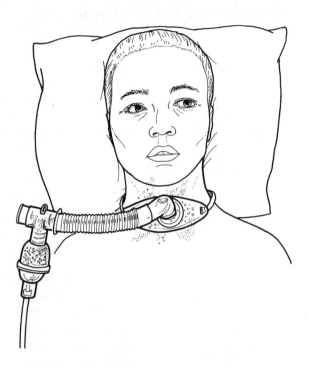

Figure 15.16. Aerosol delivery by tracheostomy collar.

EXERCISE 15.4.6 AEROSOL DELIVERY BY T-PIECE OR BRIGGS ADAPTOR

Repeat Exercise 15.4.3 using a T-piece or Briggs adaptor, as shown in Figure 15.17.

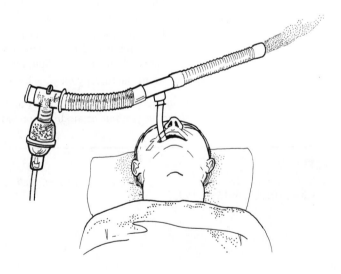

Figure 15.17. Aerosol delivery by Briggs adaptor.

EXERCISE 15.5 RESPIRGARD™/ISO-NEB™ NEBULIZERS

1. Obtain a Respirgard™ or ISO-NEB™ nebulizer and assemble the component parts.
2. Aseptically instill 3 mL of normal saline into the medication cup.
3. Turn the flow to 6 Lpm. **Record your observations of the density, particle size, and release of particles into the atmosphere on your laboratory report.**

4. Turn the flow to 10 Lpm. **Record your observations of the density, particle size, and release of particles into the atmosphere on your laboratory report.**

EXERCISE 15.6 SPUTUM INDUCTION

NOTE: For best results in inducing sputum, a 3% hypertonic saline solution is used. However, because of its irritating nature and the possibility of adverse reactions, the instructor may wish to use sterile water or saline for this exercise. Caution should always be taken with any student who has asthma or reactive airways disease.

1. Gather the necessary equipment for sputum induction via ultrasonic nebulizer: ultrasonic nebulizer, electrical outlet, aerosol mask, several lengths of large-bore corrugated aerosol tubing, bottle of sterile water or saline, watch with second hand, and stethoscope.
2. Check the "chart" for order or protocol, diagnosis, history, and other pertinent information.
3. Wash or sanitize your hands and apply standard precautions and transmission-based isolation procedures as applicable.
4. Introduce yourself and your department. Verify "patient" identification, explain the procedure, and verify "patient" understanding.
5. Position the "patient" in an upright seated position, if possible.
6. Perform pretreatment assessment by measuring heart rate and pattern, respiratory rate and pattern, and auscultation.
7. Assemble the ultrasonic nebulizer. Fill the couplant chamber with tap water. Plug the unit into an electrical outlet.
8. Attach the large-bore corrugated tubing to the nebulizer outlet and attach the aerosol mask to the end of the tubing.
9. Aseptically fill the medication chamber of the nebulizer with the ordered medication.
10. Turn the unit on and adjust the output control.
11. Place the mask comfortably on the "patient's" face and instruct the "patient" to take slow, deep breaths with occasional inspiratory hold as tolerated.
12. Periodically reassess vital signs and breath sounds throughout the treatment.
13. Modify technique and reinstruct the "patient" as needed based on "patient" response.
14. Terminate treatment after 15 to 30 minutes if significant adverse reactions occur, or when sputum specimen has been obtained.
15. Reassess vital signs and breath sounds.
16. Encourage the "patient" to cough and expectorate sputum into specimen cup. Observe for volume, color, consistency, odor, and presence or absence of blood.
17. Label the specimen container with "patient" identification and information (including name, room number, identification number, physician, antibiotic therapy, source of specimen, and date and time of collection) and deliver to the appropriate personnel.
18. **Chart the therapy on your laboratory report.**

Notify appropriate personnel of any adverse reactions or other concerns and make any necessary recommendations or modifications to the "patient" care plan.

REFERENCES

1. Woo, AH, Goetz, A, and Yu, VL: Transmission of *Legionella* by respiratory equipment and aerosol generating devices. Chest 102:1586–1589, 1992.

Laboratory Report

CHAPTER 15: AEROSOL AND MEDICATION THERAPY

Name _____ Date _____

Course/Section _____ Instructor _____

Data Collection

EXERCISE 15.1 Small-Volume Nebulizers

EXERCISE 15.1.1 IDENTIFICATION OF COMPONENT PARTS

A. _____

B. _____

C. _____

D. _____

E. _____

F. _____

G. _____

EXERCISE 15.1.2 OPERATION OF A SMALL-VOLUME NEBULIZER

OBSERVATIONS

1 mL normal saline solution (NSS)/6 Lpm:

_____

_____

3 mL NSS:

_____

_____

10 Lpm:

_____

_____

2 Lpm:

_____

_____

6 mL NSS/6 Lpm:

_____

_____

EXERCISE 15.2 Identification of Component Parts of Additional Delivery Devices

EXERCISE 15.2.1 DRY POWDERED INHALER (DPI) DEVICES AND MEDICATIONS

Available medication in DPI form:

_____

_____

_____

Nonactive and dispersal agents:

_____

_____

_____

EXERCISE 15.3 Specialty Nebulizers

Comparison of a filtered nebulizer with a small-volume nebulizer:

_____

_____

_____

Comparison of the Heart and Circulaire™ nebulizers with a small-volume nebulizer:

_____

_____

_____

Comparison of AeronebPro™ with a small-volume nebulizer:

_____

_____

_____

Comparison of the Pari™ nebulizer with a small-volume nebulizer:

_____

_____

_____

Comparison of the AeroEclipse™ BAN nebulizer with a small-volume nebulizer:

_____

_____

_____

_____

EXERCISE 15.4 Aerosol Medication Administration

EXERCISE 15.4.1 DRY POWDERED INHALER (DPI) ADMINISTRATION

Medication and device used:

_____

_____

_____

Chart your therapy:

_____

_____

_____

EXERCISE 15.4.2 METERED DOSE INHALER (MDI) ADMINISTRATION

Propellant and nonactive ingredients:

_____

_____

_____

Chart your therapy:

_____

_____

_____

_____

_____

EXERCISE 15.4.3 SMALL-VOLUME NEBULIZER (SVN) ADMINISTRATION

Chart your therapy:

_____

_____

_____

_____

_____

_____

EXERCISE 15.5 Respirgard™/ISO-NEB™ Nebulizers

OBSERVATIONS

3 mL NSS/6 Lpm—density, particle size, and release of particles into the atmosphere:

_____

_____

_____

10 Lpm—density, particle size, and release of particles into the atmosphere:

_____

_____

_____

EXERCISE 15.6 Sputum Induction

Chart your therapy:

_____

_____

_____

_____

_____

_____

Critical Thinking Questions

Mr. Sullivan is a 55-year-old man who has just arrived at the emergency room. He has a documented history of bronchitis and asthma. The physician has requested that you immediately assess the patient and make a recommendation for treatment. Your initial assessment reveals tachypnea, tachycardia, diaphoresis, audible wheezing, and the use of accessory muscles.

1. What other bedside assessments would be important to perform at this time?

2. What specific treatment(s) would you recommend for this patient?

3. Which specific medication and dosage would you suggest?

4. The physician disagrees with your suggestion and orders 5 mg of albuterol sulfate to be delivered every hour. Briefly describe how you would handle this situation. What further recommendations would you make?

5. The initial aerosol therapy treatment has been started in the emergency room and has been administered for 5 minutes. Monitoring of the patient indicates that the pulse rate has increased from 112/minute to 140/minute and the audible wheezing appears to be improving. Describe your response to this situation.

6. The patient's attending physician has been contacted and the patient is being admitted. The physician has written *additional* orders for an Atrovent, Azmacort, and Cromolyn, two puffs each, to be administered q4h. In which order should the medications be given?

7. How do the Respirgard™/Cadema, Circulaire™, and Heart nebulizers differ from small-volume nebulizers? What medication is delivered via Respirgard™/ISO-NEB™ a nebulizers?

8. Given the following clinical scenarios, select the proper aerosol generator *and* aerosol delivery device:

A. A 60-year-old obtunded black man who requires treatment with 0.5 mL Proventil and 3.0 mL NSS.

B. An AIDS patient who requires pentamidine.

C. A 35-year-old woman in the recovery room after abdominal surgery.

D. A 55-year-old man with a size 8.0 tracheostomy tube.

E. A 30-year-old patient with possible pneumonia; a sputum sample is required.

F. A 4-month-old with respiratory syncytial virus.

G. An 18-year-old asthmatic who is sensitive to the propellant in the MDI.

H. Status asthmaticus patient admitted to intensive care. The patient is not responding to q1-2h treatments. The physician requests that you administer high-dose bronchodilator therapy.

Procedural Competency Evaluation

STUDENT: **DATE:**

AEROSOL MEDICATION DELIVERY: NEBULIZED SOLUTIONS

Evaluator: ☐ Peer ☐ Instructor   **Setting:** ☐ Lab ☐ Clinical Simulation

Equipment Utilized: **Conditions (Describe):**

Performance Level:

S or ✓ = Satisfactory, no errors of omission or commission
U = Unsatisfactory Error of Omission or Commission
NA = Not applicable

Performance Rating:

5 **Independent:** Near flawless performance; minimal errors; able to perform without supervision; seeks out new learning; shows initiative; A = 4.7–5.0 average

4 **Minimally Supervised:** Few errors, able to self-correct; seeks guidance when appropriate; B = 3.7–4.65

3 **Competent:** Minimal required level; no critical errors; able to correct with coaching; meets expectations; safe; C = 3.0–3.65

2 **Marginal:** Below average; critical errors or problem areas noted; would benefit from remediation; D = 2.0–2.99

1 **Dependent:** Poor; unacceptable performance; unsafe; gross inaccuracies; potentially harmful; F = < 2.0

Two or more errors of commission or omission of mandatory or essential performance elements will terminate the procedure, and require additional practice and/or remediation and reevaluation. Student is responsible for obtaining additional evaluation forms as needed from the Director of Clinical Education (DCE).

Columns: PERFORMANCE RATING | PERFORMANCE LEVEL

EQUIPMENT AND PATIENT PREPARATION

1. Common Performance Elements Steps 1–8
2. Determines best medication delivery method (SVN, BAN, USN, Circulaire or other specialty nebulizer)
3. Checks label and verifies correct medication, dosage, and expiration date
4. Prepares medications per physician's orders
5. Determines most appropriate patient interface to achieve therapeutic goals (mouthpiece, mask spacer, T-piece, tracheostomy collar, ventilator in-line adaptor)

ASSESSMENT AND IMPLEMENTATION

6. Common Performance Elements Steps 9 and 10
7. Selects appropriate propellant gas (air or oxygen)
8. Instructs patient to breath normally with occasional slow, deep breaths and inspiratory hold as tolerated
9. Coaches and assists patient to modify technique as needed
10. Monitors vital signs throughout procedure
11. Measures peak flow before and after in asthmatic patients
12. Encourages and assists patient cough; notes sputum production
13. Assesses treatment effectiveness
14. Terminates treatment if significant adverse reaction to medication occurs

FOLLOW-UP

15. Common Performance Elements Steps 11-16
16. Ensures patient rinses mouth if aerosolized steroid administered
17. Shakes out nebulizer, rinses with sterile water only and/or dries with gas flow, and returns to treatment bag or clean container
18. Instructs patient and family on disinfection of nebulizer for home use

SIGNATURES   Student: Evaluator: Date:

Clinical Performance Evaluation

PERFORMANCE RATING:

5 **Independent:** Near flawless performance; minimal errors; able to perform without supervision; seeks out new learning; shows initiative; A = 4.7–5.0 average

4 **Minimally Supervised:** Few errors, able to self-correct; seeks guidance when appropriate; B = 3.7–4.65

3 **Competent:** Minimal required level; no critical errors; able to correct with coaching; meets expectations; safe; C = 3.0–3.65

2 **Marginal:** Below average; critical errors or problem areas noted; would benefit from remediation; D = 2.0–2.99

1 **Dependent:** Poor; unacceptable performance; unsafe; gross inaccuracies; potentially harmful; F = < 2.0

Circle the appropriate response below. Please be consistent, objective, and honest in your assessment of the student's clinical performance and ability.

PERFORMANCE CRITERIA	SCORE				
COGNITIVE DOMAIN					
1. Consistently displays knowledge, comprehension, and command of essential concepts	5	4	3	2	1
2. Demonstrates the relationship between theory and clinical practice	5	4	3	2	1
3. Able to select, review, apply, analyze, synthesize, interpret, and evaluate information; makes recommendations to modify care plan	5	4	3	2	1
PSYCHOMOTOR DOMAIN					
4. Minimal errors, no critical errors; able to self-correct; performs all steps safely and accurately	5	4	3	2	1
5. Selects, assembles, and verifies proper function and cleanliness of equipment; assures operation and corrects malfunctions; provides adequate care and maintenance	5	4	3	2	1
6. Exhibits the required manual dexterity	5	4	3	2	1
7. Performs procedure in a reasonable time frame for clinical level	5	4	3	2	1
8. Applies and maintains aseptic technique and PPE as required	5	4	3	2	1
9. Maintains concise and accurate patient and clinical records	5	4	3	2	1
10. Reports promptly on patient status/needs to appropriate personnel	5	4	3	2	1
AFFECTIVE DOMAIN					
11. Exhibits courteous and pleasant demeanor; shows consideration and respect, honesty, and integrity	5	4	3	2	1
12. Communicates verbally and in writing clearly and concisely	5	4	3	2	1
13. Preserves confidentiality and adheres to all policies	5	4	3	2	1
14. Follows directions, exhibits sound judgment, and seeks help when required	5	4	3	2	1
15. Demonstrates initiative, self-direction, responsibility, and accountability	5	4	3	2	1

TOTAL POINTS = _____ /15 = AVERAGE GRADE = _____

ADDITIONAL COMMENTS: IDENTIFY AREAS OF EXCELLENCE; LIST ERRORS OF OMISSION OR COMMISSION, CRITICAL ERRORS

SUMMARY PERFORMANCE EVALUATION AND RECOMMENDATIONS

☐ PASS: Satisfactory Performance

    ☐ Minimal supervision needed, may progress to next level provided specific skills, clinical time completed

    ☐ Minimal supervision needed, able to progress to next level without remediation

☐ FAIL: Unsatisfactory Performance (check all that apply)

    ☐ Minor reevaluation only

    ☐ Needs additional clinical practice before reevaluation

    ☐ Needs additional laboratory practice before skills performed in clinical area

    ☐ Recommend clinical probation

SIGNATURES

Evaluator (print name):   Evaluator signature: Date:

Student Signature: Date:

Student Comments:

Procedural Competency Evaluation

STUDENT: **DATE:**

AEROSOL MEDICATION DELIVERY: CONTINUOUS BRONCHODILATOR NEBULIZATION

	PERFORMANCE RATING	PERFORMANCE LEVEL
Evaluator: ☐ Peer ☐ Instructor **Setting:** ☐ Lab ☐ Clinical Simulation		
Equipment Utilized: **Conditions (Describe):**		
Performance Level: S or ✓ = Satisfactory, no errors of omission or commission U = Unsatisfactory Error of Omission or Commission NA = Not applicable		
Performance Rating: 5 **Independent:** Near flawless performance; minimal errors; able to perform without supervision; seeks out new learning; shows initiative; A = 4.7–5.0 average 4 **Minimally Supervised:** Few errors, able to self-correct; seeks guidance when appropriate; B = 3.7–4.65 3 **Competent:** Minimal required level; no critical errors; able to correct with coaching; meets expectations; safe; C = 3.0–3.65 2 **Marginal:** Below average; critical errors or problem areas noted; would benefit from remediation; D = 2.0–2.99 1 **Dependent:** Poor; unacceptable performance; unsafe; gross inaccuracies; potentially harmful; F = < 2.0 *Two or more errors of commission or omission of mandatory or essential performance elements will terminate the procedure, and require additional practice and/or remediation and reevaluation. Student is responsible for obtaining additional evaluation forms as needed from the Director of Clinical Education (DCE).*		
EQUIPMENT AND PATIENT PREPARATION		
1. Common Performance Elements Steps 1–8		
2. Checks label and verifies correct medication and expiration date		
3. Prepares medications per physician's orders		
ASSESSMENT AND IMPLEMENTATION		
4. Common Performance Elements Steps 9 and 10		
5. Selects appropriate propellant gas		
6. Assembles continuous medication delivery device		
7. Instills sufficient amount of medication and diluent		
8. Coaches and assists patient as needed		
9. Assesses treatment effectiveness		
10. Monitors vital signs throughout procedure		
11. Encourages and assists patient cough; notes sputum production		
FOLLOW-UP		
12. Common Performance Elements Steps 11–16		

SIGNATURES   Student: Evaluator: Date:

Clinical Performance Evaluation

PERFORMANCE RATING:

5 **Independent:** Near flawless performance; minimal errors; able to perform without supervision; seeks out new learning; shows initiative; A = 4.7–5.0 average

4 **Minimally Supervised:** Few errors, able to self-correct; seeks guidance when appropriate; B = 3.7–4.65

3 **Competent:** Minimal required level; no critical errors; able to correct with coaching; meets expectations; safe; C = 3.0–3.65

2 **Marginal:** Below average; critical errors or problem areas noted; would benefit from remediation; D = 2.0–2.99

1 **Dependent:** Poor; unacceptable performance; unsafe; gross inaccuracies; potentially harmful; F = < 2.0

Circle the appropriate response below. Please be consistent, objective, and honest in your assessment of the student's clinical performance and ability.

PERFORMANCE CRITERIA	SCORE				
COGNITIVE DOMAIN					
1. Consistently displays knowledge, comprehension, and command of essential concepts	5	4	3	2	1
2. Demonstrates the relationship between theory and clinical practice	5	4	3	2	1
3. Able to select, review, apply, analyze, synthesize, interpret, and evaluate information; makes recommendations to modify care plan	5	4	3	2	1
PSYCHOMOTOR DOMAIN					
4. Minimal errors, no critical errors; able to self-correct; performs all steps safely and accurately	5	4	3	2	1
5. Selects, assembles, and verifies proper function and cleanliness of equipment; assures operation and corrects malfunctions; provides adequate care and maintenance	5	4	3	2	1
6. Exhibits the required manual dexterity	5	4	3	2	1
7. Performs procedure in a reasonable time frame for clinical level	5	4	3	2	1
8. Applies and maintains aseptic technique and PPE as required	5	4	3	2	1
9. Maintains concise and accurate patient and clinical records	5	4	3	2	1
10. Reports promptly on patient status/needs to appropriate personnel	5	4	3	2	1
AFFECTIVE DOMAIN					
11. Exhibits courteous and pleasant demeanor; shows consideration and respect, honesty, and integrity	5	4	3	2	1
12. Communicates verbally and in writing clearly and concisely	5	4	3	2	1
13. Preserves confidentiality and adheres to all policies	5	4	3	2	1
14. Follows directions, exhibits sound judgment, and seeks help when required	5	4	3	2	1
15. Demonstrates initiative, self-direction, responsibility, and accountability	5	4	3	2	1

TOTAL POINTS =   /15 = AVERAGE GRADE =

ADDITIONAL COMMENTS: IDENTIFY AREAS OF EXCELLENCE; LIST ERRORS OF OMISSION OR COMMISSION, CRITICAL ERRORS

SUMMARY PERFORMANCE EVALUATION AND RECOMMENDATIONS

☐ PASS: Satisfactory Performance

    ☐ Minimal supervision needed, may progress to next level provided specific skills, clinical time completed

    ☐ Minimal supervision needed, able to progress to next level without remediation

☐ FAIL: Unsatisfactory Performance (check all that apply)

    ☐ Minor reevaluation only

    ☐ Needs additional clinical practice before reevaluation

    ☐ Needs additional laboratory practice before skills performed in clinical area

    ☐ Recommend clinical probation

SIGNATURES

Evaluator (print name):   Evaluator signature: Date:

Student Signature: Date:

Student Comments:

Procedural Competency Evaluation

STUDENT: _____ DATE: _____

AEROSOL MEDICATION DELIVERY: MDI, DPI

Evaluator: ☐ Peer ☐ Instructor	**Setting:** ☐ Lab ☐ Clinical Simulation	
Equipment Utilized:	**Conditions (Describe):**	

Performance Level:

S or ✓ = Satisfactory, no errors of omission or commission
U = Unsatisfactory Error of Omission or Commission
NA = Not applicable

Performance Rating:

5   **Independent:** Near flawless performance; minimal errors; able to perform without supervision; seeks out new learning; shows initiative; A = 4.7–5.0 average

4   **Minimally Supervised:** Few errors, able to self-correct; seeks guidance when appropriate; B = 3.7–4.65

3   **Competent:** Minimal required level; no critical errors; able to correct with coaching; meets expectations; safe; C = 3.0–3.65

2   **Marginal:** Below average; critical errors or problem areas noted; would benefit from remediation; D = 2.0–2.99

1   **Dependent:** Poor; unacceptable performance; unsafe; gross inaccuracies; potentially harmful; F = < 2.0

Two or more errors of commission or omission of mandatory or essential performance elements will terminate the procedure, and require additional practice and/or remediation and reevaluation. Student is responsible for obtaining additional evaluation forms as needed from the Director of Clinical Education (DCE).

The following items each have columns for **PERFORMANCE RATING** and **PERFORMANCE LEVEL**.

EQUIPMENT AND PATIENT PREPARATION

1. Common Performance Elements Steps 1–8
2. Determines best medication delivery method (MDI, DPI, spacer, or holding chamber)
3. Checks label and verifies correct medication, dosage, and expiration date
4. Prepares medications per physician's orders
5. Determines most appropriate patient interface to achieve therapeutic goals (mouthpiece, mask, spacer, or holding chamber with appropriate connector, ventilator, in-line adaptor)

ASSESSMENT AND IMPLEMENTATION

6. Common Performance Elements Steps 9 and 10
7. Determines patient's ability to perform procedure and follow directions
8. If MDI used, assures respiratory rate <25/min; if DPI used, verifies patient can inhale rapidly with inspiratory flow >60 lpm
9. Removes dust cap, inspects actuator mouthpiece for any foreign objects
10. Shakes MDI, actuates one puff into air if more than 24 hours has elapsed since last use
11. Attaches MDI canister to spacer or holding chamber
12. Instructs patient as follows:
    A. Exhale normally
    B. Take slow inspiration with coordination of MDI actuation
    C. Perform maximal inhalation with inspiratory hold for 5–10 seconds if possible
    D. Waits at least 1–2 minutes between puffs
    E. Instructs patient to inhale more slowly if whistling sound heard from spacer
13. If ventilator interface is used, coordinates actuation with inspiratory phase of ventilator cycle
14. Coaches and assists patient as needed
15. Assesses treatment effectiveness
    A. Monitors vital signs throughout procedure
    B. Measures peak flow in asthmatic patients
16. Encourages and assists patient cough; notes sputum production
17. Terminates treatment if significant adverse reaction to medication occurs

FOLLOW-UP

18. Common Performance Elements Steps 11–16
19. Recaps mouthpiece when finished
20. Rinses mouth if aerosolized steroids are administered
21. Rinses mouthpiece and spacer with warm water at least daily
22. Determines MDI or DPI contents remaining

SIGNATURES   Student: _____   Evaluator: _____   Date: _____

Clinical Performance Evaluation

PERFORMANCE RATING:

5   **Independent:** Near flawless performance; minimal errors; able to perform without supervision; seeks out new learning; shows initiative; A = 4.7–5.0 average

4   **Minimally Supervised:** Few errors, able to self-correct; seeks guidance when appropriate; B = 3.7–4.65

3   **Competent:** Minimal required level; no critical errors; able to correct with coaching; meets expectations; safe; C = 3.0–3.65

2   **Marginal:** Below average; critical errors or problem areas noted; would benefit from remediation; D = 2.0–2.99

1   **Dependent:** Poor; unacceptable performance; unsafe; gross inaccuracies; potentially harmful; F = < 2.0

Circle the appropriate response below. Please be consistent, objective, and honest in your assessment of the student's clinical performance and ability.

PERFORMANCE CRITERIA	SCORE				
COGNITIVE DOMAIN					
1. Consistently displays knowledge, comprehension, and command of essential concepts	5	4	3	2	1
2. Demonstrates the relationship between theory and clinical practice	5	4	3	2	1
3. Able to select, review, apply, analyze, synthesize, interpret, and evaluate information; makes recommendations to modify care plan	5	4	3	2	1
PSYCHOMOTOR DOMAIN					
4. Minimal errors, no critical errors; able to self-correct; performs all steps safely and accurately	5	4	3	2	1
5. Selects, assembles, and verifies proper function and cleanliness of equipment; assures operation and corrects malfunctions; provides adequate care and maintenance	5	4	3	2	1
6. Exhibits the required manual dexterity	5	4	3	2	1
7. Performs procedure in a reasonable time frame for clinical level	5	4	3	2	1
8. Applies and maintains aseptic technique and PPE as required	5	4	3	2	1
9. Maintains concise and accurate patient and clinical records	5	4	3	2	1
10. Reports promptly on patient status/needs to appropriate personnel	5	4	3	2	1
AFFECTIVE DOMAIN					
11. Exhibits courteous and pleasant demeanor; shows consideration and respect, honesty, and integrity	5	4	3	2	1
12. Communicates verbally and in writing clearly and concisely	5	4	3	2	1
13. Preserves confidentiality and adheres to all policies	5	4	3	2	1
14. Follows directions, exhibits sound judgment, and seeks help when required	5	4	3	2	1
15. Demonstrates initiative, self-direction, responsibility, and accountability	5	4	3	2	1

TOTAL POINTS =   /15 = AVERAGE GRADE =

ADDITIONAL COMMENTS: IDENTIFY AREAS OF EXCELLENCE; LIST ERRORS OF OMISSION OR COMMISSION, CRITICAL ERRORS

SUMMARY PERFORMANCE EVALUATION AND RECOMMENDATIONS

☐ PASS: Satisfactory Performance

     ☐ Minimal supervision needed, may progress to next level provided specific skills, clinical time completed

     ☐ Minimal supervision needed, able to progress to next level without remediation

☐ FAIL: Unsatisfactory Performance (check all that apply)

     ☐ Minor reevaluation only

     ☐ Needs additional clinical practice before reevaluation

     ☐ Needs additional laboratory practice before skills performed in clinical area

     ☐ Recommend clinical probation

SIGNATURES

Evaluator (print name):   Evaluator signature: Date:

Student Signature: Date:

Student Comments:

Procedural Competency Evaluation

STUDENT: DATE:

SPUTUM INDUCTION

		PERFORMANCE RATING	PERFORMANCE LEVEL
Evaluator: ☐ Peer ☐ Instructor **Setting:** ☐ Lab ☐ Clinical Simulation			
Equipment Utilized: **Conditions (Describe):**			

Performance Level:

S or ✓ = Satisfactory, no errors of omission or commission
U = Unsatisfactory Error of Omission or Commission
NA = Not applicable

Performance Rating:

5 **Independent:** Near flawless performance; minimal errors; able to perform without supervision; seeks out new learning; shows initiative; A = 4.7–5.0 average

4 **Minimally Supervised:** Few errors, able to self-correct; seeks guidance when appropriate; B = 3.7–4.65

3 **Competent:** Minimal required level; no critical errors; able to correct with coaching; meets expectations; safe; C = 3.0–3.65

2 **Marginal:** Below average; critical errors or problem areas noted; would benefit from remediation; D = 2.0–2.99

1 **Dependent:** Poor; unacceptable performance; unsafe; gross inaccuracies; potentially harmful; F = < 2.0

Two or more errors of commission or omission of mandatory or essential performance elements will terminate the procedure, and require additional practice and/or remediation and reevaluation. Student is responsible for obtaining additional evaluation forms as needed from the Director of Clinical Education (DCE).

EQUIPMENT AND PATIENT PREPARATION

1. Common Performance Elements Steps 1–8

ASSESSMENT AND IMPLEMENTATION

2. Common Performance Elements Steps 9 and 10

3. Selects the proper equipment for obtaining a sputum sample:
   A. USN
   B. Bland aerosol
   C. Other aerosol

4. Administers the therapy

5. Instructs the patient in the proper coughing techniques for obtaining a sputum sample

6. Instructs patient to expectorate into the sterile sputum cup

7. Ensures that the sample is from the lung and not naso/oropharynx

8. Labels the sample accurately and properly according to facility policy

9. Places the sample in biohazard bag according to facility policy

10. Ensures that the proper laboratory request form is completed

11. Ensures that the sample is sent to the laboratory

FOLLOW-UP

12. Common Performance Elements Steps 11–16

SIGNATURES Student: Evaluator: Date:

Clinical Performance Evaluation

PERFORMANCE RATING:

5   **Independent:** Near flawless performance; minimal errors; able to perform without supervision; seeks out new learning; shows initiative; A = 4.7–5.0 average

4   **Minimally Supervised:** Few errors, able to self-correct; seeks guidance when appropriate; B = 3.7–4.65

3   **Competent:** Minimal required level; no critical errors; able to correct with coaching; meets expectations; safe; C = 3.0–3.65

2   **Marginal:** Below average; critical errors or problem areas noted; would benefit from remediation; D = 2.0–2.99

1   **Dependent:** Poor; unacceptable performance; unsafe; gross inaccuracies; potentially harmful; F = < 2.0

Circle the appropriate response below. Please be consistent, objective, and honest in your assessment of the student's clinical performance and ability.

PERFORMANCE CRITERIA	SCORE				
COGNITIVE DOMAIN					
1. Consistently displays knowledge, comprehension, and command of essential concepts	5	4	3	2	1
2. Demonstrates the relationship between theory and clinical practice	5	4	3	2	1
3. Able to select, review, apply, analyze, synthesize, interpret, and evaluate information; makes recommendations to modify care plan	5	4	3	2	1
PSYCHOMOTOR DOMAIN					
4. Minimal errors, no critical errors; able to self-correct; performs all steps safely and accurately	5	4	3	2	1
5. Selects, assembles, and verifies proper function and cleanliness of equipmen; assures operation and corrects malfunctions; provides adequate care and maintenance	5	4	3	2	1
6. Exhibits the required manual dexterity	5	4	3	2	1
7. Performs procedure in a reasonable time frame for clinical level	5	4	3	2	1
8. Applies and maintains aseptic technique and PPE as required	5	4	3	2	1
9. Maintains concise and accurate patient and clinical records	5	4	3	2	1
10. Reports promptly on patient status/needs to appropriate personnel	5	4	3	2	1
AFFECTIVE DOMAIN					
11. Exhibits courteous and pleasant demeanor; shows consideration and respect, honesty, and integrity	5	4	3	2	1
12. Communicates verbally and in writing clearly and concisely	5	4	3	2	1
13. Preserves confidentiality and adheres to all policies	5	4	3	2	1
14. Follows directions, exhibits sound judgment, and seeks help when required	5	4	3	2	1
15. Demonstrates initiative, self-direction, responsibility, and accountability	5	4	3	2	1

TOTAL POINTS =   /15 = AVERAGE GRADE =

ADDITIONAL COMMENTS: IDENTIFY AREAS OF EXCELLENCE; LIST ERRORS OF OMISSION OR COMMISSION, CRITICAL ERRORS

SUMMARY PERFORMANCE EVALUATION AND RECOMMENDATIONS

☐ PASS: Satisfactory Performance

    ☐ Minimal supervision needed, may progress to next level provided specific skills, clinical time completed

    ☐ Minimal supervision needed, able to progress to next level without remediation

☐ FAIL: Unsatisfactory Performance (check all that apply)

    ☐ Minor reevaluation only

    ☐ Needs additional clinical practice before reevaluation

    ☐ Needs additional laboratory practice before skills performed in clinical area

    ☐ Recommend clinical probation

SIGNATURES

Evaluator (print name):   Evaluator signature: Date:

Student Signature: Date:

Student Comments:

16 Hyperinflation Therapy Techniques

INTRODUCTION

Hyperinflation techniques include a variety of basic respiratory care modalities, all of which are designed to promote lung expansion and thereby prevent or reverse atelectasis. This is accomplished by increasing **transpulmonary pressure** and inspiratory volumes.[1] Additional benefits of these modalities as a component of bronchial hygiene therapy include promoting a more effective cough, thereby improving mobilization of secretions.

Incentive spirometry, or sustained maximal inspiration (SMI), techniques primarily prevent atelectasis by mimicking or replacing the normal sigh mechanism and encouraging the patient to take slow, deep breaths with an inspiratory hold. Intermittent **positive pressure** breathing (IPPB) provides short-term mechanical inflation to **augment** inspiratory volumes, deliver aerosol medication, assist ventilation, and mobilize secretions.[2] IPPB may be applied to spontaneously breathing patients and to those with artificial airways. It is not the first choice for aerosol delivery or augmenting lung expansion when less expensive or less invasive techniques can reliably accomplish these clinical outcomes.[2]

OBJECTIVES

Upon completion of this chapter, the student will be able to:

1. Practice the communication skills needed for the instruction of patients in the techniques of sustained maximal inspiration and hyperinflation therapy.
2. Perform and monitor incentive spirometry therapy using both flow and volume devices.
3. Practice medical charting for the therapeutic procedures of hyperinflation.
4. Identify and compare the component parts and controls of various IPPB devices.
5. Assemble and ensure proper function of IPPB equipment.
6. Perform and monitor volume-oriented IPPB therapy.
7. Evaluate the effects of various control manipulation on the volumes, I:E ratio, and F_IO_2 delivered by IPPB devices.
8. Analyze the effect of altered lung compliance and airway resistance on the volume delivered by IPPB devices.

KEY TERMS

augment   positive pressure   transpulmonary
hyperinflation   splint   pressure

Exercises

EQUIPMENT REQUIRED

☐ 50-psi air and oxygen sources
☐ Computerized lung simulator, optional
☐ Continuous positive airway pressure (CPAP) mask and head straps
☐ Disposable IPPB circuits
☐ Disposable mouthpieces
☐ Disposable noseclips
☐ Down's Flow or Whisper Flow generator valves
☐ Flange (lip seal)
☐ Flow- and volume-based incentive spirometry devices
☐ Gloves
☐ High-pressure hoses

☐ IPPB machines—Bird and Bennett
☐ Masks
☐ One-way valve adaptors
☐ Oxygen analyzer with T-adaptor
☐ Peak flowmeter and disposable mouthpieces
☐ Positive end-expiratory pressure (PEEP) valves
☐ Pillow
☐ Respirometers
☐ Stethoscopes
☐ Stopwatch
☐ Test lungs
☐ Tissues
☐ Unit-dose normal saline vials

EXERCISE 16.1 INCENTIVE SPIROMETRY

EXERCISE 16.1.1 SUSTAINED MAXIMAL INSPIRATION (SMI) PREOPERATIVE INSTRUCTION

Your laboratory partner will play the role of a preoperative patient who must be instructed in the techniques of SMI. In clinical situations, SMI is most effective when the patient is instructed preoperatively.

1. Gather the necessary equipment for this exercise:
    Respirometer
    One-way valve adaptor
    Flow or volume incentive spirometer device
    Pillow
2. Wash or sanitize your hands and apply standard precautions and transmission-based isolation procedures as applicable.
3. Introduce yourself and your department. Explain the purpose of the therapy to the "patient" and verify patient understanding.
4. Measure the "patient's" preoperative inspiratory capacity and vital capacity using the respirometer.
5. Assemble the incentive spirometer device as shown in Figure 16.1.
6. Instruct the "patient" on the use and frequency of the incentive spirometer device in the following manner:
    A. Exhale normally.
    B. Insert the mouthpiece into your mouth and inhale *slowly* and *deeply*.
    C. Hold your breath at the end of inspiration to the count of 10 (3 to 5 seconds).
    D. Exhale normally.
    E. Repeat the procedure 6 to 10 times per hour. Allow adequate recovery time between breaths to prevent hyperventilation.
7. Instruct the "patient" on using a pillow to **splint** the incision postoperatively to minimize pain during therapy, as shown in Figure 16.2.
8. Have the "patient" demonstrate the procedure to you.
9. **Chart your "patient's" preoperative evaluation and instruction on your laboratory report.**

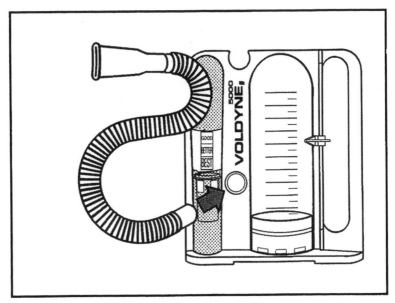

1. Remove components from package.
2. Attach open end of tubing to stem on front side of exerciser.

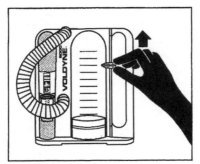

Slide the pointer of unit to prescribed volume level. Hold or stand exerciser in an upright position.

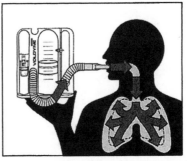

Inhale slowly to raise the white piston in the chamber. When inhaling, maintain top of yellow flow cup in the "Best" flow range.

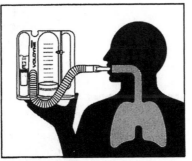

Exhale normally. Then place lips tightly around mouthpiece.

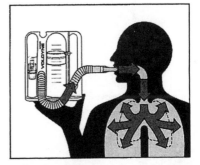

Continue inhaling and try to raise piston to prescribed level.* When inhalation is complete remove mouthpiece, hold breath as prescribed, and exhale normally. Allow piston to return to bottom of chamber, rest and repeat exercise. Frequency of use and recommended inspiratory volumes should be performed at the direction of your physician.

Figure 16.1. Assembly of **(A)** volume incentive spirometer (courtesy of Voldyne, Sherwood, Davis & Geck, St. Louis, MO) and **(B)** flow incentive spirometer (courtesy of Diemolding Corp., Diemolding Healthcare Division, Canastota, NY). *(continued)*

A

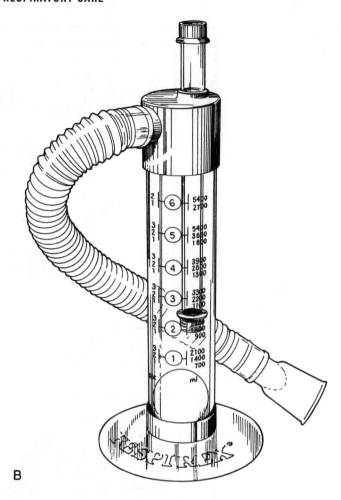

Figure 16.1. *continued*   B

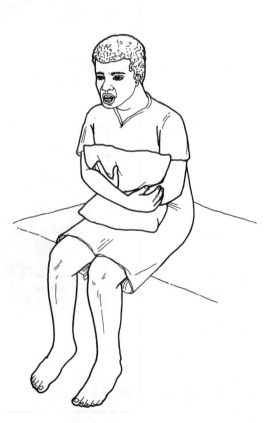

Figure 16.2. Splinting an abdominal incision.

EXERCISE 16.1.2 INCENTIVE SPIROMETRY POSTOPERATIVE THERAPY

Your laboratory partner will play the role of a postoperative thoracotomy patient who is in mild to moderate discomfort.

1. Gather the necessary equipment:

   Stethoscope

   Respirometer

   One-way valve adaptor

   Flow or volume incentive spirometer device

   Pillow

2. Wash or sanitize your hands and apply standard precautions and transmission-based isolation procedures as applicable.

3. Introduce yourself and your department.

4. Explain the purpose of the therapy to the "patient" and verify patient understanding.

5. Measure the "patient's" postoperative inspiratory capacity and vital capacity using the respirometer. Your "patient" should simulate a decreased effort for this exercise.

6. Assemble the incentive spirometer device.

7. Assess patient progress by the following:

   A. Pain medication schedule

   B. Chest x-ray report from the "chart"

   C. Change in "patient's" temperature from the chart

   D. "Patient's" pulse and respiratory rate

   E. Breath sounds on auscultation

8. Reinstruct the "patient" on the use and frequency of the incentive spirometer device in the following manner:

   A. Exhale normally.

   B. Insert the mouthpiece into your mouth and inhale *slowly* and *deeply*.

   C. Hold your breath at the end of inspiration to the count of 10 (3 to 5 seconds).

   D. Exhale normally.

   E. Repeat the procedure 6 to 10 times per hour. Allow adequate recovery time between breaths to prevent hyperventilation.

9. Assist the "patient" in using the pillow to splint the incision postoperatively to minimize pain during therapy.

10. Have the "patient" demonstrate the procedure to you.

11. Measure the achieved volume. For a volume-based device, observe the maximum inspiratory effort achieved. For a flow-based device, the volume can be measured by attaching the respirometer as shown in Figure 16.3.

12. Instruct the "patient" to cough. Observe for any sputum production. Auscultate the patient.

13. **Chart the therapy on your laboratory report.**

EXERCISE 16.2 IDENTIFICATION OF INTERMITTENT POSITIVE-PRESSURE BREATHING MACHINE COMPONENT PARTS AND CONTROLS

1. Obtain a Bird IPPB machine. Identify the component parts shown in Figure 16.4. **Record the model used and components on your laboratory report.** (If the model used is not the same as the one pictured, identify the controls of the model used and note how the controls differ.)

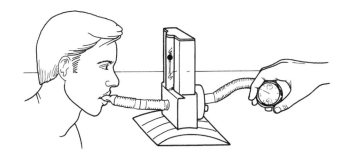

Figure 16.3. Measuring inspiratory volumes on an incentive spirometer.

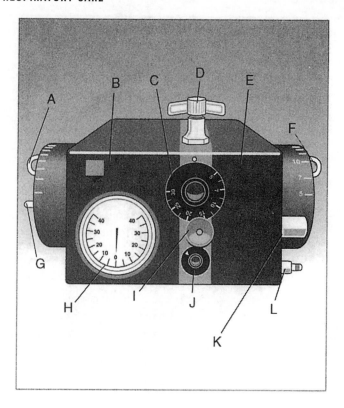

Figure 16.4. Components of a Bird intermittent positive-pressure breathing (IPPB) machine. (From Persing, G: Entry-level Respiratory Care Review, ed 2. WB Saunders, Philadelphia, 1996, p. 27, with permission.)

Expiratory (apnea) timer
Manual cycle rod
Large-bore tubing connection
Pressure chamber
Flow rate control
Gas inlet
Air-mix plunger
Pressure manometer
Sensitivity
Ambient chamber
Pressure limit
Nebulizer/exhalation valve connection

2. Obtain a Bennett IPPB device. Identify the component parts shown in Figure 16.5. **Record the model used and components on your laboratory report.**

Nebulizer—inspiration
Control pressure
Sensitivity
Air dilution
Nebulizer—expiration
System pressure
Peak flow
Pressure limit
Negative pressure
Expiratory time
Terminal flow
Rate
Bennett valve with dustcover
Accumulator

3. Remove the dustcover from the Bennett valve. Unscrew and carefully remove and examine the valve. Replace it when you have completed your observation.

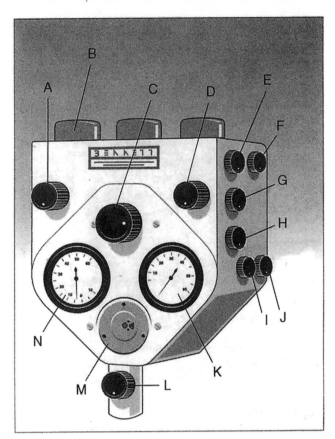

Figure 16.5. Components of a Bennett IPPB machine. (From Persing, G: Entry-level Respiratory Care Review, ed 2. WB Saunders, Philadelphia, 1996, p. 79, with permission.)

EXERCISE 16.3 INTERMITTENT POSITIVE-PRESSURE BREATHING CIRCUITRY ASSEMBLY

1. Attach the high-pressure hose to the IPPB machine and then to a 50-psi gas source.
2. Assemble an IPPB circuit as shown in Figure 16.6 and attach it to an IPPB machine.
3. Test the function of the machine by adjusting the pressure to maximum, manually cycling the machine on, and aseptically occluding the outlet with a gloved hand or gauze. Ensure that the machine cycles off. If it does not, examine it for any loose connections or a faulty exhalation valve.
4. Attach a test lung to the circuit outlet (where the mouthpiece would normally be attached). Increase the sensitivity adjustment until the machine automatically self-triggers, and then decrease it slightly until auto-triggering stops. Now squeeze the test lung. The machine should cycle on.
5. Adjust the pressure so that the machine cycles off at 20 cm H_2O.
6. Adjust the flow so that inspiration takes approximately 2 seconds.
7. Attach the respirometer to the expiratory outlet of the circuit. Measure the volume achieved and **record it on your laboratory report.**

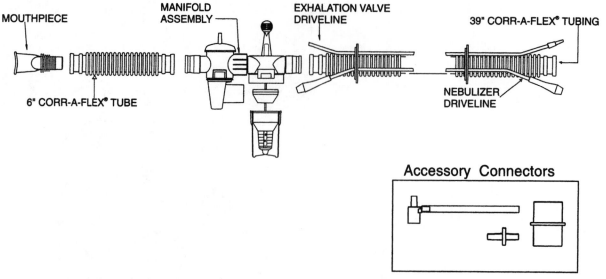

Figure 16.6. Assembly and components of an IPPB circuit. (Courtesy of Hudson Respiratory Care Inc., Temecula, CA.)

EXERCISE 16.4 MANIPULATION OF INTERMITTENT POSITIVE-PRESSURE BREATHING CONTROLS

EXERCISE 16.4.1 VOLUME AND INSPIRATION: EXPIRATION RATIO ADJUSTMENT

Using a test lung attached to the IPPB circuit, make the following adjustments and observe the results. Measure exhaled volumes using a respirometer attached to the expiratory outlet.

1. **Record the current volume, flow, and sensitivity settings on the machine on your laboratory report.** Cycle the machine on, and **record the achieved inspiratory volume on your laboratory report.**
2. Increase the pressure and cycle the machine on. Note and **record the pressure at end inspiration and any change in inspiratory volume and time on your laboratory report.**
3. Set the pressure below the original setting. Note and **record the pressure at end inspiration and any change in inspiratory volume and time on your laboratory report.**
4. Return the pressure to the original setting. Increase the flow setting. Note and **record the pressure at end inspiration and any change in inspiratory volume and time on your laboratory report.**
5. Decrease the flow setting below the original settings. Note and **record the pressure at end inspiration and any change in inspiratory volume on your laboratory report.**
6. Adjust the pressure and flow controls until a tidal volume of 500 mL is achieved. Note and **record the settings needed to achieve this volume and the inspiratory time on your laboratory report.**
7. Adjust the pressure and flow controls until a tidal volume of 700 mL is achieved. Note and **record the settings needed to achieve this volume and the inspiratory time on your laboratory report.**
8. Adjust the pressure and flow controls until a tidal volume of 300 mL is achieved. Note and **record the settings needed to achieve this volume and the inspiratory time on your laboratory report.**

EXERCISE 16.4.2 SENSITIVITY CONTROL

Set the pressure and flow to the original settings.

1. Increase the sensitivity control and note what happens when the test lung is squeezed. Note and **record the negative pressure needed to initiate inspiration on your laboratory report.**
2. Increase the sensitivity until the machine auto-triggers.
3. Decrease the sensitivity setting. Squeeze the test lung and note and **record on your laboratory report the negative pressure needed to initiate inspiration.**

EXERCISE 16.4.3 F_IO_2 CONTROL

1. Attach the IPPB machine to a 50-psi oxygen gas source.
2. Calibrate an oxygen analyzer and insert it between the inspiratory outlet and the test lung.
3. Adjust the rate control so that the machine automatically cycles on at a rate of 12 to 15 breaths per minute.
4. Adjust the oxygen control on the IPPB machine to the "in," or air-mix off, position. Allow the machine to cycle for several breaths and **record the F_IO_2 reading on the analyzer on your laboratory report.**
5. Adjust the oxygen control to the "out," or air-mix on, position. Allow the machine to cycle for several breaths and **record the F_IO_2 reading on the analyzer on your laboratory report.**
6. Increase the pressure reading. Allow the machine to cycle for several breaths and **record the F_IO_2 reading on the analyzer on your laboratory report.**
7. Decrease the pressure setting. Allow the machine to cycle for several breaths and **record the F_IO_2 reading on the analyzer on your laboratory report.**
8. Increase the flow setting. Allow the machine to cycle for several breaths and **record the F_IO_2 reading on the analyzer on your laboratory report.**
9. Decrease the flow setting. Allow the machine to cycle for several breaths and **record the F_IO_2 reading on the analyzer on your laboratory report.**

EXERCISE 16.5 INTERMITTENT POSITIVE-PRESSURE BREATHING THERAPY

In this exercise your laboratory partner will act as a patient. Because the therapy will be given with aerosolized normal saline, caution should be used for any student with hypersensitive airways.

1. Gather the necessary equipment.
2. Wash or sanitize your hands and apply standard precautions and transmission-based isolation procedures as appropriate.
3. Introduce yourself and your department, explain the procedure, and verify "patient" understanding.
4. Assess the "patient" before therapy by measuring pulse rate and pattern, respiratory rate and pattern, and auscultation.
5. Measure the "patient's" tidal volume, vital capacity, and peak flow rate.
6. Assemble the IPPB circuit with a mouthpiece and test the function. Adjust the settings initially at a low pressure (approximately 10 cm H_2O) and a moderate flow setting. Adjust the sensitivity so that the machine is not auto-triggering.
7. Aseptically fill the nebulizer with a 3- to 5-mL unit dose of normal saline solution. If a Bennett machine is used, adjust the nebulizer control to achieve a moderate mist.
8. Have the "patient" insert the mouthpiece into his or her mouth and maintain a tight seal. If the "patient" has difficulty, noseclips or a mouth flange may be used.
9. Instruct the "patient" to inhale slightly until the machine triggers on and allow the machine to augment inspiration. Note the volume achieved during inspiration.
10. Adjust the sensitivity if needed.
11. Adjust the pressure and flow until a maximum possible volume (at least two to three times the tidal volume) is achieved during inspiration without "patient" discomfort.
12. Instruct the "patient" to breathe slowly to prevent hyperventilation.
13. Monitor pulse, respirations, and breath sounds during therapy. Observe the "patient" for any adverse reactions.
14. At the end of the therapy, reassess the "patient's" vital signs, breath sounds, vital capacity, and peak flow.
15. Instruct the "patient" to cough. Note any sputum production. Assess volume, color, consistency, and odor.
16. Disassemble the equipment, dispose of any infectious waste in the appropriate containers, and wash or sanitize your hands.
17. **Chart the therapy on your laboratory report.**
18. Repeat the therapy using the mouth flange.
19. Repeat the therapy using a mask, as shown in Figure 16.7.
20. Repeat the therapy using an artificial airway, as shown in Figure 16.8.

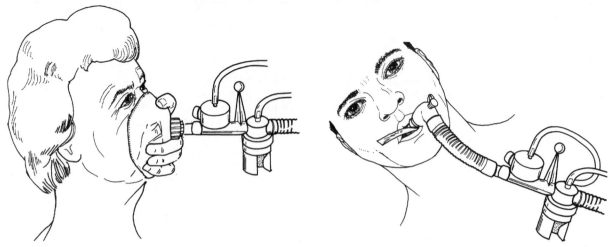

Figure 16.7. Administration of an IPPB treatment with a face mask.

Figure 16.8. Administration of an IPPB treatment via artificial airway.

EXERCISE 16.6   COMPUTERIZED LUNG SIMULATOR: EFFECT OF COMPLIANCE AND RESISTANCE CHANGES ON INTERMITTENT POSITIVE-PRESSURE BREATHING VOLUMES

The following exercise may be performed if a computerized lung simulator is available. If not, an airway management trainer can be used with endotracheal tubes of varying size to simulate resistance changes and manual manipulation of a test lung to simulate compliance changes.

1. Adjust the lung simulator for normal compliance and resistance.
2. Adjust the IPPB machine to achieve a tidal volume of 700 mL. **Record these settings on your laboratory report.**
3. Increase the airway resistance setting (or decrease the size of the endotracheal tube). **Record any changes in achieved tidal volume and inspiratory time on your laboratory report.**
4. Return the resistance to normal. Decrease the compliance below normal on the lung simulator (or manually restrict the expansion of the test lung). **Record any changes in achieved tidal volume and inspiratory time on your laboratory report.**
5. Increase the compliance above normal. **Record any changes in achieved tidal volume and inspiratory time on your laboratory report.**

REFERENCES

1. American Association for Respiratory Care: The AARC clinical practice guideline: Incentive spirometry. Respir Care 36:1402–1405, 1991.
2. American Association for Respiratory Care: The AARC clinical practice guideline: Intermittent positive pressure breathing: 2003 revision and update. Respir Care 48(5):540–546, 2003.

Laboratory Report

CHAPTER 16: HYPERINFLATION THERAPY TECHNIQUES

Name _____   Date _____

Course/Section _____   Instructor _____

Data Collection

EXERCISE 16.1 Incentive Spirometry

EXERCISE 16.1.1 SUSTAINED MAXIMAL INSPIRATION (SMI) PREOPERATIVE INSTRUCTION

"Chart" the preoperative "patient" evaluation and instruction below. Include the "patient's" preoperative inspiratory, vital capacity, and peak flow measurements.

_____

_____

_____

_____

_____

_____

EXERCISE 16.1.2 INCENTIVE SPIROMETRY POSTOPERATIVE THERAPY

"Chart" the postoperative treatment below as you would on a legal medical record.

_____

_____

_____

_____

_____

_____

_____

_____

EXERCISE 16.2 Identification of Intermittent Positive-Pressure Breathing Machine Component Parts and Controls

1. Bird controls.
Model of machine used: _____

A. _____

B. _____

C. _____

D. _____

E. _____

F. _____

G. _____

H. _____

I. _____

J. _____ (Identify which are the pressure and ambient chambers.)

K. _____

L. _____

2. Bennett controls.

Model of machine used: _____

A. _____

B. _____

C. _____

D. _____

E. _____

F. _____

G. _____

H. _____

I. _____

J. _____

K. _____

L. _____

M. _____

N. _____

Controls on other Bennett machines: _____

_____

_____

_____

_____

EXERCISE 16.3 Intermittent Positive-Pressure Breathing Circuitry Assembly

Volume achieved: _____

EXERCISE 16.4 Manipulation of Intermittent Positive-Pressure Breathing Controls

EXERCISE 16.4.1 VOLUME AND INSPIRATION: EXPIRATION RATIO ADJUSTMENT

A. Original settings:

Pressure: _____

Flow: _____

Sensitivity: _____

Volume achieved: _____

Inspiratory time: _____

B. Increased pressure setting:

Pressure: _____

Flow: _____

Sensitivity: _____

Volume achieved: _____

Inspiratory time: _____

C. Decreased pressure setting:

Pressure: _____

Flow: _____

Sensitivity: _____

Volume achieved: _____

Inspiratory time: _____

D. Increased flow setting:

Pressure: _____

Flow: _____

Sensitivity: _____

Volume achieved: _____

Inspiratory time: _____

E. Decreased flow setting:

Pressure: _____

Flow: _____

Sensitivity: _____

Volume achieved: _____

Inspiratory time: _____

F. 500 mL:

Pressure setting: _____

Flow setting: _____

Inspiratory time: _____

G. 700 mL:

Pressure setting: _____

Flow setting: _____

Inspiratory time: _____

H. 300 mL:

Pressure setting: _____

Flow setting: _____

Inspiratory time: _____

EXERCISE 16.4.2 SENSITIVITY CONTROL

1. Increased sensitivity, negative manometer pressure reading: _____

2. Decreased sensitivity, negative manometer pressure reading: _____

EXERCISE 16.4.3 F_IO_2 CONTROL

1. Air mix in; F_IO_2: _____

2. Air mix out; F_IO_2: _____

3. Increased pressure; F_IO_2: _____

4. Decreased pressure; F_IO_2: _____

5. Increased flow; F_IO_2: _____

6. Decreased flow; F_IO_2: _____

EXERCISE 16.5 Intermittent Positive-Pressure Breathing Therapy

"Chart" the IPPB therapy as you would on a legal medical record.

_____

_____

_____

_____

_____

_____

_____

EXERCISE 6.6 Computerized Lung Simulator

1. Original settings:

   Compliance: _____

   Resistance: _____

   Pressure: _____

   Flow: _____

   Volume achieved: _____

   Inspiratory time: _____

2. Increased resistance:

   Compliance: _____

   Resistance: _____

   Pressure: _____

   Flow: _____

   Volume achieved: _____

   Inspiratory time: _____

3. Decreased compliance:

   Compliance: _____

   Resistance: _____

   Pressure: _____

   Flow: _____

   Volume achieved: _____

   Inspiratory time: _____

4. Increased compliance:

   Compliance: _____

   Resistance: _____

Pressure: _____

Flow: _____

Volume achieved: _____

Inspiratory time: _____

Critical Thinking Questions

Mr. Rodriguez is a 29-year-old man with quadriplegia as a result of a spinal cord injury. He has been having episodes of recurrent atelectasis in the right lower lobe (RLL).

1. What therapeutic hyperinflation technique would you recommend as most appropriate for this patient?

2. Mr. Rodriguez is noted to have a reduced inspiratory and vital capacity.

    A. On the Bird IPPB machine, which control(s) could be adjusted to increase the volume achieved during therapy?

    B. How would you adjust the setting of these control(s) for this purpose?

    C. If a Bennett machine is used, which control(s) could be adjusted to increase the volume? How would the control(s) be adjusted?

3. Mr. Rodriguez is having difficulty initiating inspiration during IPPB. Which control should be adjusted? How should it be adjusted?

4. It is noted during IPPB therapy that the pressure gauge is rising very slowly during the first half of inspiration. What control could be adjusted to correct this situation?

5. The patient complains of light-headedness, paresthesias, and headache during incentive spirometry therapy. What is the most likely cause and how would you correct this situation?

6. A patient with COPD who is breathing on hypoxic drive is being given an IPPB treatment to prevent impending respiratory failure. How would you adjust the F_IO_2? Describe the difference in this adjustment between a Bird versus a Bennett machine.

7. A Bird IPPB device is noted to be stuck in the inspiratory position. Identify three causes of this problem and what you would need to do to correct each situation.

8. What types of patients would most benefit from incentive spirometry?

9. How can the effectiveness of incentive spirometry therapy be determined?

10. During IPPB therapy, a patient suddenly complains of a sharp, left-sided chest pain. She becomes cyanotic and dyspneic. How would you assess this patient's condition and what actions should be taken?

Procedural Competency Evaluation

STUDENT: DATE:

INCENTIVE SPIROMETRY

Evaluator: ☐ Peer ☐ Instructor	**Setting:** ☐ Lab ☐ Clinical Simulation	
Equipment Utilized:	**Conditions (Describe):**	

Performance Level:

S or ✓ = Satisfactory, no errors of omission or commission
U = Unsatisfactory Error of Omission or Commission
NA = Not applicable

Performance Rating:

5 **Independent:** Near flawless performance; minimal errors; able to perform without supervision; seeks out new learning; shows initiative; A = 4.7–5.0 average

4 **Minimally Supervised:** Few errors, able to self-correct; seeks guidance when appropriate; B = 3.7–4.65

3 **Competent:** Minimal required level; no critical errors; able to correct with coaching; meets expectations; safe; C = 3.0–3.65

2 **Marginal:** Below average; critical errors or problem areas noted; would benefit from remediation; D = 2.0–2.99

1 **Dependent:** Poor; unacceptable performance; unsafe; gross inaccuracies; potentially harmful; F = < 2.0

Two or more errors of commission or omission of mandatory or essential performance elements will terminate the procedure, and require additional practice and/or remediation and reevaluation. Student is responsible for obtaining additional evaluation forms as needed from the Director of Clinical Education (DCE).

(Right-side columns: PERFORMANCE RATING | PERFORMANCE LEVEL)

	PERFORMANCE RATING	PERFORMANCE LEVEL
EQUIPMENT AND PATIENT PREPARATION		
1. Common Performance Elements Steps 1–8		
2. Determines patient's pain medication schedule and coordinates therapy as needed		
3. Assesses and instructs patient pre-operatively if possible		
ASSESSMENT AND IMPLEMENTATION		
4. Common Performance Elements Steps 9 and 10		
5. Assesses vital signs, breath sounds, and chest x-ray		
6. Instructs patient in splinting if needed		
7. Measures VT, IC, and SVC with respirometer		
8. Instructs patient to inhale slowly to inspiratory capacity; with 5–10 second inspiratory hold if tolerated		
9. Instructs patient to repeat 6–10 times per hour		
10. Coaches and assists patient's technique		
11. Allows adequate recovery time between breaths to prevent hyperventilation		
12. Evaluates and reinstructs patient performance		
13. Sets volume or flow rate goals		
FOLLOW-UP		
14. Ensures IS device is within patient's reach		
15. Periodically reassesses and reevaluates goals		
16. Common Performance Elements Steps 11–16		

SIGNATURES   Student: Evaluator: Date:

Clinical Performance Evaluation

PERFORMANCE RATING:

5 **Independent:** Near flawless performance; minimal errors; able to perform without supervision; seeks out new learning; shows initiative; A = 4.7–5.0 average

4 **Minimally Supervised:** Few errors, able to self-correct; seeks guidance when appropriate; B = 3.7–4.65

3 **Competent:** Minimal required level; no critical errors; able to correct with coaching; meets expectations; safe; C = 3.0–3.65

2 **Marginal:** Below average; critical errors or problem areas noted; would benefit from remediation; D = 2.0–2.99

1 **Dependent:** Poor; unacceptable performance; unsafe; gross inaccuracies; potentially harmful; F = < 2.0

Circle the appropriate response below. Please be consistent, objective, and honest in your assessment of the student's clinical performance and ability.

PERFORMANCE CRITERIA	SCORE				
COGNITIVE DOMAIN					
1. Consistently displays knowledge, comprehension, and command of essential concepts	5	4	3	2	1
2. Demonstrates the relationship between theory and clinical practice	5	4	3	2	1
3. Able to select, review, apply, analyze, synthesize, interpret, and evaluate information; makes recommendations to modify care plan	5	4	3	2	1
PSYCHOMOTOR DOMAIN					
4. Minimal errors, no critical errors; able to self-correct; performs all steps safely and accurately	5	4	3	2	1
5. Selects, assembles, and verifies proper function and cleanliness of equipment; assures operation and corrects malfunctions; provides adequate care and maintenance	5	4	3	2	1
6. Exhibits the required manual dexterity	5	4	3	2	1
7. Performs procedure in a reasonable time frame for clinical level	5	4	3	2	1
8. Applies and maintains aseptic technique and PPE as required	5	4	3	2	1
9. Maintains concise and accurate patient and clinical records	5	4	3	2	1
10. Reports promptly on patient status/needs to appropriate personnel	5	4	3	2	1
AFFECTIVE DOMAIN					
11. Exhibits courteous and pleasant demeanor; shows consideration and respect, honesty, and integrity	5	4	3	2	1
12. Communicates verbally and in writing clearly and concisely	5	4	3	2	1
13. Preserves confidentiality and adheres to all policies	5	4	3	2	1
14. Follows directions, exhibits sound judgment, and seeks help when required	5	4	3	2	1
15. Demonstrates initiative, self-direction, responsibility, and accountability	5	4	3	2	1

TOTAL POINTS = _____ /15 = AVERAGE GRADE = _____

ADDITIONAL COMMENTS: IDENTIFY AREAS OF EXCELLENCE; LIST ERRORS OF OMISSION OR COMMISSION, CRITICAL ERRORS

SUMMARY PERFORMANCE EVALUATION AND RECOMMENDATIONS

☐ PASS: Satisfactory Performance

☐ Minimal supervision needed, may progress to next level provided specific skills, clinical time completed

☐ Minimal supervision needed, able to progress to next level without remediation

☐ FAIL: Unsatisfactory Performance (check all that apply)

☐ Minor reevaluation only

☐ Needs additional clinical practice before reevaluation

☐ Needs additional laboratory practice before skills performed in clinical area

☐ Recommend clinical probation

SIGNATURES

Evaluator (print name): _____   Evaluator signature: _____   Date: _____

Student Signature: _____   Date: _____

Student Comments:

Procedural Competency Evaluation

STUDENT: DATE:

INTERMITTENT POSITIVE PRESSURE BREATHING (IPPB)

					PERFORMANCE RATING	PERFORMANCE LEVEL
Evaluator: ☐ Peer ☐ Instructor		**Setting:** ☐ Lab		☐ Clinical Simulation		
Equipment Utilized:		**Conditions (Describe):**				

Performance Level:

S or ✓ = Satisfactory, no errors of omission or commission
U = Unsatisfactory Error of Omission or Commission
NA = Not applicable

Performance Rating:

5 **Independent:** Near flawless performance; minimal errors; able to perform without supervision; seeks out new learning; shows initiative; A = 4.7–5.0 average

4 **Minimally Supervised:** Few errors, able to self-correct; seeks guidance when appropriate; B = 3.7–4.65

3 **Competent:** Minimal required level; no critical errors; able to correct with coaching; meets expectations; safe; C = 3.0–3.65

2 **Marginal:** Below average; critical errors or problem areas noted; would benefit from remediation; D = 2.0–2.99

1 **Dependent:** Poor; unacceptable performance; unsafe; gross inaccuracies; potentially harmful; F = < 2.0

Two or more errors of commission or omission of mandatory or essential performance elements will terminate the procedure, and require additional practice and/or remediation and reevaluation. Student is responsible for obtaining additional evaluation forms as needed from the Director of Clinical Education (DCE).

EQUIPMENT AND PATIENT PREPARATION		
1. Common Performance Elements Steps 1–8		
2. Connects circuit to the ventilator		
3. Uses filter on machine outlet		
4. Ensures integrity of connections (leak check)		
5. Adjusts ventilator to acceptable baseline settings		
A. Sensitivity (one thumb above auto-cycle)		
B. Pressure 10–15 cm		
C. Flow 10–15 Lpm		
D. F_IO_2 or air-mix		
ASSESSMENT AND IMPLEMENTATION		
6. Common Performance Elements Steps 9 and 10		
7. Evaluates chest x-ray and breath sounds		
8. Measures tidal volume, VC, and peak flow		
9. Aseptically inserts medication into nebulizer		
10. Instructs patient in initiation of a positive pressure breath		
11. Applies noseclips, mouth flange, or mask as appropriate		
12. Adjusts ventilator to optimize treatment for VT; approx. 10–20 mL/Kg ideal body weight		
A. Instructs the patient not to exhale forcefully against exhalation valve		
B. Instructs the patient to breath slowly to prevent hyperventilation		
C. Reinstructs patient in technique as needed		
13. Monitors exhaled volumes using VentiComp™ bag or respirometer		
14. Monitors vital signs, SpO_2, and breath sounds		
15. Evaluates effectiveness of treatment		
16. Assists and encourages patient cough; examines and collects sputum		
FOLLOW-UP		
17. Common Performance Elements Steps 11–16		

SIGNATURES   Student: Evaluator: Date:

Clinical Performance Evaluation

PERFORMANCE RATING:

5 **Independent:** Near flawless performance; minimal errors; able to perform without supervision; seeks out new learning; shows initiative; A = 4.7–5.0 average

4 **Minimally Supervised:** Few errors, able to self-correct; seeks guidance when appropriate; B = 3.7–4.65

3 **Competent:** Minimal required level; no critical errors; able to correct with coaching; meets expectations; safe; C = 3.0–3.65

2 **Marginal:** Below average; critical errors or problem areas noted; would benefit from remediation; D = 2.0–2.99

1 **Dependent:** Poor; unacceptable performance; unsafe; gross inaccuracies; potentially harmful; F = < 2.0

Circle the appropriate response below. Please be consistent, objective, and honest in your assessment of the student's clinical performance and ability.

PERFORMANCE CRITERIA	SCORE				
COGNITIVE DOMAIN					
1. Consistently displays knowledge, comprehension, and command of essential concepts	5	4	3	2	1
2. Demonstrates the relationship between theory and clinical practice	5	4	3	2	1
3. Able to select, review, apply, analyze, synthesize, interpret, and evaluate information; makes recommendations to modify care plan	5	4	3	2	1
PSYCHOMOTOR DOMAIN					
4. Minimal errors, no critical errors; able to self-correct; performs all steps safely and accurately	5	4	3	2	1
5. Selects, assembles, and verifies proper function and cleanliness of equipment; assures operation and corrects malfunctions; provides adequate care and maintenance	5	4	3	2	1
6. Exhibits the required manual dexterity	5	4	3	2	1
7. Performs procedure in a reasonable time frame for clinical level	5	4	3	2	1
8. Applies and maintains aseptic technique and PPE as required	5	4	3	2	1
9. Maintains concise and accurate patient and clinical records	5	4	3	2	1
10. Reports promptly on patient status/needs to appropriate personnel	5	4	3	2	1
AFFECTIVE DOMAIN					
11. Exhibits courteous and pleasant demeanor; shows consideration and respect, honesty, and integrity	5	4	3	2	1
12. Communicates verbally and in writing clearly and concisely	5	4	3	2	1
13. Preserves confidentiality and adheres to all policies	5	4	3	2	1
14. Follows directions, exhibits sound judgment, and seeks help when required	5	4	3	2	1
15. Demonstrates initiative, self-direction, responsibility, and accountability	5	4	3	2	1

TOTAL POINTS = _____ /15 = AVERAGE GRADE = _____

ADDITIONAL COMMENTS: IDENTIFY AREAS OF EXCELLENCE; LIST ERRORS OF OMISSION OR COMMISSION, CRITICAL ERRORS

SUMMARY PERFORMANCE EVALUATION AND RECOMMENDATIONS

☐ PASS: Satisfactory Performance

　☐ Minimal supervision needed, may progress to next level provided specific skills, clinical time completed

　☐ Minimal supervision needed, able to progress to next level without remediation

☐ FAIL: Unsatisfactory Performance (check all that apply)

　☐ Minor reevaluation only

　☐ Needs additional clinical practice before reevaluation

　☐ Needs additional laboratory practice before skills performed in clinical area

　☐ Recommend clinical probation

SIGNATURES

Evaluator (print name): _____　　Evaluator signature: _____　　Date: _____

Student Signature: _____　　Date: _____

Student Comments:

17 Bronchial Hygiene: Chest Physiotherapy

INTRODUCTION

Chest physiotherapy techniques will be discussed in this chapter. Adjunct and breathing exercises will be discussed in Chapter 18.

Increased mucus production or impaired cough ability from physical limitations can overwhelm the body's normal clearance mechanisms and lead to retained secretions. Removal of retained secretions and improved cough effort are necessary to prevent atelectasis and infection. Bronchial hygiene incorporates several techniques and therapies, each with unique indications, contraindications, and hazards, to compensate for physical limitations and assist in the removal of secretions. These techniques may be performed either manually or with the use of mechanically assisted devices. By using gravity and mechanical vibration, secretions can be mobilized to a point at which they may be spontaneously expectorated. If the patient does not have an adequate cough effort, the respiratory care practitioner (RCP) must incorporate additional procedures to remove the secretions or results may be less than optimal. Responsibilities of the RCP also include instruction of patients and their families in these techniques for home administration.

Bronchial hygiene techniques include the following:

1. Chest physiotherapy (CPT)
   A. Postural drainage
   B. Chest percussion
   C. Expiratory vibration
2. Directed cough and manual-assisted cough
3. Vibratory positive expiratory pressure (PEP) therapy and similar adjuncts
4. High-frequency chest wall oscillating (HFCWO) vest
5. Breathing exercises
6. Inspiratory resistive muscle training

OBJECTIVES

Upon completion of this chapter, the student will be able to:

1. Identify each lobe and segment of the lungs and the corresponding bronchi on a lung model.
2. Properly position and perform postural drainage, percussion, and vibration techniques for all lung lobes and segments.
3. After reviewing x ray reports and assessing physical examination results, perform chest physical therapy techniques to the appropriate lobes and segments.

KEY TERMS

apices   lobe   sputum
copious   segment

Exercises

EQUIPMENT REQUIRED

☐ Adult mannequin
☐ Bed sheets
☐ Blood pressure manometer and cuffs
☐ Foam wedge
☐ Hospital bed, electrical (if available)
☐ Infant mannequin
☐ Infectious waste disposal basin
☐ Mechanical percussor
☐ Nonsterile gloves
☐ Percussion cups, various sizes

☐ Pillows and pillowcases
☐ Pulse oximeter and probes
☐ Segmented lung model and tracheobronchial tree
☐ Stethoscope
☐ Tilt table (if hospital bed is not available)
☐ Tissues
☐ Towels
☐ Watch with second hand

EXERCISE 17.1 IDENTIFICATION OF LUNG LOBES AND SEGMENTS

Using a segmented lung model and Figure 17.1, identify the lobes of the lung. Using a segmented lung model and Figure 17.2, identify all the lung segments.

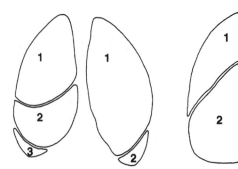

Figure 17.1. Lobes of the lung.

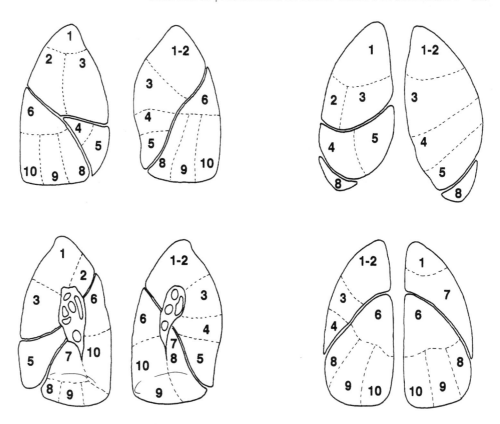

Figure 17.2. Lung segments.

RIGHT LUNG	LEFT LUNG
Right upper lobe (RUL)	**Left upper lobe (LUL)**
1 Apical	1–2 Apical posterior
2 Posterior	3 Anterior
3 Anterior	
Right middle lobe (RML)	
4 Lateral	4 Superior lingula
5 Medial	5 Inferior lingula
Right lower lobe (RLL)	**Left lower lobe (LLL)**
6 Superior	6 Superior
7 Medial basal	7–8 Anteromedial basal
8 Anterior basal	9 Lateral basal
9 Lateral basal	10 Posterior basal
10 Posterior basal	

Using the model of the tracheobronchial tree and Figure 17.3, identify the major lobar and segmental bronchi.

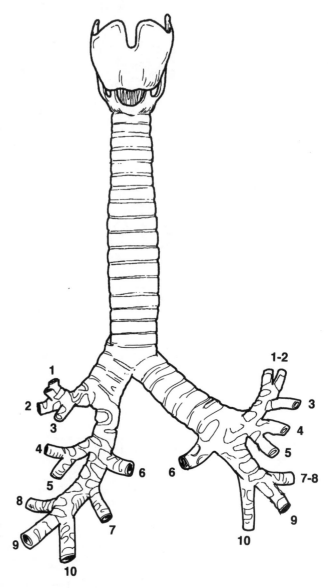

Figure 17.3. Tracheobronchial tree.

EXERCISE 17.2 POSTURAL DRAINAGE

NOTE: Because all of the following procedures for mobilization of secretions involve a patient cough effort, local exhaust ventilation and personal protective equipment may be necessary to prevent exposure to droplet nuclei in an actual clinical setting as well as in the lab with fellow students. Standard precautions and transmission-based isolation procedures should be followed.

EXERCISE 17.2.1 POSTURAL DRAINAGE POSITIONING IN INFANTS

To drain the anterior basal segments of the lower lobes, two alternative positions have been suggested by different authors.[1,2]

NOTE: The baby should always be kept facing the practitioner to provide for direct visualization and to permit a rapid response to changing levels of tolerance.

1. Using an infant mannequin, practice positioning an infant mannequin in your lab on a pillow as shown in Figure 17.4.
2. Place the "infant" in each position to drain all lobes and segments, from most dependent to least dependent lobes and segments (in infants this is **apices** to bases).

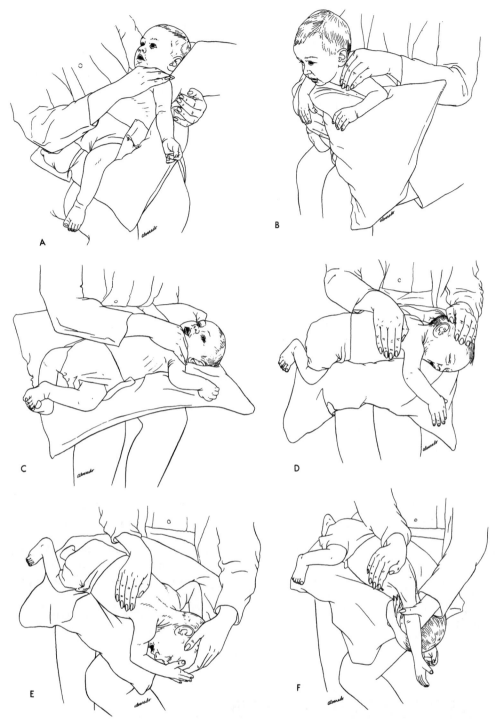

Figure 17.4. Postural drainage positions in infants. [From Waring, WW: Diagnostic and therapeutic procedures. In Chernick, V (ed): Kendig's Disorders of the Respiratory Tract in Children, ed 5. WB Saunders, Philadelphia, 1990, pp. 86–87, with permission.]

(continued)

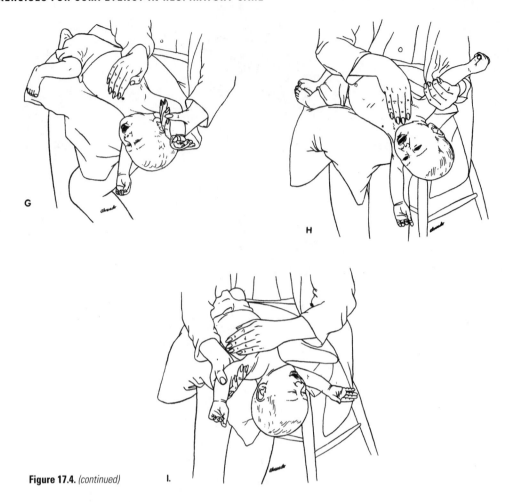

Figure 17.4. *(continued)*

EXERCISE 17.2.2 POSTURAL DRAINAGE POSITIONING IN ADULTS

NOTE: The practitioner should always be positioned facing the patient to provide for direct visualization and to permit a rapid response to changing levels of tolerance. Roll the patient toward you, not away.

1. Using a laboratory partner or an adult mannequin, practice properly positioning a patient for postural drainage on a bed or table.
2. Place the "patient" in each position to drain all lobes and segments, from most dependent to least dependent lobes and segments (in adults this is from bases to apices).
3. Use pillows and foam wedges to help maintain the proper positions.

EXERCISE 17.3 CHEST PERCUSSION

Practice the technique of chest percussion as shown in Figure 17.5, using your laboratory partner as the "patient."

1. Remove your jewelry and wash or sanitize your hands. Apply standard precautions and transmission-based isolation procedures as appropriate.
2. Cup your hands and allow for relaxed motion from the wrist. Do not stiffen your upper arms. Rhythmically strike the designated area, alternating hands.
3. Practice first on your thigh. Listen for a hollow "clapping" or "galloping" sound. This sound should be audible to someone not in the room, but should not cause pain or discomfort.
4. Position the "patient" for postural drainage (any position may be used for this exercise).
5. Perform chest percussion on the "patient" for at least 3 minutes. Remember the following precautions:
   A. Do not percuss over any buttons, zippers, or similar items that the subject may have on.

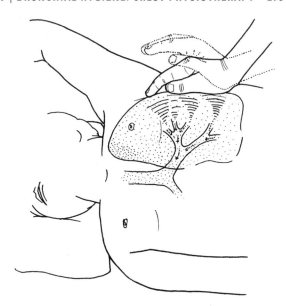

Figure 17.5. Chest percussion technique.

 B. Do not percuss on bare skin. On an actual patient, use a towel or sheet over the patient's skin.

 C. Avoid bony processes. Do not percuss on the spine, on clavicles, on scapulae, on breast tissue, over areas of incisions, over areas of rib fractures, or below the rib margins.

6. Repeat the procedure using a mechanical percussion device (Fig. 17.6). Vary the speed and force to observe the effects.

7. Repeat the procedure using percussion cups (Fig. 17.7), one in each hand. Small sizes are available for children and infants, or a small face mask may be used by sealing the opening with tape.

8. Baby G is going to be discharged tomorrow. With your laboratory partner acting as the parent, instruct the "parent" on how to perform these procedures.

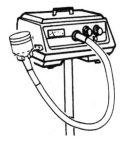

Figure 17.6. Mechanical percussor. (Courtesy of General Physiotherapy, Inc., St. Louis, MO.)

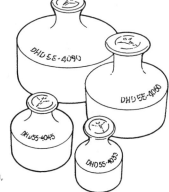

Figure 17.7. Percussion cups. (Courtesy of Diemolding Corp., Diemolding Healthcare Division, Canastota, NY.)

EXERCISE 17.4 EXPIRATORY VIBRATION

Practice the technique of expira-tory vibration, using your laboratory partner as the patient.

1. Remove jewelry and wash or sanitize your hands. Apply standard precautions and transmission-based isolation procedures as appropriate.

2. Place the "patient" in any position for postural drainage in which he or she is lying down.

3. Place one hand over the other on the area to be vibrated, as shown in Figure 17.8.

4. Instruct the "patient" to take a deep breath and exhale slowly through pursed lips.

5. Apply a gentle vibrating motion during exhalation only. Your upper arm muscles should tighten and allow transmission of the vibration to your hands. Do not shake the "patient." Repeat the vibration technique two or three times for each segment.

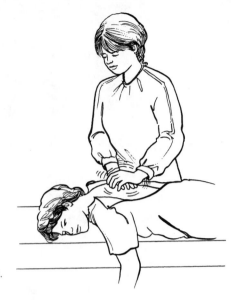

Figure 17.8. Expiratory vibration technique. (From Pierce, LNB: Guide to Mechanical Ventilation and Intensive Respiratory Care. WB Saunders, Philadelphia, 1995, p. 143, with permission.)

EXERCISE 17.5 CHEST PHYSIOTHERAPY

Perform a complete chest physiotherapy treatment with postural drainage, percussion, and vibration on your lab partner or a human patient simulator.

1. Review any pertinent data on the "patient's" chart, including physician's orders or protocol, history and physical examination, diagnosis, x-ray results, and any precautions or possible contraindications to performing the procedure.
2. Wash or sanitize your hands and apply standard precautions and transmission-based isolation procedures as appropriate.
3. Coordinate therapy before meals and tube feedings or 1½ hours after.
4. Introduce yourself to the "patient" and explain the procedure.
5. Assess the "patient" before therapy. Assessment should include the following:
   Pulse
   Respirations
   SpO_2
   Blood pressure
   Chest symmetry and expansion using palpation
   Color
   Level of dyspnea
   Level of cooperation
6. Place the "patient" in each of the positions for drainage shown in Figure 17.9. Use pillows to support the "patient" where necessary. Begin with the most dependent segments first.

NOTE: In an actual clinical situation, the patient would remain in each position for a minimum of 3 to 15 minutes as tolerated, for drainage.[3] In special circumstances, the patient may remain in drainage positions for longer periods of time.

7. Allow the "patient" to sit up and cough after each position. An immediate response does not always result. The practitioner may need to check back with the "patient" at a later time to determine any sputum production after the treatment.
8. Reassess the "patient's" tolerance in each position by evaluating the following:
   Pulse
   Respirations
   SpO_2
   Blood pressure
   Color
   Level of dyspnea
   Level of cooperation
9. Note the volume, consistency, color, and presence or absence of blood in the sputum. Note which positions are most productive.
10. **Chart the therapy on your laboratory report.**

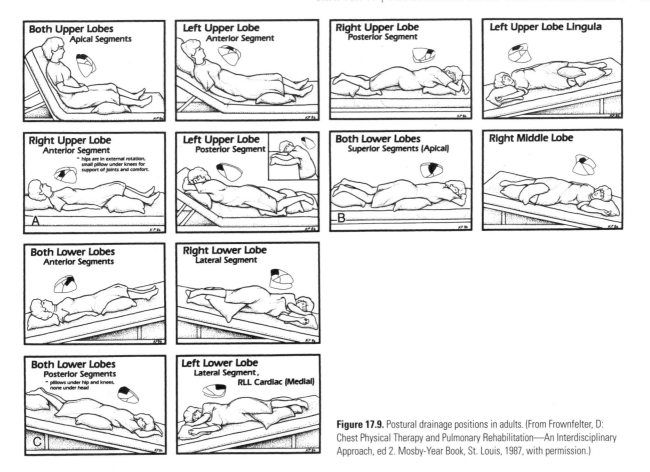

Figure 17.9. Postural drainage positions in adults. (From Frownfelter, D: Chest Physical Therapy and Pulmonary Rehabilitation—An Interdisciplinary Approach, ed 2. Mosby-Year Book, St. Louis, 1987, with permission.)

REFERENCES
1. Frownfelter, D, Dean, E: Cardiovascular and Pulmonary Physical Therapy: Evidence and Practice, ed 4. Mosby, St. Louis, 2006.
2. Wilkins, R et al. (eds): Egan's Fundamentals of Respiratory Care, ed 8. Mosby, St. Louis, 2003.
3. American Association for Respiratory Care: AARC clinical practice guideline: Postural drainage therapy. Respir Care 36:1418–1426, 1991.

Laboratory Report

CHAPTER 17: BRONCHIAL HYGIENE: CHEST PHYSIOTHERAPY

Name _____   Date _____

Course/Section _____   Instructor _____

Data Collection

EXERCISE 17.1 Identification of Lung Lobes and Segments

Right	Left
1	1
2	2
3	

Right	Left
Lobe	
1	1 and 2
2	
3	3
Lobe	
4	4
5	5
Lobe	
6	6
7	7 and 8
8	
9	9
10	10

EXERCISE 17.2   Postural Drainage

Identify the lobes and segments being drained in Figure 17.10.

A: _____

B: _____

C: _____

D: _____

E: _____

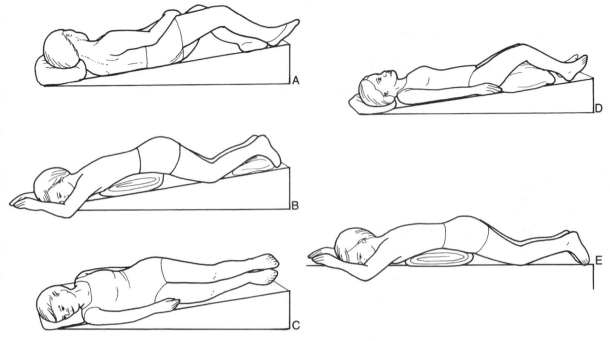

Figure 17.10. Label the segments being drained in the positions shown.

EXERCISE 17.5 Chest Physiotherapy

Chart the therapy:

_____

_____

_____

_____

_____

_____

_____

_____

Critical Thinking Questions

1. Identify normal airway clearance mechanisms in each of the following sections of the respiratory system:

    A. Upper airway

    B. Larynx

C.   Tracheobronchial tree

D.   Respiratory unit

2.   Identify at least 10 conditions that would lead to ineffective secretion clearance.

3.   Identify at least three hazards of coughing.

4.   According to the AARC clinical practice guidelines (CPGs), how much sputum needs to be produced daily to be considered copious?

5.   Explain the role of hydration in mobilization of secretions.

6.   What is meant by the expression to "keep the good lung down"?

A.   What exceptions are there to this rule?

7.   When is prone positioning indicated?

A.   Explain how it may help improve the patient condition.

8. Why is it recommended *not* to let the patient cough in the Trendelenburg position?

9. An 82-year-old woman with a history of osteoporosis who has recently undergone thoracic surgery has been producing large amounts of purulent secretions. The physician has ordered CPT. What contraindications or precautions would you need to be aware of? What recommendations or modifications would you suggest to accomplish this therapy?

10. A 17-year-old girl with cystic fibrosis who has copious sputum production complains of dyspnea and shows signs of mild cyanosis during postural drainage positioning in the Trendelenburg position.

    A. What modifications on recommendations can be made to improve the patient's tolerance of the procedure?

    B. How would you monitor the effectiveness of these modifications?

11. A 25-year-old man with quadriplegia and a tracheostomy has been experiencing recurrent atelectasis in the RML and RLL.

    A. How would you assess what positions to place the patient in for postural drainage?

    B. Describe the appropriate positioning in this situation.

    C. The patient is unable to adequately cough spontaneously after postural drainage. What techniques could be incorporated to improve his cough effort and to remove any mobilized secretions?

Procedural Competency Evaluation

STUDENT: **DATE:**

CHEST PHYSIOTHERAPYY

					PERFORMANCE RATING	PERFORMANCE LEVEL
Evaluator: ☐ Peer ☐ Instructor			**Setting:** ☐ Lab	☐ Clinical Simulation		
Equipment Utilized:			**Conditions (Describe):**			

Performance Level:

S or ✓ = Satisfactory, no errors of omission or commission
U = Unsatisfactory Error of Omission or Commission
NA = Not applicable

Performance Rating:

5 **Independent:** Near flawless performance; minimal errors; able to perform without supervision; seeks out new learning; shows initiative; A = 4.7–5.0 average

4 **Minimally Supervised:** Few errors, able to self-correct; seeks guidance when appropriate; B = 3.7–4.65

3 **Competent:** Minimal required level; no critical errors; able to correct with coaching; meets expectations; safe; C = 3.0–3.65

2 **Marginal:** Below average; critical errors or problem areas noted; would benefit from remediation; D = 2.0–2.99

1 **Dependent:** Poor; unacceptable performance; unsafe; gross inaccuracies; potentially harmful; F = < 2.0

Two or more errors of commission or omission of mandatory or essential performance elements will terminate the procedure, and require additional practice and/or remediation and reevaluation. Student is responsible for obtaining additional evaluation forms as needed from the Director of Clinical Education (DCE).

EQUIPMENT AND PATIENT PREPARATION

1. Common Performance Elements Steps 1–8

ASSESSMENT AND IMPLEMENTATION

2. Common Performance Elements Steps 9 and 10
3. Determines lobes and segments to be drained by assessing CXR, progress notes, and breath sounds
4. Verifies no relative or absolute contraindications exist; modifies procedure accordingly
5. Coordinates therapy prior to meals and tube feedings or 1 to 1 1/2 hours after meals
6. Correctly positions patient for segments to be drained, 3–15 minutes as tolerated
  A. Positions self to always be facing the patient
  B. Performs drainage beginning with dependent lung segments first (age appropriate)
7. Performs percussion in correct locations for 3–5 minutes as tolerated
  A. Uses appropriate hand position, adjuncts such as palm cups or mechanical percussors
  B. Uses appropriate light cover
  C. Produces appropriate sound
  D. Does not percuss over bone, incisions, jewelry, buttons, or below ribs
8. Performs expiratory vibration with pressure appropriate to patient tolerance
9. Assesses adequate ventilation and oxygenation during procedure; adjusts oxygen therapy as needed during therapy; checks SpO_2, pulse, respirations, and blood pressure periodically throughout therapy
10. Encourages and assists patient to cough in upright position
NOTE: patient should not be allowed to cough in Trendelenburg position
11. Repositions patient prior to departure
12. Collects, examines sputum

FOLLOW-UP

13. Evaluates, recommends alternative procedures as applicable (PEP therapy, chest oscillating vest)
14. Common Performance Elements Steps 11–16

SIGNATURES Student: Evaluator: Date:

Clinical Performance Evaluation

PERFORMANCE RATING:

5 **Independent:** Near flawless performance; minimal errors; able to perform without supervision; seeks out new learning; shows initiative; A = 4.7–5.0 average

4 **Minimally Supervised:** Few errors, able to self-correct; seeks guidance when appropriate; B = 3.7–4.65

3 **Competent:** Minimal required level; no critical errors; able to correct with coaching; meets expectations; safe; C = 3.0–3.65

2 **Marginal:** Below average; critical errors or problem areas noted; would benefit from remediation; D = 2.0–2.99

1 **Dependent:** Poor; unacceptable performance; unsafe; gross inaccuracies; potentially harmful; F = < 2.0

Circle the appropriate response below. Please be consistent, objective, and honest in your assessment of the student's clinical performance and ability.

PERFORMANCE CRITERIA	SCORE				
COGNITIVE DOMAIN					
1. Consistently displays knowledge, comprehension, and command of essential concepts	5	4	3	2	1
2. Demonstrates the relationship between theory and clinical practice	5	4	3	2	1
3. Able to select, review, apply, analyze, synthesize, interpret, and evaluate information; makes recommendations to modify care plan	5	4	3	2	1
PSYCHOMOTOR DOMAIN					
4. Minimal errors, no critical errors; able to self-correct; performs all steps safely and accurately	5	4	3	2	1
5. Selects, assembles, and verifies proper function and cleanliness of equipment; assures operation and corrects malfunctions; provides adequate care and maintenance	5	4	3	2	1
6. Exhibits the required manual dexterity	5	4	3	2	1
7. Performs procedure in a reasonable time frame for clinical level	5	4	3	2	1
8. Applies and maintains aseptic technique and PPE as required	5	4	3	2	1
9. Maintains concise and accurate patient and clinical records	5	4	3	2	1
10. Reports promptly on patient status/needs to appropriate personnel	5	4	3	2	1
AFFECTIVE DOMAIN					
11. Exhibits courteous and pleasant demeanor; shows consideration and respect, honesty, and integrity	5	4	3	2	1
12. Communicates verbally and in writing clearly and concisely	5	4	3	2	1
13. Preserves confidentiality and adheres to all policies	5	4	3	2	1
14. Follows directions, exhibits sound judgment, and seeks help when required	5	4	3	2	1
15. Demonstrates initiative, self-direction, responsibility, and accountability	5	4	3	2	1

TOTAL POINTS = _____ /15 = AVERAGE GRADE = _____

ADDITIONAL COMMENTS: IDENTIFY AREAS OF EXCELLENCE; LIST ERRORS OF OMISSION OR COMMISSION, CRITICAL ERRORS

SUMMARY PERFORMANCE EVALUATION AND RECOMMENDATIONS

☐ PASS: Satisfactory Performance

    ☐ Minimal supervision needed, may progress to next level provided specific skills, clinical time completed

    ☐ Minimal supervision needed, able to progress to next level without remediation

☐ FAIL: Unsatisfactory Performance (check all that apply)

    ☐ Minor reevaluation only

    ☐ Needs additional clinical practice before reevaluation

    ☐ Needs additional laboratory practice before skills performed in clinical area

    ☐ Recommend clinical probation

SIGNATURES

Evaluator (print name): _____ Evaluator signature: _____ Date: _____

Student Signature: _____ Date: _____

Student Comments:

18 Adjunct Techniques for Bronchial Hygiene

INTRODUCTION

Mucus clearance is an essential component of managing chronic pulmonary diseases such as cystic fibrosis, bronchiectasis, and chronic bronchitis. In addition to the pharmacologic regimen, breathing exercises, directed cough, and the use of adjunctive mucus clearance devices help with the maintenance of good pulmonary hygiene. It is essential that the respiratory care practitioner have expertise in the use of these devices as it is the role of the respiratory care practitioner to educate patients and care givers in their proper use.

OBJECTIVES

Upon completion of this chapter, the student will be able to:

1. Instruct and monitor a patient on coughing, splinting, and pursed-lip breathing.
2. Practice directed cough and manually assisted cough techniques to improve cough effectiveness according to AARC clinical practice guidelines.
3. Perform vibratory PEP therapy according to AARC clinical practice guidelines.
4. Instruct and monitor a patient on diaphragmatic, thoracic expansion, and relaxation breathing exercises.
5. Perform inspiratory muscle-training techniques.

KEY TERMS

forced expiratory technique (FET)
intracranial pressure (ICP)

intrapulmonic percussion ventilation (IPV)

positive expiratory pressure (PEP)

Exercises

EQUIPMENT REQUIRED

- [ ] 50-psi compressed air gas source
- [ ] Adult mannequin
- [ ] Disposable mouthpieces
- [ ] Flowmeter
- [ ] Infectious waste disposal basin
- [ ] Inspiratory force adaptors
- [ ] Inspiratory-resistive muscle-training devices
- [ ] Maximum inspiratory pressure manometer

- [ ] Nonsterile gloves
- [ ] Noseclips
- [ ] Pressure manometer
- [ ] Pulse oximeter and probes
- [ ] Stethoscope
- [ ] Tissues
- [ ] Vibratory PEP devices: PEP mask, Thera-Pep®, Acapella®, Flutter® valve

EXERCISE 18.1 DIRECTED COUGH

Several techniques are available to help improve the patient's cough effort. Practice patient instruction and monitoring of these techniques, using your laboratory partner as the patient. The sequence of steps in a normal cough is illustrated in Figure 18.1.

EXERCISE 18.1.1 COUGH INSTRUCTION

1. Wash or sanitize your hands and apply standard precautions and transmission-based isolation procedures as appropriate.
2. Introduce yourself to the "patient" and explain the purpose of an adequate cough effort.
3. Have the "patient" sit up in a chair or on the bed or table. Patients who cannot tolerate a sitting position can use a side-lying position with knees bent (Fig. 18.2).
4. Instruct the "patient" to take a deep breath, followed by a slight breath hold, then a cough. Have tissues and a waste receptacle readily available. Note the volume, consistency, color, and presence or absence of blood in any sputum expectorated.
5. Using a pillow or your hands, instruct the "patient" on splinting of any painful areas (Fig. 18.3). Apply gentle pressure over the involved area before deep inspiration, and increase pressure slightly during the forced expiratory phase of the cough. Use standard precautions and transmission-based isolation procedures as appropriate.

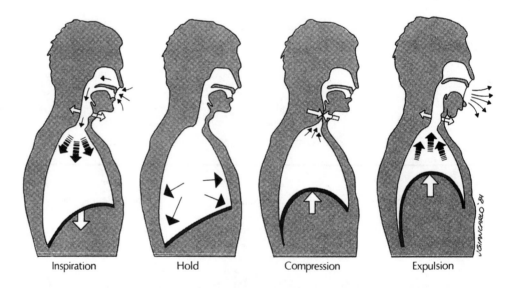

Figure 18.1. Cough reflex.

Inspiration   Hold   Compression   Expulsion

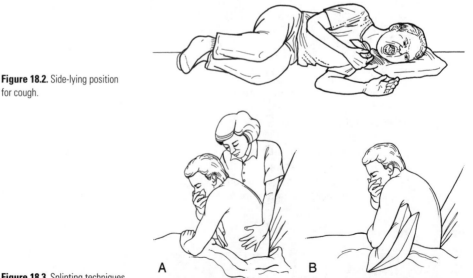

Figure 18.2. Side-lying position for cough.

Figure 18.3. Splinting techniques.

A   B

EXERCISE 18.1.2 COUGH ALTERNATIVES

Some patients do not have the capacity or tolerance for a single forceful cough. Alternative methods can be used to improve cough effectiveness, compensate for physical limitations, and provide voluntary control over the cough reflex. Instruct your laboratory partner in each of the following techniques:

1. Wash or sanitize your hands. Apply standard precautions and transmission-based isolation procedures as appropriate.

2. Introduce yourself to the "patient" and explain the purpose of the procedure. Have tissues and a waste receptacle readily available.

3. Instruct the "patient" in serial coughing techniques. Have the "patient" take a moderately deep breath, followed by a slight breath hold. Then perform two or three short coughs, one after another. Rest and repeat the procedure.

4. Instruct the "patient" in a forced expiratory technique (FET), or huffing maneuver.

   A. Have the "patient" take a moderately deep breath, followed by a short breath hold. Then perform three short forced exhalations with an open glottis. The "patient" should make a huffing or "ha ha ha" sound on exhalation. Follow this with a period of relaxed, controlled diaphragmatic breathing.

   B. This can be assisted by self-compression of the chest wall by using a brisk **adduction** movement of the upper arms[1] also known as a "chicken breath," as shown in Figure 18.4.

5. Improvement of the cough effort can be accomplished by providing a manually assisted cough, using epigastric pressure or external lateral compression of the thoracic cage[2] (Fig. 18.5).

   A. Instruct the "patient" to take a moderately deep breath, followed by a short breath hold. Apply gentle pressure to the epigastric region coordinated with the "patient's" cough effort, making sure to avoid the xiphoid area. This should not be done after meals.

   B. Instruct the "patient" to take a moderately deep breath, followed by a short breath hold. Apply pressure to the lateral thoracic cage coordinated with the "patient's" cough effort.

NOTE: In a patient with a tracheostomy, a manually assisted deep inspiration can be provided using a manual resuscitator bag in conjunction with manually assisted cough techniques, as shown in Figure 18.6.

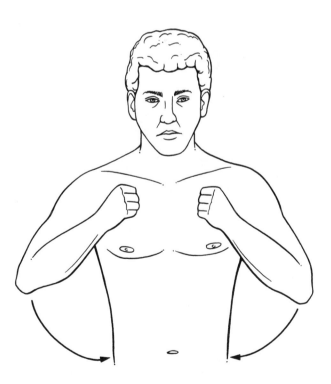

Figure 18.4. "Chicken breath" technique for use with huffing.

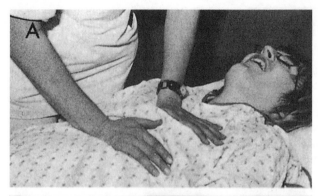

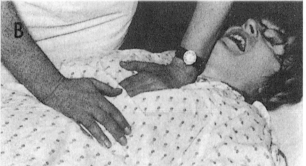

Figure 18.5. Assisted cough techniques. (From Frownfelter, D: Chest Physical Therapy and Pulmonary Rehabilitation—An Interdisciplinary Approach, ed 2. Mosby-Year Book, St. Louis, 1987, p. 264, with permission.)

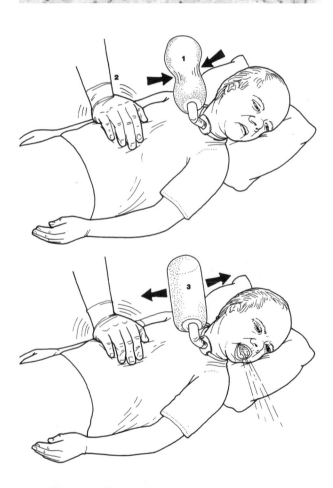

Figure 18.6. Assisted cough in a tracheostomized patient.

EXERCISE 18.2 VIBRATORY POSITIVE EXPIRATORY PRESSURE (PEP) THERAPY

PEP mask therapy has received attention as a possible adjunct or alternative to postural drainage and percussion techniques for bronchial hygiene.[3,4] Many devices are now on the market to create vibratory PEP, reverse atelectasis, and promote secretion removal.

EXERCISE 18.2.1 COMPARE VIBRATORY PEP DEVICES

1. Obtain the following devices:
   Flutter® valve (Fig. 18.7)
   PEP mask valve (Fig. 18.8)
   Thera-Pep® device (Fig. 18.9)
   Acapella® device (Fig. 18.10)
2. Assemble each device and compare the components of each.

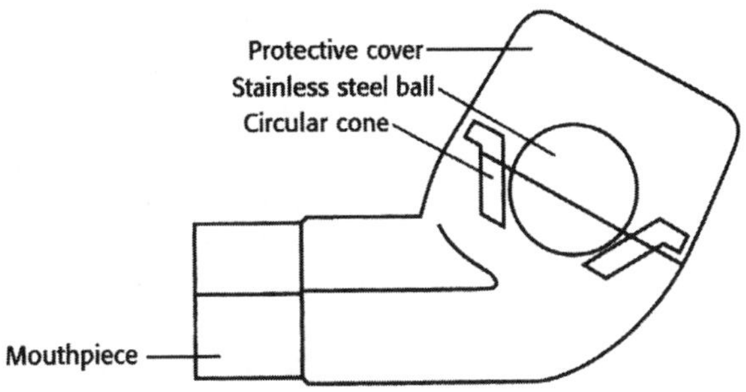

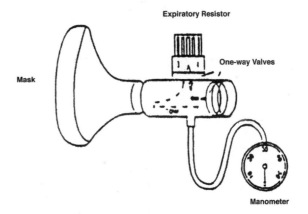

Figure 18.7. Flutter® valve. (Reprinted by permission of Nellcor Puritan Bennett, Pleasanton, CA.)

Figure 18.8. Components of a PEP mask system. (Courtesy of Resistex™, Mecury Medical, Clearwater, FL.)

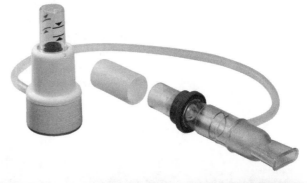

Figure 18.9. Thera-Pep® device. (Courtesy of Smiths Medical, a division of Smiths Group plc., London, UK.)

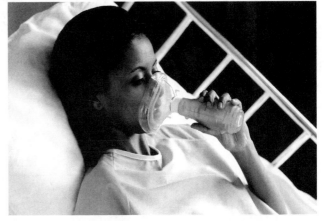

Figure 18.10. Acapella® device. (Courtesy of Smiths Medical, a division of Smiths Group plc., London, UK.)

EXERCISE 18.2.2 VIBRATORY PEP THERAPY

1. Obtain a PEP device and set it up with the pressure manometer in line.
2. Wash or sanitize your hands and apply standard precautions and transmission-based isolation procedures as appropriate.
3. Introduce yourself to the "patient" and explain the purpose of the procedure.
4. Assess the "patient's" vital signs, mental function, skin color, and breath sounds.
5. Adjust the fixed exhalation orifice to the largest setting.
6. Have the "patient" sit upright with his or her elbows resting comfortably on a table.
7. Place the mask comfortably but tightly over the nose and mouth or adjust noseclips and mouthpiece.
8. Instruct the "patient" to take a larger than normal breath (but not to total lung capacity) and exhale slowly at an I:E ratio of 1:3 or 1:4.
9. Observe the pressure generated on the manometer during exhalation. Decrease the size of the fixed orifice until 10 to 20 cm H_2O pressure is generated during exhalation. Note the "patient's" response.
10. Instruct the "patient" to take 10 to 20 breaths followed by two or three huffs (FET). In an actual clinical situation, this procedure would be repeated four to eight times for 10 to 20 minutes. Reassess the "patient" periodically.
11. Note the quantity, color, and consistency of any sputum expectorated. Note the presence or absence of blood.
12. **"Chart" the therapy on your laboratory report.**

EXERCISE 18.3 BREATHING EXERCISES

Using your laboratory partner as the patient, instruct your "patient" in the following breathing exercises:

1. Wash or sanitize your hands and apply standard precautions and transmission-based isolation procedures as appropriate.
2. Introduce yourself, and explain the procedure to the "patient."
3. Instruct the "patient" on pursed-lip breathing technique (Fig. 18.11).
   A. Have the "patient" take a deep breath through his or her nose.
   B. Instruct the "patient" to exhale through pursed lips with a slow, steady exhalation at an I:E ratio of at least 1:3.
4. Instruct the "patient" in abdominal breathing techniques.
   A. Have the "patient" lie down. For initial instruction, a slight Trendelenburg position is recommended.
   B. Place one hand on the "patient's" epigastric area and one hand on the upper chest, as shown in Figure 18.12.

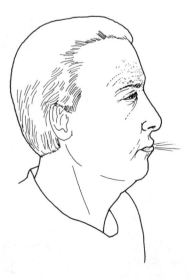

Figure 18.11. Pursed-lip breathing technique.

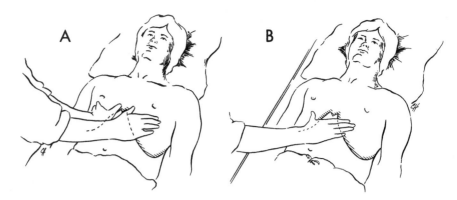

Figure 18.12. Diaphragmatic breathing. (From Frownfelter, D: Chest Physical Therapy and Pulmonary Rehabilitation—An Interdisciplinary Approach, ed 2. Mosby-Year Book, St. Louis, 1987, p. 237, with permission.)

C. Ask the "patient" to sniff or pant to feel diaphragmatic movement.

D. Instruct the "patient" to take a slow, deep breath through the mouth and exhale through pursed lips. Apply firm pressure during inspiration. The "patient" should push your hand away by protruding the abdomen. The upper chest and shoulders should expand but not move up.

E. Replace your hands with a light book or other object, and instruct the "patient" to practice moving the book up on inspiration. A bag of rice or birdseed may be used for this exercise.

F. The "patient" can eventually repeat the procedure in a more elevated position as tolerated while sitting and walking, as shown in Figures 18.13, 18.14, and 18.15.

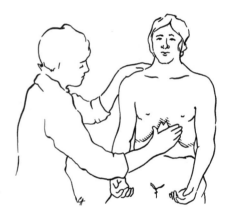

Figure 18.13. Abdominal breathing in the sitting position. (From Frownfelter, D: Chest Physical Therapy and Pulmonary Rehabilitation—An Interdisciplinary Approach, ed 2. Mosby-Year Book, St. Louis, 1987, p. 238, with permission.)

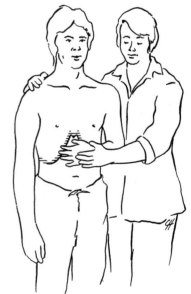

Figure 18.14. Abdominal breathing while standing. (From Frownfelter, D: Chest Physical Therapy and Pulmonary Rehabilitation—An Interdisciplinary Approach, ed 2. Mosby-Year Book, St. Louis, 1987, p. 239, with permission.)

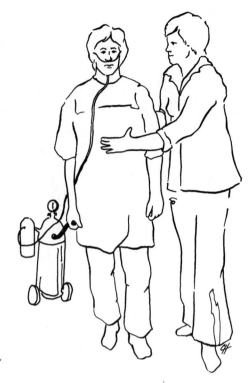

Figure 18.15. Breathing retraining while walking with oxygen. (From Frownfelter, D: Chest Physical Therapy and Pulmonary Rehabilitation—An Interdisciplinary Approach, ed 2. Mosby-Year Book, St. Louis, 1987, p. 239, with permission.)

The following relaxation techniques and exercises can be practiced at home on yourself or with a partner as the patient.

5. Have the "patient" lying in bed with head flexed slightly forward, thoracic spine straight, shoulders rotated inward slightly, elbows flexed, and hips and knees flexed.

6. Instruct the "patient" to perform the following maneuvers. The "patient" should close his or her eyes, take slow breaths, and attempt to relax the body part while holding each position for a count of 10.

    A. Turn head to right.

    B. Turn head to left.

    C. Raise head from pillow.

    D. Push head into pillow.

    E. Make a fist with both hands.

    F. Open fists.

    G. Bend wrists.

    H. Extend wrists.

    I. Bend elbows.

    J. Straighten elbows.

    K. Reach arms above head.

    L. Return arms to sides.

    M. Shrug shoulders.

    N. Raise the left leg and then lower it.

    O. Raise the right leg and then lower it.

    P. Spread legs apart.

    Q. Bring legs together.

    R. Roll knees in.

    S. Roll knees out.

    T. Flex both ankles.

    U. Extend both ankles.

    V. Curl toes.

    W. Straighten toes.

EXERCISE 18.4 INSPIRATORY-RESISTIVE MUSCLE TRAINING

Inspiratory-resistive muscle training is usually performed over a 6-week training period for approximately 30 minutes/day with a gradual increase in workload.[5]

1. Wash or sanitize your hands and apply standard precautions and transmission-based isolation procedures as appropriate.
2. Set up the device as shown in Figure 18.16 or Figure 18.17. A flow-resistive or threshold-resistive device may be used.
3. Measure the "patient's" maximum inspiratory pressure using a pressure manometer.
4. Select the inspiratory-resistive device (colored caps or dial selector) with the largest opening and apply it to the inspiratory port.
5. Attach the pressure manometer in-line to the monitoring adaptor.
6. Place noseclips comfortably on the "patient's" nose.
7. Have the "patient" make a tight seal around the mouthpiece.
8. Instruct the "patient" to inhale and exhale slowly through the mouthpiece.
9. Note the manometer pressure during inspiration. Adjust the inspiratory-resistive orifice until you are using the resistor that achieves 30% of the "patient's" MIP effort.
10. In an actual clinical situation, this would be repeated for 15 minutes twice daily.[5]
11. **"Chart" the therapy on your laboratory report.**

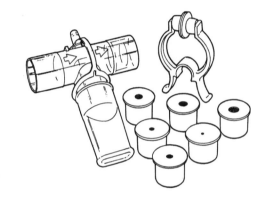

Figure 18.16. Flow-resistive inspiratory muscle-training device. (From HealthScan Products Inc., Cedar Grove, NJ, with permission.)

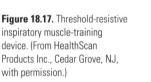

Figure 18.17. Threshold-resistive inspiratory muscle-training device. (From HealthScan Products Inc., Cedar Grove, NJ, with permission.)

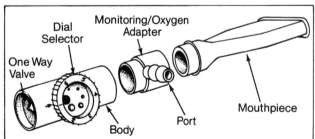

REFERENCES

1. American Association for Respiratory Care: AARC clinical practice guideline: Directed cough. Respir Care 38:495–499, 1993.
2. American Association for Respiratory Care: AARC clinical practice guideline: Postural drainage therapy. Respir Care 36:1418–1426, 1991.
3. Mahlmeister, M et al: Positive expiratory pressure mask therapy: Theoretical and practical consideration and a review of the literature. Respir Care 36:1218–1230, 1991.
4. American Association for Respiratory Care: AARC clinical practice guideline: Use of positive airway pressure adjuncts to bronchial hygiene therapy. Respir Care 38:516–521, 1993.
5. Scanlan, C et al. (eds): Egan's Fundamentals of Respiratory Care, ed 6. Mosby, St. Louis, 1995.

Laboratory Report

CHAPTER 18: ADJUNCT TECHNIQUES FOR BRONCHIAL HYGIENE

Name _____ Date _____

Course/Section _____ Instructor _____

Data Collection

EXERCISE 18.2. Vibratory Positive Expiratory Pressure (PEP) Therapy

EXERCISE 18.2.2 VIBRATORY PEP THERAPY

"Chart" the therapy given as you would on a legal medical record. Be sure to include all pertinent data and measurements.

_____
_____
_____
_____

EXERCISE 18.4 Inspiratory-Resistive Muscle Training

"Chart" the therapy given as you would on a legal medical record. Be sure to include all pertinent data and measurements.

_____
_____
_____
_____

Critical Thinking Questions

1. Identify the possible hazards of PEP mask therapy. State at least one situation in which the procedure may be contraindicated.

2. A physician has ordered chest physical therapy on a postoperative craniotomy patient whose chart indicates that the head of the bed must remain elevated 30 degrees. Identify what modifications to therapy or recommendations you believe are necessary in this situation, and explain why.

3. A 65-year-old woman with COPD has begun a breathing exercise regimen. What data (objective and subjective) would indicate beneficial effects of this program?

Procedural Competency Evaluation

STUDENT: **DATE:**

BREATHING EXERCISES

	PERFORMANCE RATING	PERFORMANCE LEVEL

Evaluator: ☐ Peer ☐ Instructor   **Setting:** ☐ Lab   ☐ Clinical Simulation

Equipment Utilized: **Conditions (Describe):**

Performance Level:

    S or ✓ = Satisfactory, no errors of omission or commission
    U = Unsatisfactory Error of Omission or Commission
    NA = Not applicable

Performance Rating:

    5   **Independent:** Near flawless performance; minimal errors; able to perform without supervision; seeks out new learning; shows initiative; A = 4.7–5.0 average

    4   **Minimally Supervised:** Few errors, able to self-correct; seeks guidance when appropriate; B = 3.7–4.65

    3   **Competent:** Minimal required level; no critical errors; able to correct with coaching; meets expectations; safe; C = 3.0–3.65

    2   **Marginal:** Below average; critical errors or problem areas noted; would benefit from remediation; D = 2.0–2.99

    1   **Dependent:** Poor; unacceptable performance; unsafe; gross inaccuracies; potentially harmful; F = < 2.0

    Two or more errors of commission or omission of mandatory or essential performance elements will terminate the procedure, and require additional practice and/or remediation and reevaluation. Student is responsible for obtaining additional evaluation forms as needed from the Director of Clinical Education (DCE).

EQUIPMENT AND PATIENT PREPARATION

1. Common Performance Elements Steps 1–8

ASSESSMENT AND IMPLEMENTATION

2. Common Performance Elements Steps 9 and 10

3. Assesses vital signs, SpO$_2$, VC, peak flow and MIP prior to instruction

4. Instructs patient on pursed-lip breathing technique (1:2 ratio, at least 1:3)

5. Performs 6-minute walk

    A. Walks with patient on level ground for six minutes as tolerated

    B. Has wheel chair and oxygen device available at all times

    C. Measures distance walked

    D. Monitors SpO$_2$, pulse, respiratory rate and blood pressure

6. Instructs the patient in abdominal breathing techniques

    A. Has patient lay down in supine or slight Trendelenburg position as tolerated

    B. Places one hand on the patient's epigastric area and one hand on the upper chest

    C. Asks patient to "sniff" or "pant" to feel diaphragmatic movement

    D. Instructs patient to take a slow deep breath through his/her mouth and exhale through pursed lips

    E. Applies firm pressure during inspiration

    F. Replaces hands with a light book or other object and instructs the patient to practice

7. Repeats the procedure in a more elevated position

8. Repeats procedure while sitting and walking, as tolerated

9. Instructs patient in relaxation techniques
    A. With patient in supine position, performs head to toe relaxation techniques

10. Instructs patient in inspiratory muscle resistive training techniques (see PCE for Muscle Training)

FOLLOW-UP

11. Common Performance Elements Steps 11–16

SIGNATURES   Student: Evaluator: Date:

Clinical Performance Evaluation

PERFORMANCE RATING:

5 Independent: Near flawless performance; minimal errors; able to perform without supervision; seeks out new learning; shows initiative; A = 4.7–5.0 average

4 Minimally Supervised: Few errors, able to self-correct; seeks guidance when appropriate; B = 3.7–4.65

3 Competent: Minimal required level; no critical errors; able to correct with coaching; meets expectations; safe; C = 3.0–3.65

2 Marginal: Below average; critical errors or problem areas noted; would benefit from remediation; D = 2.0–2.99

1 Dependent: Poor; unacceptable performance; unsafe; gross inaccuracies; potentially harmful; F = < 2.0

Circle the appropriate response below. Please be consistent, objective, and honest in your assessment of the student's clinical performance and ability.

PERFORMANCE CRITERIA

PERFORMANCE CRITERIA	SCORE				
COGNITIVE DOMAIN					
1. Consistently displays knowledge, comprehension, and command of essential concepts	5	4	3	2	1
2. Demonstrates the relationship between theory and clinical practice	5	4	3	2	1
3. Able to select, review, apply, analyze, synthesize, interpret, and evaluate information; makes recommendations to modify care plan	5	4	3	2	1
PSYCHOMOTOR DOMAIN					
4. Minimal errors, no critical errors; able to self-correct; performs all steps safely and accurately	5	4	3	2	1
5. Selects, assembles, and verifies proper function and cleanliness of equipment; assures operation and corrects malfunctions; provides adequate care and maintenance	5	4	3	2	1
6. Exhibits the required manual dexterity	5	4	3	2	1
7. Performs procedure in a reasonable time frame for clinical level	5	4	3	2	1
8. Applies and maintains aseptic technique and PPE as required	5	4	3	2	1
9. Maintains concise and accurate patient and clinical records	5	4	3	2	1
10. Reports promptly on patient status/needs to appropriate personnel	5	4	3	2	1
AFFECTIVE DOMAIN					
11. Exhibits courteous and pleasant demeanor; shows consideration and respect, honesty, and integrity	5	4	3	2	1
12. Communicates verbally and in writing clearly and concisely	5	4	3	2	1
13. Preserves confidentiality and adheres to all policies	5	4	3	2	1
14. Follows directions, exhibits sound judgment, and seeks help when required	5	4	3	2	1
15. Demonstrates initiative, self-direction, responsibility, and accountability	5	4	3	2	1

TOTAL POINTS =   /15 = AVERAGE GRADE =

ADDITIONAL COMMENTS: IDENTIFY AREAS OF EXCELLENCE; LIST ERRORS OF OMISSION OR COMMISSION, CRITICAL ERRORS

SUMMARY PERFORMANCE EVALUATION AND RECOMMENDATIONS

☐ PASS: Satisfactory Performance

  ☐ Minimal supervision needed, may progress to next level provided specific skills, clinical time completed

  ☐ Minimal supervision needed, able to progress to next level without remediation

☐ FAIL: Unsatisfactory Performance (check all that apply)

  ☐ Minor reevaluation only

  ☐ Needs additional clinical practice before reevaluation

  ☐ Needs additional laboratory practice before skills performed in clinical area

  ☐ Recommend clinical probation

SIGNATURES

Evaluator (print name):   Evaluator signature: Date:

Student Signature: Date:

Student Comments:

Procedural Competency Evaluation

STUDENT: _____   DATE: _____

DIRECTED COUGH

Evaluator: ☐ Peer ☐ Instructor	**Setting:** ☐ Lab	☐ Clinical Simulation	
Equipment Utilized:	**Conditions (Describe):**		

Performance Level:

S or ✓ = Satisfactory, no errors of omission or commission
U = Unsatisfactory Error of Omission or Commission
NA = Not applicable

Performance Rating:

5 **Independent:** Near flawless performance; minimal errors; able to perform without supervision; seeks out new learning; shows initiative; A = 4.7–5.0 average

4 **Minimally Supervised:** Few errors, able to self-correct; seeks guidance when appropriate; B = 3.7–4.65

3 **Competent:** Minimal required level; no critical errors; able to correct with coaching; meets expectations; safe; C = 3.0–3.65

2 **Marginal:** Below average; critical errors or problem areas noted; would benefit from remediation; D = 2.0–2.99

1 **Dependent:** Poor; unacceptable performance; unsafe; gross inaccuracies; potentially harmful; F = < 2.0

Two or more errors of commission or omission of mandatory or essential performance elements will terminate the procedure, and require additional practice and/or remediation and reevaluation. Student is responsible for obtaining additional evaluation forms as needed from the Director of Clinical Education (DCE).

	PERFORMANCE RATING	PERFORMANCE LEVEL
EQUIPMENT AND PATIENT PREPARATION		
1. Common Performance Elements Steps 1–8		
ASSESSMENT AND IMPLEMENTATION		
2. Common Performance Elements Steps 9 and 10		
3. Instructs patient in vibratory PEP therapy (See PCE for PEP Therapy)		
A. Repeats 4 to 8 times for 10–20 minutes		
4. Instructs patient in effective use of diaphragm and cough		
5. Assures forceful contraction of abdominal muscles		
6. Instructs the patient in serial coughing techniques		
7. Instructs patient on forced expiratory technique (FET), or huffing		
8. Provides manually assisted cough		
9. Applies pressure to the lateral thoracic cage coordinated with the patient's cough effort		
10. With tracheostomy, provides manually assisted deep inspiration utilizing a manual resuscitator bag in conjunction with manually assisted cough techniques (quad cough)		
11. Repeats procedures as indicated/tolerated		
12. Collects and examines sputum		
FOLLOW-UP		
13. Common Performance Elements Steps 11–16		

SIGNATURES   Student: _____   Evaluator: _____   Date: _____

Clinical Performance Evaluation

PERFORMANCE RATING:

5 **Independent:** Near flawless performance; minimal errors; able to perform without supervision; seeks out new learning; shows initiative; A = 4.7–5.0 average

4 **Minimally Supervised:** Few errors, able to self-correct; seeks guidance when appropriate; B = 3.7–4.65

3 **Competent:** Minimal required level; no critical errors; able to correct with coaching; meets expectations; safe; C = 3.0–3.65

2 **Marginal:** Below average; critical errors or problem areas noted; would benefit from remediation; D = 2.0–2.99

1 **Dependent:** Poor; unacceptable performance; unsafe; gross inaccuracies; potentially harmful; F = < 2.0

Circle the appropriate response below. Please be consistent, objective, and honest in your assessment of the student's clinical performance and ability.

PERFORMANCE CRITERIA	SCORE				
COGNITIVE DOMAIN					
1. Consistently displays knowledge, comprehension, and command of essential concepts	5	4	3	2	1
2. Demonstrates the relationship between theory and clinical practice	5	4	3	2	1
3. Able to select, review, apply, analyze, synthesize, interpret, and evaluate information; makes recommendations to modify care plan	5	4	3	2	1
PSYCHOMOTOR DOMAIN					
4. Minimal errors, no critical errors; able to self-correct; performs all steps safely and accurately	5	4	3	2	1
5. Selects, assembles, and verifies proper function and cleanliness of equipment; assures operation and corrects malfunctions; provides adequate care and maintenance	5	4	3	2	1
6. Exhibits the required manual dexterity	5	4	3	2	1
7. Performs procedure in a reasonable time frame for clinical level	5	4	3	2	1
8. Applies and maintains aseptic technique and PPE as required	5	4	3	2	1
9. Maintains concise and accurate patient and clinical records	5	4	3	2	1
10. Reports promptly on patient status/needs to appropriate personnel	5	4	3	2	1
AFFECTIVE DOMAIN					
11. Exhibits courteous and pleasant demeanor; shows consideration and respect, honesty, and integrity	5	4	3	2	1
12. Communicates verbally and in writing clearly and concisely	5	4	3	2	1
13. Preserves confidentiality and adheres to all policies	5	4	3	2	1
14. Follows directions, exhibits sound judgment, and seeks help when required	5	4	3	2	1
15. Demonstrates initiative, self-direction, responsibility, and accountability	5	4	3	2	1

TOTAL POINTS = _____ /15 = AVERAGE GRADE = _____

ADDITIONAL COMMENTS: IDENTIFY AREAS OF EXCELLENCE; LIST ERRORS OF OMISSION OR COMMISSION, CRITICAL ERRORS

SUMMARY PERFORMANCE EVALUATION AND RECOMMENDATIONS

☐ PASS: Satisfactory Performance

    ☐ Minimal supervision needed, may progress to next level provided specific skills, clinical time completed

    ☐ Minimal supervision needed, able to progress to next level without remediation

☐ FAIL: Unsatisfactory Performance (check all that apply)

    ☐ Minor reevaluation only

    ☐ Needs additional clinical practice before reevaluation

    ☐ Needs additional laboratory practice before skills performed in clinical area

    ☐ Recommend clinical probation

SIGNATURES

Evaluator (print name): _____ Evaluator signature: _____ Date: _____

Student Signature: _____ Date: _____

Student Comments:

Procedural Competency Evaluation

STUDENT: _____   DATE: _____

POSITIVE EXPIRATORY PRESSURE (PEP) THERAPY/VIBRATORY PEP

Evaluator:	☐ Peer	☐ Instructor		**Setting:**	☐ Lab	☐ Clinical Simulation	

Equipment Utilized: _____   **Conditions (Describe):** _____

Performance Level:

S or ✓ = Satisfactory, no errors of omission or commission
U = Unsatisfactory Error of Omission or Commission
NA = Not applicable

Performance Rating:

5   **Independent:** Near flawless performance; minimal errors; able to perform without supervision; seeks out new learning; shows initiative; A = 4.7–5.0 average

4   **Minimally Supervised:** Few errors, able to self-correct; seeks guidance when appropriate; B = 3.7–4.65

3   **Competent:** Minimal required level; no critical errors; able to correct with coaching; meets expectations; safe; C = 3.0–3.65

2   **Marginal:** Below average; critical errors or problem areas noted; would benefit from remediation; D = 2.0–2.99

1   **Dependent:** Poor; unacceptable performance; unsafe; gross inaccuracies; potentially harmful; F = < 2.0

Two or more errors of commission or omission of mandatory or essential performance elements will terminate the procedure, and require additional practice and/or remediation and reevaluation. Student is responsible for obtaining additional evaluation forms as needed from the Director of Clinical Education (DCE).

(Columns: PERFORMANCE RATING | PERFORMANCE LEVEL)

EQUIPMENT AND PATIENT PREPARATION

1. Common Performance Elements Steps 1–8

2. Differentiates between different PEP and vibratory PEP devices (Flutter®, Acapella®, PEP, Thera-PeP®, EZPAP™)

ASSESSMENT AND IMPLEMENTATION

3. Common Performance Elements Steps 9 and 10

4. Adjusts exhalation orifice (PEP device) to the largest setting; adjusts pressure reading (TheraPeP®); adjusts compressed gas flow (EZPAP™) or hold Flutter® level; for Acapella®, adjusts flow control to open position

5. Positions patient upright with elbows resting comfortably on a table

6. Places mask comfortably but tightly over the nose and mouth or adjusts noseclips and mouthpiece

7. Instructs patient to take a larger than normal breath and exhale slowly at an I:E ratio of 1:3 or 1:4

8. Observes pressure generated on manometer or gauge during exhalation; increases the pressure and/or vibration until 10 or 20 cm H_2O is generated during exhalation, or until audible vibration can be heard

9. Instructs patient to take 10 to 30 breaths followed by 2 or 3 huffs (FET); repeats 4 to 8 times for 10 to 20 minutes

10. Reassesses patient periodically and reinstructs if necessary

11. Encourages cough periodically; collects and examines sputum

FOLLOW-UP

12. Common Performance Elements Steps 11–16

SIGNATURES   Student: _____   Evaluator: _____   Date: _____

Clinical Performance Evaluation

PERFORMANCE RATING:

5 **Independent:** Near flawless performance; minimal errors; able to perform without supervision; seeks out new learning; shows initiative; A = 4.7–5.0 average

4 **Minimally Supervised:** Few errors, able to self-correct; seeks guidance when appropriate; B = 3.7–4.65

3 **Competent:** Minimal required level; no critical errors; able to correct with coaching; meets expectations; safe; C = 3.0–3.65

2 **Marginal:** Below average; critical errors or problem areas noted; would benefit from remediation; D = 2.0–2.99

1 **Dependent:** Poor; unacceptable performance; unsafe; gross inaccuracies; potentially harmful; F = < 2.0

Circle the appropriate response below. Please be consistent, objective, and honest in your assessment of the student's clinical performance and ability.

PERFORMANCE CRITERIA	SCORE				
COGNITIVE DOMAIN					
1. Consistently displays knowledge, comprehension, and command of essential concepts	5	4	3	2	1
2. Demonstrates the relationship between theory and clinical practice	5	4	3	2	1
3. Able to select, review, apply, analyze, synthesize, interpret, and evaluate information; makes recommendations to modify care plan	5	4	3	2	1
PSYCHOMOTOR DOMAIN					
4. Minimal errors, no critical errors; able to self-correct; performs all steps safely and accurately	5	4	3	2	1
5. Selects, assembles, and verifies proper function and cleanliness of equipment; assures operation and corrects malfunctions; provides adequate care and maintenance	5	4	3	2	1
6. Exhibits the required manual dexterity	5	4	3	2	1
7. Performs procedure in a reasonable time frame for clinical level	5	4	3	2	1
8. Applies and maintains aseptic technique and PPE as required	5	4	3	2	1
9. Maintains concise and accurate patient and clinical records	5	4	3	2	1
10. Reports promptly on patient status/needs to appropriate personnel	5	4	3	2	1
AFFECTIVE DOMAIN					
11. Exhibits courteous and pleasant demeanor; shows consideration and respect, honesty, and integrity	5	4	3	2	1
12. Communicates verbally and in writing clearly and concisely	5	4	3	2	1
13. Preserves confidentiality and adheres to all policies	5	4	3	2	1
14. Follows directions, exhibits sound judgment, and seeks help when required	5	4	3	2	1
15. Demonstrates initiative, self-direction, responsibility, and accountability	5	4	3	2	1

TOTAL POINTS =   /15 = AVERAGE GRADE =

ADDITIONAL COMMENTS: IDENTIFY AREAS OF EXCELLENCE; LIST ERRORS OF OMISSION OR COMMISSION, CRITICAL ERRORS

SUMMARY PERFORMANCE EVALUATION AND RECOMMENDATIONS

☐ PASS: Satisfactory Performance

　　☐ Minimal supervision needed, may progress to next level provided specific skills, clinical time completed

　　☐ Minimal supervision needed, able to progress to next level without remediation

☐ FAIL: Unsatisfactory Performance (check all that apply)

　　☐ Minor reevaluation only

　　☐ Needs additional clinical practice before reevaluation

　　☐ Needs additional laboratory practice before skills performed in clinical area

　　☐ Recommend clinical probation

SIGNATURES

Evaluator (print name):　　　　　　Evaluator signature:　　　　　　Date:

Student Signature:　　　　　　Date:

Student Comments:

Procedural Competency Evaluation

STUDENT: DATE:

INSPIRATORY RESISTIVE MUSCLE TRAINING

	PERFORMANCE RATING	PERFORMANCE LEVEL

Evaluator: ☐ Peer ☐ Instructor **Setting:** ☐ Lab ☐ Clinical Simulation

Equipment Utilized: **Conditions (Describe):**

Performance Level:

S or ✓ = Satisfactory, no errors of omission or commission
U = Unsatisfactory Error of Omission or Commission
NA = Not applicable

Performance Rating:

5 **Independent:** Near flawless performance; minimal errors; able to perform without supervision; seeks out new learning; shows initiative; A = 4.7–5.0 average

4 **Minimally Supervised:** Few errors, able to self-correct; seeks guidance when appropriate; B = 3.7–4.65

3 **Competent:** Minimal required level; no critical errors; able to correct with coaching; meets expectations; safe; C = 3.0–3.65

2 **Marginal:** Below average; critical errors or problem areas noted; would benefit from remediation; D = 2.0–2.99

1 **Dependent:** Poor; unacceptable performance; unsafe; gross inaccuracies; potentially harmful; F = < 2.0

Two or more errors of commission or omission of mandatory or essential performance elements will terminate the procedure, and require additional practice and/or remediation and reevaluation. Student is responsible for obtaining additional evaluation forms as needed from the Director of Clinical Education (DCE).

EQUIPMENT AND PATIENT PREPARATION		
1. Common Performance Elements Steps 1–8		
ASSESSMENT AND IMPLEMENTATION		
2. Common Performance Elements Steps 9 and 10		
3. Measures maximum inspiratory pressure and vital capacity		
4. Selects inspiratory-resistive device or dial selector with least resistance		
5. Attaches pressure manometer in-line		
6. Comfortably places noseclips		
7. Instructs patient to exhale slowly through the mouthpiece, maintaining a tight seal		
8. Notes manometer pressure during inspiration, adjusts inspiratory-resistive orifice to achieve 30% of MIP		
9. Instructs patient to repeat exercise for 15 minutes, twice a day		
10. Reassesses and reinstructs as necessary		
11. Encourages cough periodically; examine and collects sputum if applicable		
FOLLOW-UP		
12. Common Performance Elements Steps 11–16		

SIGNATURES Student: Evaluator: Date:

Clinical Performance Evaluation

PERFORMANCE RATING:

5   **Independent:** Near flawless performance; minimal errors; able to perform without supervision; seeks out new learning; shows initiative; A = 4.7–5.0 average

4   **Minimally Supervised:** Few errors, able to self-correct; seeks guidance when appropriate; B = 3.7–4.65

3   **Competent:** Minimal required level; no critical errors; able to correct with coaching; meets expectations; safe; C = 3.0–3.65

2   **Marginal:** Below average; critical errors or problem areas noted; would benefit from remediation; D = 2.0–2.99

1   **Dependent:** Poor; unacceptable performance; unsafe; gross inaccuracies; potentially harmful; F = < 2.0

Circle the appropriate response below. Please be consistent, objective, and honest in your assessment of the student's clinical performance and ability.

PERFORMANCE CRITERIA	SCORE				
COGNITIVE DOMAIN					
1. Consistently displays knowledge, comprehension, and command of essential concepts	5	4	3	2	1
2. Demonstrates the relationship between theory and clinical practice	5	4	3	2	1
3. Able to select, review, apply, analyze, synthesize, interpret, and evaluate information; makes recommendations to modify care plan	5	4	3	2	1
PSYCHOMOTOR DOMAIN					
4. Minimal errors, no critical errors; able to self-correct; performs all steps safely and accurately	5	4	3	2	1
5. Selects, assembles, and verifies proper function and cleanliness of equipment; assures operation and corrects malfunctions; provides adequate care and maintenance	5	4	3	2	1
6. Exhibits the required manual dexterity	5	4	3	2	1
7. Performs procedure in a reasonable time frame for clinical level	5	4	3	2	1
8. Applies and maintains aseptic technique and PPE as required	5	4	3	2	1
9. Maintains concise and accurate patient and clinical records	5	4	3	2	1
10. Reports promptly on patient status/needs to appropriate personnel	5	4	3	2	1
AFFECTIVE DOMAIN					
11. Exhibits courteous and pleasant demeanor; shows consideration and respect, honesty, and integrity	5	4	3	2	1
12. Communicates verbally and in writing clearly and concisely	5	4	3	2	1
13. Preserves confidentiality and adheres to all policies	5	4	3	2	1
14. Follows directions, exhibits sound judgment, and seeks help when required	5	4	3	2	1
15. Demonstrates initiative, self-direction, responsibility, and accountability	5	4	3	2	1

TOTAL POINTS =   /15 = AVERAGE GRADE =

ADDITIONAL COMMENTS: IDENTIFY AREAS OF EXCELLENCE; LIST ERRORS OF OMISSION OR COMMISSION, CRITICAL ERRORS

SUMMARY PERFORMANCE EVALUATION AND RECOMMENDATIONS

☐ PASS: Satisfactory Performance

    ☐ Minimal supervision needed, may progress to next level provided specific skills, clinical time completed

    ☐ Minimal supervision needed, able to progress to next level without remediation

☐ FAIL: Unsatisfactory Performance (check all that apply)

    ☐ Minor reevaluation only

    ☐ Needs additional clinical practice before reevaluation

    ☐ Needs additional laboratory practice before skills performed in clinical area

    ☐ Recommend clinical probation

SIGNATURES

Evaluator (print name):   Evaluator signature: Date:

Student Signature: Date:

Student Comments:

Procedural Competency Evaluation

STUDENT: _____   DATE: _____

INTRAPULMONIC PERCUSSION VENTILATION (IPV)

		PERFORMANCE RATING	PERFORMANCE LEVEL
Evaluator: ☐ Peer ☐ Instructor **Setting:** ☐ Lab ☐ Clinical Simulation			
Equipment Utilized: _____ **Conditions (Describe):** _____			
Performance Level:			
S or ✓ = Satisfactory, no errors of omission or commission U = Unsatisfactory Error of Omission or Commission NA = Not applicable			
Performance Rating:			
5	**Independent:** Near flawless performance; minimal errors; able to perform without supervision; seeks out new learning; shows initiative; A = 4.7–5.0 average		
4	**Minimally Supervised:** Few errors, able to self-correct; seeks guidance when appropriate; B = 3.7–4.65		
3	**Competent:** Minimal required level; no critical errors; able to correct with coaching; meets expectations; safe; C = 3.0–3.65		
2	**Marginal:** Below average; critical errors or problem areas noted; would benefit from remediation; D = 2.0–2.99		
1	**Dependent:** Poor; unacceptable performance; unsafe; gross inaccuracies; potentially harmful; F = < 2.0		
	Two or more errors of commission or omission of mandatory or essential performance elements will terminate the procedure, and require additional practice and/or remediation and reevaluation. Student is responsible for obtaining additional evaluation forms as needed from the Director of Clinical Education (DCE).		

EQUIPMENT AND PATIENT PREPARATION

1.	Common Performance Elements Steps 1–8		
2.	Assembles equipment and verifies function		

ASSESSMENT AND IMPLEMENTATION

3.	Common Performance Elements Steps 9 and 10		
4.	Selects appropriate interface		
5.	Fills reservoir with the prescribed solution or medication		
6.	Plugs in unit, turns on the unit, and adjusts the amplification and frequency to generate sufficient percussion and mist for effectiveness		
7.	Attaches the delivery device to the patient and ensures patient comfort		
8.	Reassesses the patient after application of the aerosol device		
9.	Collects sputum, labels, and sends to lab if indicated		

FOLLOW-UP

10.	Common Performance Elements Steps 11–16		

SIGNATURES   Student: _____   Evaluator: _____   Date: _____

Clinical Performance Evaluation

PERFORMANCE RATING:

5 **Independent:** Near flawless performance; minimal errors; able to perform without supervision; seeks out new learning; shows initiative; A = 4.7–5.0 average

4 **Minimally Supervised:** Few errors, able to self-correct; seeks guidance when appropriate; B = 3.7–4.65

3 **Competent:** Minimal required level; no critical errors; able to correct with coaching; meets expectations; safe; C = 3.0–3.65

2 **Marginal:** Below average; critical errors or problem areas noted; would benefit from remediation; D = 2.0–2.99

1 **Dependent:** Poor; unacceptable performance; unsafe; gross inaccuracies; potentially harmful; F = < 2.0

Circle the appropriate response below. Please be consistent, objective, and honest in your assessment of the student's clinical performance and ability.

PERFORMANCE CRITERIA	SCORE				
COGNITIVE DOMAIN					
1. Consistently displays knowledge, comprehension, and command of essential concepts	5	4	3	2	1
2. Demonstrates the relationship between theory and clinical practice	5	4	3	2	1
3. Able to select, review, apply, analyze, synthesize, interpret, and evaluate information; makes recommendations to modify care plan	5	4	3	2	1
PSYCHOMOTOR DOMAIN					
4. Minimal errors, no critical errors; able to self-correct; performs all steps safely and accurately	5	4	3	2	1
5. Selects, assembles, and verifies proper function and cleanliness of equipment; assures operation and corrects malfunctions; provides adequate care and maintenance	5	4	3	2	1
6. Exhibits the required manual dexterity	5	4	3	2	1
7. Performs procedure in a reasonable time frame for clinical level	5	4	3	2	1
8. Applies and maintains aseptic technique and PPE as required	5	4	3	2	1
9. Maintains concise and accurate patient and clinical records	5	4	3	2	1
10. Reports promptly on patient status/needs to appropriate personnel	5	4	3	2	1
AFFECTIVE DOMAIN					
11. Exhibits courteous and pleasant demeanor; shows consideration and respect, honesty, and integrity	5	4	3	2	1
12. Communicates verbally and in writing clearly and concisely	5	4	3	2	1
13. Preserves confidentiality and adheres to all policies	5	4	3	2	1
14. Follows directions, exhibits sound judgment, and seeks help when required	5	4	3	2	1
15. Demonstrates initiative, self-direction, responsibility, and accountability	5	4	3	2	1

TOTAL POINTS = _____ /15 = AVERAGE GRADE = _____

ADDITIONAL COMMENTS: IDENTIFY AREAS OF EXCELLENCE; LIST ERRORS OF OMISSION OR COMMISSION, CRITICAL ERRORS

SUMMARY PERFORMANCE EVALUATION AND RECOMMENDATIONS

☐ PASS: Satisfactory Performance

    ☐ Minimal supervision needed, may progress to next level provided specific skills, clinical time completed

    ☐ Minimal supervision needed, able to progress to next level without remediation

☐ FAIL: Unsatisfactory Performance (check all that apply)

    ☐ Minor reevaluation only

    ☐ Needs additional clinical practice before reevaluation

    ☐ Needs additional laboratory practice before skills performed in clinical area

    ☐ Recommend clinical probation

SIGNATURES

Evaluator (print name): _____ Evaluator signature: _____ Date: _____

Student Signature: _____ Date: _____

Student Comments:

CHAPTER 19 Manual Resuscitators and Manual Ventilation

INTRODUCTION

Manual resuscitators are adjunctive devices used to support short-term artificial ventilation. Situations that may require their use include transport of ventilated patients, application of positive-pressure breaths for hyperinflation and oxygenation during suctioning, ventilator malfunction, and cough assisting. These devices can be used to assist the spontaneously breathing patient and to fully support the apneic patient.

One of the most important uses of these devices is to support ventilation during a respiratory or cardiac arrest. The respiratory care practitioner is often one of the first members of the healthcare team to arrive at a **resuscitation** event and is usually responsible for airway maintenance and ventilation. It is imperative, therefore, that the respiratory care practitioner understand the capabilities and functioning of manual resuscitation devices and be able to troubleshoot them in an emergency situation.

In basic life support procedures, rescue breathing is accomplished by mouth-to-mouth ventilation. In the healthcare environment, mouth-to-mask ventilation and bag-valve-mask ventilation are used. Bag-valve-mask devices, or manual resuscitators, have changed over the years. Standards for these devices are published by the American Society for Testing and Materials[1] and in the *Journal of the American Medical Association*.[2] These standards include the following:

- Criteria for F_IO_2 delivery
- Prevention of valve malfunction up to flows of 30 Lpm
- A valve that is easily cleaned (within 20 seconds) if vomitus prevents proper functioning
- A universal 15-/22-mm adaptor for the patient connection
- Durability and ability to withstand shock
- An override capability of the pressure relief valve
- A maximum of 40 cm H_2O pressure relief valve for neonatal (± 5%) and pediatric (± 10%) bags
- Pressure relief valves are not required for adult bags

Considerations for the practitioner in selecting a resuscitation device should include the following:

- Good "feel" to determine patient's lung compliance
- Quick inflation and refill response
- Adequate ventilating volumes
- Ease of valve opening with the patient's spontaneous breathing efforts
- Durability (if nondisposable)
- Ease of assembly/disassembly

OBJECTIVES

Upon completion of this chapter, the student will be able to:

1. Identify and differentiate the types of patient valves and how each operates during inspiration and expiration.
2. Identify and discuss the advantages and disadvantages of self-filling and flow-filling bags.
3. Assemble and disassemble each type of device.
4. Demonstrate effective manual ventilation techniques with mouth-to-mask devices, bag-valve-mask devices, and bag-valve resuscitators to an artificial airway and a spontaneously breathing subject.
5. Explain the purpose of a pressure relief valve on a manual resuscitator and demonstrate its operation.
6. Discuss the relationship between resistance, compliance, and the amount of positive pressure necessary to accomplish ventilation.
7. Compare the variability in positive pressure, volume delivery, and F_IO_2 using different ventilation techniques.

KEY TERMS

capnometer   pop-off
hyperextend   resuscitation

Exercises

EQUIPMENT REQUIRED

☐ Adaptors and connectors
☐ Computerized lung simulator or test lungs
☐ End-tidal P_ECO_2 devices (colorimetric **cap-nometers**), adult and pediatric
☐ Intubated and nonintubated mannequins (adult, child, and infant)
☐ Masks of various sizes
☐ Mouth-valve-mask resuscitation unit (pocket mask)
☐ Laryngoscopes and blades

☐ Oxygen analyzers
☐ Oxygen connecting tubing
☐ Oxygen gas source
☐ Oxygen nipple adapters
☐ Pressure manometers (disposable or nondisposable)
☐ Respirometers
☐ Spring-loaded, duckbill/diaphragm, and diaphragm/leaf types of adult and neonatal/pediatric resuscitators

EXERCISE 19.1 ASSEMBLY AND DISASSEMBLY OF RESUSCITATORS

1. Select one of each type of resuscitator, as available: spring-loaded, duckbill/diaphragm, and diaphragm/leaf (Fig. 19.1). Study the type of valves and identify the manufacturers. **Record these on your laboratory report.**
2. Disassemble the unit completely. This step will depend on which bag you are disassembling. See the manufacturer's specifications or refer to an equipment text if needed.
3. Reassemble the units. Make sure there are no leftover parts.
4. Test the unit for proper function by occluding the outlet and squeezing the bag. The bag should hold pressure and volume until released. **Record your observations on your laboratory report.**
5. Carefully observe the operation of the patient valve and oxygen inlet during inspiration and expiration. Compare schematic representations of the operation of the valves during inspiration vs. expiration.
6. Repeat steps 2 through 5 for each bag selected.
7. Obtain a flow-filling ventilation device and assemble. **Describe how this differs from self-inflating bags on your laboratory report.**

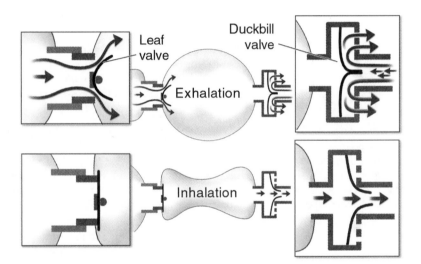

Figure 19.1. Nonbreathing valves commonly used with manual resuscitators.

EXERCISE 19.2 PRESSURE RELIEF VALVES

1. Examine the pressure relief pop-off on the infant resuscitator. **Record the set pressure release, if available, on your laboratory report.**
2. Occlude the outlet of the bag while squeezing it. Observe the function of the pressure pop-off, and **record your observations on your laboratory report.**
3. Attach the bag to a lung simulator with a pressure manometer. Squeeze the bag slowly and gently and note the highest pressure obtained during inspiration. **Record this pressure on your laboratory report.**
4. With the bag still attached to the lung simulator with pressure manometer, squeeze the bag forcefully and rapidly. Note the highest pressure obtained during inspiration. **Record this pressure on your laboratory report.** How do these pressures compare to the ATSM standards?
5. Bypass the pressure relief mechanism so that it is nonfunctional. According to standards, it should be obvious how to do this. Refer to the manufacturer's literature or your instructor if you have any questions.
6. Occlude the outlet of the bag while squeezing it. Observe the function of the pressure pop-off, and **record your observations on your laboratory report.**
7. With the pressure relief disabled, attach the bag to a lung simulator with a pressure manometer. Squeeze the bag slowly and gently and note the highest pressure obtained during inspiration. **Record this pressure on your laboratory report.**

8. With the bag still attached to the lung simulator with pressure manometer, squeeze the bag forcefully and rapidly. Note the highest pressure obtained during inspiration. **Record this pressure on your laboratory report.**

EXERCISE 19.3 MEASUREMENT OF PRESSURES, STROKE VOLUMES, AND F_IO_2

1. Attach a pressure manometer, respirometer, and oxygen analyzer in-line between the patient valve and the endotracheal tube connection, as shown in Figure 19.2. Make sure you have the oxygen turned up to 15 Lpm before proceeding to step 2.

2. Squeeze the bag gently with one hand several times, allowing for sufficient exhalation between breaths. **Record the pressure generated, the F_IO_2, and the volume delivered on your laboratory report.**

3. Repeat the exercise, except this time squeeze the bag vigorously with *both hands*. **Record the pressure generated, F_IO_2, and the volume delivered on your laboratory report.**

4. Disconnect the reservoir and repeat the measurement.

5. Reattach the reservoir.

6. Turn the liter flow down to 8 Lpm and repeat the one-handed squeeze and the two-handed squeeze. **Record the F_IO_2 delivered on your laboratory report.**

7. Disconnect the reservoir and repeat the measurement. **Record the F_IO_2 delivered on your laboratory report.**

8. Place a positive end-expiratory pressure (PEEP) valve on the exhalation valve of the resuscitator (see Fig. 19.2) and repeat the measurements. Depending on the type of bag being used, a special adaptor may be required. The PEEP valve may be preset or adjustable. **Record the type of valve used and the pressure setting on your laboratory report.**

The following exercises should be done using a lung simulator, if available. If not, a test lung can be adapted to approximate the resistance and compliance changes.

1. Set the resistance at R = 5 (normal resistance) and the compliance at 0.10 L/cm H_2O. Deliver three breaths and **record the pressures and volumes on your laboratory report.** If a lung simulator is not available, use a standard test lung with an 8-mm endotracheal tube.

   Increase the resistance to R = 50 (high resistance). Deliver three breaths and **record the pressures and volumes on your laboratory report.** If a lung simulator is not available, use a standard test lung with a 3-mm endotracheal tube.

2. Return the resistance to R = 5 (normal resistance) and change the compliance to 0.01 L/cm H_2O. Deliver three breaths and **record the pressures and volumes on your laboratory report.** If a lung simulator is not available, use a standard test lung with an 8-mm endotracheal tube. Place a rubber band around the center of the test lung.

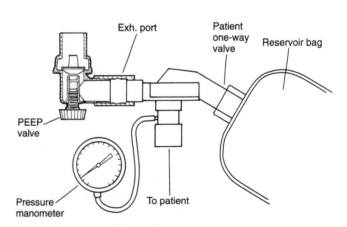

Figure 19.2. Monitoring equipment and PEEP valve in-line with manual resuscitator. (Courtesy of Instrumentation Industries Inc., Bethel Park, PA.)

EXERCISE 19.4 MOUTH-TO-MASK VENTILATION

1. Select a mouth-valve mask breathing device.

2. Select an adult, unintubated mannequin.

3. Place the head in the proper position using the head-tilt/chin-lift technique learned in BLS, as shown in Figure 19.3.

4. Grasp the mask properly, as shown in Figure 19.4. Place your thumb over the bridge of the mask. Use the index and middle or middle and ring fingers to grasp just above the mask cushion. Seal the mask over the mouth and nose, placing the mask on the bridge of the nose first (Fig. 19.5). Using both hands, tilt the head back to reopen the airway, as shown in Figure 19.6.

5. Administer two breaths. Make sure you allow time for exhalation. Observe to see if the chest rises and falls. Repeat until chest rise is achieved consistently.

6. Seal the mask over the nose using one hand only, without applying pressure on the mask over the chin. Administer three breaths. Observe to see if the chest rises and falls. Repeat until chest rise is achieved consistently. **Record your observations on your laboratory report.**

7. Place the head in a neutral position without using any airway opening techniques. Attempt to ventilate. Reposition the head and repeat attempt to ventilate. Repeat until chest rise is achieved consistently. **Record your observations on your laboratory report.**

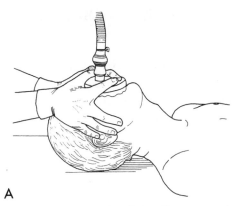

A

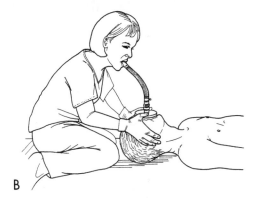

B

Figure 19.3. Mouth-to-mask ventilation with a one-way valve.

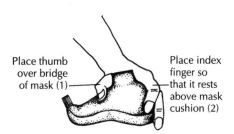

Place thumb over bridge of mask (1)

Place index finger so that it rests above mask cushion (2)

Figure 19.4. Proper hand position for resuscitator mask. (From Eubanks, DH and Bone, RC: Comprehensive Respiratory Care: A Learning System. Mosby-Year Book, St. Louis, 1990, p. 642, with permission.)

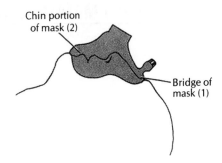

Chin portion of mask (2)

Bridge of mask (1)

Figure 19.5. Mask position on face. (From Eubanks, DH and Bone, RC: Comprehensive Respiratory Care: A Learning System. Mosby-Year Book, St. Louis, 1990, p. 642, with permission.)

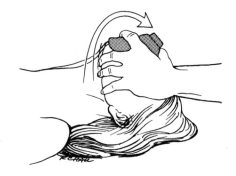

Figure 19.6. Performing head-tilt maneuver with mask in place. (From Eubanks, DH and Bone, RC: Comprehensive Respiratory Care: A Learning System. Mosby-Year Book, St. Louis, 1990, p. 136, with permission.)

EXERCISE 19.5 MANUAL VENTILATION WITH MASK

1. Select adult, pediatric, and infant bag-valve-mask resuscitators.
2. Select infant, pediatric, and adult unintubated mannequins.
3. Attach the oxygen supply tubing to the oxygen source and turn to 15 Lpm.
4. Place the head of the adult mannequin in the proper position, using the head-tilt/chin-lift technique.
5. Place the mask over the mouth and nose, using one hand to achieve a seal while maintaining proper head position. This can be accomplished by using the last three fingers of your nondominant hand to seal the lower portion of the mask while lifting up on the jaw and using your thumb and index finger to secure the mask over the mouth and nose.
6. Administer ventilations at a rate of 12 to 20 breaths per minute for at least 1 minute. Make sure to maintain a good seal and verify that the chest rises and falls with each breath, but *do not hyperinflate.* Attempt ventilation with different masks and mannequins.
7. Repeat these steps using the child and infant mannequins and resuscitator at a rate of at least 20 breaths per minute for 1 minute. Avoid gastric insufflation. *Remember: Do not hyperextend the infant's head to open the airway! Do not overventilate.*
8. **Record your observations on your laboratory report.**

EXERCISE 19.6 MANUAL VENTILATION WITH AN INTUBATED MANNEQUIN

1. Select adult, child, and infant bag-valve-mask resuscitators.
2. Select adult, child, and infant intubated mannequins.
3. Attach the oxygen supply tubing to the oxygen source and turn to 15 Lpm.
4. Using the adult mannequin, connect the patient connector on the resuscitator to the 22/15 connector on the endotracheal tube.
5. Squeeze the bag and give the mannequin three breaths, allowing for sufficient exhalation after each breath. **Record your observations on your laboratory report.**
6. Repeat these steps using the child and infant mannequins and resuscitators.

EXERCISE 19.7 MANUAL VENTILATION WHILE COMPRESSIONS ARE PERFORMED

1. Select adult, child, and infant nonintubated mannequins.
2. Select an adult bag-valve-mask resuscitator and the adult mannequin.
3. Go through the ABCs:
   A. Determine responsiveness
   B. Call for help
   C. Check for breathing
   D. Give two manual ventilations
   E. Check pulse
3. With pulse present, continue rescue breathing at a rate of 12 to 10 per minute.
4. With no pulse present, have a partner perform cardiac compressions at a rate of 80 to 100 per minute.
5. Ventilate at 12 to 20 per minute in between the compressions for at least 1 minute.
6. Repeat these steps using the child and infant mannequins and resuscitators.

EXERCISE 19.8 ASSISTED MANUAL VENTILATION IN A SPONTANEOUSLY BREATHING SUBJECT

1. Select an adult bag-valve-mask resuscitator. Apply standard precautions and transmission-based isolation procedures as appropriate.

2. Attach the oxygen supply tubing to the oxygen source and turn to 15 Lpm.

3. If human patient simulator is available, set the respiratory rate at 5 to 10 breaths per minute.

4. Using your laboratory partner as the subject, or a human patient simulator if available, place the head in the proper position using the head-tilt/chin-lift technique.

5. Place the mask over the mouth and nose, using one hand to achieve a seal while maintaining proper head position.

6. Allow your partner or human patient simulator to breath spontaneously through the bag. Observe the valve operation.

7. Assist your partner's or human patient simulator's spontaneous ventilations. This is accomplished by timing when you squeeze the bag to synchronize with the early inspiratory phase. Administer moderately deep ventilations to achieve adequate chest rise. For your laboratory partner's comfort, do this only for every second or third breath.

8. If a simulator is used, assist all breaths and attempt to ventilate in between assisted breaths to achieve a total rate of 15 to 20 per minute.

9. Place the bags and masks in the designated dirty equipment area when this exercise is completed.

REFERENCES

1. American Society for Testing and Materials: Standard Specifications for Performance and Safety Requirements for Resuscitators Intended for Use with Humans (F 920 85). American Society for Testing and Materials, Philadelphia, 1985.

2. American Heart Association: Guidelines for cardiopulmonary resuscitation and emergency cardiac care: Recommendations of the 1992 national conference. JAMA 268:2200, 1992.

Laboratory Report

CHAPTER 19: MANUAL RESUSCITATORS AND MANUAL VENTILATION

Name _____ Date _____

Course/Section _____ Instructor _____

Data Collection

EXERCISE 19.1 Assembly and Disassembly of Resuscitators

BAG 1

    Type of valve: _____

    Name and manufacturer: _____

    Test function observations: _____

BAG 2

    Type of valve: _____

    Name and manufacturer: _____

    Test function observations: _____

BAG 3

    Type of valve: _____

    Name and manufacturer: _____

    Test function observations: _____

BAG 4

    Flow filling: _____

    Differences from self-inflating bag: _____

EXERCISE 19.2 Pressure Relief Valves

Set pressure: _____ Observations while occluded: _____

Pressure achieved squeezing slowly: _____

Pressure achieved squeezing forcefully: _____

Compare pressures achieved to standards: _____

Observations with pressure relief disabled: _____

Pressure achieved with pressure relief disabled (slow): _____

Pressure achieved with pressure relief disabled (forceful): _____

EXERCISE 19.3 Measurement of Pressures, Stroke Volumes, and F_IO_2

ONE-HANDED SQUEEZE, GENTLE

Pressure: _____ Volume: _____

F_IO_2 with reservoir: _____

ONE-HANDED SQUEEZE, VIGOROUS

Pressure: _____ Volume: _____

F_IO_2 with reservoir: _____

F_IO_2 without reservoir: _____

TWO-HANDED SQUEEZE

Pressure: _____ Volume: _____

F_IO_2: _____

F_IO_2 without reservoir: _____

FLOW AT 8 LPM

F_IO_2 with one-handed squeeze: _____

F_IO_2 with two-handed squeeze: _____

F_IO_2 without reservoir: _____

PEEP VALVE ATTACHMENT

Type of valve: _____ PEEP: _____ Pressure: _____ Volume: _____

LUNG SIMULATOR

Normal resistance (Rp = 5)/Normal compliance (0.10 L/cm H_2O): _____

Pressure: _____ Volume: _____

Increased resistance (Rp = 50): _____

Pressure: _____ Volume: _____

Resistance (Rp = 5)/Decreased compliance (0.01 L/cm H_2O): _____

Pressure: _____ Volume: _____

EXERCISE 19.4 Mouth-to-Mask Ventilation

Observation of one-handed, nose seal only: _____

_____

Observations with head in neutral position: _____

_____

EXERCISE 19.5 Manual Ventilation with Mask

Observations: _____

_____

_____

EXERCISE 19.6 Manual Ventilation with an Intubated Mannequin

Observations: _____

_____

Pressure relief setting: _____

Observations with occluded outlet: _____

_____

Observations with pressure relief bypassed: _____

_____

Critical Thinking Questions

1. Based on your observations in Exercise 19.1, how do you know that you assembled the device properly?

2. Identify at least three ways to increase the F_IO_2 delivered by a manual resuscitator.

3. Identify at least two additional techniques that could be used to improve the patient's PaO_2 during manual ventilation.

4. What are the complications of manual ventilation?

5. Compare and contrast adult ventilation with that of a neonate.

6. Identify at least three ways to initially assess the adequacy of manual ventilation.

7. What limitations are there to ventilating with (a) a mask and (b) an artificial airway?

8. What effect did changes in compliance and resistance have on the volumes and pressures delivered?

   A. Increased compliance, decreased resistance

   B. Increased compliance, increased resistance

   C. Decreased compliance, increased resistance

   D. Decreased compliance, decreased resistance

9. Identify possible clinical situations/disorders that would imitate the changes in compliance and resistance as demonstrated on the lung simulator in a patient requiring manual ventilation.

   A. Normal compliance, normal resistance

   B. Increased compliance, decreased resistance

   C. Increased compliance, increased resistance

   D. Decreased compliance, increased resistance

   E. Decreased compliance, decreased resistance

Procedural Competency Evaluation

STUDENT: _____ DATE: _____

MANUAL VENTILATION

			PERFORMANCE RATING	PERFORMANCE LEVEL
Evaluator: ☐ Peer ☐ Instructor	**Setting:** ☐ Lab	☐ Clinical Simulation		
Equipment Utilized:	**Conditions (Describe):**			

Performance Level:

S or ✓ = Satisfactory, no errors of omission or commission
U = Unsatisfactory Error of Omission or Commission
NA = Not applicable

Performance Rating:

5 **Independent:** Near flawless performance; minimal errors; able to perform without supervision; seeks out new learning; shows initiative; A = 4.7–5.0 average

4 **Minimally Supervised:** Few errors, able to self-correct; seeks guidance when appropriate; B = 3.7–4.65

3 **Competent:** Minimal required level; no critical errors; able to correct with coaching; meets expectations; safe; C = 3.0–3.65

2 **Marginal:** Below average; critical errors or problem areas noted; would benefit from remediation; D = 2.0–2.99

1 **Dependent:** Poor; unacceptable performance; unsafe; gross inaccuracies; potentially harmful; F = < 2.0

Two or more errors of commission or omission of mandatory or essential performance elements will terminate the procedure, and require additional practice and/or remediation and reevaluation. Student is responsible for obtaining additional evaluation forms as needed from the Director of Clinical Education (DCE).

	PERFORMANCE RATING	PERFORMANCE LEVEL
EQUIPMENT AND PATIENT PREPARATION		
1. Common Performance Elements Steps 1–8		
ASSESSMENT AND IMPLEMENTATION		
2. Common Performance Elements Steps 9 and 10		
3. Positions patient's head with head-tilt/chin-lift or modified jaw thrust		
4. Checks breathing and pulse		
5. Inserts pharyngeal airway when available		
6. Adjusts liter flow to ≥15 Lpm or flush and connects oxygen tubing to BVM reservoir		
7. Applies mask to face or 22-/15-mm adaptor to artificial airway		
8. Squeezes the bag to administer breaths, synchronizes with spontaneous breath if present		
9. Assesses adequacy of ventilation and oxygenation by chest expansion, auscultation, vital signs, and SpO_2		
10. Repositions head/mask as necessary		
11. Reassesses adequacy of ventilation and oxygenation and presence of pulse periodically		
12. Manually ventilates 12–20 breaths per minute		
FOLLOW-UP		
13. Common Performance Elements Steps 11–16		

SIGNATURES   Student: _____   Evaluator: _____   Date: _____

Clinical Performance Evaluation

PERFORMANCE RATING:

5 **Independent:** Near flawless performance; minimal errors; able to perform without supervision; seeks out new learning; shows initiative; A = 4.7–5.0 average

4 **Minimally Supervised:** Few errors, able to self-correct; seeks guidance when appropriate; B = 3.7–4.65

3 **Competent:** Minimal required level; no critical errors; able to correct with coaching; meets expectations; safe; C = 3.0–3.65

2 **Marginal:** Below average; critical errors or problem areas noted; would benefit from remediation; D = 2.0–2.99

1 **Dependent:** Poor; unacceptable performance; unsafe; gross inaccuracies; potentially harmful; F = < 2.0

Circle the appropriate response below. Please be consistent, objective, and honest in your assessment of the student's clinical performance and ability.

PERFORMANCE CRITERIA	SCORE				
COGNITIVE DOMAIN					
1. Consistently displays knowledge, comprehension, and command of essential concepts	5	4	3	2	1
2. Demonstrates the relationship between theory and clinical practice	5	4	3	2	1
3. Able to select, review, apply, analyze, synthesize, interpret, and evaluate information; makes recommendations to modify care plan	5	4	3	2	1
PSYCHOMOTOR DOMAIN					
4. Minimal errors, no critical errors; able to self-correct; performs all steps safely and accurately	5	4	3	2	1
5. Selects, assembles, and verifies proper function and cleanliness of equipment; assures operation and corrects malfunctions; provides adequate care and maintenance	5	4	3	2	1
6. Exhibits the required manual dexterity	5	4	3	2	1
7. Performs procedure in a reasonable time frame for clinical level	5	4	3	2	1
8. Applies and maintains aseptic technique and PPE as required	5	4	3	2	1
9. Maintains concise and accurate patient and clinical records	5	4	3	2	1
10. Reports promptly on patient status/needs to appropriate personnel	5	4	3	2	1
AFFECTIVE DOMAIN					
11. Exhibits courteous and pleasant demeanor; shows consideration and respect, honesty, and integrity	5	4	3	2	1
12. Communicates verbally and in writing clearly and concisely	5	4	3	2	1
13. Preserves confidentiality and adheres to all policies	5	4	3	2	1
14. Follows directions, exhibits sound judgment, and seeks help when required	5	4	3	2	1
15. Demonstrates initiative, self-direction, responsibility, and accountability	5	4	3	2	1

TOTAL POINTS = _____ /15 = AVERAGE GRADE = _____

ADDITIONAL COMMENTS: IDENTIFY AREAS OF EXCELLENCE; LIST ERRORS OF OMISSION OR COMMISSION, CRITICAL ERRORS

SUMMARY PERFORMANCE EVALUATION AND RECOMMENDATIONS

☐ PASS: Satisfactory Performance

　☐ Minimal supervision needed, may progress to next level provided specific skills, clinical time completed

　☐ Minimal supervision needed, able to progress to next level without remediation

☐ FAIL: Unsatisfactory Performance (check all that apply)

　☐ Minor reevaluation only

　☐ Needs additional clinical practice before reevaluation

　☐ Needs additional laboratory practice before skills performed in clinical area

　☐ Recommend clinical probation

SIGNATURES

Evaluator (print name): _____　Evaluator signature: _____　Date: _____

Student Signature: _____　Date: _____

Student Comments:

CHAPTER 20

Pharyngeal Airways

INTRODUCTION

Artificial airways are devices that are used to establish and maintain airway patency, facilitate ventilation, and assist in the removal of secretions. These include nasopharyngeal and oropharyngeal airways, laryngeal mask airways (LMAs), and endotracheal and tracheostomy tubes. The respiratory care practitioner must be able to select the appropriate airway, properly size and insert the airway, and maintain the airway and ventilation.

Nasopharyngeal airways, sometimes called nasal airways or trumpets, are chiefly used to facilitate the suctioning procedure. If the tube is too long it can interfere with the opening of the epiglottis. Even proper placement can lead to **epistaxis**, **otitis media**, or **sinusitis**.

Oropharyngeal airways are used to prevent the tongue from falling back into the oropharynx and blocking the airway. They are chiefly used to facilitate bag-valve-mask ventilation. They may also be used to maintain airway patency in patients who have adequate respiratory effort but inadequate muscle tone or airway protection reflexes. If the airway selected is too large it can interfere with the epiglottis. If the airway is too small it can push the tongue back into the pharynx. According to the AARC practice guideline on resuscitation, the oropharyngeal airway design should incorporate a **flange** and a short bite-block segment.[1] Tubes, such as the Esophageal-Tracheal Combitube™ (ETC), are being used occasionally by prehospital providers for difficult intubations.[2] The LMA has become increasingly popular as an alternative for difficult intubations in the operating room as well as emergency room and prehospital settings. This device provides a low-pressure seal around the glottis and may cause less trauma than endotracheal intubation. However, it does not reliably prevent aspiration.[2,3] It is contraindicated in nonfasting patients and in patients at high risk for aspiration. Its usefulness in an emergency setting has not yet been completely evaluated. Disposable versions in various sizes by different manufacturers are now available.

Endotracheal intubation and tracheostomy tubes are discussed in Chapters 22 and 23.

OBJECTIVES

Upon completion of this chapter, the student will be able to:

1. Identify various types of airway adjuncts, including oropharyngeal and nasopharyngeal airways, LMAs, ETC, and accessories such as bite blocks, tongue blades, and oropharyngeal suction devices.
2. Given a clinical scenario, select the most appropriate airway.
3. Measure a subject for the appropriate size airway.
4. Insert nasopharyngeal, oropharyngeal, LMA, and ETC airways into a mannequin or human patient simulator.

KEY TERMS

epistaxis	mandible	sinusitis
flange	naris	tragus
incisors	otitis media	uvula

Exercises

EQUIPMENT REQUIRED

- ☐ 4×4 gauze
- ☐ 50-psi gas source
- ☐ Airway management trainers—adult, pediatric, and infant
- ☐ Alcohol prep pads
- ☐ Brigg's adapter
- ☐ Cloth tape
- ☐ Esophageal-Tracheal Combitube™
- ☐ Flowmeter
- ☐ Gloves—nonsterile, latex-free, various sizes
- ☐ Goggles or face shields
- ☐ Hand sanitizer
- ☐ Human patient simulator (if available)
- ☐ Large-bore tubing

- ☐ Large-volume nebulizer
- ☐ Laryngeal mask airways (LMAs), various sizes
- ☐ Manual resuscitators with masks, various sizes
- ☐ Nasopharyngeal airways, various sizes and styles
- ☐ Oropharyngeal airways—Guedal and Berman styles, various sizes
- ☐ Silicone spray lubricant
- ☐ Suction source and connection tubing
- ☐ Tonsillar tip rigid catheter holder
- ☐ Water-soluble lubricant
- ☐ Yankauer (tonsillar tip) catheters, various styles

EXERCISE 20.1 IDENTIFICATION OF AIRWAY ADJUNCTS

Compare Figures 20.1 through 20.6 with the airways provided in the laboratory. **Identify the type of airway shown from the following list and record on your laboratory report.**

- Esophageal-Tracheal Combitube™
- Laryngeal mask airway
- Nasal airway—Rusch style
- Nasal trumpet
- Oropharyngeal airway—Berman style
- Oropharyngeal airway—Guedal style

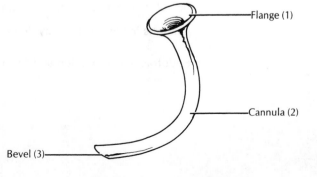

Figure 20.1. A. (Adapted from Eubanks, DH and Bone, RC: Comprehensive Respiratory Care: A Learning System. Mosby-Year Book, St. Louis, 1990, p. 548, with permission.)

Flange (1)

Cannula (2)

Bevel (3)

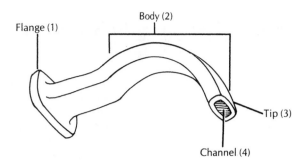

Figure 20.2. B. (From Eubanks, DH and Bone, RC: Comprehensive Respiratory Care: A Learning System. Mosby-Year Book, St. Louis, 1990, p. 548, with permission.)

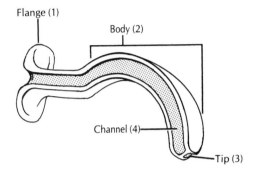

Figure 20.3. C. (From Eubanks, DH and Bone, RC: Comprehensive Respiratory Care: A Learning System. Mosby-Year Book, St. Louis, 1990, p. 548, with permission.)

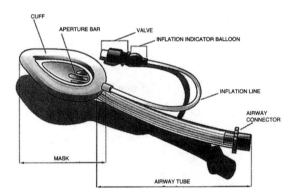

Figure 20.4. D. [Courtesy of Gensia, Inc., San Diego, CA. Gensia, Inc. is the exclusive distributor of the Laryngeal Mask Airway (LMA) in the United States.]

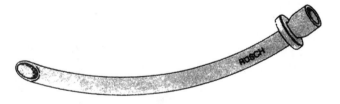

Figure 20.5. E. (Courtesy of Rusch Inc., Duluth, GA.)

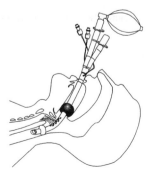

Figure 20.6. F. (Courtesy of Kendall Healthcare Products Company, Mansfield, MA.)

EXERCISE 20.2 SELECTION AND INSERTION OF A NASOPHARYNGEAL AIRWAY

1.   Select several sizes and styles of nasopharyngeal airways.
2.   Determine the proper size airway to use on your laboratory partner, as shown in Figure 20.7, by placing one end of the airway at the tip of the nose of your partner. Now pull the tube toward the ear. If the tube goes past the opening of the ear, it is too large. The tube length should equal the distance from the tip of the nose to the tragus of the ear plus 1 inch.[4] **Record the size selected on your laboratory report.**
3.   Wash or sanitize your hands and apply standard precautions and transmission-based isolation procedures as appropriate. Put on nonsterile gloves.
4.   Lubricate the airway of the airway management training mannequin with the silicone spray. NOTE: When inserting an airway into a patient, use a water-soluble lubricant.
5.   Insert the airway into the external naris of the airway management trainer and push the airway gently into place, following the anatomical curve as shown in Figure 20.8. Never force an airway into place. If an obstruction is met, try the other naris.
6.   The tip of the airway should be just past the uvula, as shown in Figure 20.9.

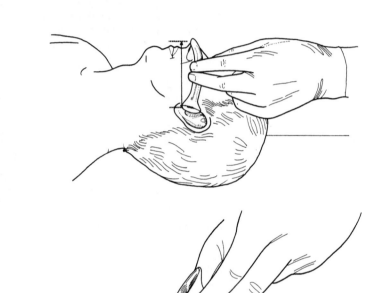

Figure 20.7. Sizing of a nasopharyngeal airway.

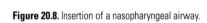

Figure 20.8. Insertion of a nasopharyngeal airway.

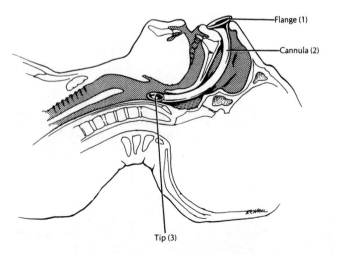

Figure 20.9. Placement of nasopharyngeal airway. (Adapted from Eubanks, DH and Bone, RC: Comprehensive Respiratory Care: A Learning System. Mosby-Year Book, St. Louis, 1990, p. 136, with permission.)

Flange (1)

Cannula (2)

Tip (3)

EXERCISE 20.3 SELECTION AND INSERTION OF AN OROPHARYNGEAL AIRWAY

1. Select several sizes of oropharyngeal airways.
2. Determine the proper size airway for your laboratory partner, as shown in Figure 20.10, by approximating the distance from the central incisors (front teeth) to the angle of the mandible.[1] **Record the size and type selected on your laboratory report.**
3. Wash your hands and apply standard precautions and transmission-based isolation procedures as appropriate. Put on nonsterile gloves.
4. Insert the airway into the airway management trainer (Fig. 20.11). Open the mouth using a cross-finger technique, and insert the airway into the mouth rotated 180 degrees (upside-down). Continue to advance the airway until it is past the hard palate to the level of the uvula. When it is almost completely in, rotate the airway into its final position so that the curvature of the airway follows the natural curvature of the tongue, keeping it in place. The end of the airway should be just beyond the base of the tongue, as shown in Figure 20.12.
5. Using a bag-valve-mask device, manually ventilate the mannequin with the airway in place for at least 5 minutes. Ensure that the chest is rising and falling.

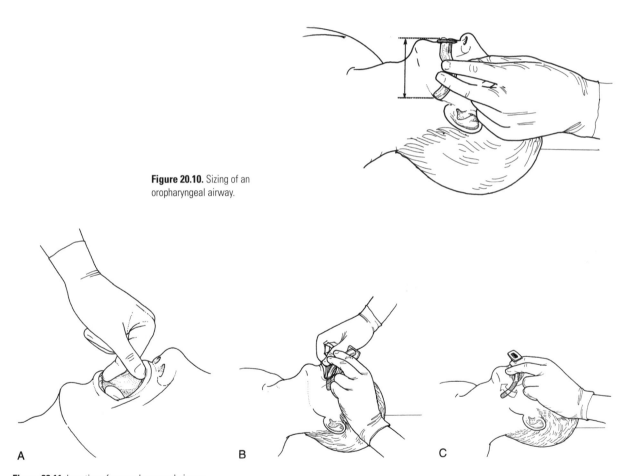

Figure 20.10. Sizing of an oropharyngeal airway.

A   B   C

Figure 20.11. Insertion of an oropharyngeal airway.

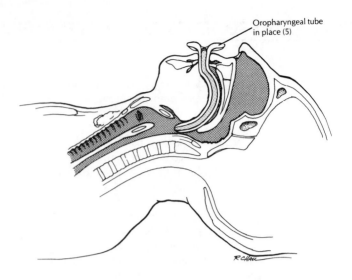

Oropharyngeal tube in place (5)

Figure 20.12. Placement of an oropharyngeal airway. (Adapted from Eubanks, DH and Bone, RC: Comprehensive Respiratory Care: A Learning System. Mosby-Year Book, St. Louis, 1990, p. 548, with permission.)

REFERENCES

1. American Association for Respiratory Care: Clinical practice guideline: Resuscitation in acute care hospitals. Respir Care 38:1169–1200, 1993.
2. American Association for Respiratory Care: AARC clinical practice guideline: Management of airway emergencies. Respir Care 40:749–760, 1995.
3. Sofair, E: Preanesthetic assessment: The professional singer with a difficult airway. Anesthesiology News 1:9, 40, 1993.
4. McPherson, S: Respiratory Care Equipment, ed 5. Mosby, St. Louis, 1995, p. 117.

Laboratory Report

CHAPTER 20: PHARYNGEAL AIRWAYS

Name _____ Date _____

Course/Section _____ Instructor _____

Data Collection

EXERCISE 20.1 Identification of Airway Adjuncts

A. Figure 20.1: _____

B. Figure 20.2: _____

C. Figure 20.3: _____

D. Figure 20.4: _____

E. Figure 20.5: _____

F. Figure 20.6: _____

EXERCISE 20.2 Selection and Insertion of a Nasopharyngeal Airway

Size selected: _____

EXERCISE 20.3 Selection and Insertion of an Oropharyngeal Airway

Size selected: _____ Type selected: _____

Critical Thinking Questions

1.   Why is a water-soluble lubricant used for inserting a nasal airway?

2.   What complications might arise from the use of a nasopharyngeal airway?

3. What complications might arise from an improperly sized oropharyngeal airway?

4. What complications might arise from an improperly sized nasopharyngeal airway?

5. For each of the following scenarios, indicate what type of airway should be used. State your rationale.

   A. Semiconscious patient in the recovery room:

   B. An elderly, nonintubated patient who requires frequent suctioning:

   C. A patient in cardiac arrest in the emergency room receiving basic life support (BLS):

6. A patient is brought into the emergency room with an Esophageal-Tracheal Combitube™ (ETC) in place. The physician wants you to intubate the patient with an endotracheal tube. What is the proper sequence of actions for replacing the ETC?

7. You are called to the recovery room to administer 40% oxygen to a patient with a laryngeal airway in place. Describe the equipment setup you would employ, including all connectors and adaptors needed.

8. The patient in question 7 has regained consciousness and the laryngeal airway has been removed. What should you do with the device at this time?

Procedural Competency Evaluation

STUDENT: DATE:

PHARYNGEAL AIRWAY INSERTION

Evaluator: ☐ Peer ☐ Instructor   **Setting:** ☐ Lab   ☐ Clinical Simulation

Equipment Utilized: **Conditions (Describe):**

Performance Level:

   S or ✓ = Satisfactory, no errors of omission or commission
   U = Unsatisfactory Error of Omission or Commission
   NA = Not applicable

Performance Rating:

  5   **Independent:** Near flawless performance; minimal errors; able to perform without supervision; seeks out new learning; shows initiative; A = 4.7–5.0 average

  4   **Minimally Supervised:** Few errors, able to self-correct; seeks guidance when appropriate; B = 3.7–4.65

  3   **Competent:** Minimal required level; no critical errors; able to correct with coaching; meets expectations; safe; C = 3.0–3.65

  2   **Marginal:** Below average; critical errors or problem areas noted; would benefit from remediation; D = 2.0–2.99

  1   **Dependent:** Poor; unacceptable performance; unsafe; gross inaccuracies; potentially harmful; F = < 2.0

  Two or more errors of commission or omission of mandatory or essential performance elements will terminate the procedure, and require additional practice and/or remediation and reevaluation. Student is responsible for obtaining additional evaluation forms as needed from the Director of Clinical Education (DCE).

(Columns: PERFORMANCE RATING, PERFORMANCE LEVEL)

EQUIPMENT AND PATIENT PREPARATION

1. Common Performance Elements Steps 1–8

ASSESSMENT AND IMPLEMENTATION

2. Common Performance Elements Steps 9 and 10
3. Assesses patient for the appropriate airway type [nasopharyngeal, oropharyngeal, Esophageal-Tracheal Combitube™ (ETC), LMA]
4. Measures the patient for the appropriate size airway
5. Lubricates the airway if necessary
6. Positions patient
7. Inserts the airway correctly
8. Assesses the patient for proper airway placement
9. Reinserts and adjusts airway if necessary
10. Inflates cuff if applicable
11. Reassesses as needed
12. Secures airway

FOLLOW-UP

13. Assures ventilation and oxygenation
14. Common Performance Elements Steps 11–16

SIGNATURES   Student: Evaluator: Date:

Clinical Performance Evaluation

PERFORMANCE RATING:

5 **Independent:** Near flawless performance; minimal errors; able to perform without supervision; seeks out new learning; shows initiative; A = 4.7–5.0 average

4 **Minimally Supervised:** Few errors, able to self-correct; seeks guidance when appropriate; B = 3.7–4.65

3 **Competent:** Minimal required level; no critical errors; able to correct with coaching; meets expectations; safe; C = 3.0–3.65

2 **Marginal:** Below average; critical errors or problem areas noted; would benefit from remediation; D = 2.0–2.99

1 **Dependent:** Poor; unacceptable performance; unsafe; gross inaccuracies; potentially harmful; F = < 2.0

Circle the appropriate response below. Please be consistent, objective, and honest in your assessment of the student's clinical performance and ability.

PERFORMANCE CRITERIA	SCORE				
COGNITIVE DOMAIN					
1. Consistently displays knowledge, comprehension, and command of essential concepts	5	4	3	2	1
2. Demonstrates the relationship between theory and clinical practice	5	4	3	2	1
3. Able to select, review, apply, analyze, synthesize, interpret, and evaluate information; makes recommendations to modify care plan	5	4	3	2	1
PSYCHOMOTOR DOMAIN					
4. Minimal errors, no critical errors; able to self-correct; performs all steps safely and accurately	5	4	3	2	1
5. Selects, assembles, and verifies proper function and cleanliness of equipment; assures operation and corrects malfunctions; provides adequate care and maintenance	5	4	3	2	1
6. Exhibits the required manual dexterity	5	4	3	2	1
7. Performs procedure in a reasonable time frame for clinical level	5	4	3	2	1
8. Applies and maintains aseptic technique and PPE as required	5	4	3	2	1
9. Maintains concise and accurate patient and clinical records	5	4	3	2	1
10. Reports promptly on patient status/needs to appropriate personnel	5	4	3	2	1
AFFECTIVE DOMAIN					
11. Exhibits courteous and pleasant demeanor; shows consideration and respect, honesty, and integrity	5	4	3	2	1
12. Communicates verbally and in writing clearly and concisely	5	4	3	2	1
13. Preserves confidentiality and adheres to all policies	5	4	3	2	1
14. Follows directions, exhibits sound judgment, and seeks help when required	5	4	3	2	1
15. Demonstrates initiative, self-direction, responsibility, and accountability	5	4	3	2	1

TOTAL POINTS = _____ /15 = AVERAGE GRADE = _____

ADDITIONAL COMMENTS: IDENTIFY AREAS OF EXCELLENCE; LIST ERRORS OF OMISSION OR COMMISSION, CRITICAL ERRORS

SUMMARY PERFORMANCE EVALUATION AND RECOMMENDATIONS

☐ PASS: Satisfactory Performance

    ☐ Minimal supervision needed, may progress to next level provided specific skills, clinical time completed

    ☐ Minimal supervision needed, able to progress to next level without remediation

☐ FAIL: Unsatisfactory Performance (check all that apply)

    ☐ Minor reevaluation only

    ☐ Needs additional clinical practice before reevaluation

    ☐ Needs additional laboratory practice before skills performed in clinical area

    ☐ Recommend clinical probation

SIGNATURES

Evaluator (print name): _____ Evaluator signature: _____ Date: _____

Student Signature: _____ Date: _____

Student Comments:

21 Suctioning

INTRODUCTION

Suctioning is one of the most frequent procedures performed by the respiratory care practitioner. It may be achieved by insertion of a suction catheter through the nasal passages (nasotracheal suction), by oral suctioning of the pharynx, or via an endotracheal tube. Unfortunately, it is too often treated as a benign procedure, which it most definitely is not. Hypoxemia, cardiac dysrhythmias, nosocomial infection, atelectasis, mucosal trauma, bronchospasm, pulmonary hemorrhage, elevated intracranial pressure, and patient discomfort are some of the more frequently encountered complications of this procedure, even when it is performed properly.[1,2] Respiratory or cardiac arrest is always a distinct possibility. Nasotracheal suctioning without an artificial airway may be one of the most dangerous procedures performed by respiratory care practitioners.

It is necessary to perform proper patient assessment before suctioning a patient. Assessing the need for suctioning can be accomplished by auscultation and palpation. Suctioning should be performed PRN only. Endotracheal suctioning may be required at some minimum frequency to ensure artificial airway patency.[1]

Practitioners should always be aware of the possible hazards and complications of these procedures. Care should be taken to ensure patient safety. Considerations include using the proper size catheter, maintenance of aseptic technique, patient preparation (including adequate preoxygenation before any suctioning event), and appropriate pressure and time limitations.

OBJECTIVES

Upon completion of this chapter, the student will be able to:

1. Identify the various types of suction devices and accessories, including Yankauer (tonsillar) catheter, Coudé or Bronchitrach-L angle-tip endobronchial catheters, closed suction system devices, and sputum traps.
2. Determine the proper suction catheter size for a given airway.
3. Demonstrate the proper aseptic donning of gloves and handling of the sterile contents of a suction kit.
4. Aseptically perform nasotracheal suctioning on an airway management trainer using appropriate personal protective equipment.
5. Perform endotracheal suctioning on an intubated airway management trainer using appropriate personal protective equipment.
6. Perform tracheobronchial lavage during suctioning.
7. Collect a sputum specimen during suctioning.
8. Demonstrate the proper disposal of contaminated suction equipment.
9. Correlate the physical principles involved in suctioning, such as Poiseuille's law, to suction equipment and procedures.

KEY TERMS

aspiration	instillation	soluble
flush	lavage	tenacious
irrigation	lubricant	vacuum

Exercises

EQUIPMENT REQUIRED

- ☐ Airway management trainers (intubated and nonintubated)
- ☐ Basins
- ☐ Biohazard transport bags
- ☐ Closed suction catheter systems, various sizes
- ☐ Coudé or Bronchitrach-L angle-tip endobronchial catheter
- ☐ Disposal bags
- ☐ Goggles or face shields
- ☐ Human patient simulator (if available)
- ☐ Manual resuscitator with mask
- ☐ Nonrebreathing masks
- ☐ Nonsterile disposable nonlatex gloves, various sizes
- ☐ Oxygen connecting tubing and nipple adaptors

- ☐ Oxygen gas source and flowmeter
- ☐ Pulse oximeter and probes
- ☐ Silicone spray for mannequins or **water-soluble lubricant**
- ☐ Sputum traps: Lukens and Dee Lee types
- ☐ Sterile gloves
- ☐ Sterile water or normal saline
- ☐ Sterile water-soluble lubricant
- ☐ Stethoscopes
- ☐ Suction catheter kits
- ☐ Suction source
- ☐ T-piece and large-bore corrugated tubing
- ☐ Unit-dose saline
- ☐ Yankauer (tonsillar tip) suction device

EXERCISE 21.1 SUCTION EQUIPMENT IDENTIFICATION

Compare the equipment provided in the laboratory with Figures 21.1 through 21.8. **Identify each item and record it on your laboratory report.**

Beaded-tip catheter

Bronchitrach-L angle-tip endobronchial catheter

Closed suction systems

Dee Lee sputum trap

Lukens sputum trap

Murphy-tip catheter

Suction connecting tubing

Thumb port or "Y" connector

Yankauer catheter, adult and pediatric

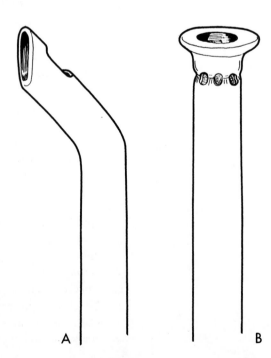

Figure 21.1. A and B

A

B

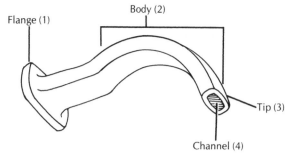

Flange (1)   Body (2)   Tip (3)   Channel (4)

Figure 21.2. C.

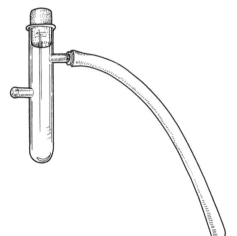

Figure 21.3. D.

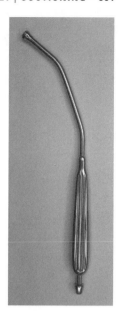

Figure 21.5. F.

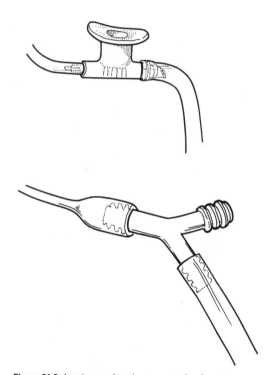

Figure 21.6. G. (Courtesy of Ballard Medical Products, Draper UT.)

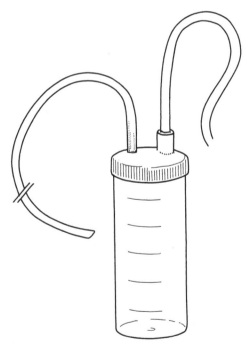

Figure 21.4. E.

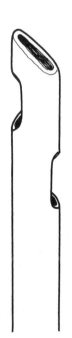

Figure 21.7. H.

Figure 21.8. Attachment of suction source to thumb-port connection or Y-connector of suction catheter.

EXERCISE 21.2 OROPHARYNGEAL SUCTIONING

1. Wash or sanitize your hands and apply standard precautions and transmission-based isolation procedures as appropriate.
2. Select a Yankauer (tonsillar) suction unit.
3. Put on nonsterile gloves.
4. Attach the Yankauer suction device to the end of the suction connecting tube.
5. Fill a basin with sterile water or normal saline.
6. Turn on the suction unit.
7. Test the unit by suctioning some of the sterile water or normal saline.
8. Introduce the Yankauer suction unit into the mouth of the mannequin and "suction" the mouth of the mannequin.
9. Remove the unit from the mouth of the mannequin and clean it by flushing the unit and the tubing.
10. Disconnect the unit and shut off the machine.
11. Cover the unit with the wrapper.
12. Remove your gloves and wash or sanitize your hands.
13. Dispose of all infectious waste in the proper receptacles.

EXERCISE 21.3 SUCTION KITS

This section is designed to practice aseptic technique in handling suction equipment. The actual suctioning procedure will be practiced in the next exercise.

1. Select a suction kit.
2. Open the kit, making sure to maintain the sterility of the contents.
3. Identify the components in the kit by visual inspection. *Do not touch the contents.*
   A. **Record the brand used and contents contained on your laboratory report.**
   B. Depending on the brand of suction kit used, additional items may need to be obtained to complete the procedure. Compare the contents of your kit with the following list, and obtain any additional items needed.
      i. Two sterile gloves
      ii. Sterile drape or other surface on which to place equipment
      iii. Sterile basin
      iv. Sterile water or saline
      v. Sterile suction catheter
4. Put on the gloves using the procedure practiced in Chapter 1.
5. Open the sterile basin and fill the basin with the sterile solution using your nondominant hand, if the basin is not prefilled. Keep in mind that if you are using a separate supply of sterile solution, the container must also be handled aseptically. The bottle of sterile solution should be marked with the date and time when first opened. Solution should be discarded after 24 hours. When opening the solution, the bottle cap should be placed upside down aseptically on a clean surface.
6. Pick up the catheter with your dominant hand, keeping the catheter coiled. Remember that this hand is considered to be the sterile hand and must touch nothing but the catheter.
7. While grasping the catheter in the palm of your hand, remove the glove from your dominant hand by pulling the glove down and completely over the catheter.
8. Remove the other glove and discard the gloves into the proper garbage receptacle.

NOTE: For the purpose of laboratory practice, you may be reusing the suction kit and supplies. If so, you should attempt to reorganize the kit in the way in which it was originally found.

EXERCISE 21.4 NASOTRACHEAL SUCTIONING

1. Wash or sanitize your hands and apply personal protective equipment as appropriate.
2. Gather the necessary equipment: oxygen gas source, nonrebreathing mask, suction kit, water-soluble lubricant, sterile water or normal saline, and suction machine.
3. Place the mannequin or human patient simulator in the Fowler's position. In an actual clinical situation, you should remove the pillow from behind the patient's head and place the head in a neutral position, avoiding hyperextension.
4. Assemble the nonrebreathing mask and oxygen.
5. Place the mask on the mannequin to hyperoxygenate the "patient" before suctioning. Instruct the "patient" to take several deep breaths. Patients should be hyperoxygenated before the suction event for at least 30 seconds.[1]
6. Assess the "patient" for adequate oxygenation, including color, respiratory rate and pattern, heart rate and rhythm, and pulse oximetry.
7. Size, lubricate, and insert a nasopharyngeal airway into one naris (as performed in Chapter 19).
8. Turn on the suction unit.
9. Adjust the suction to the appropriate suction pressure (Table 21.1).
10. Open the water-soluble lubricant.
11. Open the suction kit and put on the gloves as in Exercise 21.2.
12. Connect the suction tubing to the thumb port connection or "Y" connector of the suction catheter, as shown in Figure 21.8.
13. Test the suction by placing the catheter into the sterile solution and occluding the thumb port with the thumb of your nondominant hand. Readjust the suction pressure if necessary.
14. Apply the lubricant to the catheter by either squeezing the tube or packet into the palm of your sterile hand and then pulling the catheter through the jelly to achieve lubrication, or applying the lubricant to the sterile interior of the suction kit and then rotating the catheter through it.
15. Without applying the suction, introduce the catheter into one of the nares, slowly and gently pushing the catheter until it advances into the oropharynx. Never force the catheter. If an obstruction is met, attempt to pass the catheter through the other naris.
16. When you notice "fogging" of the catheter (condensation from exhaled air) or you hear a change in the patient's voice, you are entering the trachea. Obviously this will not be apparent on a mannequin. Continue introducing the catheter until an obstruction is met.
17. Once the obstruction is met, withdraw the catheter about one-half inch and apply the suction with your thumb on the thumb port.
18. Continue to withdraw the catheter until it is removed. The withdrawal procedure and application of suction should not take longer than 10 seconds.[1,2] Frequently assess the "patient" during the procedure.
19. Reapply the nonrebreathing mask with your nonsterile hand to reoxygenate the "patient." Patients should be reoxygenated for at least 1 minute before repeating the suction event.[2]
20. Flush the catheter and the tubing to clean it by suctioning the sterile solution through the catheter.
21. Reassess the "patient" and repeat the procedure if needed after a sufficient time for recovery.
22. Remove the nonrebreathing mask.
23. Turn the suction off.
24. Remove gloves and dispose of all equipment properly.
25. Wash or sanitize your hands.

Table 21.1 Recommended Suction Vacuum Pressures

	Wall Unit	Portable Unit
Adult	−100 to −120 mm Hg (−150 mm Hg maximum may be used)	10–15 in. Hg
Child	−80 to −100 mm Hg	5–10 in. Hg
Infant	−60 to −80 mm Hg	3–5 in. Hg

EXERCISE 21.5 ENDOTRACHEAL SUCTIONING

1. Select an intubated mannequin. Note the size of the endotracheal tube (ETT) being used by looking at the underside of the 15-mm endotracheal tube adaptor. **Record the size of the endotracheal tube on your laboratory report.**

2. Determine the size of the suction catheter to use. The outer diameter (OD) of the suction catheter should not exceed one-half the size of the inner diameter (ID) of the airway.[1] Because the airway is usually measured in millimeters and suction catheters are usually measured in even-numbered French (Fr) sizes, a conversion is necessary. The following formula will result in the maximum recommended catheter size:

   $$[(0.5\ ID\ mm \times 3) + 2] = Fr\ suction\ catheter\ size$$

   Alternatively, the following can be used:

   $$[(ETT\ ID\ mm \times 2) - 2]$$

3. **Record the size of the catheter selected on your laboratory report.**

4. Wash or sanitize your hands and apply personal protective equipment as appropriate. Goggles, gloves, and gown are recommended.[3,4]

5. Gather the necessary equipment: oxygen gas source, manual resuscitator, suction kit, sterile water or normal saline, unit-dose saline, and suction machine.

6. Assemble the manual resuscitator and oxygen. The "patient" should receive hyperoxygenation by 100% oxygen for at least 30 seconds before the suction procedure.[1] This may be accomplished by several methods.

7. Increase the F_IO_2 to 100% on the oxygen delivery device, if possible.

8. A manual resuscitator may be used with maximum F_IO_2. Practitioners should ensure that PEEP levels are maintained.[1]

9. If the "patient" is on a mechanical ventilator, the F_IO_2 can be adjusted to 100% or, alternatively, some ventilators have a temporary oxygen enrichment mode available. This method may be more effective than using a manual resuscitator.[1] If this method is used, sufficient time must be allowed for the circuit to be flushed with the 100% oxygen before the suction event.

10. Regardless of the method selected, the practitioner must allow sufficient time for pre- and postoxygenation so that the SpO_2 nears 100%. Be sure to return the F_IO_2 to the original setting when the procedure is completed.

11. Adjust the suction to the appropriate suction pressure.

12. Loosen the oxygen delivery device connected to the endotracheal tube.

13. Open the suction kit and put on the gloves as described in Exercise 21.2.

14. Connect the suction tubing to the other end of the suction catheter.

15. Test the suction unit as described in Exercise 21.3.

16. With your nonsterile hand, disconnect the oxygen delivery device attached to the endotracheal tube and connect the manual resuscitator. Make sure that you place the oxygen delivery device on a sterile field so as not to contaminate the device.

17. Hyperinflate and hyperoxygenate for at least 30 seconds. Assess the "patient" for adequate oxygenation, including color, respiratory rate and pattern, heart rate and rhythm, electrocardiogram (ECG), and pulse oximetry.

18. Quickly disconnect the oxygen source with your nondominant hand. Be sure not to place the device in a soiled area.

19. Without applying the suction, quickly introduce the catheter into the tube, advancing the catheter until it meets an obstruction.

20. Upon meeting an obstruction, withdraw the catheter about one-half inch and apply the suction with your thumb on the thumb port.

21. Continue to withdraw the catheter, rotating it between your fingers, until it is removed. The entire procedure should not take longer than 15 seconds. The withdrawal procedure and application of suction should not take longer than 10 seconds. Frequently reassess the "patient" during the procedure. Suction may be applied continuously. Intermittent suction has not demonstrated any significant beneficial effect.[5,6]

22. Reconnect the bag and hyperinflate and hyperoxygenate for at least 1 minute.

23. With your nonsterile hand, open one or two unit-dose saline vials. NOTE: If secretions are particularly tenacious or difficult to remove, the "patient" may be lavaged with saline to facilitate secretion removal. Recent studies suggest that a potential for dislodging bacteria

into the lower airway and causing nosocomial infection may exist,[4,7] and continued practice is an unresolved issue. At this time, the procedure is still recommended when necessary but should be abandoned as a routine procedure.[1,8]

24. Disconnect the bag and aseptically instill the saline into the tube.
25. Reconnect and hyperinflate and hyperoxygenate for at least 1 minute.
26. Repeat the suction procedure.
27. Reconnect and hyperinflate and hyperoxygenate for at least 1 minute.
28. Return the "patient" to the proper oxygen delivery device and F_IO_2.
29. Flush the catheter and the tubing.
30. Disconnect the catheter from the connecting tubing. Remove gloves around the catheter as previously described, and dispose of all equipment properly.
31. Turn the suction off.
32. Dispose of infectious waste. Wash or sanitize your hands.

EXERCISE 21.6 ENDOTRACHEAL SUCTIONING WITH A CLOSED SYSTEM

1. Select an intubated mannequin.
2. Wash or sanitize your hands and then put on nonsterile gloves.
3. Assemble the closed suction system, as shown in Figure 21.9, and attach to the patient connection.

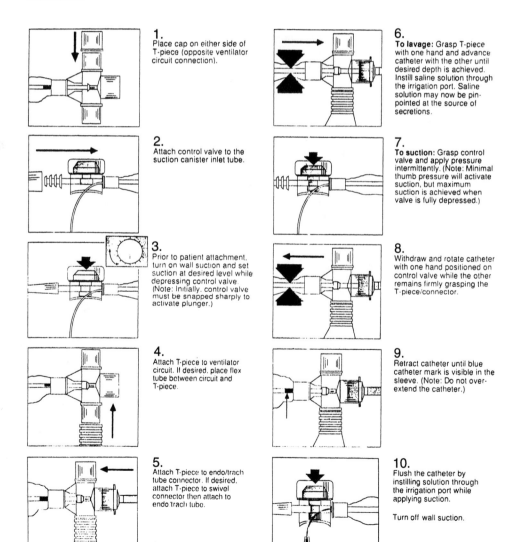

1. Place cap on either side of T-piece (opposite ventilator circuit connection).

2. Attach control valve to the suction canister inlet tube.

3. Prior to patient attachment, turn on wall suction and set suction at desired level while depressing control valve. (Note: Initially, control valve must be snapped sharply to activate plunger.)

4. Attach T-piece to ventilator circuit. If desired, place flex tube between circuit and T-piece.

5. Attach T-piece to endo/trach tube connector. If desired, attach T-piece to swivel connector then attach to endo/trach tube.

6. **To lavage:** Grasp T-piece with one hand and advance catheter with the other until desired depth is achieved. Instill saline solution through the irrigation port. Saline solution may now be pin-pointed at the source of secretions.

7. **To suction:** Grasp control valve and apply pressure intermittently. (Note: Minimal thumb pressure will activate suction, but maximum suction is achieved when valve is fully depressed.)

8. Withdraw and rotate catheter with one hand positioned on control valve while the other remains firmly grasping the T-piece/connector.

9. Retract catheter until blue catheter mark is visible in the sleeve. (Note: Do not over-extend the catheter.)

10. Flush the catheter by instilling solution through the irrigation port while applying suction.

Turn off wall suction.

Figure 21.9. Assembly of a closed suction system. (Courtesy of Smiths Industries Medical Systems, Keene, NH.)

4. Connect the end of the system to the suction tubing.
5. Turn the suction unit on.
6. Turn the thumb control for suction to the "on" position.
7. Hyperoxygenate and hyperinflate the "patient" for at least 30 seconds. (Note that because these units are most commonly used with a ventilator, hyperinflation and hyperoxygenation are achieved through the ventilator before this step.)
8. Assess the "patient" for adequate oxygenation, including color, respiratory rate and pattern, heart rate and rhythm, ECG (if available), and pulse oximetry.
9. Introduce the catheter into the airway by sliding it through the plastic sheath until resistance is met.
10. Withdraw the catheter about one-half inch and apply suction as you withdraw the catheter completely, pulling it straight out. Make sure that the tip is visible past the T connection. Reassess the "patient" frequently during the procedure.
11. Reoxygenate and hyperinflate for at least 1 minute. Repeat the procedure if necessary.
12. Clean the catheter. Some brands have an irrigation port that allows you to inject saline and flush the catheter. Refer to the manufacturer's package insert for brand specific instructions.
13. Make sure the thumb suction control is returned to the "off" or locked position when finished.
14. Turn the suction off.

EXERCISE 21.7 OBTAINING A SPUTUM SAMPLE

1. Repeat all the steps in Exercise 21.4, except make sure that you have put a sputum trap in line as shown in Figure 21.10. Do not perform the lavage procedure.
2. After completing the procedure, disconnect the trap from the suction connecting tube. Seal it by interconnecting the tubing to the trap inlet.
3. Label the sample with the appropriate information, and **record this information on your laboratory report.**
   A. "Patient" name and identification number
   B. Room number
   C. Date and time
   D. Type or source of sample
4. Place in biohazard transport bag with the "lab slip."
5. Notify the "nurse" that the sample has been obtained.

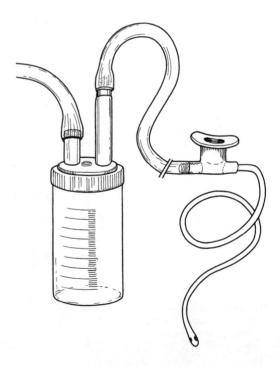

Figure 21.10. Assembly of
suction-sputum trap equipment.

REFERENCES

1. American Association for Respiratory Care: AARC clinical practice guideline: Endotracheal suctioning of mechanically ventilated adults and children with artificial airways. Respir Care 36:500–504, 1991.
2. American Association for Respiratory Care: AARC clinical practice guideline: Nasotracheal suctioning. Respir Care 36:898–901, 1991.
3. Centers for Disease Control and Prevention: Update: Universal precautions for prevention of transmission of human immunodeficiency virus, hepatitis B virus, and other blood-borne pathogens in the health care setting. MMWR 37:377–399, 1988.
4. Centers for Disease Control and Prevention: Guideline for prevention of nosocomial pneumonia. Respir Care 39:1191–1236, 1994.
5. Czarni, R et al: Differential effects of continuous versus intermittent suction on tracheal tissue. Heart Lung 202:144, 1991.
6. Kleiber, C, Krutzfield, N and Rose, E: Acute histologic changes in the tracheobronchial tree associated with different suction catheter insertion techniques. Heart Lung 17:12, 1988.
7. Hagler, DA and Traver, GA: Endotracheal saline and suction catheters: Sources of lower airway contamination. Am J Crit Care 3:444, 1993.
8. Ackerman, MH: The effect of saline lavage prior to suctioning. Am J Crit Care 2:326–330, 1993.

Laboratory Report

CHAPTER 21: SUCTIONING

Name _____   Date _____

Course/Section _____   Instructor _____

Data Collection

EXERCISE 21.1 Suction Equipment Identification

A. _____

B. _____

C. _____

D. _____

E. _____

F. _____

G. _____

H. _____

EXERCISE 21.3 Suction Kits

Brand used: _____

Contents: _____

EXERCISE 21.5 Endotracheal Suctioning

Size of endotracheal tube: _____

Size of the suction catheter (**show your work!**): _____
_____

EXERCISE 21.7 Obtaining a Sputum Sample

LABEL INFORMATION

Patient name:_____ ID#:_____

Date:_____ Time:_____

Type of sample:_____ Site:_____

Critical Thinking Questions

1. Identify at least three hazards and complications of suctioning that are unique to the nasotracheal route.

2. Contrast the dysrhythmias one would expect as a result of vagal stimulation during the suctioning procedure versus those that would result from hypoxemia.

3. Differentiate between mucus, sputum, and phlegm.

4. Is sputum normally considered a high-risk fluid for the transmission of bloodborne pathogens? Why or why not?

5. What is the rationale for personal protective equipment use while performing suctioning?

6. Given the following scenarios, identify all possible causes of the problem and offer at least two alternative solutions to correct each problem.

   A. You turn on an electrical suction machine and it does not work.

   B. In the middle of suctioning a patient, the suction is lost.

   C. You cannot get suction from a wall suction regulator.

D.   While attempting to suction an adult patient with an endotracheal tube, you cannot advance the catheter more than 5 inches.

E.   After suctioning a patient, you hear a honking or high-pitched sound coming from the endotracheal tube.

7.   Calculate the maximum catheter sizes that can be used (**show your work!**):

A.   ID 4.0-mm tracheostomy tube

B.   ID 6.0-mm endotracheal tube

C.   ID 7.5-mm endotracheal tube

D.   ID 10-mm tracheostomy tube

8.   A patient is suffering from hypoxemia, dysrhythmias, and bronchospasm during suctioning. Identify what methods you would use to assess the patient's status during suctioning and describe what precautions should be taken to prevent each of the hazards mentioned.

Procedural Competency Evaluation

STUDENT: _____   **DATE:** _____

	PERFORMANCE RATING	PERFORMANCE LEVEL
ENDOTRACHEAL SUCTIONING		
Evaluator: ☐ Peer ☐ Instructor **Setting:** ☐ Lab ☐ Clinical Simulation		
Equipment Utilized: _____ **Conditions (Describe):** _____		
Performance Level: S or ✓ = Satisfactory, no errors of omission or commission U = Unsatisfactory Error of Omission or Commission NA = Not applicable		
Performance Rating: **5** **Independent:** Near flawless performance; minimal errors; able to perform without supervision; seeks out new learning; shows initiative; A = 4.7–5.0 average **4** **Minimally Supervised:** Few errors, able to self-correct; seeks guidance when appropriate; B = 3.7–4.65 **3** **Competent:** Minimal required level; no critical errors; able to correct with coaching; meets expectations; safe; C = 3.0–3.65 **2** **Marginal:** Below average; critical errors or problem areas noted; would benefit from remediation; D = 2.0–2.99 **1** **Dependent:** Poor; unacceptable performance; unsafe; gross inaccuracies; potentially harmful; F = < 2.0 *Two or more errors of commission or omission of mandatory or essential performance elements will terminate the procedure, and require additional practice and/or remediation and reevaluation. Student is responsible for obtaining additional evaluation forms as needed from the Director of Clinical Education (DCE).*		
EQUIPMENT AND PATIENT PREPARATION		
1. Common Performance Elements Steps 1–8		
ASSESSMENT AND IMPLEMENTATION		
2. Common Performance Elements Steps 9 and 10		
3. Adjusts vacuum pressure to age-appropriate level		
4. Attaches sputum trap, if required		
5. Preoxygenates/hyperinflates patient using manual resuscitation bag, ventilator set to 100% suction, or nonrebreathing mask (spontaneously breathing patient without airway) for 30–60 seconds until SpO_2 100%		
6. Inserts catheter in airway; withdraws slightly if resistance met		
7. Aspirates the airway on withdrawal only with a gentle rotating motion (continuous or intermittent suction may be applied)		
8. Ensures aspiration lasts no longer than 10 seconds		
9. Maintains aseptic technique throughout procedure		
10. Monitors for adverse reactions		
11. Oxygenates patient following aspiration until stabilized		
12. Repeats as necessary		
13. Returns O_2 therapy to previous level		
FOLLOW-UP		
14. Common Performance Elements Steps 11–16		
15. If in-line closed suction used, ensures black line is pulled out of airway adaptor and locks thumb port device		
16. Turns off suction gauge		

SIGNATURES   Student: _____   Evaluator: _____   Date: _____

Clinical Performance Evaluation

PERFORMANCE RATING:

5 **Independent:** Near flawless performance; minimal errors; able to perform without supervision; seeks out new learning; shows initiative; A = 4.7–5.0 average

4 **Minimally Supervised:** Few errors, able to self-correct; seeks guidance when appropriate; B = 3.7–4.65

3 **Competent:** Minimal required level; no critical errors; able to correct with coaching; meets expectations; safe; C = 3.0–3.65

2 **Marginal:** Below average; critical errors or problem areas noted; would benefit from remediation; D = 2.0–2.99

1 **Dependent:** Poor; unacceptable performance; unsafe; gross inaccuracies; potentially harmful; F = < 2.0

Circle the appropriate response below. Please be consistent, objective, and honest in your assessment of the student's clinical performance and ability.

PERFORMANCE CRITERIA | SCORE

PERFORMANCE CRITERIA					
COGNITIVE DOMAIN					
1. Consistently displays knowledge, comprehension, and command of essential concepts	5	4	3	2	1
2. Demonstrates the relationship between theory and clinical practice	5	4	3	2	1
3. Able to select, review, apply, analyze, synthesize, interpret, and evaluate information; makes recommendations to modify care plan	5	4	3	2	1
PSYCHOMOTOR DOMAIN					
4. Minimal errors, no critical errors; able to self-correct; performs all steps safely and accurately	5	4	3	2	1
5. Selects, assembles, and verifies proper function and cleanliness of equipment; assures operation and corrects malfunctions; provides adequate care and maintenance	5	4	3	2	1
6. Exhibits the required manual dexterity	5	4	3	2	1
7. Performs procedure in a reasonable time frame for clinical level	5	4	3	2	1
8. Applies and maintains aseptic technique and PPE as required	5	4	3	2	1
9. Maintains concise and accurate patient and clinical records	5	4	3	2	1
10. Reports promptly on patient status/needs to appropriate personnel	5	4	3	2	1
AFFECTIVE DOMAIN					
11. Exhibits courteous and pleasant demeanor; shows consideration and respect, honesty, and integrity	5	4	3	2	1
12. Communicates verbally and in writing clearly and concisely	5	4	3	2	1
13. Preserves confidentiality and adheres to all policies	5	4	3	2	1
14. Follows directions, exhibits sound judgment, and seeks help when required	5	4	3	2	1
15. Demonstrates initiative, self-direction, responsibility, and accountability	5	4	3	2	1

TOTAL POINTS = /15 = AVERAGE GRADE =

ADDITIONAL COMMENTS: IDENTIFY AREAS OF EXCELLENCE; LIST ERRORS OF OMISSION OR COMMISSION, CRITICAL ERRORS

SUMMARY PERFORMANCE EVALUATION AND RECOMMENDATIONS

☐ PASS: Satisfactory Performance

☐ Minimal supervision needed, may progress to next level provided specific skills, clinical time completed

☐ Minimal supervision needed, able to progress to next level without remediation

☐ FAIL: Unsatisfactory Performance (check all that apply)

☐ Minor reevaluation only

☐ Needs additional clinical practice before reevaluation

☐ Needs additional laboratory practice before skills performed in clinical area

☐ Recommend clinical probation

SIGNATURES

Evaluator (print name): Evaluator signature: Date:

Student Signature: Date:

Student Comments:

Procedural Competency Evaluation

STUDENT: DATE:

NASOTRACHEAL SUCTIONING

		PERFORMANCE RATING	PERFORMANCE LEVEL
Evaluator: ☐ Peer ☐ Instructor **Setting:** ☐ Lab ☐ Clinical Simulation			
Equipment Utilized: **Conditions (Describe):**			
Performance Level: S or ✓ = Satisfactory, no errors of omission or commission U = Unsatisfactory Error of Omission or Commission NA = Not applicable			
Performance Rating: **5** **Independent:** Near flawless performance; minimal errors; able to perform without supervision; seeks out new learning; shows initiative; A = 4.7–5.0 average **4** **Minimally Supervised:** Few errors, able to self-correct; seeks guidance when appropriate; B = 3.7–4.65 **3** **Competent:** Minimal required level; no critical errors; able to correct with coaching; meets expectations; safe; C = 3.0–3.65 **2** **Marginal:** Below average; critical errors or problem areas noted; would benefit from remediation; D = 2.0–2.99 **1** **Dependent:** Poor; unacceptable performance; unsafe; gross inaccuracies; potentially harmful; F = < 2.0 *Two or more errors of commission or omission of mandatory or essential performance elements will terminate the procedure, and require additional practice and/or remediation and reevaluation. Student is responsible for obtaining additional evaluation forms as needed from the Director of Clinical Education (DCE).*			
EQUIPMENT AND PATIENT PREPARATION			
1. Common Performance Elements Steps 1–8			
2. Adjusts vacuum pressure to age-appropriate level			
3. Ensures oxygenation device is available			
ASSESSMENT AND IMPLEMENTATION			
4. Common Performance Elements Steps 9 and 10			
5. Positions patient appropriately (Fowler's, pillow removed, head in "sniffing" position)			
6. Preoxygenates/hyperinflates the patient with BVM or nonrebreathing mask for at least 30 seconds			
7. Lubricates nasal airway and inserts into patent naris			
8. Lubricates suction catheter and inserts catheter into nasal airway at appropriate distance			
9. Assesses catheter entry into the trachea (cough, change in voice, fogging)			
10. Applies suction <10 seconds upon withdrawal with gentle rotating motion, 15 seconds max for entire event			
11. Reoxygenates patient following aspiration for at least 1 minute			
12. Monitors for adverse reactions and stops procedure if necessary			
13. If laryngospasm occurs, attaches suction catheter to oxygen source (does not remove) and applies manual ventilation			
14. Examines sputum, collects if indicated			
15. Repeats as necessary			
FOLLOW-UP			
16. Repositions patient			
17. Returns O$_2$ therapy to previous level			
18. Turns off suction gauge when finished			
19. Common Performance Elements Steps 11–16			

SIGNATURES   Student: Evaluator: Date:

Clinical Performance Evaluation

PERFORMANCE RATING:

5 **Independent:** Near flawless performance; minimal errors; able to perform without supervision; seeks out new learning; shows initiative; A = 4.7–5.0 average

4 **Minimally Supervised:** Few errors, able to self-correct; seeks guidance when appropriate; B = 3.7–4.65

3 **Competent:** Minimal required level; no critical errors; able to correct with coaching; meets expectations; safe; C = 3.0–3.65

2 **Marginal:** Below average; critical errors or problem areas noted; would benefit from remediation; D = 2.0–2.99

1 **Dependent:** Poor; unacceptable performance; unsafe; gross inaccuracies; potentially harmful; F = < 2.0

Circle the appropriate response below. Please be consistent, objective, and honest in your assessment of the student's clinical performance and ability.

PERFORMANCE CRITERIA	SCORE				
COGNITIVE DOMAIN					
1. Consistently displays knowledge, comprehension, and command of essential concepts	5	4	3	2	1
2. Demonstrates the relationship between theory and clinical practice	5	4	3	2	1
3. Able to select, review, apply, analyze, synthesize, interpret, and evaluate information; makes recommendations to modify care plan	5	4	3	2	1
PSYCHOMOTOR DOMAIN					
4. Minimal errors, no critical errors; able to self-correct; performs all steps safely and accurately	5	4	3	2	1
5. Selects, assembles, and verifies proper function and cleanliness of equipment; assures operation and corrects malfunctions; provides adequate care and maintenance	5	4	3	2	1
6. Exhibits the required manual dexterity	5	4	3	2	1
7. Performs procedure in a reasonable time frame for clinical level	5	4	3	2	1
8. Applies and maintains aseptic technique and PPE as required	5	4	3	2	1
9. Maintains concise and accurate patient and clinical records	5	4	3	2	1
10. Reports promptly on patient status/needs to appropriate personnel	5	4	3	2	1
AFFECTIVE DOMAIN					
11. Exhibits courteous and pleasant demeanor; shows consideration and respect, honesty, and integrity	5	4	3	2	1
12. Communicates verbally and in writing clearly and concisely	5	4	3	2	1
13. Preserves confidentiality and adheres to all policies	5	4	3	2	1
14. Follows directions, exhibits sound judgment, and seeks help when required	5	4	3	2	1
15. Demonstrates initiative, self-direction, responsibility, and accountability	5	4	3	2	1

TOTAL POINTS = _____ /15 = AVERAGE GRADE = _____

ADDITIONAL COMMENTS: IDENTIFY AREAS OF EXCELLENCE; LIST ERRORS OF OMISSION OR COMMISSION, CRITICAL ERRORS

SUMMARY PERFORMANCE EVALUATION AND RECOMMENDATIONS

☐ PASS: Satisfactory Performance

　☐ Minimal supervision needed, may progress to next level provided specific skills, clinical time completed

　☐ Minimal supervision needed, able to progress to next level without remediation

☐ FAIL: Unsatisfactory Performance (check all that apply)

　☐ Minor reevaluation only

　☐ Needs additional clinical practice before reevaluation

　☐ Needs additional laboratory practice before skills performed in clinical area

　☐ Recommend clinical probation

SIGNATURES

Evaluator (print name): _____　　Evaluator signature: _____　　Date: _____

Student Signature: _____　　Date: _____

Student Comments:

22 Endotracheal Intubation

INTRODUCTION

In previous chapters you have learned how to manage the airway without inserting an artificial airway into the trachea. A patient's life may depend on the ability of an individual to recognize the need for intubation of the trachea and to place and manage that airway properly. That individual is often the respiratory care practitioner. The practitioner must be able to place the airway properly and must be able to recognize the clinical situations in which one airway is preferred over another.[1] The AARC clinical practice guideline for management of airway emergencies emphasizes the need for the practitioner to be able to identify, use, and maintain the equipment necessary for intubation. Intubation of the trachea is an advanced skill that requires extensive practice. One does not become proficient in intubation by completing these exercises. Further practice in an environment such as an operating room is required.

OBJECTIVES

Upon completion of this chapter, the student will be able to:

1. Identify, select, prepare, and correct malfunctions of equipment necessary for endotracheal intubation of the infant and adult.
2. Identify the different types of endotracheal tubes, component parts, and tube markings.
3. Assess the potential difficulty of intubation using the Mallampati classification.[2,3]
4. Test an artificial airway for cuff leaks.
5. Insert an orotracheal tube into an infant, a pediatric, and an adult airway management trainer.
6. Remove an esophageal or tracheal Combitube™ tube airway after intubation.
7. Manage and remove a laryngeal mask airway (LMA) in a postoperative recovery situation.
8. Insert a nasotracheal tube into an adult airway management trainer using direct vision and blind technique.
9. Verify the proper positioning of an artificial airway and secure it in place.
10. Apply infection control guidelines and standards according to OSHA regulations and CDC guidelines while performing endotracheal intubation.

KEY TERMS

Mallampati classification   Sellick maneuver   vallecula

Exercises

EQUIPMENT REQUIRED

- [ ] 10-mL syringes
- [ ] Adhesive removal pads
- [ ] Airway management trainers—adult, pediatric, and infant
- [ ] Atomizer
- [ ] Basins
- [ ] Batteries for laryngoscopes
- [ ] Cloth tape
- [ ] Colorimetric capnometer (EasyCap™) or other spot-check capnography device
- [ ] Commercial endotracheal tube holders
- [ ] Cook airway exchange catheter
- [ ] Curved (MacIntosh) laryngoscope blades, adult and pediatric sizes
- [ ] Endotracheal tubes: adult cuffed
- [ ] Endotracheal tubes: Carlen's catheter or double-lumen endotracheal tube (DLET)
- [ ] Endotracheal tubes: Cole catheter
- [ ] Endotracheal tubes: Emergency Medicine Tube (EMT®)
- [ ] Endotracheal tubes: Endotrol (built-in stylet)
- [ ] Endotracheal tubes: Hi-Lo Evac Tube™ (continuous cuff suction)
- [ ] Endotracheal tubes: infant uncuffed
- [ ] Endotracheal tubes: nasal or oral Ring-Adair-Elwyn (RAE)
- [ ] Endotracheal tubes: pediatric size, cuffed and uncuffed
- [ ] Endotracheal tubes: wire-reinforced (anode or armored)

- [ ] Esophageal-Tracheal Combitube™ (ETC)
- [ ] Goggles or face shields
- [ ] Hand sanitizer
- [ ] In-line suction catheters, various sizes
- [ ] Laryngeal mask airways (LMAs), various sizes
- [ ] Laryngoscope handles
- [ ] Magill forceps
- [ ] Manual resuscitators with masks, adult and infant
- [ ] Nasopharyngeal airways, various sizes
- [ ] Oropharyngeal airways, various sizes
- [ ] Oxygen connecting tubing and nipple adaptors
- [ ] Oxygen gas source and flowmeter
- [ ] Replacement laryngoscope bulbs
- [ ] Scissors
- [ ] Silicone spray
- [ ] Sterile and nonsterile disposable latex and vinyl gloves, various sizes
- [ ] Sterile water or normal saline
- [ ] Stethoscopes
- [ ] Straight (Miller) laryngoscope blades—adult, pediatric, and infant sizes
- [ ] Stylets, adult and pediatric sizes
- [ ] Suction catheter kits
- [ ] Suction source and connecting tubing
- [ ] Tincture of benzoin application pads
- [ ] Tongue blades
- [ ] Towels
- [ ] Water-soluble lubricant
- [ ] Yankauer catheter

EXERCISE 22.1 INTUBATION EQUIPMENT AND PREPARATION

EXERCISE 22.1.1 IDENTIFICATION OF INTUBATION EQUIPMENT

Compare the equipment provided in the laboratory with Figures 22.1 through 22.14. **Identify the items and record them on your laboratory report.**

Cook airway exchange catheter

Curved (MacIntosh) laryngoscope blades

Endotracheal tube: adult cuffed

Endotracheal tube: Carlen's catheter or double-lumen endotracheal tube (DLET)

Endotracheal tube: Cole catheter

Endotracheal tube: Emergency Medicine Tube (EMT®)

Endotracheal tube: Endotrol (built-in stylet)

Endotracheal tube: Hi-Lo Evac Tube™ (continuous cuff suction)

Endotracheal tube: infant uncuffed

Endotracheal tube: nasal or oral RAE

Endotracheal tube: wire-reinforced (anode or armored)

Magill forceps

Straight (Miller) laryngoscope

Stylet

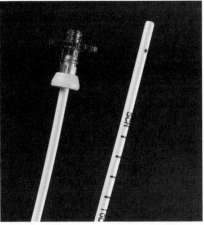

Figure 22.1. A. (Courtesy of Cook Medical Incorporated, Bloomington, Indiana)

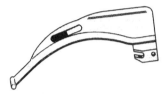

Figure 22.2. B. (Courtesy of Rüsch Inc., Duluth, GA.)

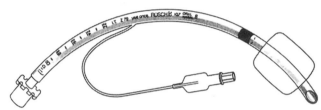

Figure 22.3. C. (Courtesy of Rüsch Inc., Duluth, GA.)

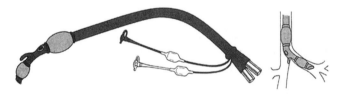

Figure 22.4. D. (Courtesy of Rüsch Inc., Duluth, GA.)

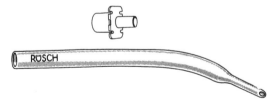

Figure 22.5. E. (Courtesy of Rüsch Inc., Duluth, GA.)

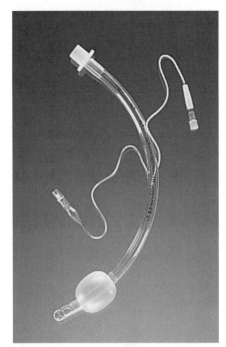

Figure 22.6. F. (Courtesy of Nellcor Puritan Bennett LLC, Boulder, CO, part of Covidien.)

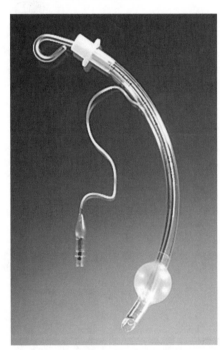

Figure 22.7. G. (Courtesy of Nellcor Puritan Bennett LLC, Boulder, CO, part of Covidien.)

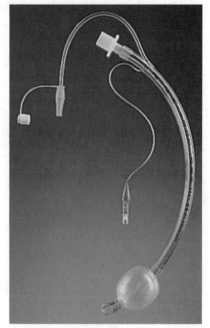

Figure 22.8. H. (Courtesy of Nellcor Puritan Bennett LLC, Boulder, CO, part of Covidien.)

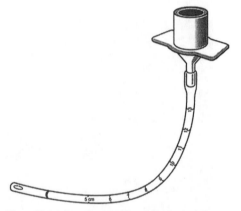

Figure 22.9. I. (From Barnhart, SL and Czervinske, MP: Perinatal and Pediatric Respiratory Care. WB Saunders, Philadelphia, 1995, p. 241, with permission.)

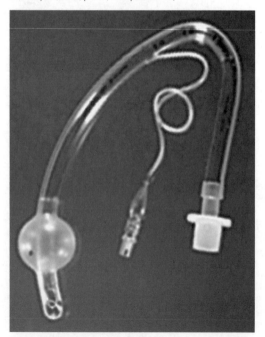

Figure 22.10. J. (Courtesy of Nellcor Puritan Bennett LLC, Boulder, CO, part of Covidien.)

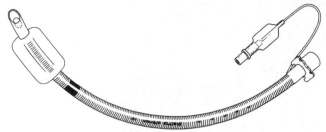

Figure 22.11. K. (Courtesy of Rüsch Inc., Duluth, GA.)

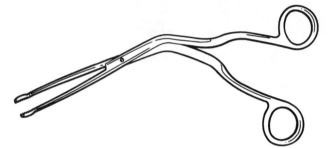

Figure 22.12. L. (Courtesy of Rüsch Inc., Duluth, GA.)

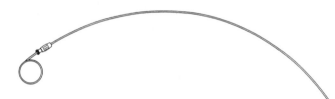

Figure 22.13. M. (Courtesy of Rüsch Inc., Duluth, GA.)

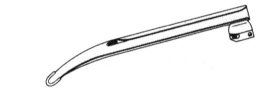

Figure 22.14. N. (Courtesy of Rüsch Inc., Duluth, GA.)

EXERCISE 22.1.2 IDENTIFICATION OF THE COMPONENTS OF AN ENDOTRACHEAL TUBE

Select an endotracheal tube and compare it with Figure 22.15. **Identify the components and record them on your laboratory report.**

Vendor or brand
15-mm connector
Spring-loaded pilot valve or balloon
Cuff
Inflation or pilot tube
Internal diameter in mm
Radiopaque line
Murphy tip with lateral eye
Distance markings in cm
Test markings (IT or Z-79)

EXERCISE 22.1.3 EQUIPMENT TESTING

1. Gather the necessary equipment:
   10-mL syringe
   Basins
   Batteries
   Bulbs
   Endotracheal tube
   Laryngoscope handles and blades
   Sterile water or saline solution
2. Assemble the laryngoscope as shown in Figure 22.16.
3. Open the blade and observe whether the light is lit. **Record this observation on your laboratory report.** Loosen the bulb (if not using a fiberoptic system) and observe whether the light goes on. **Record this observation on your laboratory report.** Retighten the bulb.

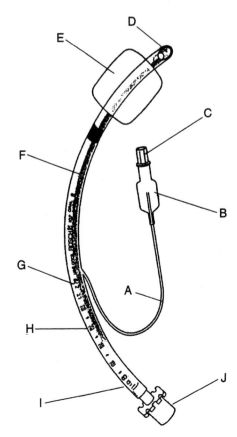

Figure 22.15. Components of an endotracheal tube. (Courtesy of Rüsch Inc., Duluth, GA.)

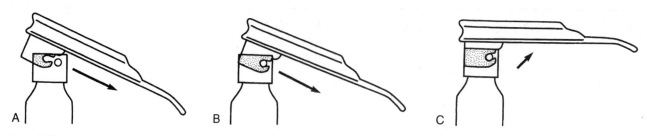

Figure 22.16. Assembly of a laryngoscope.

4. Unscrew the base of the laryngoscope handle and remove the batteries. **Note the size of the batteries on your laboratory report.**

5. Open the blade and observe whether the light is lit. **Record this observation on your laboratory report.**

6. Fill a basin with water or saline solution.

7. Put 5 mL of air into the 10-mL syringe and connect it to the valve on the pilot balloon.

8. Inject the air into the pilot balloon and observe the cuff inflation.

9. Submerge the cuffed end of the endotracheal tube in the basin. Observe the solution for any air bubbles and **record your observations on your laboratory report.**

10. Add 5 mL more into the cuff. Squeeze the cuff gently and observe the pilot balloon. Record this observation on your laboratory report. Place the syringe into the Luer-Lok™ of the pilot valve. Squeeze the cuff gently and observe the pilot balloon and syringe. **Record this observation on your laboratory report.**

11. Remove the tube and deflate the cuff completely.

EXERCISE 22.1.4 ASSIGNMENT OF MALLAMPATI CLASSIFICATION

*Frequently, the **Mallampati classification** is employed to help anticipate the difficulty of orotracheal intubation. This is usually done for elective intubations but it may be of help in an emergency intubation as well. It is not, however, a sole predictor of difficulty.[2,3]*

1. Using your laboratory partner as the patient, explain the purpose of this assessment.

2. With your "patient" seated and head placed in a neutral position, instruct him or her to open the mouth widely and put the tongue out as far as possible. Use tongue blade if needed.

3. Visually inspect the oropharynx and classify it by comparing your observations with Figure 22.17.

4. **Record the Mallampati classification for your "patient" on your laboratory report.**

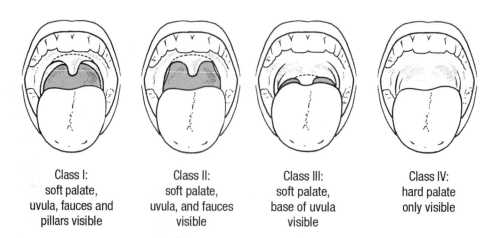

Figure 22.17. Mallampati classification.

Class I: soft palate, uvula, fauces and pillars visible

Class II: soft palate, uvula, and fauces visible

Class III: soft palate, base of uvula visible

Class IV: hard palate only visible

EXERCISE 22.2 OROTRACHEAL INTUBATION

EXERCISE 22.2.1 OROTRACHEAL INTUBATION WITH A MACINTOSH BLADE

In this exercise, two students are to work as partners; one will intubate and the other will prepare the equipment and assist. The student who is to intubate should manually resuscitate the mannequin while the other student gets all equipment ready. After successful intubation, the students should switch roles. Remember, in the clinical sites in most cases your role will be as the assistant, not the intubator! It is imperative that you know how to be a good assistant.

1. Gather the necessary equipment to intubate an adult airway management trainer using the MacIntosh (curved) blade (make sure the trainer is properly lubricated with the silicone spray). The proper endotracheal tube and blade sizes are shown in Table 22.1.

2. Wash or sanitize your hands and apply standard precautions and transmission-based isolation procedures as appropriate. The use of goggles or face shield is recommended in an actual clinical situation.

3. Prepare all equipment first while one student ventilates the "patient" with a manual resuscitator.

4. Open the endotracheal tube package halfway, leaving the cuffed end aseptically protected in the wrapper. Insert a stylet into the tube, making sure the tip does not protrude from the other end, as shown in Figure 22.18. Bend the top of the stylet (if necessary) over the top of the tube to prevent it from slipping down. Shape the tube so that the curve is maintained.

5. Using the manual resuscitator with bag-valve-mask, preoxygenate the patient.

6. Suction the oropharynx.

7. Remove the oropharyngeal airway if one is present.

8. Position the head in the *sniffing position*, as shown in Figure 22.19, by flexing the neck and tilting the head backward. Do not hyperextend. This allows alignment of the mouth, pharynx, and larynx. One or two towels can be used under the neck and shoulders to help achieve this position.

9. Ensure that all equipment is functioning and readily available.

10. Open the mouth using the crossed-finger, or scissor, technique.

11. Holding the laryngoscope in your *left hand* (regardless of which is your dominant hand), insert the blade into the mouth, as shown in Figure 22.20.

12. Pushing aside the tongue to the left, as shown in Figure 22.21, advance the blade until the epiglottis is visualized, as shown in Figure 22.22. **Identify the anatomic landmarks and record the corresponding letters on your laboratory report.**

Table 22.1 Endotracheal Tubes, Tracheostomy Tubes, and Laryngoscope Blades[a]

Approximate Age or Weight	Endotracheal Tubes[b]		
	Internal Diameter (ID, in mm)	Outer Diameter (OD, in mm)	Length (cm) (avg OD)
Premature infants (2–5 lb)	2.0–3.0	3.7–4.5	8
Newborn infants (5.0–5.5 lb)	3.0	4.5	9
Newborn infants to 3 mo (5.5–11 lb)	3.5–4.0	5.0–5.5	9
3–10 mo (11–18 lb)	4.3	5.7	10
10–12 mo (19–20 lb)	4.5	6.0	11
13–24 mo (20–25 lb)	5.0	6.5	12
2–3 yr (25–33 lb)	5.5	7.0	13
4–5 yr (33–44 lb)	6.0	8.0	14
6–7 yr (44–55 lb)	6.5	8.5	15
8–9 yr (55–70 lb)	7.0	9.0	16
9–10 yr (55–70 lb)	7.0	9.0	16
10–12 yr (70–85 lb)	7.5	9.5	17
12–16 yr (85–130 lb)	7.5	9.5	22.5
Adult females	8.0–9.0	10.0–12.0	19–24
Adult males	8.5–10.0	8.0–9.0	20–28

(continued)

Table 22.1 Endotracheal Tubes, Tracheostomy Tubes, and Laryngoscope Blades[a] *(continued)*

Age	Tracheostomy Tubes	
	Jackson Tube Size	OD
Premature to newborn	00	4.5
Newborn to 3 mo	0	5.0
Up to 1 yr	1	5.5
1–3 yr	2	6.0
3–6 yr	3	7.0
6–12 yr	1	8.0
12 yr to adult	5–9	9.0–13.0
Age	**Laryngoscope Blades (Type and Size)**	
Premature	Miller (0)	
Infant to 3 mo	Miller (1)	
3–12 mo	Miller or MacIntosh (1½)	
3–9 yr	MacIntosh (2)	
9 yr to adult	MacIntosh (3)	

[a]Tube thickness may vary with manufacturer.
[b]Conversion to French scale: 4 × ID or 3 × OD.
(From Pilbeam, SP: Mechanical Ventilation: Physiological and Clinical Applications, ed 2. Mosby-Year Book, St. Louis, p. 603, with permission.)

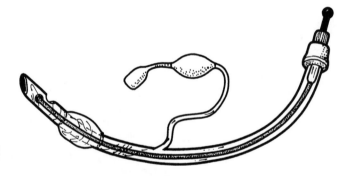

Figure 22.18. Insertion of a stylet into an endotracheal tube.

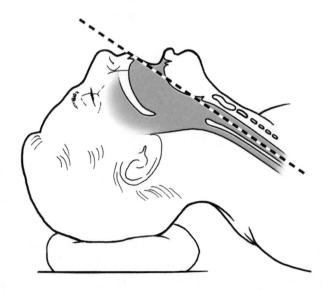

Figure 22.19. "Sniffing" position for intubation.

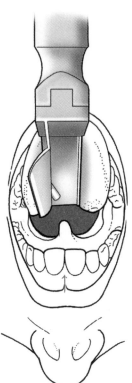

Figure 22.20. Insertion of laryngoscope blade into the mouth.

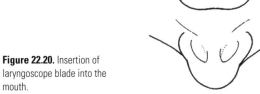

Figure 22.21. Displacement of the tongue.

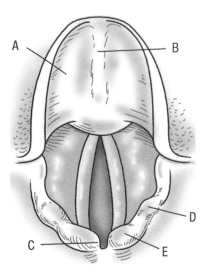

Figure 22.22. Visualization of the landmarks for intubation.

13. Continue to advance the tip of the blade into the **vallecula,** as shown in Figure 22.23, and indirectly expose the glottis by applying an upward and forward lift with your wrist kept straight, as shown in Figure 22.24. Do not use the blade as a lever by resting it on the upper teeth. This prying motion will result in cracked or broken teeth. The Sellick maneuver (the application of pressure on the cricoid cartilage by an assistant) is sometimes beneficial in visualization, as shown in Figure 22.25. The glottis is now exposed.

14. No intubation attempt should last longer than 30 seconds. If problems are encountered with the visualization procedure, stop the intubation attempt and reoxygenate the patient with 100% oxygen between attempts for at least 1 minute.

15. Have your assistant remove the tube from the wrapper without contaminating the cuffed end. Without taking your eyes off the glottis, insert the endotracheal tube into the right side of the mouth, advancing it until the cuff goes just beyond the vocal cords.

16. Holding the tube securely in position, quickly but gently remove the laryngoscope blade from the mouth. The assistant will help remove the stylet and inflate the cuff with 5 to 10 mL of air.

17. Ventilate and oxygenate the patient. Observe for bilateral symmetrical chest expansion.

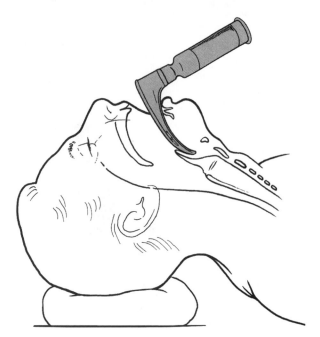

Figure 22.23. Tip of the Macintosh blade in the vallecula.

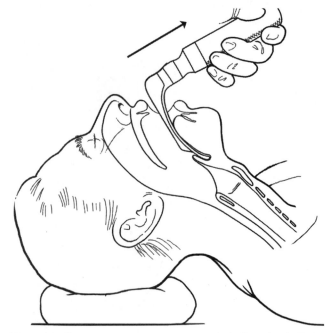

Figure 22.24. The upward, forward tilt to expose the glottis. Notice that the blade is not resting on the teeth.

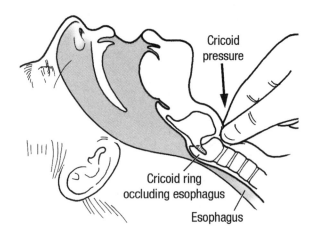

Figure 22.25. Applying cricoid pressure.

18. Have your assistant place an end-tidal colorimetric capnometer (e.g., EasyCap™) between the 15-mm adapter endotracheal and the resuscitator bag connection.
19. Auscultate for bilateral breath sounds.
20. Auscultate the epigastric region to listen for air in the stomach.
21. If no breath sounds are heard, deflate the cuff, remove the tube, and ventilate with a bag-valve-mask until the procedure is attempted again.
22. If unilateral sounds are heard, deflate the cuff and withdraw the tube gently while continuing to bag the patient until bilateral sounds are heard. Then reinflate the cuff.
23. Secure the tube with tape, as shown in Figure 22.26, or with a commercial orotracheal tube holder.
24. Attach the patient to an oxygenation or ventilation device.
25. Remove your gloves and other personal protective equipment.
26. Wash your hands and dispose of waste.

EXERCISE 22.2.2 OROTRACHEAL INTUBATION WITH A MILLER BLADE

1. Replace the MacIntosh blade used in the previous exercise with a Miller blade.
2. Repeat all of the steps in the previous exercise.

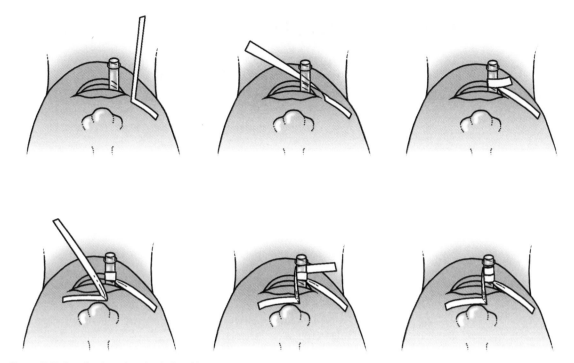

Figure 22.26. Securing the endotracheal tube with tape.

3. Directly expose the glottis by picking up the epiglottis with the tip of the blade, as shown in Figure 22.27.
4. Continue the remaining steps in the previous exercise.

EXERCISE 22.2.3 INTUBATION WHEN AN ESOPHAGEAL-TRACHEAL COMBITUBE™ (ETC) AIRWAY IS IN PLACE

1. Select an airway management trainer that has an ETC tube airway in place.
2. Intubate the trainer as previously described, moving the ETC out of the way without removing it.
3. Once the endotracheal tube (ETT) is in place, deflate the ETC cuffs.
4. Remove the ETC once the ETT is in place.
5. Attach the oxygenation or ventilation device to the 15-mm ETT adapter.

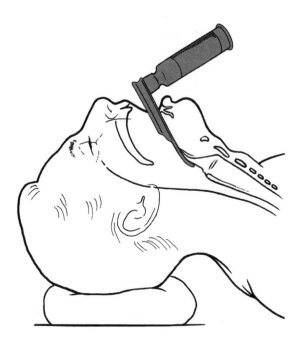

Figure 22.27. Exposure of the glottis using the Miller blade.

EXERCISE 22.2.4 INTUBATION WHEN A LARYNGEAL MASK AIRWAY (LMA) IS IN PLACE

1. Select an airway management trainer that has an LMA tube airway in place.
2. Intubate the trainer by inserting the ETT through the LMA.
3. Deflate the LMA cuff.
4. Remove the LMA once the ETT is in place.
5. Attach the oxygenation or ventilation device to the 15-mm ETT adapter.

EXERCISE 22.2.5 NASOTRACHEAL INTUBATION

1. Gather the necessary equipment.
2. Lubricate the nose of the adult airway management trainer with silicon spray. In the clinical setting a water-soluble jelly is used to lubricate the nasotracheal tube.
3. Wash or sanitize hands and apply standard precautions and transmission-based isolation procedures as appropriate.
4. Prepare the patient as in Exercise 22.2.1.
5. Insert the tube into one of the nares.
6. Advance the tube into the oropharynx. Never force a tube. If an obstruction is met, attempt to pass the tube through the other naris.
7. When the tube is in the oropharynx, insert the laryngoscope blade into the mouth as previously described and expose the glottis.
8. Using the Magill forceps, pick up the tip of the nasotracheal tube before the cuff.
9. Ask your laboratory partner to push on the tube as you direct the tip into the glottis. Steps 8 and 9 are shown in Figure 22.28.
10. Once the tube is in the trachea, gently remove the equipment from the mouth and continue as in the previous exercises.

Blind nasotracheal intubation is sometimes attempted. It is difficult to practice in the laboratory setting because the passing of the tube requires a spontaneously breathing subject.[4] The procedure is basically the same for nasotracheal intubation except that a laryngoscope and forceps are not used. The practitioner must time the insertion of the tube with the opening of the epiglottis. Successful attempts are often indicated by an emission of a harsh sound as the tube passes the vocal cords, the inability of the patient to speak, and the feel of moist air coming from the tube on exhalation.

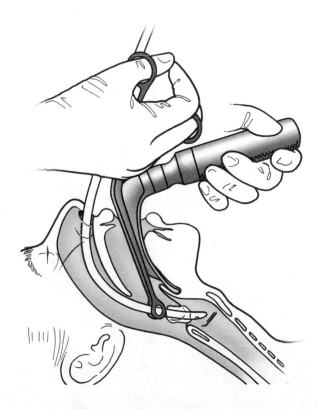

Figure 22.28. Nasal intubation using Magill forceps.

EXERCISE 22.2.6 INFANT INTUBATION

1. Gather the necessary equipment. Refer to Table 22.1 for the proper size tubes and blades.
2. Select an infant airway management trainer and lubricate the pharynx with silicone spray. (In a clinical setting, tubes would not be lubricated.)
3. Preoxygenate.
4. Position the head in the neutral, or "sniffing," position.
5. Intubate the trainer using the techniques learned in Exercise 22.2.1.
6. Continue the steps as described in Exercise 22.2.1.

EXERCISE 22.3 SECURING AN ENDOTRACHEAL TUBE

Using the intubated mannequins from the previous exercises, do the following:

1. Both you and your laboratory partner wash or sanitize your hands, apply standard precautions and transmission-based isolation procedures as appropriate, and have your partner hold the endotracheal tube securely in position while you perform the following steps. Note the position of the endotracheal tube.
2. Do not apply gloves until the tape is prepared. Prepare the cloth tape for use to secure the endotracheal tube. Several methods may be used, as shown in Figures 22.29 and 22.30.
3. Put on your gloves.

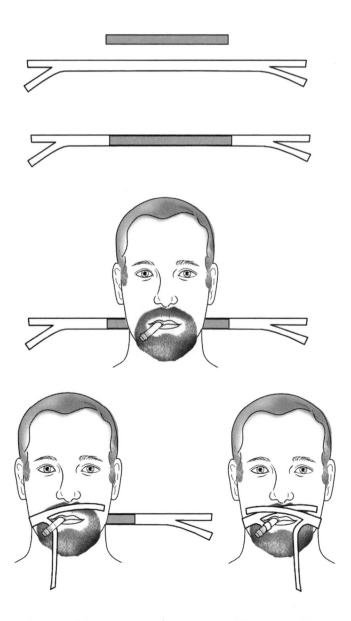

Figure 22.29. Securing the tube in a bearded patient.

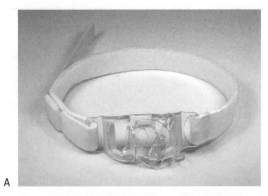

A

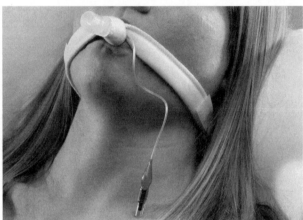

Figure 22.30. (A), (B) Securing an endotracheal tube using a commercial endotracheal tube holder. (Courtesy of Cardinal Health, Dublin, OH.)

B

4. *The following should NOT be done to the mannequin or patient simulator!* To enhance the adhesiveness of the tape, tincture of benzoin may be applied to the "patient's" skin using a 4×4 gauze pad or commercial prep pads. Do not spray or apply the liquid directly to the "patient's" face.

5. Apply the tape using one of the previously shown methods. Ensure that the tube position is correct. Secure the tape around the oropharyngeal airway to serve as a bite block. Reassess correct tube placement when finished. **"Chart" the procedure on your laboratory report.**

6. Repeat the exercise using a nasotracheally intubated mannequin.

7. Repeat the exercise using an infant mannequin.

REFERENCES

1. American Association for Respiratory Care: AARC clinical practice guideline: Management of airway emergencies. Respir Care 40:749–760, 1995.
2. Sofair, E: Preanesthetic assessment: The professional singer with a difficult airway. Anesthesiology News 1:40, 1993.
3. Whitten, CE: Anyone Can Intubate. KW Publications, San Diego, 1996, p. 41.
4. Finucane, BT and Santora, AH: Principles of Airway Management, ed 2. Mosby, St. Louis, 1996.

Laboratory Report

CHAPTER 22: ENDOTRACHEAL INTUBATION

Name _____   Date _____

Course/Section _____   Instructor _____

Data Collection

EXERCISE 22.1 Intubation Equipment and Preparation

EXERCISE 22.1.1 IDENTIFICATION OF INTUBATION EQUIPMENT

A. _____

B. _____

C. _____

D. _____

E. _____

F. _____

G. _____

H. _____

I. _____

J. _____

K. _____

L. _____

M. _____

N. _____

EXERCISE 22.1.2 IDENTIFICATION OF THE COMPONENTS OF AN ENDOTRACHEAL TUBE

A. _____

B. _____

C. _____

D. _____

E. _____

F. _____

G. _____

H. _____

I. _____

J. _____

EXERCISE 22.1.3 EQUIPMENT TESTING

Light observation: _____

Light observation with loosened bulb: _____

If the lamp failed to light, list the items you would check in the order in which you would check them:

_____

_____

_____

Size of batteries: _____

Light observation with blade open: _____

Observations of endotracheal tube cuff testing in solution:

_____

Observations of cuff and pilot balloon:

_____

Observations of the cuff and pilot balloon with syringe in place: _____

EXERCISE 22.1.4 ASSIGNMENT OF MALLAMPATI CLASSIFICATION

Mallampati classification: _____

EXERCISE 22.2 Orotracheal Intubation

EXERCISE 22.2.1 OROTRACHEAL INTUBATION WITH A MACINTOSH BLADE

Identify the anatomic landmarks:

A. _____

B. _____

C. _____

D. _____

E. _____

EXERCISE 22.3 Securing an Endotracheal Tube

Chart the intubation procedure, your assessment of tube placement, and the securing of the endotracheal tube:

_____

_____

_____

_____

_____

_____

_____

Critical Thinking Questions

1. You have been asked by the nursing supervisor to supply an adult intubation tray for the emergency room. List all the equipment that you would recommend.

2. When would a topical anesthetic be indicated during the intubation procedure? What anesthetics can be used?

3. In a restless, fighting patient requiring immediate oral intubation, what pharmacological agent(s) could be used to facilitate intubation?

4. Describe in specific radiologic terms the proper location of an endotracheal tube.

5. The emergency medical technicians have brought in a 65-year-old victim in cardiac arrest. The patient had been ventilated with a manual resuscitator and mask. As you attempt to ventilate, the patient vomits.

    A. What would be your immediate actions?

    B. During your next attempt to intubate, you observe a large piece of undigested steak blocking your view of the glottis. How would you clear the airway, and what equipment would be needed?

Procedural Competency Evaluation

STUDENT: **DATE:**

ORAL ENDOTRACHEAL INTUBATION

Evaluator: ☐ Peer ☐ Instructor	**Setting:** ☐ Lab	☐ Clinical Simulation

Equipment Utilized: **Conditions (Describe):**

Performance Level:

S or ✓ = Satisfactory, no errors of omission or commission
U = Unsatisfactory Error of Omission or Commission
NA = Not applicable

Performance Rating:

5   **Independent:** Near flawless performance; minimal errors; able to perform without supervision; seeks out new learning; shows initiative; A = 4.7–5.0 average

4   **Minimally Supervised:** Few errors, able to self-correct; seeks guidance when appropriate; B = 3.7–4.65

3   **Competent:** Minimal required level; no critical errors; able to correct with coaching; meets expectations; safe; C = 3.0–3.65

2   **Marginal:** Below average; critical errors or problem areas noted; would benefit from remediation; D = 2.0–2.99

1   **Dependent:** Poor; unacceptable performance; unsafe; gross inaccuracies; potentially harmful; F = < 2.0

Two or more errors of commission or omission of mandatory or essential performance elements will terminate the procedure, and require additional practice and/or remediation and reevaluation. Student is responsible for obtaining additional evaluation forms as needed from the Director of Clinical Education (DCE).

(Right side columns: PERFORMANCE RATING | PERFORMANCE LEVEL)

	PERFORMANCE RATING	PERFORMANCE LEVEL
EQUIPMENT AND PATIENT PREPARATION		
1. Common Performance Elements Steps 1–8		
ASSESSMENT AND IMPLEMENTATION		
2. Common Performance Elements Steps 9 and 10		
3. Hyperoxygenates/hyperventilates the patient with 100% BVM and oral airway		
4. Performs or has assistant perform the following:		
A. Selects appropriate laryngoscope blade and ETT size		
B. Tests function of lamp		
C. Checks function of cuff; lubricates tube with water-soluble lubricant		
D. Inserts stylet into tube; ensures it is not protruding from end or lateral eye		
5. Inserts and manipulates blade appropriately; suctions if needed		
6. Inserts ETT under direct visualization within 15 seconds		
7. Immediately ventilates following insertion		
8. Inflates cuff with maximum of 10 cc air		
9. Stabilizes ETT until secured with tape/ETT stabilizer		
10. Verifies ETT position by chest rise, auscultation, and capnometry		
11. Correctly secures ETT with tape or commercial tube stabilizer		
FOLLOW-UP		
12. Measures cuff volume, pressure		
13. Confirms tube position on CXR		
14. Common Performance Elements Steps 11–16		

SIGNATURES   Student: Evaluator: Date:

Clinical Performance Evaluation

PERFORMANCE RATING:

5 **Independent:** Near flawless performance; minimal errors; able to perform without supervision; seeks out new learning; shows initiative; A = 4.7–5.0 average

4 **Minimally Supervised:** Few errors, able to self-correct; seeks guidance when appropriate; B = 3.7–4.65

3 **Competent:** Minimal required level; no critical errors; able to correct with coaching; meets expectations; safe; C = 3.0–3.65

2 **Marginal:** Below average; critical errors or problem areas noted; would benefit from remediation; D = 2.0–2.99

1 **Dependent:** Poor; unacceptable performance; unsafe; gross inaccuracies; potentially harmful; F = < 2.0

Circle the appropriate response below. Please be consistent, objective, and honest in your assessment of the student's clinical performance and ability.

PERFORMANCE CRITERIA	SCORE				
COGNITIVE DOMAIN					
1. Consistently displays knowledge, comprehension, and command of essential concepts	5	4	3	2	1
2. Demonstrates the relationship between theory and clinical practice	5	4	3	2	1
3. Able to select, review, apply, analyze, synthesize, interpret, and evaluate information; makes recommendations to modify care plan	5	4	3	2	1
PSYCHOMOTOR DOMAIN					
4. Minimal errors, no critical errors; able to self-correct; performs all steps safely and accurately	5	4	3	2	1
5. Selects, assembles, and verifies proper function and cleanliness of equipment; assures operation and corrects malfunctions; provides adequate care and maintenance	5	4	3	2	1
6. Exhibits the required manual dexterity	5	4	3	2	1
7. Performs procedure in a reasonable time frame for clinical level	5	4	3	2	1
8. Applies and maintains aseptic technique and PPE as required	5	4	3	2	1
9. Maintains concise and accurate patient and clinical records	5	4	3	2	1
10. Reports promptly on patient status/needs to appropriate personnel	5	4	3	2	1
AFFECTIVE DOMAIN					
11. Exhibits courteous and pleasant demeanor; shows consideration and respect, honesty, and integrity	5	4	3	2	1
12. Communicates verbally and in writing clearly and concisely	5	4	3	2	1
13. Preserves confidentiality and adheres to all policies	5	4	3	2	1
14. Follows directions, exhibits sound judgment, and seeks help when required	5	4	3	2	1
15. Demonstrates initiative, self-direction, responsibility, and accountability	5	4	3	2	1

TOTAL POINTS = _____ /15 = AVERAGE GRADE = _____

ADDITIONAL COMMENTS: IDENTIFY AREAS OF EXCELLENCE; LIST ERRORS OF OMISSION OR COMMISSION, CRITICAL ERRORS

SUMMARY PERFORMANCE EVALUATION AND RECOMMENDATIONS

☐ PASS: Satisfactory Performance

    ☐ Minimal supervision needed, may progress to next level provided specific skills, clinical time completed

    ☐ Minimal supervision needed, able to progress to next level without remediation

☐ FAIL: Unsatisfactory Performance (check all that apply)

    ☐ Minor reevaluation only

    ☐ Needs additional clinical practice before reevaluation

    ☐ Needs additional laboratory practice before skills performed in clinical area

    ☐ Recommend clinical probation

SIGNATURES

Evaluator (print name): _____　　　Evaluator signature: _____　　　Date: _____

Student Signature: _____　　　Date: _____

Student Comments:

23 Tracheostomy Care

INTRODUCTION

For long-term artificial airway availability, the tracheostomy tube is the airway of choice. Maintenance of the tracheostomy tube is essential and is the responsibility of the respiratory care practitioner (RCP). These responsibilities include securing the tube, adequate humidification and secretion clearance, provision for patient communication, providing cuff and **stoma** care, changing **tracheostomy** tubes, and troubleshooting airway-related problems.[1] Although an RCP is not responsible for the actual **tracheotomy** procedure, the practitioner may be called on to assist with the procedure, replace a displaced tracheostomy tube, or change it from one type of tube to another. Detailed knowledge of these tubes is also an essential part of the responsibility of the RCP.

OBJECTIVES

Upon completion of this chapter, the student will be able to:

1. Practice communication skills needed for assessing the level of patient comprehension while instructing patients in airway care procedures.
2. Practice medical charting for airway care procedures.
3. Apply infection control guidelines and standards associated with equipment and procedures, according to OSHA regulations and CDC guidelines.
4. Secure a tracheostomy tube by changing twill tape and commercial tracheostomy tube holders.
5. Identify the various types of tracheostomy tubes, buttons, and adjuncts and their component parts.
6. Perform tracheostomy care, including equipment cleaning and stoma care.
7. Change a tracheostomy tube on an adult airway management trainer.
8. Provide for adequate patient communication with an artificial airway in place.

KEY TERMS

decannulation
obturator

stoma
tracheostomy

tracheotomy

Exercises

EQUIPMENT REQUIRED

- ☐ Airway management trainer
- ☐ Silicone spray
- ☐ Water-soluble lubricant
- ☐ Goggles or face shields
- ☐ Sterile and nonsterile disposable latex and vinyl gloves, various sizes
- ☐ Oxygen gas source and flowmeter
- ☐ Oxygen connecting tubing and nipple adaptors
- ☐ Tracheostomy tubes, various sizes and styles:
  - ☐ Jackson metal
  - ☐ Cuffed and cuffless
  - ☐ Cuffed and cuffless fenestrated
- ☐ Disposable and nondisposable inner cannulas
- ☐ Fenestrated and nonfenestrated cannulas
- ☐ Bivona or Kamen-Wilkinson Fome-Cuff tubes
- ☐ Lanz-Maguiness cuff tubes
- ☐ Montgomery tubes
- ☐ Shiley speaking valve with oxygen port
- ☐ Tracheal buttons
- ☐ Stethoscopes
- ☐ Manual resuscitators with masks—adult and infant
- ☐ Suction catheter kits

- ☐ Yankauer catheter
- ☐ Basins
- ☐ Suction machines
- ☐ Sterile water or normal saline
- ☐ Hydrogen peroxide
- ☐ Tracheostomy care kits
- ☐ Tracheostomy collars
- ☐ Briggs adaptors (T-piece)
- ☐ Passy-Muir, Shiley, or other brand of speaking valves
- ☐ Letter board or pad and pen/pencil
- ☐ Tracheostomy communication devices
- ☐ Twill tape
- ☐ Cloth tape
- ☐ Tracheostomy tube holders
- ☐ 10-mL syringes
- ☐ Towels
- ☐ Scissors
- ☐ Cotton swabs
- ☐ 4×4 sterile gauze
- ☐ Large-volume nebulizer
- ☐ Large-bore corrugated tubing
- ☐ Pulse oximeter

EXERCISE 23.1 TRACHEOSTOMY TUBES

EXERCISE 23.1.1 COMPONENTS OF TRACHEOSTOMY TUBES

1. Compare the various components of the tracheostomy tube provided in the laboratory and compare it with Figure 23.1. **Identify the components and record them on your laboratory report.**

   Disposable inner cannula

   Nondisposable inner cannula

   Outer cannula

   Pilot balloon

   Pilot valve

   Cuff

   Fenestration

   Cannula cap

   Obturator

   15-mm connector

   Neck plate

   Inflation line

2. Open a tracheostomy tube box. Examine the contents and the manner in which they are packed. Pay close attention to what is sterile and what is not. **Record the contents of the box on your laboratory report. Include the manufacturer, size, and style of the tube.**

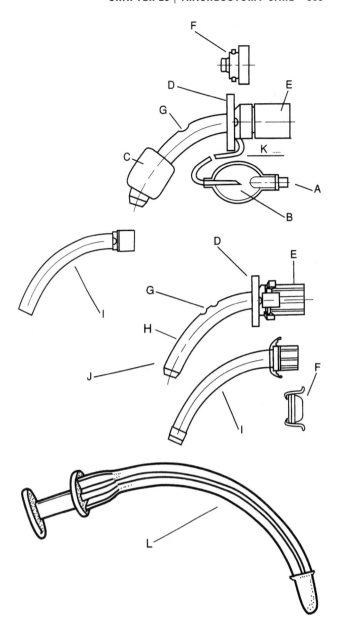

Figure 23.1. Components of tracheostomy tubes. (Adapted from Shiley Tracheostomy Products, courtesy of Mallinckrodt Medical, St. Louis, MO, with permission.)

EXERCISE 23.1.2 TYPES OF TRACHEOSTOMY TUBES AND DEVICES

Compare the various types of tracheostomy tubes and devices provided in the laboratory and compare them with Figures 23.2 through 23.9. **Identify the type of tube or device and record it on your laboratory report.**

Montgomery tube

Tracheostomy button

Lanz-Maguinness cuff

Bivona or Kamen-Wilkinson Fome-Cuff

Passy-Muir valve

Pitt speaking tube

Olympic Trach-Talk

Jackson tracheostomy tube

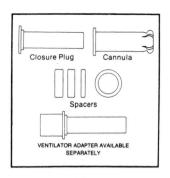
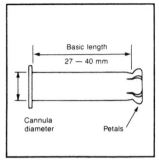
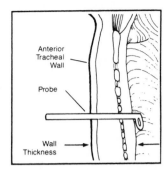

Figure 23.2. A. (Courtesy of Olympic Medical, Seattle, WA.)

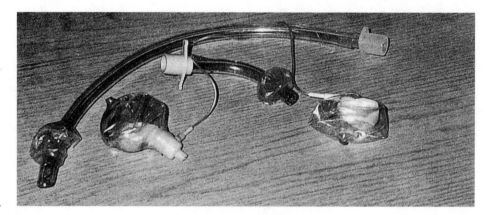

Figure 23.3. B.

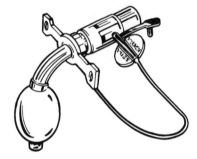

Figure 23.4. C. (Courtesy of
Bivona Medical Technologies,
Gary, IN.)

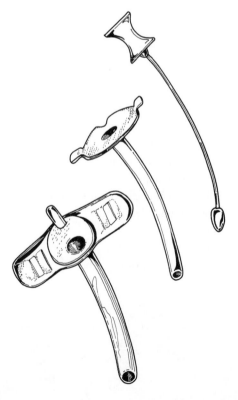

Figure 23.5. D.

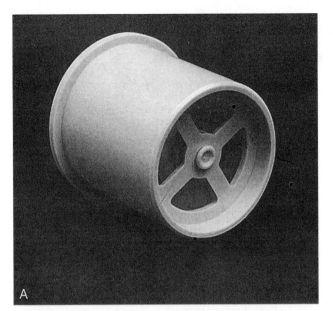

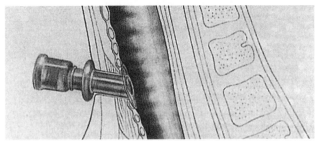

Figure 23.7. F. (Courtesy of Boston Medical Products, Westborough, MA.)

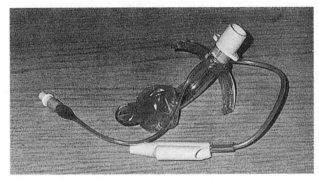

Figure 23.8. G.

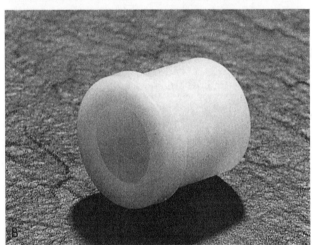

Figure 23.6. E. [Courtesy of (A) Passy
Muir Inc., Irvine, CA; (B) Boston
Medical Products, Westborough, MA.]

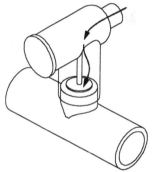

Figure 23.9. H. (Courtesy of Olympic Medical, Seattle, WA.)

EXERCISE 23.2 TRACHEOSTOMY TUBE CARE

EXERCISE 23.2.1 TRACHEOSTOMY CARE AND CLEANING

NOTE: Tracheostomy patients should always have a replacement tracheostomy tube at the bedside in case an emergency replacement becomes necessary.

1. Wash your hands and apply standard precautions and transmission-based isolation procedures as appropriate.

2. Gather the necessary equipment:

   Tracheostomy care kit

   Suction kit

   Gloves

   Peroxide

   Sterile water or saline

   Spare inner cannula or disposable cannula

3. Explain the procedure and confirm patient understanding.

4. Suction thoroughly.

5. Remove the old dressing and discard in an infectious waste container.

6. Remove the inner cannula and replace with the spare red-top cannula if a nondisposable cannula is in place.

7. Open the tracheostomy care kit and fill one basin with hydrogen peroxide and the other with sterile saline.

8. Scrub the cannula with a brush in the peroxide and rinse with the sterile saline.

9. Replace the permanent cannula.

10. If a disposable cannula is used, remove the dirty cannula, dispose of it properly, and replace it with a clean disposable cannula.

11. Clean the stoma site and exterior portions of the tube using peroxide, cotton-tipped applicators, and pipe cleaner for the tube crevices.

12. Replace the dressing using a precut 4×4 gauze pad.

13. Remove the old ties by cutting them with a scissor. *Be careful not to cut the pilot tube.* Commercial tracheostomy tube holders can be removed and replaced by following the manufacturer's instructions.

14. Attach the tracheostomy twill tape to one end of the tube by making a loop and inserting it into one of the holes on the neck plate. Bring the other end back through the loop and pull. Bring the tape around the patient's neck and insert one end of the tape into the other hole. Tie the tube in place by making a square knot on the side of the neck. Avoid overtightening by placing one finger between the tape and the patient's neck (Fig. 23.10).

15. Ensure that the tube is in the proper position, and reassess the patient.

16. Ensure that all equipment is disposed of in the proper waste container.

17. Remove gloves and wash your hands.

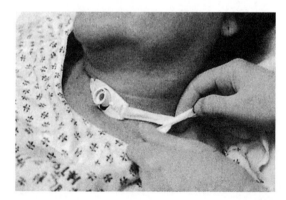

Figure 23.10. Retying tracheostomy tapes. (Courtesy of Shiley Tracheostomy Products, Mallinckrodt Medical, St. Louis, MO.)

EXERCISE 23.2.2   TRACHEOSTOMY TUBE INSERTION

1. Select a tracheostomized adult airway management trainer.
2. Gather the necessary equipment:
   Tracheostomy tube and components
   Tracheostomy ties or holder
   Suction equipment
   Water-soluble lubricant (silicone spray)
   Sterile water or saline
   Basin
   Sterile gloves
3. Using your laboratory partner as the patient, explain the procedure for changing the tracheostomy tube.
4. Suction the trachea based on "patient" assessment.
5. Wash your hands, put on sterile gloves, and use other standard precautions and transmission-based isolation procedures as appropriate.
6. Your laboratory partner will now serve as your assistant. Have your partner open the new tracheostomy tube box, remove the tube, and place it on a sterile field.
7. Have your partner fill a basin with sterile solution.
8. While you hold the new tube in your sterile hand, instruct your partner to inject 5 mL of air into the cuff. Remember that your partner *cannot* touch the tube.
9. Check the tube for cuff leaks.
10. If no leaks are present, deflate the cuff completely.
11. Have your partner attach the new, clean tracheostomy ties or holder.
12. Remove the inner cannula and insert the obturator.
13. Lubricate the tip of the tracheostomy tube/obturator.
14. Reassure your "patient" and position the "patient's" head. The "patient" should be seated in a semi-Fowler's position with the neck slightly extended.
15. Have your partner loosen or untie the old tracheostomy ties and deflate the cuff if it is inflated.
16. Remove the oxygen or humidity therapy device and place aseptically.
17. With one hand, remove the old tracheostomy tube.
18. Visually inspect the stoma for bleeding or infection.
19. Insert the new tube as shown in Figure 23.11. Gently introduce the tip of the obturator into the stoma and advance the tube into the trachea with a slightly downward motion. Do not force if resistance is met.
20. Quickly remove the obturator and insert the inner cannula. Make sure that one finger keeps the tracheostomy tube in place until it is secured.
21. Inflate the cuff if ordered.
22. Ensure proper placement by auscultation, feeling airflow through the tube and chest expansion.
23. Tie the tube into place. Remember to place one finger under the tie to prevent overtightening. Velcro tube holders may also be employed.
24. Restore the "patient" to the previous oxygen or humidity therapy device.
25. Dispose of the dirty tube, ties, and gloves in the proper receptacle.
26. Wash your hands.

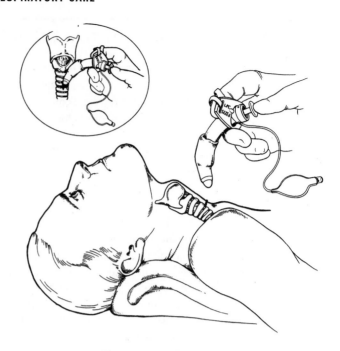

Figure 23.11. Insertion of replacement tracheostomy tube. (Courtesy of Shiley Tracheostomy Products, Mallinckrodt Medical, St. Louis, MO.)

EXERCISE 23.2.3 TRACHEOSTOMY TUBE DECANNULATION

1. Select a tracheostomized adult airway management trainer.
2. Gather the necessary equipment:
   - 4×4 sterile gauze dressings
   - Cloth tape
   - Suction equipment
   - Sterile water or saline
   - Gloves
3. Using your laboratory partner as the patient, explain the procedure for removing the tracheostomy tube.
4. Suction the trachea based on "patient" assessment.
5. Wash your hands, put on sterile gloves, and use other standard precautions and transmission-based isolation procedures as appropriate.
6. If the tube is cuffed, ensure that the cuff is deflated. If the cuff is inflated, deflate it completely.
7. Undo the tracheostomy tube holder or untie the twill tape.
8. Remove the tracheostomy tube.
9. Clean the stoma with sterile gauze damp with sterile water or normal saline.
10. Dry the area thoroughly.
11. Fold sterile gauze in quarters and place it over the stoma.
12. Tape the gauze over the stoma.
13. Instruct the "patient" that it is important to support the gauze by putting several fingers and applying slight pressure when speaking and coughing.
14. Observe the "patient" supporting the dressing during speaking and coughing to confirm the "patient's" understanding. Reinstruct if necessary.
15. Dispose of all waste in the appropriate canister.

REFERENCES
1. Scanlan, C et al. (eds): Egan's Fundamentals of Respiratory Care, ed 6. Mosby, St. Louis, 1995, p. 565.

Laboratory Report

CHAPTER 23: TRACHEOSTOMY CARE

Name _____   Date _____

Course/Section _____   Instructor _____

Data Collection

EXERCISE 23.1 Tracheostomy Tubes

EXERCISE 23.1.1 COMPONENTS OF TRACHEOSTOMY TUBES

A. _____

B. _____

C. _____

D. _____

E. _____

F. _____

G. _____

H. _____

I. _____

J. _____

K. _____

L. _____

Manufacturer: _____

Size of tube: _____

Type of tube: _____

Box contents: _____

_____

EXERCISE 23.1.2 TYPES OF TRACHEOSTOMY TUBES AND DEVICES

A. _____

B. _____

C. _____

D. _____

E. _____

F. _____

G. _____

H. _____

Critical Thinking Questions

1. You are changing a tracheostomy tube in a patient with no spontaneous respirations who is being mechanically ventilated. You cannot get the new tube in. Describe in detail what you would do.

2. Al Strachen is a 16-year-old quadriplegic with a C7 fracture caused by a diving accident. He is currently in a rehabilitation facility. He has a size 6 nonfenestrated cuffed tracheostomy tube in place. The physiatrist has requested that the nurse provide a tracheostomy adjunct to allow the patient to speak. The nurse obtained a Passy-Muir valve and attached it to the 15-mm adaptor of the inner cannula. You were then called stat to evaluate the patient for severe respiratory distress. Explain why the patient did not tolerate the procedure and what you would need to do to correct the situation.

Procedural Competency Evaluation

STUDENT: **DATE:**

TRACHEOSTOMY CARE

	PERFORMANCE RATING	PERFORMANCE LEVEL
Evaluator: ☐ Peer ☐ Instructor **Setting:** ☐ Lab ☐ Clinical Simulation		
Equipment Utilized: **Conditions (Describe):**		
Performance Level: S or ✓ = Satisfactory, no errors of omission or commission U = Unsatisfactory Error of Omission or Commission NA = Not applicable		
Performance Rating: **5** **Independent:** Near flawless performance; minimal errors; able to perform without supervision; seeks out new learning; shows initiative; A = 4.7–5.0 average **4** **Minimally Supervised:** Few errors, able to self-correct; seeks guidance when appropriate; B = 3.7–4.65 **3** **Competent:** Minimal required level; no critical errors; able to correct with coaching; meets expectations; safe; C = 3.0–3.65 **2** **Marginal:** Below average; critical errors or problem areas noted; would benefit from remediation; D = 2.0–2.99 **1** **Dependent:** Poor; unacceptable performance; unsafe; gross inaccuracies; potentially harmful; F = < 2.0 *Two or more errors of commission or omission of mandatory or essential performance elements will terminate the procedure, and require additional practice and/or remediation and reevaluation. Student is responsible for obtaining additional evaluation forms as needed from the Director of Clinical Education (DCE).*		
EQUIPMENT AND PATIENT PREPARATION		
1. Common Performance Elements Steps 1–8		
ASSESSMENT AND IMPLEMENTATION		
2. Common Performance Elements Steps 9 and 10		
3. Verifies size and type of airway		
4. Opens and prepares tracheostomy care kit; fills basins with hydrogen peroxide and sterile normal saline; applies sterile drape		
5. Suctions trachea		
6. Removes and discards old tracheostomy dressing		
7. Removes inner cannula and replaces with spare if available; discards if disposable		
8. Scrubs inner cannula with peroxide; rinses with saline if non-disposable is being used		
9. Replaces inner cannula; if disposable, replaces inner cannula with new one		
10. Cleans stoma site and exterior portions of the tube using peroxide, sterile cotton-tipped applicators, and pipe cleaners		
11. Replaces dressing with a sterile precut 4x4 gauze		
12. Removes old ties or commercial tube holder and replaces with clean ones		
13. Ensures tube is secured in proper position; verifies airway patency, ventilation, and oxygenation		
FOLLOW-UP		
14. Common Performance Elements Steps 11–16		

SIGNATURES   Student: Evaluator: Date:

Clinical Performance Evaluation

PERFORMANCE RATING:

5 **Independent:** Near flawless performance; minimal errors; able to perform without supervision; seeks out new learning; shows initiative; A = 4.7–5.0 average

4 **Minimally Supervised:** Few errors, able to self-correct; seeks guidance when appropriate; B = 3.7–4.65

3 **Competent:** Minimal required level; no critical errors; able to correct with coaching; meets expectations; safe; C = 3.0–3.65

2 **Marginal:** Below average; critical errors or problem areas noted; would benefit from remediation; D = 2.0–2.99

1 **Dependent:** Poor; unacceptable performance; unsafe; gross inaccuracies; potentially harmful; F = < 2.0

Circle the appropriate response below. Please be consistent, objective, and honest in your assessment of the student's clinical performance and ability.

PERFORMANCE CRITERIA	SCORE				
COGNITIVE DOMAIN					
1. Consistently displays knowledge, comprehension, and command of essential concepts	5	4	3	2	1
2. Demonstrates the relationship between theory and clinical practice	5	4	3	2	1
3. Able to select, review, apply, analyze, synthesize, interpret, and evaluate information; makes recommendations to modify care plan	5	4	3	2	1
PSYCHOMOTOR DOMAIN					
4. Minimal errors, no critical errors; able to self-correct; performs all steps safely and accurately	5	4	3	2	1
5. Selects, assembles, and verifies proper function and cleanliness of equipment; assures operation and corrects malfunctions; provides adequate care and maintenance	5	4	3	2	1
6. Exhibits the required manual dexterity	5	4	3	2	1
7. Performs procedure in a reasonable time frame for clinical level	5	4	3	2	1
8. Applies and maintains aseptic technique and PPE as required	5	4	3	2	1
9. Maintains concise and accurate patient and clinical records	5	4	3	2	1
10. Reports promptly on patient status/needs to appropriate personnel	5	4	3	2	1
AFFECTIVE DOMAIN					
11. Exhibits courteous and pleasant demeanor; shows consideration and respect, honesty, and integrity	5	4	3	2	1
12. Communicates verbally and in writing clearly and concisely	5	4	3	2	1
13. Preserves confidentiality and adheres to all policies	5	4	3	2	1
14. Follows directions, exhibits sound judgment, and seeks help when required	5	4	3	2	1
15. Demonstrates initiative, self-direction, responsibility, and accountability	5	4	3	2	1

TOTAL POINTS = /15 = AVERAGE GRADE =

ADDITIONAL COMMENTS: IDENTIFY AREAS OF EXCELLENCE; LIST ERRORS OF OMISSION OR COMMISSION, CRITICAL ERRORS

SUMMARY PERFORMANCE EVALUATION AND RECOMMENDATIONS

☐ PASS: Satisfactory Performance

☐ Minimal supervision needed, may progress to next level provided specific skills, clinical time completed

☐ Minimal supervision needed, able to progress to next level without remediation

☐ FAIL: Unsatisfactory Performance (check all that apply)

☐ Minor reevaluation only

☐ Needs additional clinical practice before reevaluation

☐ Needs additional laboratory practice before skills performed in clinical area

☐ Recommend clinical probation

SIGNATURES

Evaluator (print name): Evaluator signature: Date:

Student Signature: Date:

Student Comments:

Procedural Competency Evaluation

STUDENT: DATE:

TRACHEOSTOMY TUBE CHANGE

	PERFORMANCE RATING	PERFORMANCE LEVEL
Evaluator: ☐ Peer ☐ Instructor **Setting:** ☐ Lab ☐ Clinical Simulation		
Equipment Utilized: **Conditions (Describe):**		
Performance Level: S or ✓ = Satisfactory, no errors of omission or commission U = Unsatisfactory Error of Omission or Commission NA = Not applicable		
Performance Rating: **5** **Independent:** Near flawless performance; minimal errors; able to perform without supervision; seeks out new learning; shows initiative; A = 4.7–5.0 average **4** **Minimally Supervised:** Few errors, able to self-correct; seeks guidance when appropriate; B = 3.7–4.65 **3** **Competent:** Minimal required level; no critical errors; able to correct with coaching; meets expectations; safe; C = 3.0–3.65 **2** **Marginal:** Below average; critical errors or problem areas noted; would benefit from remediation; D = 2.0–2.99 **1** **Dependent:** Poor; unacceptable performance; unsafe; gross inaccuracies; potentially harmful; F = < 2.0 *Two or more errors of commission or omission of mandatory or essential performance elements will terminate the procedure, and require additional practice and/or remediation and reevaluation. Student is responsible for obtaining additional evaluation forms as needed from the Director of Clinical Education (DCE).*		
EQUIPMENT AND PATIENT PREPARATION		
1. Common Performance Elements Steps 1–8		
2. Sedates if needed; allows adequate time for sedation to take effect		
ASSESSMENT AND IMPLEMENTATION		
3. Common Performance Elements Steps 9 and 10		
4. Suctions trachea		
5. Performs stoma care; visually inspects for bleeding, erosion, or signs of infection		
6. Positions patient in semi-Fowler's position with head slightly extended		
7. Opens new tracheostomy tube box; places tube on sterile field		
8. Checks cuff for leaks if applicable; deflates cuff		
9. Attaches new ties or commercial tube holder		
10. Lubricates tip of obturator with sterile, water-soluble lubricant		
11. Removes inner cannula and inserts obturator into new tube		
12. Loosens or unties old tracheostomy ties and deflates cuff if applicable		
13. Removes oxygen or humidity device		
14. Removes old tracheostomy tube		
15. Inserts new tube		
16. Removes obturator and inserts inner cannula; inflates cuff, if necessary		
17. Ensures correct tube placement; verifies patent airway; assesses patient's ventilation and oxygenation		
18. Reapplies oxygen or humidity device		
19. Secures tube in place		
20. Replaces soiled tracheostomy dressing with sterile, pre-cut dressing if needed		
FOLLOW-UP		
21. Common Performance Elements Steps 11–16		
22. Ensures spare tracheostomy tube of same size and type is available at patient bedside		
23. Soaks old tracheostomy tube in peroxide for 20 minutes		
24. Uses pipe cleaners and brushes to remove organic debris from inner and outer cannula		
25. Soaks tracheostomy tube in soapy water		
26. Rinses, disinfects, or sterilizes tracheostomy tube according to department policy		

SIGNATURES   Student: Evaluator: Date:

Clinical Performance Evaluation

PERFORMANCE RATING:

5   **Independent:** Near flawless performance; minimal errors; able to perform without supervision; seeks out new learning; shows initiative; A = 4.7–5.0 average

4   **Minimally Supervised:** Few errors, able to self-correct; seeks guidance when appropriate; B = 3.7–4.65

3   **Competent:** Minimal required level; no critical errors; able to correct with coaching; meets expectations; safe; C = 3.0–3.65

2   **Marginal:** Below average; critical errors or problem areas noted; would benefit from remediation; D = 2.0–2.99

1   **Dependent:** Poor; unacceptable performance; unsafe; gross inaccuracies; potentially harmful; F = < 2.0

Circle the appropriate response below. Please be consistent, objective, and honest in your assessment of the student's clinical performance and ability.

PERFORMANCE CRITERIA	SCORE				
COGNITIVE DOMAIN					
1. Consistently displays knowledge, comprehension, and command of essential concepts	5	4	3	2	1
2. Demonstrates the relationship between theory and clinical practice	5	4	3	2	1
3. Able to select, review, apply, analyze, synthesize, interpret, and evaluate information; makes recommendations to modify care plan	5	4	3	2	1
PSYCHOMOTOR DOMAIN					
4. Minimal errors, no critical errors; able to self-correct; performs all steps safely and accurately	5	4	3	2	1
5. Selects, assembles, and verifies proper function and cleanliness of equipment; assures operation and corrects malfunctions; provides adequate care and maintenance	5	4	3	2	1
6. Exhibits the required manual dexterity	5	4	3	2	1
7. Performs procedure in a reasonable time frame for clinical level	5	4	3	2	1
8. Applies and maintains aseptic technique and PPE as required	5	4	3	2	1
9. Maintains concise and accurate patient and clinical records	5	4	3	2	1
10. Reports promptly on patient status/needs to appropriate personnel	5	4	3	2	1
AFFECTIVE DOMAIN					
11. Exhibits courteous and pleasant demeanor; shows consideration and respect, honesty, and integrity	5	4	3	2	1
12. Communicates verbally and in writing clearly and concisely	5	4	3	2	1
13. Preserves confidentiality and adheres to all policies	5	4	3	2	1
14. Follows directions, exhibits sound judgment, and seeks help when required	5	4	3	2	1
15. Demonstrates initiative, self-direction, responsibility, and accountability	5	4	3	2	1

TOTAL POINTS = _____ /15 = AVERAGE GRADE = _____

ADDITIONAL COMMENTS: IDENTIFY AREAS OF EXCELLENCE; LIST ERRORS OF OMISSION OR COMMISSION, CRITICAL ERRORS

SUMMARY PERFORMANCE EVALUATION AND RECOMMENDATIONS

☐ PASS: Satisfactory Performance

    ☐ Minimal supervision needed, may progress to next level provided specific skills, clinical time completed

    ☐ Minimal supervision needed, able to progress to next level without remediation

☐ FAIL: Unsatisfactory Performance (check all that apply)

    ☐ Minor reevaluation only

    ☐ Needs additional clinical practice before reevaluation

    ☐ Needs additional laboratory practice before skills performed in clinical area

    ☐ Recommend clinical probation

SIGNATURES

Evaluator (print name): _____   Evaluator signature: _____   Date: _____

Student Signature: _____   Date: _____

Student Comments:

24
Artificial Airway Care and Maintenance

INTRODUCTION

Once an artificial tracheal airway is in place, meticulous maintenance and care are needed to prevent infection, airway emergencies, and other complications of prolonged intubation.

The respiratory care practitioner qualified to intubate may also extubate patients. The patient must be assessed after **extubation** for laryngeal edema and vocal cord injury. Appropriate oxygenation and humidification must be provided. Administration of racemic epinephrine or steroids may help relieve airway obstruction caused by edema.

Lack of appropriate airway care can lead to short- and long-term complications ranging from minor bleeding or edema to permanent anatomical airway changes or life-threatening emergencies.[1] Airway emergencies include inadvertent extubation, cuff leak, and obstructed airway with failure to provide adequate ventilation. Injuries associated with airway placement include tissue pressure **necrosis**, **granulomas**, tracheoesophageal or arterial **fistula**, **tracheomalacia**, tracheal **stenosis**, laryngotracheal web formation, vocal cord paralysis, and **paresis**.

OBJECTIVES

Upon completion of this chapter, the student will be able to:

1. Practice communication skills needed for assessing the level of patient comprehension while instructing patients in airway care procedures.
2. Practice medical charting for airway care procedures.
3. Apply infection control guidelines and standards associated with equipment and procedures, according to OSHA regulations and CDC guidelines.
4. Resecure an endotracheal tube in place by changing cloth tape and commercial endotracheal tube holders.
5. Reposition an endotracheal tube and assess the proper size and placement.
6. Perform minimum occluding volume (MOV) and minimal leak technique (MLT) cuff inflation procedures.
7. Measure airway cuff pressures with aneroid pressure manometers.
8. Extubate a patient and evaluate the patient's respiratory status after extubation.
9. Provide appropriate postextubation airway care, including oxygenation, humidification, and pharmacological treatment.
10. Identify airway emergencies and take appropriate actions to ensure patient ventilation and oxygenation, as well as troubleshoot equipment, including cuff leaks, tube obstructions, tube malpositions, and inadvertent extubation.

KEY TERMS

extubation granulomas paresis tracheomalacia
fistula necrosis stenosis

Exercises

EQUIPMENT REQUIRED

- ☐ Oropharyngeal airways, various sizes
- ☐ Airway management trainers
- ☐ Silicone spray
- ☐ Water-soluble lubricant
- ☐ Goggles or face shields
- ☐ Sterile and nonsterile disposable latex and vinyl gloves, various sizes
- ☐ Oxygen gas source and flowmeter
- ☐ Oxygen connecting tubing and nipple adaptors
- ☐ Endotracheal tubes, various sizes
- ☐ Stethoscopes
- ☐ Colorimetric capnometry (Easy Cap™) or other spot-check capnography device
- ☐ Manual resuscitators with masks, adult and infant
- ☐ Laryngoscope blades and handles:
  - ☐ Miller (various sizes)
  - ☐ MacIntosh (various sizes)
- ☐ Batteries for laryngoscopes
- ☐ Replacement laryngoscope bulbs
- ☐ Stylets
- ☐ Suction catheter kits
- ☐ Yankauer catheter
- ☐ Basins
- ☐ Suction machines
- ☐ Sterile water or normal saline
- ☐ Swivel adaptor and deadspace tubing
- ☐ Tracheostomy collars
- ☐ Briggs adaptors (T-piece)
- ☐ Letter board or pad and pen/pencil
- ☐ Cloth tape
- ☐ Tincture of benzoin
- ☐ Endotracheal tube holders
- ☐ 10-mL syringes
- ☐ Towels
- ☐ Scissors
- ☐ Lemon glycerine swabs
- ☐ Toothbrush and toothpaste
- ☐ Razor and shaving cream
- ☐ Cotton swabs
- ☐ 4×4 sterile gauze
- ☐ Hemostats
- ☐ Needles, various sizes
- ☐ Pressure manometers
- ☐ Three-way stopcocks
- ☐ Posey Cufflator™ cuff inflation device
- ☐ Large-volume nebulizer
- ☐ Large-bore corrugated tubing
- ☐ Aerosol masks
- ☐ Endotracheal tubes with ruptured cuff, malfunctioning pilot balloon, cut pilot tube
- ☐ Endotracheal tubes obstructed by Silly Putty®, Play-Doh®, or material of similar consistency
- ☐ Pulse oximeter

EXERCISE 24.1 CUFF CARE

EXERCISE 24.1.1 MINIMAL LEAK TECHNIQUE

1. Orally intubate an airway management trainer.
2. Verify correct tube placement as practiced in Chapter 22. **Record the endotracheal tube size and centimeter mark to the mouth on your laboratory report.**
3. While your laboratory partner is manually ventilating the mannequin, use a 10-mL syringe to slowly inject air into the pilot balloon of the endotracheal tube.
4. Continue to inflate the cuff until no leak is heard while auscultating the lateral neck (this will have to be simulated on the mannequin). Withdraw a slight amount of air from the cuff until a small leak is heard above the cuff on the lateral neck during peak inspiration. If air leakage is felt from the nose or mouth, too large a leak has been created.
5. Note the total volume of air used to inflate the cuff, and **record the volume on your laboratory report.**

EXERCISE 24.1.2 MINIMUM OCCLUDING VOLUME

1. Orally intubate an airway management trainer.
2. Verify correct tube placement as practiced in Chapter 22. **Record the endotracheal tube size and centimeter mark to the mouth on your laboratory report.**
3. While your laboratory partner is manually ventilating the mannequin, use a 10-mL syringe to slowly inject air into the pilot balloon of the endotracheal tube.
4. Continue to inflate the cuff until no leak is heard while auscultating the lateral neck (this will have to be simulated on the mannequin). Maximum inflation should be done during peak inspiration of positive pressure breath where the seal is needed most.
5. Note the total volume of air used to inflate the cuff, and **record the volume on your laboratory report.**

EXERCISE 24.1.3 CUFF PRESSURE MEASUREMENT

1. Inflate the cuff of an orally intubated mannequin to MOV.
2. Obtain a three-way stopcock (Fig. 24.1). Turn the valve stem so that it is off to the Luer-Lok™. Observe all three of the openings to determine which two of the ports are open. This would allow air to flow in that particular direction.
3. Turn the valve stem so that it is off to the left port of the three-way stopcock. Observe all three of the openings to determine which two of the ports are open. This would allow air to flow in that particular direction.
4. Turn the valve stem so that it is off to the right port of the three-way stopcock. Observe all three of the openings to determine which two of the ports are open. This would allow air to flow in that particular direction.
5. Set up a cuff pressure measurement system using the aneroid manometer, as shown in Figure 24.2.
6. Suction any secretions in the pharynx and above the cuff thoroughly.
7. Attach the measurement system to the valve connection on the pilot balloon with the three-way stopcock open to all directions. The cuff will automatically deflate. This will allow equilibration between the manometer, the pilot tube, and the cuff.
8. Pull the syringe barrel back to 10 mL and attach it to the three-way stopcock.
9. Slowly inflate the cuff to MOV during peak inspiration. **Record the peak pressure achieved on the manometer during expiration on your laboratory report.**
10. The maximum cuff pressure should be maintained at less than 20 to 25 mm Hg or 25 to 33 cm H_2O. The pressure increases during exhalation when the tracheal diameter is narrower. Maximum cuff pressures should not be exceeded during the exhalation phase.
11. Turn the stopcock off to the pilot tube. Detach the manometer system.
12. Attach the 10-mL syringe to the pilot tube. Remove the air from the cuff, measure it, and **record the volume on your laboratory report.** Reinsert the air slowly back into the cuff.
13. Repeat steps 6 through 12 using MLT.
14. Repeat steps 6 through 12 using a Posey Cufflator™ (Fig 24.3).

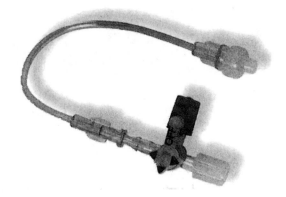

Figure 24.1. Three way stopcock. (Courtesy of Smith Industries Medical Systems, Keene, NH.)

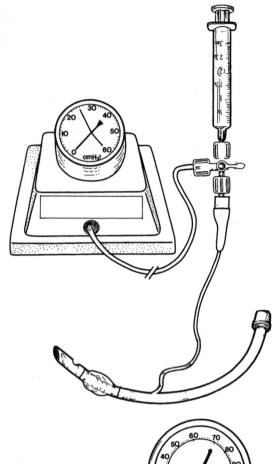

Figure 24.2. Cuff pressure measurements using an aneroid manometer.

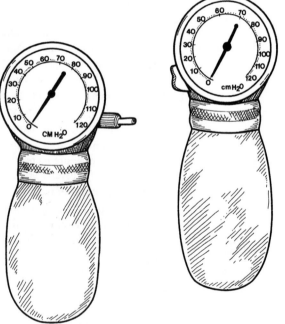

Figure 24.3. Cuff pressure measurements using a Posey Cufflator™.

EXERCISE 24.2 RESECURING AND REPOSITIONING OF AN ENDOTRACHEAL TUBE AND ORAL HYGEINE

To perform this exercise, you will need an intubated mannequin with a Briggs adaptor and large-bore tubing attached to simulate a clinical situation. The tube should be secured with tape before the exercise.

1. Have your laboratory partner wash his or her hands, apply standard precautions and transmission-based isolation procedures as appropriate, and hold the endotracheal tube securely in position while you perform the following steps. Note the position of the endotracheal tube.

2. Wash your hands. Apply standard precautions and transmission-based isolation procedures as appropriate. Do not apply gloves until the tape is prepared. Prepare the cloth tape for use to secure the endotracheal tube.

3. Put on your gloves. Carefully cut and remove the tape currently securing the endotracheal tube. *Do not cut the pilot tube.* Make sure it is out of your way. Discard the used tape in an infectious waste container.

4. Oral hygiene is crucial in an intubated patient. Brush the teeth, rinsing out the mouth with sterile water. Suction with a Yankauer suction apparatus. Lemon glycerine swabs may be used to clean the mouth. Male patients may also be shaved at this time.

5. Move the endotracheal tube to the opposite side of the mouth. A tongue depressor may be used to assist if the tongue prevents easy repositioning. Insert an oropharyngeal airway into the mouth medially to the endotracheal tube.

6. Clean the patient's face using a wet 4×4 gauze pad, removing as much of the previous adhesive as possible.

7. Dry the skin with a clean towel or 4×4 gauze pad.

8. To enhance the adhesiveness of the tape, tincture of benzoin may be applied using a 4×4 gauze pad to the patient's skin. Do not spray or apply the liquid directly to the patient's face.

9. Apply the tape using one of the methods practiced in Chapter 22. Ensure that the tube position is correct. Secure the tape around the oropharyngeal airway to serve as a bite block. Reassess correct tube placement when finished. **"Chart" the procedure on your laboratory report.**

10. Repeat the exercise using a commercial endotracheal tube holder to secure the tube.

EXERCISE 24.3   EXTUBATION

1. Verify a physician's order or protocol or assess "patient's" readiness for extubation. Check the chart or protocol for the appropriate F_IO_2 after extubation.

2. Gather the necessary equipment:

   Suction and suction kits

   Large-volume nebulizer

   Large-bore corrugated tubing

   Aerosol mask

   Scissors

   10-mL syringe

   Intubation tray (see Chapter 22)

3. Assemble the equipment to deliver the appropriate F_IO_2.

4. Using your lab partner as the patient, explain the procedure and confirm the "patient's" understanding.

5. Wash your hands and apply standard precautions and transmission-based isolation procedures as appropriate.

6. Assess the "patient," including pulse oximetry.

7. Place the "patient" in a high Fowler's position.

8. Suction the "patient's" endotracheal tube and pharynx thoroughly, as described in Chapter 21.

9. Remove the endotracheal tube tape or securing device and deflate the cuff completely. Alternatively, the pilot tube may then be cut to ensure easy removal of any remaining air during tube withdrawal.

10. Instruct the "patient" to take a maximum inspiration and remove the tube at peak inspiration so that the vocal cords are completely abducted. An alternative method is to have the "patient" cough, which will also maximally abduct the vocal cords.

11. Apply the oxygen and humidity device on the "patient."

12. Assess the "patient." Determine the adequacy of spontaneous ventilation. Make particular note of hoarseness or stridor. If stridor is present, racemic epinephrine aerosol may be administered. If stridor worsens and the "patient's" clinical situation deteriorates, reintubation may be necessary.

13. **Chart the procedure on your laboratory report.**

EXERCISE 24.4   AIRWAY EMERGENCIES

Your instructor will provide you with an orally intubated mannequin attached to a ventilator swivel adaptor and tubing connection. The mannequin has one of the following airway emergencies simulated:

Cuff rupture

Tube obstruction

Pilot tube leak

Pilot valve leak

1. Remove the ventilator adaptor and manually ventilate the mannequin. Can you ventilate the mannequin? Does the air go in easily? Is there an air leak around the mouth or nose? **Record your observations on your laboratory report.**

2. Your action plan will depend on the cause of the airway emergency.

    A. If you cannot ventilate or air cannot enter easily and there does *not* appear to be an air leak, the tube is most likely obstructed. Troubleshooting steps for an obstructed airway should be followed:

        (1) Attempt to pass a suction catheter. Suction and lavage the airway to clear the obstruction. Attempt to ventilate. Assess the adequacy of ventilation.

        (2) If it is not possible to clear the obstruction, notify the appropriate personnel. Emergency extubation is a last resort and should not be performed unless all other attempts have failed. The next step in a spontaneously breathing patient is to deflate the cuff and assess for adequate ventilation. If ventilation is adequate, the situation is less emergent and the proper equipment and personnel can be assembled to reintubate under more controlled circumstances.

        (3) If the patient cannot be adequately ventilated, an emergent situation is at hand. The nurse and physician should be notified of the situation and the patient should be extubated. Extubate and manually ventilate the mannequin with a mask while preparations for reintubation are made.

    B. If you are able to squeeze the manual resuscitator without difficulty but a leak is noted from the mouth or nose, there is a problem with the cuff or the pilot tube or valve. In an actual clinical situation a conscious patient may even be able to vocalize. Troubleshooting steps for a cuff leak should be followed:

        (1) Attempt to reinflate the cuff as previously practiced. If successful, measure the cuff pressure.

        (2) Ventilate and assess for leaks.

        (3) If the leak persists, visually inspect the pilot tube, balloon, and valve for any cuts, nicks, or other signs of damage. If the pilot tube is damaged, refer to step (7).

        (4) Reinflate the cuff and apply a hemostat to the pilot tube as shown in Figure 24.4. Be cautious not to apply excessive pressure so that the tube is not permanently crimped or damaged.

        (5) Ventilate and assess for leaks.

        (6) If clamping the pilot tube in step (4) eliminated the leak, most likely the pilot valve is damaged. Gather the equipment and assemble a temporary inflating device as shown in Figure 24.5 by using an appropriate size needle, three-way stopcock, and syringe. Cut the pilot valve and inflating tube past the point of any damage. Insert the needle into the remaining portion of the pilot tube and attach the inflating device. Tape the entire assembly to a tongue depressor to prevent accidental needle-stick injuries or dislodging of the needle. Reinflate the cuff, measure the cuff pressure, and reassess ventilation.

        (7) If the leak persists, it is likely that the cuff is ruptured. This is the most emergent situation if you cannot achieve adequate ventilation. The nurse and physician should be notified of the situation and the patient should be extubated. Extubate and manually ventilate the mannequin with a mask while preparations for reintubation are made.

3. **Chart your assessment of the cause of the airway emergency and the corrective actions taken on your laboratory report.**

4. Repeat steps 1 and 2 for the other three airway emergencies.

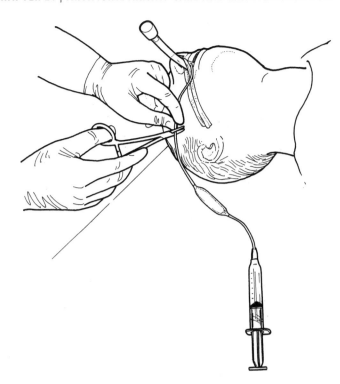

Figure 24.4. Clamping the pilot tube.

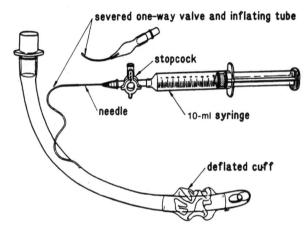

Figure 24.5. Temporary inflation device for a damaged pilot valve.

REFERENCES

1. American Association for Respiratory Care: AARC clinical practice guideline: Management of airway emergencies. Respir Care 40:749–760, 1995.

Laboratory Report

CHAPTER 24: ARTIFICIAL AIRWAY CARE AND MAINTENANCE

Name _____   Date _____

Course/Section _____   Instructor _____

Data Collection

EXERCISE 24.1 Cuff Care

EXERCISE 24.1.1 MINIMAL LEAK TECHNIQUE

Endotracheal tube size: _____

Position: _____ cm

Cuff volume: _____

EXERCISE 24.1.2 MINIMAL OCCLUDING VOLUME

Endotracheal tube size: _____

Position: _____ cm

Cuff volume: _____

EXERCISE 24.1.3 CUFF PRESSURE MEASUREMENT

Cuff pressure at MOV: _____

Volume at MOV: _____

Cuff pressure at MLT: _____

Volume at MLT: _____

Cuff pressure using Posey Cufflator™: _____

Volume using Posey Cufflator™: _____

EXERCISE 24.2 Resecuring and Repositioning of an Endotracheal Tube and Oral Hygiene

Chart the procedure:

_____

_____

_____

_____

EXERCISE 24.3 Extubation

Chart the procedure:

_____

_____

_____

_____

EXERCISE 24.4 Airway Emergencies

Can you ventilate? _____

Does air go in easily? _____

Is there an air leak around the mouth and nose? _____

Chart your assessment of the airway emergency and corrective actions taken:

_____

_____

_____

_____

_____

_____

_____

_____

_____

Critical Thinking Questions

1. For the following clinical situations, what type of artificial tracheal airway should be used? If more than one option is indicated, include all appropriate choices with an explanation.

    A. Cardiac arrest

    B. Suspected C-1 fracture

    C. 3-year-old patient with epiglottitis

    D. Patient with paralyzed vocal cords

E.   Patient with dysphagia and chronic aspiration

F.   Fractured jaw

G.   An alert stroke patient who cannot cough

2.   Describe the safety precautions that should be taken during oral hygiene of the intubated patient. What emergency equipment should be readily available?

3.   You are called to the surgical ICU to assess Mrs. King, who had open heart surgery and is 20 hours postop. Describe how you would assess her readiness for extubation.

4.   Mr. Kee is intubated with a 7.5-mm orotracheal tube. He is in the ICU on a ventilator. The low-exhaled-volume alarm is sounding and Mr. Kee is phonating. His respiratory rate is 32/minute, the heart rate is 122/minute, and the pulse oximeter is 89%. You measure the cuff pressure to be 30 cm H_2O, and the pilot tube and valve are intact. What would be your recommendations to remedy this situation?

Procedural Competency Evaluation

STUDENT: _____   **DATE:** _____

EXTUBATION

Evaluator: ☐ Peer ☐ Instructor	**Setting:** ☐ Lab ☐ Clinical Simulation	
Equipment Utilized:	**Conditions (Describe):**	

Performance Level:

S or ✓ = Satisfactory, no errors of omission or commission
U = Unsatisfactory Error of Omission or Commission
NA = Not applicable

Performance Rating:

5   **Independent:** Near flawless performance; minimal errors; able to perform without supervision; seeks out new learning; shows initiative; A = 4.7–5.0 average

4   **Minimally Supervised:** Few errors, able to self-correct; seeks guidance when appropriate; B = 3.7–4.65

3   **Competent:** Minimal required level; no critical errors; able to correct with coaching; meets expectations; safe; C = 3.0–3.65

2   **Marginal:** Below average; critical errors or problem areas noted; would benefit from remediation; D = 2.0–2.99

1   **Dependent:** Poor; unacceptable performance; unsafe; gross inaccuracies; potentially harmful; F = < 2.0

Two or more errors of commission or omission of mandatory or essential performance elements will terminate the procedure, and require additional practice and/or remediation and reevaluation. Student is responsible for obtaining additional evaluation forms as needed from the Director of Clinical Education (DCE).

(Columns at right: **PERFORMANCE RATING** | **PERFORMANCE LEVEL**)

EQUIPMENT AND PATIENT PREPARATION

1. Common Performance Elements Steps 1–8

2. Assembles and verifies function of oxygen and humidification device to be used post-extubation

ASSESSMENT AND IMPLEMENTATION

3. Common Performance Elements Steps 9 and 10

4. Positions patient in a high Fowler's position

5. Suctions patient's endotracheal tube and pharyngeal area thoroughly

6. Deflates cuff and assesses cuff leak (>30% VT) and vocalization

7. Removes ET tube tape or securing device

8. Instructs patient to take maximum inspiration and removes tube at peak inspiration (or alternatively during maximal cough); NOTE: do not remove tube during suctioning

9. Applies oxygen and humidification device

10. Reassesses patient to determine adequacy of spontaneous ventilation and airway patency; verifies comfort and attends needs

11. Encourages patient to cough; periodically reassesses

FOLLOW-UP

12. Recommends cool mist, steroids, or racemic epinephrine as indicated

13. Common Performance Elements Steps 11–16

SIGNATURES   Student: _____   Evaluator: _____   Date: _____

Clinical Performance Evaluation

PERFORMANCE RATING:

5 **Independent:** Near flawless performance; minimal errors; able to perform without supervision; seeks out new learning; shows initiative; A = 4.7–5.0 average

4 **Minimally Supervised:** Few errors, able to self-correct; seeks guidance when appropriate; B = 3.7–4.65

3 **Competent:** Minimal required level; no critical errors; able to correct with coaching; meets expectations; safe; C = 3.0–3.65

2 **Marginal:** Below average; critical errors or problem areas noted; would benefit from remediation; D = 2.0–2.99

1 **Dependent:** Poor; unacceptable performance; unsafe; gross inaccuracies; potentially harmful; F = < 2.0

Circle the appropriate response below. Please be consistent, objective, and honest in your assessment of the student's clinical performance and ability.

PERFORMANCE CRITERIA | SCORE

PERFORMANCE CRITERIA	SCORE				
COGNITIVE DOMAIN					
1. Consistently displays knowledge, comprehension, and command of essential concepts	5	4	3	2	1
2. Demonstrates the relationship between theory and clinical practice	5	4	3	2	1
3. Able to select, review, apply, analyze, synthesize, interpret, and evaluate information; makes recommendations to modify care plan	5	4	3	2	1
PSYCHOMOTOR DOMAIN					
4. Minimal errors, no critical errors; able to self-correct; performs all steps safely and accurately	5	4	3	2	1
5. Selects, assembles, and verifies proper function and cleanliness of equipment; assures operation and corrects malfunctions; provides adequate care and maintenance	5	4	3	2	1
6. Exhibits the required manual dexterity	5	4	3	2	1
7. Performs procedure in a reasonable time frame for clinical level	5	4	3	2	1
8. Applies and maintains aseptic technique and PPE as required	5	4	3	2	1
9. Maintains concise and accurate patient and clinical records	5	4	3	2	1
10. Reports promptly on patient status/needs to appropriate personnel	5	4	3	2	1
AFFECTIVE DOMAIN					
11. Exhibits courteous and pleasant demeanor; shows consideration and respect, honesty, and integrity	5	4	3	2	1
12. Communicates verbally and in writing clearly and concisely	5	4	3	2	1
13. Preserves confidentiality and adheres to all policies	5	4	3	2	1
14. Follows directions, exhibits sound judgment, and seeks help when required	5	4	3	2	1
15. Demonstrates initiative, self-direction, responsibility, and accountability	5	4	3	2	1

TOTAL POINTS = ____ /15 = AVERAGE GRADE = ____

ADDITIONAL COMMENTS: IDENTIFY AREAS OF EXCELLENCE; LIST ERRORS OF OMISSION OR COMMISSION, CRITICAL ERRORS

SUMMARY PERFORMANCE EVALUATION AND RECOMMENDATIONS

☐ PASS: Satisfactory Performance

   ☐ Minimal supervision needed, may progress to next level provided specific skills, clinical time completed

   ☐ Minimal supervision needed, able to progress to next level without remediation

☐ FAIL: Unsatisfactory Performance (check all that apply)

   ☐ Minor reevaluation only

   ☐ Needs additional clinical practice before reevaluation

   ☐ Needs additional laboratory practice before skills performed in clinical area

   ☐ Recommend clinical probation

SIGNATURES

Evaluator (print name): ____ Evaluator signature: ____ Date: ____

Student Signature: ____ Date: ____

Student Comments:

Procedural Competency Evaluation

STUDENT: **DATE:**

ARTIFICIAL AIRWAY CARE

	PERFORMANCE RATING	PERFORMANCE LEVEL
Evaluator: ☐ Peer ☐ Instructor **Setting:** ☐ Lab ☐ Clinical Simulation		
Equipment Utilized: **Conditions (Describe):**		
Performance Level: S or ✓ = Satisfactory, no errors of omission or commission U = Unsatisfactory Error of Omission or Commission NA = Not applicable		
Performance Rating: **5** **Independent:** Near flawless performance; minimal errors; able to perform without supervision; seeks out new learning; shows initiative; A = 4.7–5.0 average **4** **Minimally Supervised:** Few errors, able to self-correct; seeks guidance when appropriate; B = 3.7–4.65 **3** **Competent:** Minimal required level; no critical errors; able to correct with coaching; meets expectations; safe; C = 3.0–3.65 **2** **Marginal:** Below average; critical errors or problem areas noted; would benefit from remediation; D = 2.0–2.99 **1** **Dependent:** Poor; unacceptable performance; unsafe; gross inaccuracies; potentially harmful; F = < 2.0 *Two or more errors of commission or omission of mandatory or essential performance elements will terminate the procedure, and require additional practice and/or remediation and reevaluation. Student is responsible for obtaining additional evaluation forms as needed from the Director of Clinical Education (DCE).*		

EQUIPMENT AND PATIENT PREPARATION		
1. Common Performance Elements Steps 1–8		
2. Ensures emergency replacement airway of same size and type is available at bedside		
ASSESSMENT AND IMPLEMENTATION		
3. Common Performance Elements Steps 9 and 10		
4. Verifies size, type, and position of airway		
5. Suctions tube and pharynx thoroughly		
6. Performs mouth or stoma care		
7. Stabilizes airway while removing fastenings		
8. Cleans and dries patient's face; uses adhesive removal product if needed		
9. Moves tube to new location (ETT) (right, left, or center)		
10. Reinflates cuff with maximum volume of 10 mL		
11. Applies new ties/tape/commercial tube holder; applies tincture of benzoin or similar skin protection product if indicated		
12. Verifies appropriate position by auscultation and tube markings		
13. Demonstrates cuff inflation to minimum occluding volume (MOV) or minimum leak technique (MLT)		
14. Demonstrates cuff pressure measurement and adjusts to 20 mm Hg to minimize VAP		
FOLLOW-UP		
15. Common Performance Elements Steps 11–16		

SIGNATURES   Student: Evaluator: Date:

Clinical Performance Evaluation

PERFORMANCE RATING:

5 **Independent:** Near flawless performance; minimal errors; able to perform without supervision; seeks out new learning; shows initiative; A = 4.7–5.0 average

4 **Minimally Supervised:** Few errors, able to self-correct; seeks guidance when appropriate; B = 3.7–4.65

3 **Competent:** Minimal required level; no critical errors; able to correct with coaching; meets expectations; safe; C = 3.0–3.65

2 **Marginal:** Below average; critical errors or problem areas noted; would benefit from remediation; D = 2.0–2.99

1 **Dependent:** Poor; unacceptable performance; unsafe; gross inaccuracies; potentially harmful; F = < 2.0

Circle the appropriate response below. Please be consistent, objective, and honest in your assessment of the student's clinical performance and ability.

PERFORMANCE CRITERIA	SCORE				
COGNITIVE DOMAIN					
1. Consistently displays knowledge, comprehension, and command of essential concepts	5	4	3	2	1
2. Demonstrates the relationship between theory and clinical practice	5	4	3	2	1
3. Able to select, review, apply, analyze, synthesize, interpret, and evaluate information; makes recommendations to modify care plan	5	4	3	2	1
PSYCHOMOTOR DOMAIN					
4. Minimal errors, no critical errors; able to self-correct; performs all steps safely and accurately	5	4	3	2	1
5. Selects, assembles, and verifies proper function and cleanliness of equipment; assures operation and corrects malfunctions; provides adequate care and maintenance	5	4	3	2	1
6. Exhibits the required manual dexterity	5	4	3	2	1
7. Performs procedure in a reasonable time frame for clinical level	5	4	3	2	1
8. Applies and maintains aseptic technique and PPE as required	5	4	3	2	1
9. Maintains concise and accurate patient and clinical records	5	4	3	2	1
10. Reports promptly on patient status/needs to appropriate personnel	5	4	3	2	1
AFFECTIVE DOMAIN					
11. Exhibits courteous and pleasant demeanor; shows consideration and respect, honesty, and integrity	5	4	3	2	1
12. Communicates verbally and in writing clearly and concisely	5	4	3	2	1
13. Preserves confidentiality and adheres to all policies	5	4	3	2	1
14. Follows directions, exhibits sound judgment, and seeks help when required	5	4	3	2	1
15. Demonstrates initiative, self-direction, responsibility, and accountability	5	4	3	2	1

TOTAL POINTS = _____ /15 = AVERAGE GRADE = _____

ADDITIONAL COMMENTS: IDENTIFY AREAS OF EXCELLENCE; LIST ERRORS OF OMISSION OR COMMISSION, CRITICAL ERRORS

SUMMARY PERFORMANCE EVALUATION AND RECOMMENDATIONS

☐ PASS: Satisfactory Performance

    ☐ Minimal supervision needed, may progress to next level provided specific skills, clinical time completed

    ☐ Minimal supervision needed, able to progress to next level without remediation

☐ FAIL: Unsatisfactory Performance (check all that apply)

    ☐ Minor reevaluation only

    ☐ Needs additional clinical practice before reevaluation

    ☐ Needs additional laboratory practice before skills performed in clinical area

    ☐ Recommend clinical probation

SIGNATURES

Evaluator (print name): _____   Evaluator signature: _____   Date: _____

Student Signature: _____   Date: _____

Student Comments: _____

Procedural Competency Evaluation

STUDENT: **DATE:**

CUFF CARE

Evaluator: ☐ Peer ☐ Instructor	Setting: ☐ Lab ☐ Clinical Simulation

Equipment Utilized: **Conditions (Describe):**

Performance Level:

S or ✓ = Satisfactory, no errors of omission or commission
U = Unsatisfactory Error of Omission or Commission
NA = Not applicable

Performance Rating:

5 **Independent:** Near flawless performance; minimal errors; able to perform without supervision; seeks out new learning; shows initiative; A = 4.7–5.0 average

4 **Minimally Supervised:** Few errors, able to self-correct; seeks guidance when appropriate; B = 3.7–4.65

3 **Competent:** Minimal required level; no critical errors; able to correct with coaching; meets expectations; safe; C = 3.0–3.65

2 **Marginal:** Below average; critical errors or problem areas noted; would benefit from remediation; D = 2.0–2.99

1 **Dependent:** Poor; unacceptable performance; unsafe; gross inaccuracies; potentially harmful; F = < 2.0

Two or more errors of commission or omission of mandatory or essential performance elements will terminate the procedure, and require additional practice and/or remediation and reevaluation. Student is responsible for obtaining additional evaluation forms as needed from the Director of Clinical Education (DCE).

(Columns: PERFORMANCE RATING | PERFORMANCE LEVEL)

EQUIPMENT AND PATIENT PREPARATION

1. Common Performance Elements Steps 1–8

ASSESSMENT AND IMPLEMENTATION

2. Common Performance Elements Steps 9 and 10
3. Verifies size, type, and position of airway
4. Stabilizes airway while removing fastenings
5. Performs mouth or stoma care
6. Moves tube to new location (ETT) (right, left, or center)
7. Applies new ties/tape holder/precut dressing (for tracheostomy) as indicated
8. Verifies appropriate position by auscultation, tube markings
9. Demonstrates cuff inflation to minimum occluding volume (MOV)
10. Demonstrates cuff inflation to minimum leak technique (MLT)
11. Demonstrates cuff pressure measurement using manometer and/or commercial cuff inflation device

FOLLOW-UP

12. Common Performance Elements Steps 11–16
13. Identifies appropriate range for cuff pressure to minimize tracheal damage, prevent VAP

SIGNATURES   Student: Evaluator: Date:

Clinical Performance Evaluation

PERFORMANCE RATING:

5 **Independent:** Near flawless performance; minimal errors; able to perform without supervision; seeks out new learning; shows initiative; A = 4.7–5.0 average

4 **Minimally Supervised:** Few errors, able to self-correct; seeks guidance when appropriate; B = 3.7–4.65

3 **Competent:** Minimal required level; no critical errors; able to correct with coaching; meets expectations; safe; C = 3.0–3.65

2 **Marginal:** Below average; critical errors or problem areas noted; would benefit from remediation; D = 2.0–2.99

1 **Dependent:** Poor; unacceptable performance; unsafe; gross inaccuracies; potentially harmful; F = < 2.0

Circle the appropriate response below. Please be consistent, objective, and honest in your assessment of the student's clinical performance and ability.

PERFORMANCE CRITERIA	SCORE				
COGNITIVE DOMAIN					
1. Consistently displays knowledge, comprehension, and command of essential concepts	5	4	3	2	1
2. Demonstrates the relationship between theory and clinical practice	5	4	3	2	1
3. Able to select, review, apply, analyze, synthesize, interpret, and evaluate information; makes recommendations to modify care plan	5	4	3	2	1
PSYCHOMOTOR DOMAIN					
4. Minimal errors, no critical errors; able to self-correct; performs all steps safely and accurately	5	4	3	2	1
5. Selects, assembles, and verifies proper function and cleanliness of equipment; assures operation and corrects malfunctions; provides adequate care and maintenance	5	4	3	2	1
6. Exhibits the required manual dexterity	5	4	3	2	1
7. Performs procedure in a reasonable time frame for clinical level	5	4	3	2	1
8. Applies and maintains aseptic technique and PPE as required	5	4	3	2	1
9. Maintains concise and accurate patient and clinical records	5	4	3	2	1
10. Reports promptly on patient status/needs to appropriate personnel	5	4	3	2	1
AFFECTIVE DOMAIN					
11. Exhibits courteous and pleasant demeanor; shows consideration and respect, honesty, and integrity	5	4	3	2	1
12. Communicates verbally and in writing clearly and concisely	5	4	3	2	1
13. Preserves confidentiality and adheres to all policies	5	4	3	2	1
14. Follows directions, exhibits sound judgment, and seeks help when required	5	4	3	2	1
15. Demonstrates initiative, self-direction, responsibility, and accountability	5	4	3	2	1

TOTAL POINTS = _____ /15 = AVERAGE GRADE = _____

ADDITIONAL COMMENTS: IDENTIFY AREAS OF EXCELLENCE; LIST ERRORS OF OMISSION OR COMMISSION, CRITICAL ERRORS

SUMMARY PERFORMANCE EVALUATION AND RECOMMENDATIONS

☐ PASS: Satisfactory Performance

　　☐ Minimal supervision needed, may progress to next level provided specific skills, clinical time completed

　　☐ Minimal supervision needed, able to progress to next level without remediation

☐ FAIL: Unsatisfactory Performance (check all that apply)

　　☐ Minor reevaluation only

　　☐ Needs additional clinical practice before reevaluation

　　☐ Needs additional laboratory practice before skills performed in clinical area

　　☐ Recommend clinical probation

SIGNATURES

Evaluator (print name): _____ Evaluator signature: _____ Date: _____

Student Signature: _____ Date: _____

Student Comments: _____

25

Noninvasive Blood Gas Monitoring

INTRODUCTION

Monitoring devices are used to observe or record physiologic phenomena and to provide information on an ongoing basis without the need for removal of body fluids or tissue.[1] The use of noninvasive technology to monitor blood gases and trends has increased exponentially over the last decade. Devices such as pulse oximeters, **transcutaneous** monitors, and capnometers and capnographs can provide useful data for clinical decisions. Their use is associated with less risk to the practitioner from infectious hazards and fewer risks to the patient than invasive techniques.

However, the data provided by these devices should not replace invasive blood gas analysis. They only provide an indirect measurement of blood gas parameters. A baseline arterial blood gas should be obtained to correlate with the noninvasive data. Noninvasive devices have significant limitations that must be thoroughly understood. False-negative or false-positive findings may lead to inappropriate treatment of the patient.[2,3] When used appropriately, noninvasive monitors can be cost-effective and time-saving additions to patient assessment.

OBJECTIVES

Upon completion of this chapter, the student will be able to:

1. Practice communication skills needed to explain noninvasive monitoring procedures to the patient and confirm understanding.
2. Apply infection control guidelines and standards associated with equipment and procedures, according to OSHA regulations and CDC guidelines.
3. Select, assemble, operate, and maintain the appropriate monitoring device for a given clinical situation.
4. Assess and correct malfunctions of noninvasive monitoring equipment.
5. Identify limitations of noninvasive monitoring devices and differentiate false-negative and false-positive readings from reliable clinical data.
6. Interpret data obtained from noninvasive monitors and correlate the results to the patient's condition.
7. Practice medical charting of noninvasive monitoring procedures and data obtained.
8. Practice verbal communication skills needed to report results of data collection and make recommendations or modifications to the patient care plan.

KEY TERMS

capnography   colorimetric   phlebotomy   tourniquet
capnometry   monitoring   sensor   transcutaneous

Exercises

EQUIPMENT REQUIRED

☐ Pulse oximeter
☐ Finger Phantoms or FingerSim® (pulse oximeter accuracy-checking devices)
☐ Disposable and nondisposable oximeter probes
☐ Nail polish: red, black, and green
☐ Nail polish remover
☐ Cotton balls
☐ 4×4 gauze
☐ Oxygen gas source and regulator
☐ Nonrebreathing masks
☐ Bucket or large basin
☐ Ice water
☐ Elastic **phlebotomy tourniquet** or blood pressure cuff
☐ Barometer (mercury or aneroid)
☐ Capnograph

☐ Mainstream or sidestream **sensor** and connectors
☐ Calibration gas source for capnograph
☐ Disposable **colorimetric** capnometer (Easy Cap II, Pedi-Cap)
☐ Disposable cannula probe
☐ Alcohol prep pads
☐ Intubated airway management trainer
☐ Swivel ventilator adaptor and 50-mL corrugated tubing
☐ Transcutaneous oxygen/carbon dioxide monitor
☐ Zero solution
☐ Transcutaneous electrodes
☐ Calibration gas source for transcutaneous monitor
☐ Adhesive tape
☐ Intubated airway management trainer

EXERCISE 25.1 PULSE OXIMETRY

EXERCISE 25.1.1 MEASUREMENT OF SATURATION AND PULSE

1. Gather the necessary equipment:
   Pulse oximeter
   Probe
   Electrical power cord
   Alcohol prep pads
   Finger Phantoms or FingerSim® (pulse oximeter accuracy-checking devices)
2. Visually inspect the power cord (if applicable), and probe the cable for any frayed or exposed wires.
3. Plug the power cord into a three-prong electrical outlet, if applicable. If a battery-operated oximeter is used, continuous monitoring could run down the battery and render the unit inoperative.
4. Determine the accuracy of the pulse oximeter by using Finger Phantom or FingerSim® pulse oximeter accuracy-checking devices, if available, as shown in Figure 25.1A,B. These come preset with three levels of saturation (97%, 90%, and 80%). Place the Finger Phantom or FingerSim® in the holder and insert it into the pulse oximeter probe. Rhythmically squeeze tip of the Phantom or simulator to simulate pulse. **Record the saturation reading on the pulse oximeter for each level on your laboratory report.**
5. Using your laboratory partner as the patient, introduce yourself to your "patient," explain the procedure, and confirm understanding.

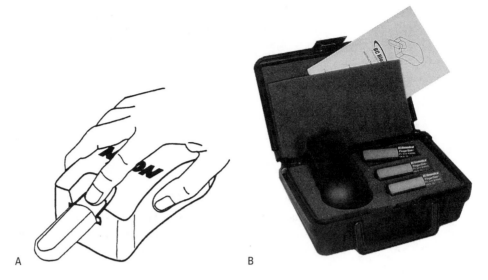

Figure 25.1. (A) Finger Phantoms pulse oximeter accuracy-checking device (courtesy of Nonin Medical, Inc., Plymouth, MN); **(B)** FingerSim® (BC Group International, Inc., St. Louis, MO).

A   B

6. With the "patient" seated comfortably, measure the "patient's" pulse rate manually. **Record it on your laboratory report.**
7. Select a site for the probe application. Clean it with an alcohol prep pad. Possible application sites are shown in Figure 25.2.
8. Turn on the oximeter.
9. Disinfect the probe if a nondisposable probe is used. Attach the probe to the selected site. If a digit is selected, place the probe so that the light source is over the nail bed as shown in Figure 25.3.
10. Measure the time required for equilibration and **record it on your laboratory report.**
11. Observe the pulse rate on the oximeter and correlate it with the manually measured rate. **Record any difference on your laboratory report.**
12. **Record the saturation on your laboratory report.**
13. If you are not able to obtain a reading, assess the capillary refill on the selected area. **Record your assessment on your laboratory report.**

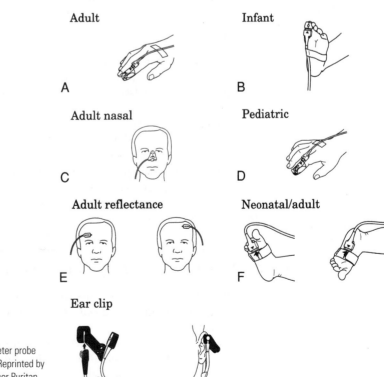

Adult   Infant

A   B

Adult nasal   Pediatric

C   D

Adult reflectance   Neonatal/adult

E   F

Ear clip

Figure 25.2. Oximeter probe application sites. (Reprinted by permission of Nellcor Puritan Bennett, Pleasanton, CA.)

G

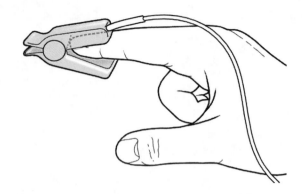

Figure 25.3. Proper orientation of oximeter finger probe.

14. Remove the probe and disinfect it.
15. **"Chart" the procedure on your laboratory report.**
16. Using your laboratory partner as the nurse, report the results obtained and explain what they mean.
17. Using your laboratory partner as the physician, report the results obtained and make any necessary recommendations or modifications to the patient care plan.

EXERCISE 25.1.2 EFFECT OF NAIL POLISH ON SATURATION

1. Polish three fingernails, each with two coats of each of the following colors:
   Black
   Red
   Green
2. Allow the nail polish to dry thoroughly.
3. Using the procedure outlined in Exercise 25.1.1, **record the manual pulse, oximeter pulse, and saturation level for each color on your laboratory report.**
4. Remove and disinfect the probe.
5. Remove the nail polish if desired.

EXERCISE 25.1.3 EFFECTS OF PERFUSION CHANGES ON PULSE OXIMETRY

Before performing these exercises, perform a modified Allen's test, as performed in Chapter 26, on your laboratory partner. **Note the result on your laboratory report.**

1. Place ice water in a basin. Soak your hand in the ice water for several minutes.
2. Using the procedure outlined in Exercise 25.1.1, **record which hand was used, the manual pulse, oximeter pulse, and saturation level obtained on your laboratory report.**
3. Using the opposite hand from that used in step 2, place an elastic phlebotomy tourniquet or blood pressure cuff snugly around the biceps of the upper arm. If a cuff is used, inflate the bladder until a radial pulse cannot be felt.
4. Using the procedure outlined in Exercise 25.1.1, **record which hand was used, the manual pulse, oximeter pulse, and saturation level obtained on your laboratory report.**
5. Deflate the cuff or remove the elastic phlebotomy tourniquet as soon as you complete the measurements.
6. Remove and disinfect the probe.

EXERCISE 25.1.4 METABOLIC EFFECTS ON PULSE OXIMETRY

1. With the pulse oximeter probe attached, hold your breath as long as possible. **Record the time of the breath hold, manual pulse, oximeter pulse, and saturation level obtained on your laboratory report.**
2. Apply oxygen via a nonrebreathing mask for 5 to 10 minutes. **Record the manual pulse, oximeter pulse, and saturation level obtained on your laboratory report.**
3. Remove the oxygen mask. Run in place for several minutes. **Record the time of the exercise, manual pulse, oximeter pulse, and saturation level obtained on your laboratory report.**
4. Remove and disinfect the probe.

EXERCISE 25.2 CAPNOGRAPHY

EXERCISE 25.2.1 DISPOSABLE CAPNOMETER (EASY CAP II OR PEDI-CAP)

1. Obtain a disposable colorimetric capnometer and remove it from the wrapper.
2. Observe the face of the capnometer and note the ranges indicated, as shown in Figure 25.4. **Record the color of the capnometer on your laboratory report.**
3. Have your laboratory partner place the adaptor in his or her mouth and breathe normally through the device. Note the change in color. **Record the color changes and the range observed on your laboratory report.**
4. Identify the amount of dead space of the device. **Record on your laboratory report.**

EXERCISE 25.2.2 CONTINUOUS CAPNOGRAPHIC MONITORING

1. Obtain the manual for the specific capnograph available in your laboratory.
2. Follow the instructions for the setup and calibration of the device. This usually requires a zero-point calibration on room air and a high-point (slope) calibration gas of 5% carbon dioxide (CO_2). The calibration is usually performed every 12 to 24 hours, and the accuracy should be within 12% or 4 mm Hg.[4] **Record the following on your laboratory report:**
   Barometric pressure
   Percent CO_2 used
   Calculation of slope calibration point (**show your work!**)
   Adjust the readings to the calibration points calculated.
3. Note the location of the sensor placement relative to the patient's airway. Is this a mainstream or sidestream sampling system? Examples of these two types of setups are shown in Figures 25.5 and 25.6. **Record your answer on your laboratory report.**
4. Attach a cannula sensing device to the capnograph (Fig. 25.7).
5. Using your laboratory partner as the patient, explain the procedure and confirm understanding.
6. Place the cannula on your "patient."
7. Instruct the "patient" to breathe normally through the nose. Observe the time required for the reading to stabilize. If the device has printer capabilities, **obtain a capnogram and attach**

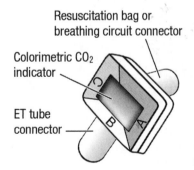

Figure 25.4. Colorimetric capnometer.

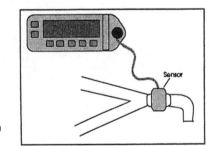

Figure 25.5. Mainstream capnography.

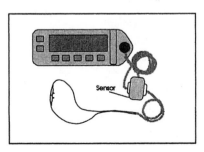

Figure 25.6. Sidestream capnography.

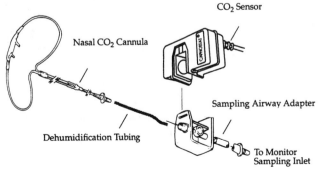

Figure 25.7. Cannula for capnography monitoring electrodes.

it to your laboratory report. If the unit does not have a printer, **observe the shape of the capnograph wave and draw a facsimile of the observed tracing on your laboratory report.**

8. Instruct your partner to breathe through the mouth. Observe the reading and **record any changes in the reading on your laboratory report.**

9. Instruct your partner to breathe slowly and shallowly. **Obtain a capnogram and attach it to your laboratory report.** If the unit does not have a printer, **observe the shape of the capnograph wave and draw a facsimile of the observed tracing on your laboratory report.**

10. Instruct your partner to breathe quickly and deeply. **Obtain a capnogram and attach it to your laboratory report.** If the unit does not have a printer, **observe the shape of the capnograph wave and draw a facsimile of the observed tracing on your laboratory report.**

11. Instruct your partner to hold his or her breath. Record the length of the breath hold and the CO_2 level once the breath is released. **Obtain a capnogram and attach it to your laboratory report.** If the unit does not have a printer, **observe the shape of the capnograph wave and draw a facsimile of the observed tracing on your laboratory report.**

12. Dispose of the cannula in the proper receptacle.

13. Set up the device on an intubated mannequin (Fig. 25.8).

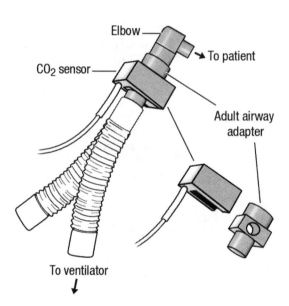

Figure 25.8. Application of a capnograph sensor to an artificial airway.

EXERCISE 25.3 TRANSCUTANEOUS MONITORS

1. Obtain a transcutaneous monitor and electrodes (Fig. 25.9).

2. Read the manual and determine whether the monitor is a P_{TCCO_2}, P_{TCO_2}, or a combined unit. **Record the type of unit on your laboratory report.**

3. Following the manufacturer's instructions, calibrate the unit using the appropriate zero solution and slope gas.

4. Select an electrode site that is away from flat, bony areas, large veins, or thick skin. Possible site selections are shown in Figure 25.10.

5. Cleanse the selected site with an alcohol prep pad and dry it.

6. Using your laboratory partner as the patient, explain the procedure and confirm understanding.

7. Attach the electrode as directed in the manual. **Record the location on your laboratory report.**

8. Adjust the temperature to 44 to 45°C.

9. Observe the length of time required for equilibration.

10. **Record the P_{TCCO_2} and P_{TCO_2} readings on your laboratory report.**

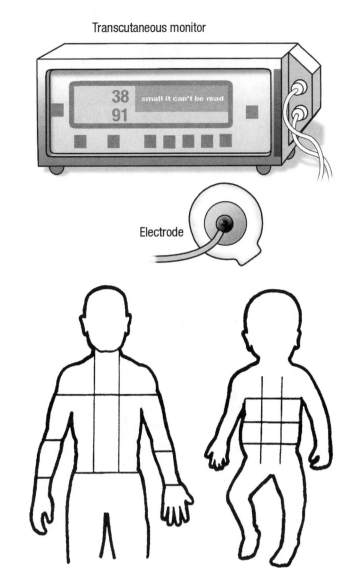

Transcutaneous monitor

Electrode

Figure 25.9. Transcutaneous monitor, and electrode.

Figure 25.10. Site selection for transcutaneous monitor placement. (Courtesy of Novametrix Medical Systems Inc., Wallingford, CT.)

Adult   **Neonate**

11. With the electrode still in place, place your laboratory partner on a nonrebreathing mask and **record the P_{TCCO_2} and P_{TCO_2} readings on your laboratory report.**

12. With the electrode still in place, instruct your laboratory partner to hold his or her breath. **Record the P_{TCCO_2} and P_{TCO_2} readings on your laboratory report.**

13. Repeat the exercise, placing the electrode in one of the following locations:

 Palm of the hand

 Sole of the foot

 Underside of the forearm

 Clavicle

 Record the site selected on your laboratory report. Observe the length of time required for equilibration and any differences in readings. **Record the P_{TCCO_2} and P_{TCO_2} readings on your laboratory report.**

14. Detach the electrode and clean it as instructed in the manufacturer's manual.

15. Shut off the unit and clean it as required.

REFERENCES

1. Peruzzi, WT and Shapiro, BA: Blood gas monitors. Respir Care Clin North Am 1:143, 1995.
2. American Association for Respiratory Care: AARC clinical practice guideline: Pulse oximetry. Respir Care 36:1406–1409, 1991.
3. American Association for Respiratory Care: AARC clinical practice guideline: Transcutaneous blood gas monitoring for neonatal & pediatric patients—2004 revision & update. Respir Care 49:1069–1072, 2004.
4. Eubanks, DH and Bone, RC: Principles and Applications of Cardiorespiratory Care Equipment. Mosby, St. Louis, 1994, p. 312.

Laboratory Report

CHAPTER 25: NONVASIVE BLOOD GAS MONITORING

Name _____ Date _____

Course/Section _____ Instructor _____

Data Collection

EXERCISE 25.1 Pulse Oximetry

EXERCISE 25.1.1 MEASUREMENT OF SATURATION AND PULSE

PULSE OXIMETRY ACCURACY CHECK

97% Phantom or FingerSim® reading: _____

90% Phantom or FingerSim® reading: _____

80% Phantom or FingerSim® reading: _____

Resting pulse rate: _____

Oximeter equilibration time: _____

Pulse difference: _____

SpO_2: _____

Capillary refill: _____

Charting: _____
_____
_____
_____

EXERCISE 25.1.2 EFFECT OF NAIL POLISH ON SATURATION

BLACK NAIL POLISH

SpO_2: _____

Pulse: _____

Manual pulse measurement: _____

RED NAIL POLISH

SpO_2: _____

Pulse: _____

Manual pulse measurement: _____

GREEN NAIL POLISH

SpO_2: _____

Pulse: _____

Manual pulse measurement: _____

EXERCISE 25.1.3 EFFECTS OF PERFUSION CHANGES ON PULSE OXIMETRY

Modified Allen's test result: _____

ICED HAND

Hand used: _____

SpO_2: _____

Pulse: _____

Manual pulse measurement: _____

TOURNIQUET OR BLOOD PRESSURE CUFF

Hand used: _____

SpO_2: _____

Pulse: _____

Manual pulse measurement: _____

EXERCISE 25.1.4 METABOLIC EFFECTS ON PULSE OXIMETRY

PULSE OXIMETER READINGS WITH BREATH HOLD

Time of breath hold: _____

SpO_2: _____

Pulse: _____

Manual pulse measurement: _____

PULSE OXIMETER READINGS WITH 100% OXYGEN

SpO_2: _____

Pulse: _____

Manual pulse measurement: _____

PULSE OXIMETER READING AFTER EXERCISE

Duration of exercise: _____

SpO_2: _____

Pulse: _____

Manual pulse measurement: _____

EXERCISE 25.2 Capnography

EXERCISE 25.2.1 DISPOSABLE CAPNOMETER (EASY CAPII OR PEDI-CAP)

Initial color: _____

Ranges available: _____

Color change: _____

Range measured: _____

Dead space: _____

EXERCISE 25.2.2 CONTINUOUS CAPNOGRAPHIC MONITORING

Barometric pressure: _____

Percent CO_2 used: _____

Calculation of slope calibration point: _____

Mainstream or sidestream? _____

Tracing of tidal breathing: _____

Observed differences between nose and mouth breathing: _____

_____

_____

Tracing of hypoventilation: CO_2 level = _____

Tracing of hyperventilation: CO_2 level = _____

Tracing of breath hold: CO_2 level = _____

EXERCISE 25.3 Transcutaneous Monitors

Type of device used: _____

Electrode placement site: _____

P_{TCCO_2}: _____

P_{TCO_2}: _____

NONREBREATHER

P_{TCCO_2}: _____

P_{TCO_2}: _____

BREATH HOLD

P_{TCCO_2}: _____

P_{TCO_2}: _____

New electrode placement site: _____

P_{TCCO_2}: _____

P_{TCO_2}: _____

Differences observed: _____

_____

Critical Thinking Questions

1. Explain the principle of operation of a pulse oximeter.

2. Identify four limitations to the use of a pulse oximeter compared with a co-oximeter, and explain how each would affect the accuracy or reliability of the reading.

3. Describe how a pulse oximeter could be used to wean a patient from oxygen.

4. What complications are associated with the use of pulse oximetry?

5. Explain the use of capnography for trending in mechanically ventilated patients. What factors might affect the trends, related to false-negative or false-positive findings?

6. Identify three conditions in which the capnography reading is lower than the $PaCO_2$.

7. In what conditions would the capnography reading be most comparable with the $PaCO_2$ in a mechanically ventilated patient?

8. Calculate the V_D/V_T ratio and the dead space (in milliliters) for the following:

    A. A COPD patient
        $P_ECO_2 = 30$ mm Hg
        $PaCO_2 = 60$ mm Hg
        $V_T = 400$ mL

    B. A drug overdose patient
        $P_ECO_2 = 55$ mm Hg
        $PaCO_2 = 60$ mm Hg
        $V_T = 500$ mL

    C. A head injury patient
        $P_ECO_2 = 28$ mm Hg
        $PaCO_2 = 30$ mm Hg
        $V_T = 800$ mL

    D. A patient with pulmonary emboli
        $P_ECO_2 = 20$ mm Hg
        $PaCO_2 = 45$ mm Hg
        $V_T = 600$ mL

9. What are the complications of capnography?

10. Identify four factors that would make the reading for $P\text{TCO}_2$ monitoring unreliable.

11. What complications are associated with transcutaneous monitoring?

12. How often and when should calibration of a transcutaneous monitor be performed?

Procedural Competency Evaluation

STUDENT: **DATE:**

PULSE OXIMETRY

		PERFORMANCE RATING	PERFORMANCE LEVEL
Evaluator: ☐ Peer ☐ Instructor **Setting:** ☐ Lab ☐ Clinical Simulation			
Equipment Utilized: **Conditions (Describe):**			

Performance Level:

S or ✓ = Satisfactory, no errors of omission or commission
U = Unsatisfactory Error of Omission or Commission
NA = Not applicable

Performance Rating:

5 **Independent:** Near flawless performance; minimal errors; able to perform without supervision; seeks out new learning; shows initiative; A = 4.7–5.0 average

4 **Minimally Supervised:** Few errors, able to self-correct; seeks guidance when appropriate; B = 3.7–4.65

3 **Competent:** Minimal required level; no critical errors; able to correct with coaching; meets expectations; safe; C = 3.0–3.65

2 **Marginal:** Below average; critical errors or problem areas noted; would benefit from remediation; D = 2.0–2.99

1 **Dependent:** Poor; unacceptable performance; unsafe; gross inaccuracies; potentially harmful; F = < 2.0

Two or more errors of commission or omission of mandatory or essential performance elements will terminate the procedure, and require additional practice and/or remediation and reevaluation. Student is responsible for obtaining additional evaluation forms as needed from the Director of Clinical Education (DCE).

EQUIPMENT AND PATIENT PREPARATION

1. Common Performance Elements Steps 1–8

2. Determines F_IO_2 and/or ventilator settings

3. Visually inspects the power cord (if applicable) and probe cable for any frayed or exposed wires

ASSESSMENT AND IMPLEMENTATION

4. Common Performance Elements Steps 9 and 10

5. Assesses patient by measuring the patient's pulse rate manually and/or by verifying the heart rate displayed on ECG monitor (if applicable)

6. Confirms the F_IO_2 and/or ventilator settings in the patient's room

7. Turns on the oximeter and allows for appropriate warm-up

8. Selects a site for the probe application and checks for adequate perfusion; removes nail polish or artificial nails if necessary

9. Cleans site and non-disposable probe with alcohol prep pad

10. Attaches probe to the selected site and secures

11. Allows for proper stabilization

12. Observes the pulse rate on the oximeter and correlates it with the manually measured rate and/or ECG rate

13. Records the pulse rate, saturation, respiratory rate, and pattern

FOLLOW-UP

14. Common Performance Elements Steps 11–16

15. Disconnects and turns unit off if not a continuous monitoring situation

16. Disinfects probe if non-disposable

SIGNATURES   Student: Evaluator: Date:

Clinical Performance Evaluation

PERFORMANCE RATING:

5 Independent: Near flawless performance; minimal errors; able to perform without supervision; seeks out new learning; shows initiative; A = 4.7–5.0 average

4 Minimally Supervised: Few errors, able to self-correct; seeks guidance when appropriate; B = 3.7–4.65

3 Competent: Minimal required level; no critical errors; able to correct with coaching; meets expectations; safe; C = 3.0–3.65

2 Marginal: Below average; critical errors or problem areas noted; would benefit from remediation; D = 2.0–2.99

1 Dependent: Poor; unacceptable performance; unsafe; gross inaccuracies; potentially harmful; F = < 2.0

Circle the appropriate response below. Please be consistent, objective, and honest in your assessment of the student's clinical performance and ability.

PERFORMANCE CRITERIA	SCORE				
COGNITIVE DOMAIN					
1. Consistently displays knowledge, comprehension, and command of essential concepts	5	4	3	2	1
2. Demonstrates the relationship between theory and clinical practice	5	4	3	2	1
3. Able to select, review, apply, analyze, synthesize, interpret, and evaluate information; makes recommendations to modify care plan	5	4	3	2	1
PSYCHOMOTOR DOMAIN					
4. Minimal errors, no critical errors; able to self-correct; performs all steps safely and accurately	5	4	3	2	1
5. Selects, assembles, and verifies proper function and cleanliness of equipment; assures operation and corrects malfunctions; provides adequate care and maintenance	5	4	3	2	1
6. Exhibits the required manual dexterity	5	4	3	2	1
7. Performs procedure in a reasonable time frame for clinical level	5	4	3	2	1
8. Applies and maintains aseptic technique and PPE as required	5	4	3	2	1
9. Maintains concise and accurate patient and clinical records	5	4	3	2	1
10. Reports promptly on patient status/needs to appropriate personnel	5	4	3	2	1
AFFECTIVE DOMAIN					
11. Exhibits courteous and pleasant demeanor; shows consideration and respect, honesty, and integrity	5	4	3	2	1
12. Communicates verbally and in writing clearly and concisely	5	4	3	2	1
13. Preserves confidentiality and adheres to all policies	5	4	3	2	1
14. Follows directions, exhibits sound judgment, and seeks help when required	5	4	3	2	1
15. Demonstrates initiative, self-direction, responsibility, and accountability	5	4	3	2	1

TOTAL POINTS =   /15 = AVERAGE GRADE =

ADDITIONAL COMMENTS: IDENTIFY AREAS OF EXCELLENCE; LIST ERRORS OF OMISSION OR COMMISSION, CRITICAL ERRORS

SUMMARY PERFORMANCE EVALUATION AND RECOMMENDATIONS

☐ PASS: Satisfactory Performance

    ☐ Minimal supervision needed, may progress to next level provided specific skills, clinical time completed

    ☐ Minimal supervision needed, able to progress to next level without remediation

☐ FAIL: Unsatisfactory Performance (check all that apply)

    ☐ Minor reevaluation only

    ☐ Needs additional clinical practice before reevaluation

    ☐ Needs additional laboratory practice before skills performed in clinical area

    ☐ Recommend clinical probation

SIGNATURES

Evaluator (print name):   Evaluator signature: Date:

Student Signature: Date:

Student Comments:

Procedural Competency Evaluation

STUDENT: **DATE:**

CAPNOGRAPHY/CAPNOMETRY

			PERFORMANCE RATING	PERFORMANCE LEVEL
Evaluator: ☐ Peer ☐ Instructor	**Setting:** ☐ Lab	☐ Clinical Simulation		

Equipment Utilized: **Conditions (Describe):**

Performance Level:

    S or ✓ = Satisfactory, no errors of omission or commission
    U = Unsatisfactory Error of Omission or Commission
    NA = Not applicable

Performance Rating:

    5   **Independent:** Near flawless performance; minimal errors; able to perform without supervision; seeks out new learning; shows initiative; A = 4.7–5.0 average

    4   **Minimally Supervised:** Few errors, able to self-correct; seeks guidance when appropriate; B = 3.7–4.65

    3   **Competent:** Minimal required level; no critical errors; able to correct with coaching; meets expectations; safe; C = 3.0–3.65

    2   **Marginal:** Below average; critical errors or problem areas noted; would benefit from remediation; D = 2.0–2.99

    1   **Dependent:** Poor; unacceptable performance; unsafe; gross inaccuracies; potentially harmful; F = < 2.0

    Two or more errors of commission or omission of mandatory or essential performance elements will terminate the proce-dure, and require additional practice and/or remediation and reevaluation. Student is responsible for obtaining additional evaluation forms as needed from the Director of Clinical Education (DCE).

EQUIPMENT PREPARATION

1. Common Performance Elements Steps 1–8

2. Determines and verifies F_IO_2 and ventilator settings

3. Calibrates capnograph with 3% or 5% CO_2 gas if required by procedure manual

PATIENT ASSESSMENT AND IMPLEMENTATION

4. Common Performance Elements Steps 9 and 10

5. For colorimetric capnometer, attaches to 15-mmETT adaptor and notes color change and percent CO_2 range; **NOTE:** Most devices may be used up to 2 hours, do NOT discard after one measurement

6. For spot check or continuous capnograph monitors, turns unit on and allows warm-up time

7. Connects clean sampling sensor to patient's nose or in-line to ventilator circuit with proper adaptor

    A. Ensures that there is no excess pull on airway

    B. Records highest P_{ETCO_2} after 3 minutes and compares to recent $PaCO_2$

8. Analyzes and prints capnograph wave if applicable and determines ventilatory status

9. Calculates VD/VD ratio ($PaCO_2 - P_{ETCO_2}/PaCO_2$) and approximate deadspace volume (VT x VD/VT)

10. Interprets results

FOLLOW-UP

11. If continuous monitoring performed, checks sensor or sampling line and water trap for moisture or debris and clears or replaces if needed

12. Common Performance Elements Steps 11–16

SIGNATURES   Student: Evaluator: Date:

Clinical Performance Evaluation

PERFORMANCE RATING:

5 **Independent:** Near flawless performance; minimal errors; able to perform without supervision; seeks out new learning; shows initiative; A = 4.7–5.0 average

4 **Minimally Supervised:** Few errors, able to self-correct; seeks guidance when appropriate; B = 3.7–4.65

3 **Competent:** Minimal required level; no critical errors; able to correct with coaching; meets expectations; safe; C = 3.0–3.65

2 **Marginal:** Below average; critical errors or problem areas noted; would benefit from remediation; D = 2.0–2.99

1 **Dependent:** Poor; unacceptable performance; unsafe; gross inaccuracies; potentially harmful; F = < 2.0

Circle the appropriate response below. Please be consistent, objective, and honest in your assessment of the student's clinical performance and ability.

PERFORMANCE CRITERIA	SCORE				
COGNITIVE DOMAIN					
1. Consistently displays knowledge, comprehension, and command of essential concepts	5	4	3	2	1
2. Demonstrates the relationship between theory and clinical practice	5	4	3	2	1
3. Able to select, review, apply, analyze, synthesize, interpret, and evaluate information; makes recommendations to modify care plan	5	4	3	2	1
PSYCHOMOTOR DOMAIN					
4. Minimal errors, no critical errors; able to self-correct; performs all steps safely and accurately	5	4	3	2	1
5. Selects, assembles, and verifies proper function and cleanliness of equipment; assures operation and corrects malfunctions; provides adequate care and maintenance	5	4	3	2	1
6. Exhibits the required manual dexterity	5	4	3	2	1
7. Performs procedure in a reasonable time frame for clinical level	5	4	3	2	1
8. Applies and maintains aseptic technique and PPE as required	5	4	3	2	1
9. Maintains concise and accurate patient and clinical records	5	4	3	2	1
10. Reports promptly on patient status/needs to appropriate personnel	5	4	3	2	1
AFFECTIVE DOMAIN					
11. Exhibits courteous and pleasant demeanor; shows consideration and respect, honesty, and integrity	5	4	3	2	1
12. Communicates verbally and in writing clearly and concisely	5	4	3	2	1
13. Preserves confidentiality and adheres to all policies	5	4	3	2	1
14. Follows directions, exhibits sound judgment, and seeks help when required	5	4	3	2	1
15. Demonstrates initiative, self-direction, responsibility, and accountability	5	4	3	2	1

TOTAL POINTS = _____ /15 = AVERAGE GRADE = _____

ADDITIONAL COMMENTS: IDENTIFY AREAS OF EXCELLENCE; LIST ERRORS OF OMISSION OR COMMISSION, CRITICAL ERRORS

SUMMARY PERFORMANCE EVALUATION AND RECOMMENDATIONS

☐ PASS: Satisfactory Performance

  ☐ Minimal supervision needed, may progress to next level provided specific skills, clinical time completed

  ☐ Minimal supervision needed, able to progress to next level without remediation

☐ FAIL: Unsatisfactory Performance (check all that apply)

  ☐ Minor reevaluation only

  ☐ Needs additional clinical practice before reevaluation

  ☐ Needs additional laboratory practice before skills performed in clinical area

  ☐ Recommend clinical probation

SIGNATURES

Evaluator (print name): _____   Evaluator signature: _____   Date: _____

Student Signature: _____   Date: _____

Student Comments:

Procedural Competency Evaluation

STUDENT: **DATE:**

TRANSCUTANEOUS MONITORING

	PERFORMANCE RATING	PERFORMANCE LEVEL
Evaluator: ☐ Peer ☐ Instructor **Setting:** ☐ Lab ☐ Clinical Simulation		
Equipment Utilized: **Conditions (Describe):**		
Performance Level:		
S or ✓ = Satisfactory, no errors of omission or commission		
U = Unsatisfactory Error of Omission or Commission		
NA = Not applicable		
Performance Rating:		
5 **Independent:** Near flawless performance; minimal errors; able to perform without supervision; seeks out new learning; shows initiative; A = 4.7–5.0 average		
4 **Minimally Supervised:** Few errors, able to self-correct; seeks guidance when appropriate; B = 3.7–4.65		
3 **Competent:** Minimal required level; no critical errors; able to correct with coaching; meets expectations; safe; C = 3.0–3.65		
2 **Marginal:** Below average; critical errors or problem areas noted; would benefit from remediation; D = 2.0–2.99		
1 **Dependent:** Poor; unacceptable performance; unsafe; gross inaccuracies; potentially harmful; F = < 2.0		
Two or more errors of commission or omission of mandatory or essential performance elements will terminate the procedure, and require additional practice and/or remediation and reevaluation. Student is responsible for obtaining additional evaluation forms as needed from the Director of Clinical Education (DCE).		

EQUIPMENT AND PATIENT PREPARATION		
1. Common Performance Elements Steps 1–8		
2. Calibrates the unit using the appropriate zero solution and slope gas		
ASSESSMENT AND IMPLEMENTATION		
3. Common Performance Elements Steps 9 and 10		
4. Assesses patient and confirms F_IO_2 and ventilator settings		
5. Selects an electrode site away from flat, boney areas, large veins, or thick skin		
6. Cleanses the selected site with an alcohol prep pad and dries it		
7. Adjusts the temperature to 43–45°C as appropriate for patient's age		
8. Allows for equilibration		
9. Records the P_{TCCO_2} and P_{TCO_2} readings as applicable		
10. Reassesses patient and electrode site periodically; changes electrode placement every 2 to 6 hours as indicated		
FOLLOW-UP		
11. Common Performance Elements Steps 11–16		

SIGNATURES   Student: Evaluator: Date:

Clinical Performance Evaluation

PERFORMANCE RATING:

5 **Independent:** Near flawless performance; minimal errors; able to perform without supervision; seeks out new learning; shows initiative; A = 4.7–5.0 average

4 **Minimally Supervised:** Few errors, able to self-correct; seeks guidance when appropriate; B = 3.7–4.65

3 **Competent:** Minimal required level; no critical errors; able to correct with coaching; meets expectations; safe; C = 3.0–3.65

2 **Marginal:** Below average; critical errors or problem areas noted; would benefit from remediation; D = 2.0–2.99

1 **Dependent:** Poor; unacceptable performance; unsafe; gross inaccuracies; potentially harmful; F = < 2.0

Circle the appropriate response below. Please be consistent, objective, and honest in your assessment of the student's clinical performance and ability.

PERFORMANCE CRITERIA	SCORE				
COGNITIVE DOMAIN					
1. Consistently displays knowledge, comprehension, and command of essential concepts	5	4	3	2	1
2. Demonstrates the relationship between theory and clinical practice	5	4	3	2	1
3. Able to select, review, apply, analyze, synthesize, interpret, and evaluate information; makes recommendations to modify care plan	5	4	3	2	1
PSYCHOMOTOR DOMAIN					
4. Minimal errors, no critical errors; able to self-correct; performs all steps safely and accurately	5	4	3	2	1
5. Selects, assembles, and verifies proper function and cleanliness of equipment; assures operation and corrects malfunctions; provides adequate care and maintenance	5	4	3	2	1
6. Exhibits the required manual dexterity	5	4	3	2	1
7. Performs procedure in a reasonable time frame for clinical level	5	4	3	2	1
8. Applies and maintains aseptic technique and PPE as required	5	4	3	2	1
9. Maintains concise and accurate patient and clinical records	5	4	3	2	1
10. Reports promptly on patient status/needs to appropriate personnel	5	4	3	2	1
AFFECTIVE DOMAIN					
11. Exhibits courteous and pleasant demeanor; shows consideration and respect, honesty, and integrity	5	4	3	2	1
12. Communicates verbally and in writing clearly and concisely	5	4	3	2	1
13. Preserves confidentiality and adheres to all policies	5	4	3	2	1
14. Follows directions, exhibits sound judgment, and seeks help when required	5	4	3	2	1
15. Demonstrates initiative, self-direction, responsibility, and accountability	5	4	3	2	1

TOTAL POINTS = _____ /15 = AVERAGE GRADE = _____

ADDITIONAL COMMENTS: IDENTIFY AREAS OF EXCELLENCE; LIST ERRORS OF OMISSION OR COMMISSION, CRITICAL ERRORS

SUMMARY PERFORMANCE EVALUATION AND RECOMMENDATIONS

☐ PASS: Satisfactory Performance

    ☐ Minimal supervision needed, may progress to next level provided specific skills, clinical time completed

    ☐ Minimal supervision needed, able to progress to next level without remediation

☐ FAIL: Unsatisfactory Performance (check all that apply)

    ☐ Minor reevaluation only

    ☐ Needs additional clinical practice before reevaluation

    ☐ Needs additional laboratory practice before skills performed in clinical area

    ☐ Recommend clinical probation

SIGNATURES

Evaluator (print name): _____ Evaluator signature: _____ Date: _____

Student Signature: _____ Date: _____

Student Comments:

26 Arterial Blood Gas Sampling

INTRODUCTION

Arterial blood gas sampling is a quick and reliable tool for patient assessment. Blood sampling from a peripheral artery or an indwelling **catheter** provides a specimen for the measurement of pH and partial pressure of carbon dioxide and oxygen. When coupled with co-oximetry, additional diagnostic indicators can be obtained such as total hemoglobin, hemoglobin saturation, and abnormal hemoglobins. Analysis of these values helps evaluate the adequacy of ventilation and oxygenation, as well as the ability of the blood to carry oxygen. They are used to assess a patient's response to therapeutic interventions, for diagnostic evaluations, and to monitor the severity and progression of a disease process.[1]

Arterial blood sampling is an invasive procedure and is not without risk to both the patient and the respiratory care practitioner. It is essential that the skills required to perform these procedures be practiced until proficiency is achieved before performing these procedures in the clinical setting. Knowledge of anatomy and infection control practices is an integral part of the requirements for safe technique. It should also be noted that although this chapter primarily covers arterial blood gas sampling, in some instances respiratory therapists may be involved in obtaining capillary samples from young patients or analyzing venous blood samples.

OBJECTIVES

Upon completion of this chapter, the student will be able to:

1. Practice communication skills needed to explain blood sampling procedures to patients.
2. Review medical charting and documentation of performance of blood gas sampling procedures.
3. Apply infection control guidelines and standards associated with equipment and procedures, according to OSHA regulations and CDC guidelines.
4. Assemble and prepare the equipment necessary for performance of arterial puncture and arterial line sampling.
5. Review the medical record for information essential to the safe performance of arterial sampling.
6. Demonstrate the safe performance of arterial puncture and arterial line sampling.
7. Demonstrate safe postpuncture care.
8. Prepare an anaerobic blood gas sample for transport.
9. Identify the equipment and steps necessary to perform a capillary sample for blood gas analysis.

KEY TERMS

acid	catheter	iodophor	point-of-service
anticoagulant	coagulopathy	lancet	valve stem
base	collateral	latex	
bevel	intraflow	Luer-Lok™	

Exercises

EQUIPMENT REQUIRED

- ☐ Arterial arm simulators
- ☐ Sterile water
- ☐ Red dye
- ☐ Arterial blood gas kits or component parts:
- ☐ Preheparinized syringes, 1, 3, or 5 mL
- ☐ 1000-U/mL heparin vials (optional)
- ☐ Various size needles: 20, 22, 23, and 25 gauge
- ☐ Syringe caps and rubber stopper
- ☐ Air bubble venting devices (optional)
- ☐ Self-capping syringes (optional)
- ☐ Sterile drape (optional)
- ☐ Biohazard bags
- ☐ **Iodophor** or alcohol-based disinfectant pads
- ☐ Patient label
- ☐ Disposable **latex** and vinyl gloves, various sizes
- ☐ Gauze, 4×4 and 2×2
- ☐ Band-Aids®
- ☐ Cloth tape

- ☐ Goggles
- ☐ Disposable gowns (optional)
- ☐ Sharps containers
- ☐ Arterial line setup:
  - ☐ IV tubing
  - ☐ Two 1000-mL IV solution bags
  - ☐ Three-way stopcocks
  - ☐ 20-gauge intracath needle
  - ☐ Blood pressure cuff or pressure infuser
  - ☐ **Intraflow** flush device
  - ☐ Heparin 1% solution
- ☐ Towels
- ☐ Ice
- ☐ Sample blood gas analysis slips
- ☐ Heparinized capillary tubes
- ☐ Rubber capillary tube stoppers
- ☐ Metal mixing "fleas" and magnet
- ☐ **Lancets**

EXERCISE 26.1 PREPARATION OF BLOOD GAS KIT COMPONENTS

1. Obtain an arterial blood gas kit. If preprepared kits are not available, gather the necessary items and identify the following components:

   Syringe. **Record the size syringe on your laboratory report.**

   Needles, various sizes. **Record the needle gauges available in your kit on your laboratory report.**

   Iodophor or alcohol prep pads

   Band-Aids®

   Label

   Biohazard transport bag

   Syringe cap and rubber stoppers

   Self-capping device (optional)

   Sterile or clean drape (optional)

   Gauze

   Liquid heparin vial (optional). Syringes may already be preheparinized with liquid sodium heparin or dry litholized lithium heparin. **Record the type of heparin used in your blood gas kit.**

   Air bubble removal device/cap (optional). This may be available with kits that contain self-capping needle protection devices (Fig. 26.1).

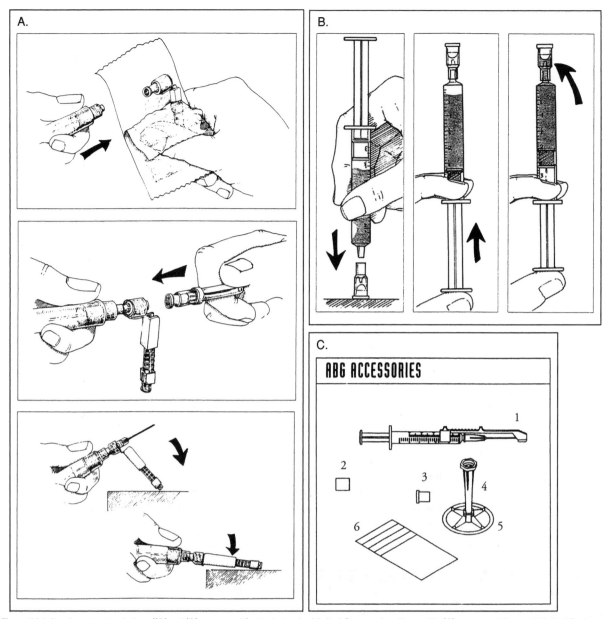

Figure 26.1. Needle protection devices. [**(A)** and **(B)** courtesy of Smiths Industries Medical Systems, Inc., Keene, NH; **(C)** courtesy of Marquest Medical Products, Inc., Englewood, CO.]

2. Wash your hands and apply latex or vinyl gloves. NOTE: Some people have or may develop severe latex allergies.[2] Vinyl gloves are recommended in this case.

3. Select the smallest needle available in your kit for performing a radial puncture. **Record the gauge selected on your laboratory report.**

4. Secure the needle on the syringe by twisting it onto the Luer-Lok™ (see Fig. 26.1).

5. If a preheparinized dry heparin syringe is used, draw back the plunger to preset the desired sample amount to be obtained. In most modern blood gas analyzers, as little as 0.5 mL is needed, but it is advisable to draw some extra blood in case repeat analysis is required.

6. If a liquid heparin preheparinized plastic syringe is used, pull back the barrel of the syringe about halfway. Then turn the syringe so that the needle is pointing straight up (Fig. 26.2). To eject any excess air, slowly push the barrel back up to the point at which the heparin enters the needle. Turn the needle and syringe downward and safely discard any excess solution. Leave only the amount of heparin needed to fill the hub of the syringe and the needle. If a glass syringe is used, the barrel of the syringe must be lubricated with the heparin before ejecting the excess. This can be accomplished by sliding the barrel of the syringe up and down until it slides freely on its own.

7. Gently loosen the needle cap but do not remove it.

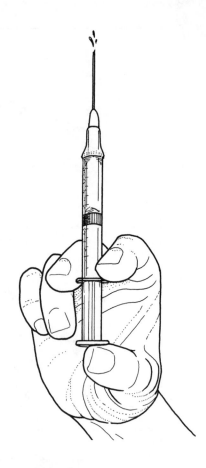

Figure 26.2. Ejecting liquid heparin from liquid heparin syringe.

8. Your instructor will give you a patient scenario. Fill out the patient label, charge slip, or both. Include the "patient" name, identification number and type of sample (e.g., arterial versus venous). Also **note and record the "patient's" temperature.**

9. Before doing the procedure, take a moment and confirm that you are doing the correct procedure on the appropriate "patient."

EXERCISE 26.2 MODIFIED ALLEN'S TEST

An arterial puncture can be performed via the radial, brachial, or femoral artery (Fig. 26.3). In general, respiratory therapists are only permitted to perform radial and brachial punctures. However, the radial artery is the most common site chosen. It is the most accessible, is easiest to stabilize, and has the best **collateral** *circulation. A modified Allen's test is used to determine the presence of collateral circulation via the ulnar artery.*

Perform the following steps on your laboratory partner:

1. Identify your "patient." Introduce yourself and your department. Explain to your partner in nonmedical terms that you are going to perform an arterial blood gas and what is involved. Confirm your partner's understanding and answer any questions or concerns. The partner should simulate a patient's concern and fears about having this invasive procedure performed and about the fact that laboratory personnel were just here drawing blood. You should respond appropriately.

2. Confirm through chart review that there are no contraindications (e.g., vascular abnormalities) to drawing the sample from either hand.

3. Determine which hand is the "patient's" dominant hand. Palpate both radial arteries and select the one with the strongest pulse. The nondominant hand is the preferred choice. The radial artery pulse can be found by placing your index finger, middle finger, or both on the lateral aspect of the wrist on the thumb side between the second and third wrist folds, then sliding your fingers into the groove between the bones and tendons.

4. Palpate the ulnar artery if possible. It is located on the lateral side of the wrist (closest to the little finger) in the groove between the tendons and the ulnar bone.

5. Have your partner hold his or her hand palm up. Using two hands, occlude both the radial and ulnar arteries as shown in Figure 26.4.

6. Instruct your partner to open and close his or her fist at least three times until you observe the palm of the hand blanching (turning pale).

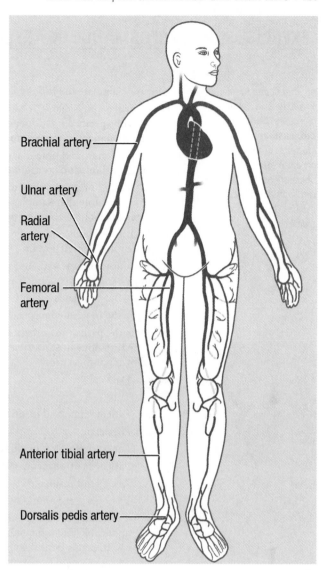

Figure 26.3. Sites available for arterial puncture.

7. Release the ulnar artery only (pinky side of partner's hand). The palm should flush within 3 to 5 seconds (10- to 15-second maximum).[3] If not, repeat the test on the other arm.

8. **Record the results of the Allen's test on your laboratory report.**

9. Practice the technique for performing a modified Allen's test on an unconscious patient. Hold the radial and ulnar arteries with one hand and raise the "patient's" arm. Keep the arm raised until the palm blanches. Lower the arm. Release the ulnar artery and look for the palm flushing as in the preceding steps.

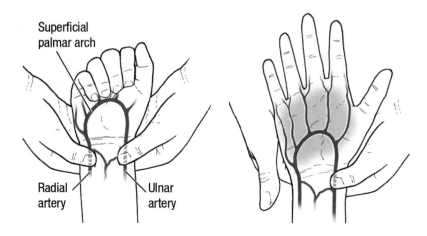

Figure 26.4. Performing the modified Allen's test.

EXERCISE 26.3 PERFORMANCE OF ARTERIAL PUNCTURE

*An arterial arm simulator should be used for this procedure. **Under no circumstances should students draw blood on each other.** Iodophor preparations will stain the simulator and should be avoided during laboratory practice*

Perform or simulate the following steps:

1. Verify the "physician's" order or protocol. Check for time and special instructions (on room air, with specified F_IO_2, immediately after ambulation, and/or special position). Also **note and record "patient's" temperature.**

2. Scan the chart and note diagnosis, order, coagulopathies, anticoagulant therapy, oxygen concentration, and contraindications such as vascular abnormalities.

3. Gather and prepare the required equipment as in Exercise 26.1. Fill the bag with ice and water, but note that samples should not be iced for certain point-of-service blood gas analysis systems. Obtain a towel to use as a support for the "patient's" wrist.

4. Wash your hands and apply standard precautions and transmission-based isolation procedures as appropriate.

5. Introduce yourself and your department, and explain the procedure. Confirm the "patient's" understanding. Reassure as needed.

6. Verify the "patient's" identity by checking the identification band.

7. Verify the oxygen concentration or ventilator settings by double-checking in the room.

8. Fill in the patient information label, charge slip, or other appropriate documentation. In some situations this information may be input directly into a computer system. Include the following information:[4]

   Date

   Time

   Patient name and identification

   Physician

   Puncture site (left or right radial artery, arterial line, brachial artery, etc.)

   Patient's current temperature (obtained from the chart or nurses flow sheet)

   Allen's test results

   F_IO_2: percent and modality

   Ventilatory status: spontaneous respiratory frequency or ventilator settings, if applicable, including machine tidal volume, machine frequency, mode of ventilation, any spontaneous tidal volume, and frequency noted

   Therapist signature

   Record this information on your laboratory report. In a clinical situation, the label may be filled out after the puncture procedure. However, ventilatory status and F_IO_2 should be verified before the puncture.

9. Select the appropriate size needle and secure it to the syringe Luer-Lok™.

10. Heparinize the syringe or set the barrel on the preheparinized syringe as in Exercise 26.1.

11. Palpate both radial arteries. Choose the best site.

12. Perform the modified Allen's test for the presence of collateral circulation as in Exercise 26.2.

13. Position the "patient's" arm so that it is extended and supported on a firm surface, palm up. Place a towel or similar item to support the wrist (Fig. 26.5). Place a sterile or clean field under the wrist if available.

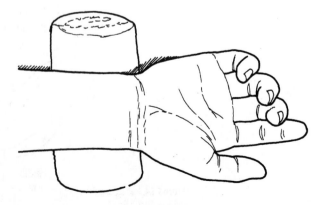

Figure 26.5. Positioning of wrist for radial artery puncture.

14. Take a moment and confirm that you are doing the correct procedure on the appropriate "patient."

15. Prepare the intended puncture site by rubbing vigorously with antiseptic solution for at least 30 seconds in a circular motion away from the puncture site. Allow it to dry. Disinfect the gloved fingers that you will be using to palpate the pulse.

16. Repalpate the puncture site and determine the path of the artery.

17. Correctly perform the puncture.

    A. Place your hand in the palm of the patient's hand to stabilize it.

    B. With the bevel of the needle facing upward, enter the artery with the syringe at a 45-degree angle (Fig. 26.6). The puncture should be performed within 2 to 3 cm of the wrist skin folds (Fig. 26.7). Insert the tip of the needle quickly just through the skin, and then pause to verify the needle angle.

    C. *Slowly* advance the needle until a flash of blood is seen in the hub, indicating that the artery has been entered. Once the flash is seen and blood begins to fill the syringe, maintain your position until blood fills the syringe to the desired amount. The amount needed will vary with the size of the syringe and the type of blood gas analyzer being used. For most automated blood gas analyzers, 0.5 to 1 mL of blood is sufficient. More may be obtained if more than one analysis will be performed on the sample. If need be, slowly withdraw the needle to just below the surface of the skin. Do not completely withdraw it. Redirect the needle angle until the blood is obtained. *Do not* re-angle the syringe while it is in the wrist. There is no set rule as to how many times repositioning the needle is acceptable. However, patient comfort and the availability of another competent person to attempt the puncture should be considered. If more than two or three repositions are needed, a beginning student should terminate the procedure and seek assistance.

    NOTE: Arterial blood can be recognized by color, pulsation into syringe, self-filling, and data results as compared with clinical condition.

    D. Remove the syringe and immediately compress the artery with the gauze.

    E. Using the rubber stopper or self-capping needle protection device, plug the needle.

    NOTE: *Never recap the needle manually using two hands.*

18. Continue to apply firm pressure to the site for 3 to 5 minutes or at least 10 minutes if the "patient" has any bleeding disorders or is receiving anticoagulant therapy.

19. If a self-venting syringe is used, expel any air from the sample by pushing the barrel toward the plugged needle. Otherwise, remove the needle from the Luer-Lok™ and expel the air into a gauze pad. Venting devices may also be available. Once all air bubbles have been removed, cap the syringe and label it.

20. Mix blood and heparin by rolling the syringe in your palms.

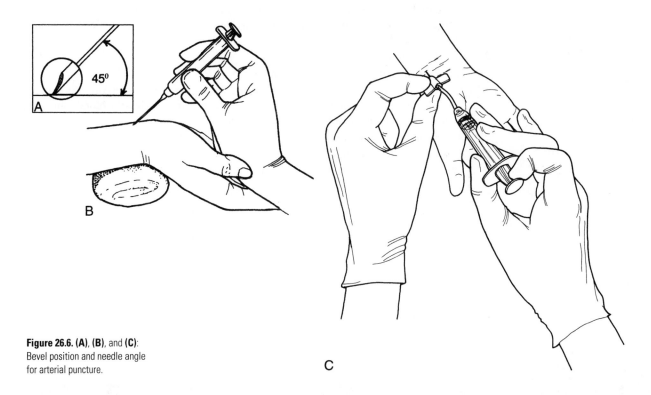

Figure 26.6. (A), (B), and **(C)**: Bevel position and needle angle for arterial puncture.

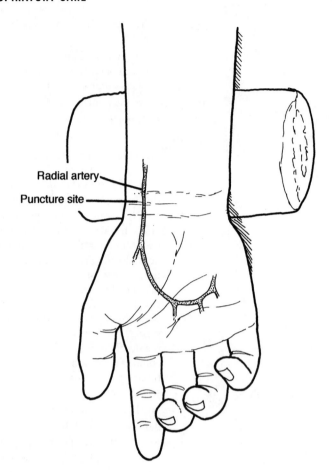

Radial artery

Puncture site

Figure 26.7. Location of radial artery puncture.

21. Place the sample on ice if analysis will be delayed by more than 15 minutes.[1] Place the sample in a biohazard bag for transport. Note that for certain point-of-service blood gas analysis systems, samples should not be iced and must be run within 5 minutes of being drawn.

22. Check the circulation distal to the puncture site. Continue to compress the artery until there is a return of pulses proximal and distal to the site and there is no evidence of bleeding, swelling, or discoloration.

23. Ensure "patient" safety and comfort.

24. Clean up. Discard needle in sharps container and dispose of any infectious waste in the appropriate receptacle. Immediately clean any blood spills according to OSHA regulations with a sodium hypochlorite (bleach) solution.

25. Remove your gloves and wash your hands.

26. Transport the sample in the sealed container.

27. Record the procedure on the chart and on appropriate departmental records, as applicable. **"Chart" the procedure on your laboratory report. Indicate whether the blood sample was obtained and how many attempts were necessary.**

28. Notify the "nurse" and raise bed rail if originally lowered.

29. Repeat the exercise for brachial artery puncture.

EXERCISE 26.4 ARTERIAL LINE SAMPLING

EXERCISE 26.4.1 ARTERIAL LINE SETUP

In this exercise, you are simulating entering the room of a patient in contact isolation to discard disposable infectious waste and safely remove a piece of reusable respiratory equipment for transport to the disinfection area. The instructor will have the "room" prepared with equipment to be discarded and to be transported.

Identify the components of the arterial line setup shown in Figure 26.8 and **record the corresponding letters on your laboratory report.**

Proximal three-way stopcock

Luer-Lok™

Intraflow flush device

Monitor

Pressure tubing

Arterial catheter

Pressure infuser

IV bag with heparinized solution

Transducer

Valve stem

Flush activator

EXERCISE 26.4.2 ARTERIAL LINE SAMPLING

An arterial arm simulator should be used for this procedure. Perform or simulate the following steps:

1. Verify the "physician's" order. Check for time and special instructions (on room air, with specified F_IO_2, and/or special position). Also **note and record "patient's" temperature.**
2. Scan the chart and note the diagnosis, anticoagulant therapy, F_IO_2 and modality, and ventilator settings.
3. Gather and prepare the required equipment:
   Discard or waste syringe, 5 mL or 10 mL, nonheparinized
   Heparinized syringe, 1, 3, or 5 mL
   Syringe cap
   4×4 gauze

Figure 26.8. Identification of arterial line components.

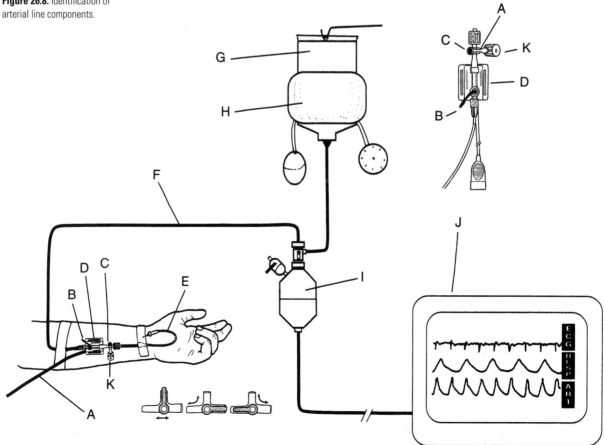

Sterile field or towel

Alcohol prep pads

Patient label

Biohazard transport bag filled with ice and water, but note that samples should not be iced for certain point-of-service blood gas analysis systems.

4. Wash your hands and apply standard precautions and transmission-based isolation procedures as appropriate.

5. Introduce yourself and your department, and explain the procedure. Confirm the "patient's" understanding if possible and reassure.

6. Verify the "patient's" identity by checking the identification band.

7. Verify the F_IO_2 or ventilator settings by double-checking in the room.

8. Heparinize one syringe or set the barrel on the preheparinized syringe as in Exercise 26.1.

9. Place a sterile field or towel under the sampling site to prevent infection and soiling.

10. Check waveform and pressure readings on the monitor to verify line function.

11. Alert the "nurse" that you are about to draw the blood and temporarily silence the arterial line alarm.

12. Remove the Luer-Lok™ cap from the three-way stopcock closest to the catheter insertion site. Place it aseptically on the sterile field or on a sterile gauze pad.

13. Wipe the Luer-Lok™ of the three-way stopcock with an alcohol prep pad.

14. Attach the nonheparinized discard syringe on the Luer-Lok™ of the three-way stopcock and twist to secure (Fig. 26.9).

15. Turn the valve stem of the stopcock toward the intraflow flush device (Fig. 26.10).

16. Fill the discard syringe until all flush solution has been removed from the catheter and whole blood begins to appear in the syringe.

17. Turn the valve stem of the stopcock back toward the Luer-Lok™, as shown in Figure 26.11, and then remove the discard syringe.

18. Attach the heparinized sample syringe on the Luer-Lok™ of the three-way stopcock and twist to secure. Turn the stopcock toward the intraflow flush device (Fig. 26.12). Fill it with the desired amount of blood for the sample.

19. Turn the valve stem of the stopcock back toward the Luer-Lok™ and then remove the sample syringe.

20. If a self-venting syringe is used, expel any air from the sample by pushing the barrel toward the plugged needle. Otherwise, remove the needle from the Luer-Lok™ and expel the air into a gauze pad. Venting devices may also be available. Cap the syringe.

21. Activate the intraflow flush device and flush the arterial line catheter until no blood is seen in the catheter (Fig. 26.13).

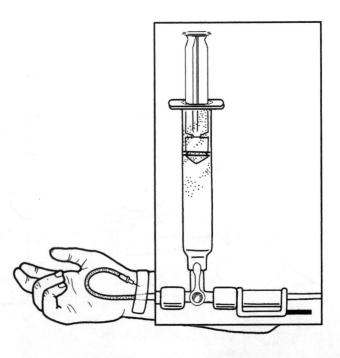

Figure 26.9. Attachment of waste syringe to stopcock.

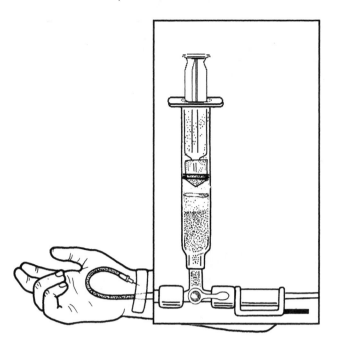

Figure 26.10. Draw waste solution into syringe until blood is obtained.

22. Turn the valve stem of the stopcock toward the catheter (off to the "patient"). Place a 4×4 gauze pad under the Luer-Lok™ and activate the intraflow flush device to flush the Luer-Lok™ clean (Fig. 26.14). Wipe the Luer-Lok™ and cap with alcohol and then recap the Luer-Lok™ (Fig. 26.15).

23. Mix blood and heparin in the syringe by rolling the syringe in your palms.

24. Label the syringe. Place the sample on ice if analysis will be delayed by more than 15 minutes.[3] Note that for certain point-of-service blood gas analysis systems, samples should not be iced and must be run within 5 minutes of being drawn.

25. Ensure "patient" safety and comfort.

26. Notify the "nurse" and raise the bed rail if originally lowered.

27. Clean up. Dispose of any infectious waste in the appropriate receptacle. Dispose of the discard syringe in a sharps container. Immediately clean any blood spills according to OSHA regulations with a bleach solution.

28. Fill in the patient information label, charge slip, and other appropriate documentation. In some situations this information may be input directly into a computer system. Include the following information:

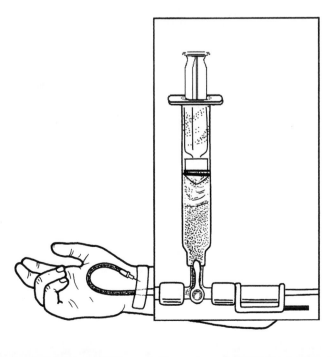

Figure 26.11. Removal of the waste syringe

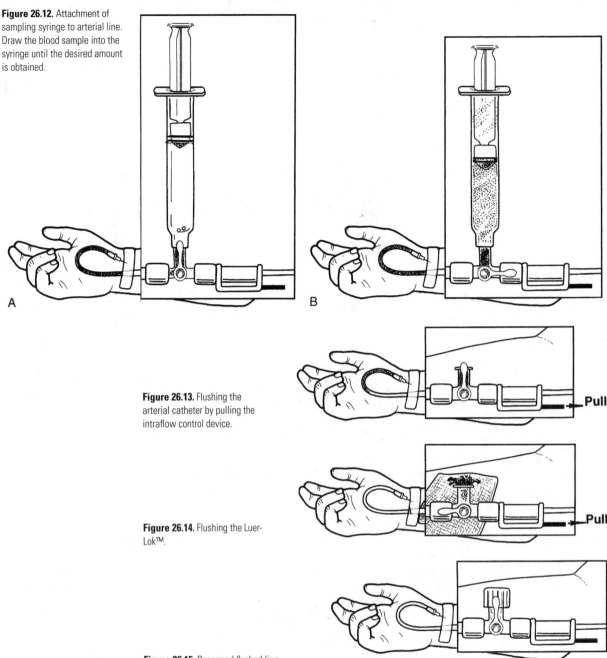

Figure 26.12. Attachment of sampling syringe to arterial line. Draw the blood sample into the syringe until the desired amount is obtained.

Figure 26.13. Flushing the arterial catheter by pulling the intraflow control device.

Figure 26.14. Flushing the Luer-Lok™.

Figure 26.15. Recapped flushed line.

Date

Time

Patient name and identification

Sample site (left or right radial, brachial, or femoral line)

F_IO_2: percent and modality

Patient temperature

Ventilatory status: spontaneous respiratory frequency or ventilator settings, if applicable, including machine tidal volume, machine frequency, mode of ventilation, any spontaneous tidal volume, and frequency noted

Technician or therapist signature

29. Reactivate the arterial line alarm and check waveform and pressure readings to verify line function.

30. Remove your gloves and wash your hands.

31. Transport the sample in a sealed biohazard container.

32. **Record the procedure on the chart and on appropriate departmental records** as applicable.

EXERCISE 26.5 CAPILLARY SAMPLING

Capillary sticks may be used in infants and children to approximate pH and PCO_2 values. The sample may be taken from areas with large capillary surface area such as the fingertip, earlobe, or (most commonly) on the lateral aspect of the heel of the foot in infants only. Values obtained for PO_2 are generally less reliable. For acid–base balance and carbon dioxide tension to be reliable, the heel must be "arterialized" by warming before capillary sampling. The procedure is difficult to simulate in the laboratory setting. Students should identify the equipment needed for capillary heel sampling and review the procedure. Practice of the procedure will be reserved for the clinical setting.

1. Gather the necessary equipment:
   Disposable latex and vinyl gloves, various sizes
   2×2 gauze
   Iodophor or alcohol prep pads
   Band-Aids®
   Cloth tape
   Biohazard bag
   Sharps containers
   Towels or warm packs
   Ice
   Heparinized capillary tubes
   Rubber capillary tube stoppers
   Metal mixing "fleas" and magnet
   Lancets
   Sample blood gas analysis slips

2. Wash your hands and apply standard precautions and transmission-based isolation procedures as appropriate.

3. Warm the heel area for 5 to 10 minutes before the procedure to arterialize by wrapping the heel in a warm soak. The heel should turn pink or red before you obtain the sample.

4. Prep the site by vigorously rubbing with betadine or an alcohol prep pad to disinfect it before puncture.

5. The acceptable locations for heel sticks are shown in Figure 26.16. Quickly puncture the lateral or medial aspect of the heel with the lancet (Fig. 26.17). The lancet should penetrate approximately 3 mm to ensure adequate blood flow.

6. Do not squeeze the heel. The result will be less accurate because of venous and interstitial fluid contaminating the sample. Blood should be flowing freely.

7. The initial drop of blood should be wiped away with gauze and discarded. Using the heparinized capillary tube, draw the sample into the tube up to the red line, making sure that no air bubbles are introduced.

8. Compress the puncture site with gauze until bleeding has stopped. An adhesive bandage may then be applied.

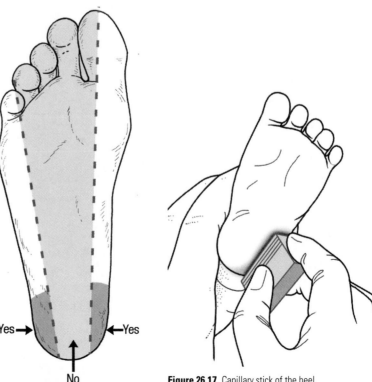

Yes→   ←Yes

No

Figure 26.16. Acceptable heel puncture sites.

Figure 26.17. Capillary stick of the heel.

9. Seal one end of the capillary tube with a rubber stopper. Introduce the metal flea into the tube, and place the circular magnet over the tube. Cap the other end of the tube as shown in Figure 26.18.

10. Mix the blood and heparin by sliding the magnet up and down the tube, thereby moving the metal flea.

11. Label the sample as in previous exercises.

12. Ice the sample if analysis will be delayed, but note that samples should not be iced for certain point-of-service blood gas analysis systems. Place the sample in a biohazard bag or container for transport.

13. Raise bed rails if originally lowered to facilitate the procedure and notify the "nurse" that you are done.

14. Remove your gloves and wash your hands.

15. Make sure to remove the metal flea before analysis of the sample.

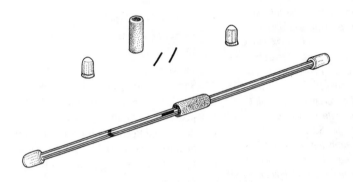

Figure 26.18. Capillary tube with metal flea and magnet.

REFERENCES

1. American Association for Respiratory Care: AARC clinical practice guideline: Sampling for arterial blood gas analysis. Respir Care 37:913–917, 1992.
2. Reines, HD and Seifert, PC: Patient safety: Latex allergy. Surg Clin North Am 85:1329–1340, 2005.
3. Wilkins, R, Sheldon, R, and Krider, S: Clinical Assessment in Respiratory Care, ed 5. Mosby, St. Louis, 2005.
4. Cairo, JM and Pilbeam, SP: Mosby's Respiratory Care Equipment. Mosby, St. Louis, 2004.

Laboratory Report

CHAPTER 26: ARTERIAL BLOOD GAS SAMPLING

Name _____   Date _____

Course/Section _____   Instructor _____

Data Collection

EXERCISE 26.1 Preparation of Blood Gas Kit Components

Syringe size used: _____

Needle sizes available: _____

Type of heparin: _____

Needle gauge selected for radial puncture: _____

EXERCISE 26.2 Modified Allen's Test

Allen's test result: _____

EXERCISE 26.3 Performance of Arterial Puncture

Patient label/charge slip information:

_____

_____

_____

_____

Chart the arterial puncture:

_____

_____

_____

_____

EXERCISE 26.4 Arterial Line Sampling

EXERCISE 26.4.1 ARTERIAL LINE SETUP

A. _____

B. _____

C. _____

D. _____

E. _____

F. _____

G. _____

H. _____

I. _____

J. _____

K. _____

Critical Thinking Questions

1. Identify three conditions that would require compression of the artery for longer than 10 minutes during postpuncture care. Identify one condition that would require compression of the artery for less than 5 minutes.

2. Identify at least four complications of arterial line sampling and state how each can be prevented.

3. You are performing a modified Allen's test to the right arm on Ms. Gordon, a 22-year-old African American woman. You notice that her fingertips are cold to the touch. After release of the ulnar artery, it takes 12 seconds for color to return to the palm. What actions should you take at this time? What are the possible causes of a negative Allen's test in this patient?

4. While performing an arterial puncture on Ms. Gordon, the patient in Critical Thinking Question 3, you encounter the following difficulties. Describe all possible solutions for each problem.

    A. The tip of the needle touches the bedside table before insertion into the patient.

    B. The artery seems to roll away from the needle each time you approach it.

    C. You are having difficulty feeling a pulse in the right (nondominant) arm.

    D. You observe a blood flash in the hub of the needle, and then blood flow stops.

E.   The patient attempts to jerk her arm away as you are inserting the needle.

F.   You have re-angled the needle three times and are still unable to get the blood sample.

G.   You notice swelling under the puncture site when you remove the needle.

H.   As you are corking the needle, you puncture your fingertip.

---

5.   Why does the IV bag in an arterial line setup need to be pressurized?

---

6.   Identify at least five complications of arterial puncture and state how each can be prevented.

---

7.   You are attempting to obtain a sample from an arterial line and encounter the following difficulties. Identify the probable cause(s), if applicable, and describe all possible solutions to the problems.

A.   You observe a blood backup halfway between the point of entrance of the catheter into the patient's arm and the sampling port.

B.   You drop the Luer-Lok™ cap on the floor.

C.   After removing the discard syringe from the Luer-Lok™, blood continues to flow onto the bed sheets.

D.   As you are withdrawing the blood sample, the patient is moving her arm and blood is filling the syringe intermittently.

E.   After removal of the sample, you are unable to flush the catheter.

Procedural Competency Evaluation

STUDENT: **DATE:**

ARTERIAL PUNCTURE

Evaluator: ☐ Peer ☐ Instructor	**Setting:** ☐ Lab	☐ Clinical Simulation

Equipment Utilized: **Conditions (Describe):**

Performance Level:

S or ✓ = Satisfactory, no errors of omission or commission
U = Unsatisfactory Error of Omission or Commission
NA = Not applicable

Performance Rating:

5   **Independent:** Near flawless performance; minimal errors; able to perform without supervision; seeks out new learning; shows initiative; A = 4.7–5.0 average

4   **Minimally Supervised:** Few errors, able to self-correct; seeks guidance when appropriate; B = 3.7–4.65

3   **Competent:** Minimal required level; no critical errors; able to correct with coaching; meets expectations; safe; C = 3.0–3.65

2   **Marginal:** Below average; critical errors or problem areas noted; would benefit from remediation; D = 2.0–2.99

1   **Dependent:** Poor; unacceptable performance; unsafe; gross inaccuracies; potentially harmful; F = < 2.0

Two or more errors of commission or omission of mandatory or essential performance elements will terminate the procedure, and require additional practice and/or remediation and reevaluation. Student is responsible for obtaining additional evaluation forms as needed from the Director of Clinical Education (DCE).

(Right side columns: PERFORMANCE RATING | PERFORMANCE LEVEL)

PATIENT AND EQUIPMENT PREPARATION

1. Common Performance Elements Steps 1–8; **Note: Never recap needle; any needle stick must be reported**

2. Confirms diagnosis, anticoagulant therapy, coagulopathies, oxygen delivery device and F_IO_2, ventilator settings, patient allergies, and if using local anesthetic

ASSESSMENT AND IMPLEMENTATION

3. Common Performance Elements Steps 9 and 10

4. Palpates pulse on both arms to determine best puncture site; uses nondominant arm, if possible

5. Performs modified Allen's test; if negative, repeats on other arm

6. Prepares the puncture site by rubbing vigorously in circular motion away from puncture site with an antiseptic solution for at least 30 seconds; disinfects gloved fingers used for palpation

7. Administers anesthetic if ordered

8. Correctly performs the puncture:

A. Sets the plunger on a self-venting syringe to obtain the desired amount of blood (enough for repeated analysis)

B. Holds the syringe at 45-degree angle, needle bevel up

C. Slowly inserts needle between second and third skin fold on wrist; safely adjusts angle needle if necessary

9. Obtains sample; removes needle and immediately applies pressure with sterile gauze

A. Maintains pressure on the puncture site for a minimum of 3–5 minutes; 10 minutes or longer if patient has bleeding disorder or uses anticoagulants

B. Checks puncture site for bleeding, swelling, discoloration, and return of pulse proximal and distal to puncture site

10. Corks needle with rubber stopper or automatic capping device

11. Ensures anaerobic sample; removes air bubbles with venting device or according to OSHA guidelines

FOLLOW-UP

12. Common Performance Elements Steps 11 and 16

13. Labels sample; places in iced, sealed biohazard container for transport

14. Documents date, time, F_IO_2, puncture site, Allen's test results, oxygen and ventilatory settings (if applicable), and therapist signature

15. Cleans any blood spills with sodium hypochlorite (bleach) solution

SIGNATURES   Student: Evaluator: Date:

Clinical Performance Evaluation

PERFORMANCE RATING:

5 **Independent:** Near flawless performance; minimal errors; able to perform without supervision; seeks out new learning; shows initiative; A = 4.7–5.0 average

4 **Minimally Supervised:** Few errors, able to self-correct; seeks guidance when appropriate; B = 3.7–4.65

3 **Competent:** Minimal required level; no critical errors; able to correct with coaching; meets expectations; safe; C = 3.0–3.65

2 **Marginal:** Below average; critical errors or problem areas noted; would benefit from remediation; D = 2.0–2.99

1 **Dependent:** Poor; unacceptable performance; unsafe; gross inaccuracies; potentially harmful; F = < 2.0

Circle the appropriate response below. Please be consistent, objective, and honest in your assessment of the student's clinical performance and ability.

PERFORMANCE CRITERIA	SCORE				
COGNITIVE DOMAIN					
1. Consistently displays knowledge, comprehension, and command of essential concepts	5	4	3	2	1
2. Demonstrates the relationship between theory and clinical practice	5	4	3	2	1
3. Able to select, review, apply, analyze, synthesize, interpret, and evaluate information; makes recommendations to modify care plan	5	4	3	2	1
PSYCHOMOTOR DOMAIN					
4. Minimal errors, no critical errors; able to self-correct; performs all steps safely and accurately	5	4	3	2	1
5. Selects, assembles, and verifies proper function and cleanliness of equipment; assures operation and corrects malfunctions; provides adequate care and maintenance	5	4	3	2	1
6. Exhibits the required manual dexterity	5	4	3	2	1
7. Performs procedure in a reasonable time frame for clinical level	5	4	3	2	1
8. Applies and maintains aseptic technique and PPE as required	5	4	3	2	1
9. Maintains concise and accurate patient and clinical records	5	4	3	2	1
10. Reports promptly on patient status/needs to appropriate personnel	5	4	3	2	1
AFFECTIVE DOMAIN					
11. Exhibits courteous and pleasant demeanor; shows consideration and respect, honesty, and integrity	5	4	3	2	1
12. Communicates verbally and in writing clearly and concisely	5	4	3	2	1
13. Preserves confidentiality and adheres to all policies	5	4	3	2	1
14. Follows directions, exhibits sound judgment, and seeks help when required	5	4	3	2	1
15. Demonstrates initiative, self-direction, responsibility, and accountability	5	4	3	2	1

TOTAL POINTS = _____ /15 = AVERAGE GRADE = _____

ADDITIONAL COMMENTS: IDENTIFY AREAS OF EXCELLENCE; LIST ERRORS OF OMISSION OR COMMISSION, CRITICAL ERRORS

SUMMARY PERFORMANCE EVALUATION AND RECOMMENDATIONS

☐ PASS: Satisfactory Performance

    ☐ Minimal supervision needed, may progress to next level provided specific skills, clinical time completed

    ☐ Minimal supervision needed, able to progress to next level without remediation

☐ FAIL: Unsatisfactory Performance (check all that apply)

    ☐ Minor reevaluation only

    ☐ Needs additional clinical practice before reevaluation

    ☐ Needs additional laboratory practice before skills performed in clinical area

    ☐ Recommend clinical probation

SIGNATURES

Evaluator (print name): _____ Evaluator signature: _____ Date: _____

Student Signature: _____ Date: _____

Student Comments:

Procedural Competency Evaluation

STUDENT: _____   DATE: _____

ARTERIAL LINE SAMPLING

	PERFORMANCE RATING	PERFORMANCE LEVEL
Evaluator: ☐ Peer ☐ Instructor **Setting:** ☐ Lab ☐ Clinical Simulation		
Equipment Utilized: _____ **Conditions (Describe):** _____		
Performance Level: S or ✓ = Satisfactory, no errors of omission or commission U = Unsatisfactory Error of Omission or Commission NA = Not applicable		
Performance Rating: **5 Independent:** Near flawless performance; minimal errors; able to perform without supervision; seeks out new learning; shows initiative; A = 4.7–5.0 average **4 Minimally Supervised:** Few errors, able to self-correct; seeks guidance when appropriate; B = 3.7–4.65 **3 Competent:** Minimal required level; no critical errors; able to correct with coaching; meets expectations; safe; C = 3.0–3.65 **2 Marginal:** Below average; critical errors or problem areas noted; would benefit from remediation; D = 2.0–2.99 **1 Dependent:** Poor; unacceptable performance; unsafe; gross inaccuracies; potentially harmful; F = < 2.0 *Two or more errors of commission or omission of mandatory or essential performance elements will terminate the procedure, and require additional practice and/or remediation and reevaluation. Student is responsible for obtaining additional evaluation forms as needed from the Director of Clinical Education (DCE).*		
PATIENT AND EQUIPMENT PREPARATION		
1. Common Performance Elements Steps 1–8		
2. Verifies F_IO_2, oxygen delivery device, and/or ventilator settings		
3. Confirms diagnosis, previous blood gas results if available		
ASSESSMENT AND IMPLEMENTATION		
4. Common Performance Elements Steps 9 and 10		
5. Confirms oxygen and/or ventilator settings; assesses oxygenation and ventilatory status		
6. Observes cardiac monitor for shape and height of arterial waveform		
7. Identifies line/intraflow device		
8. Aspirates flush into waste syringe, if applicable		
A. Removes cap from stopcock hub; disinfects and places aseptically on clean gauze or drape		
B. Attaches unheparinized syringe and turns stopcock off to intraflow device		
C. Places gauze under the stopcock while aspirating approximately 3–5 mL until flush solution removed and whole blood appears in syringe from the patient line		
D. Turns stopcock off to syringe; removes syringe and disposes in sharps container		
9. Aspirates sample:		
A. Sets plunger of self-venting syringe for desired amount of blood (enough for repeat analysis)		
B. Secures heparinized syringe on Luer-Lok hub		
C. Re-opens stopcock; collects sample		
D. Turns stopcock off to syringe and removes syringe		
10. Caps syringe; removes air bubbles following OSHA guidelines		
11. Mixes and labels sample; places in sealed biohazard container; sends blood to be analyzed		
12. Maintains line:		
A. Using intraflow, with stopcock turned toward Luer-Lok, flushes the line to the patient for one pass of the screen		
B. Turns stopcock off to the patient; places gauze under hub; pulls the intraflow to flush the stopcock hub		
C. Turns the stopcock off to the Luer-Lok; disinfects hub and cap with alcohol and replaces cap on hub		
13. Checks waveform and verifies line function		
FOLLOW-UP		
14. Common Performance Elements Steps 11–16		
A. Discards all disposables; disposes of sharps in puncture-proof container		
B. Documents date, time, F_IO_2 or delivery device, site, ventilation settings and status, therapist signature		

SIGNATURES   Student: _____   Evaluator: _____   Date: _____

Clinical Performance Evaluation

PERFORMANCE RATING:

5 **Independent:** Near flawless performance; minimal errors; able to perform without supervision; seeks out new learning; shows initiative; A = 4.7–5.0 average

4 **Minimally Supervised:** Few errors, able to self-correct; seeks guidance when appropriate; B = 3.7–4.65

3 **Competent:** Minimal required level; no critical errors; able to correct with coaching; meets expectations; safe; C = 3.0–3.65

2 **Marginal:** Below average; critical errors or problem areas noted; would benefit from remediation; D = 2.0–2.99

1 **Dependent:** Poor; unacceptable performance; unsafe; gross inaccuracies; potentially harmful; F = < 2.0

Circle the appropriate response below. Please be consistent, objective, and honest in your assessment of the student's clinical performance and ability.

PERFORMANCE CRITERIA	SCORE				
COGNITIVE DOMAIN					
1. Consistently displays knowledge, comprehension, and command of essential concepts	5	4	3	2	1
2. Demonstrates the relationship between theory and clinical practice	5	4	3	2	1
3. Able to select, review, apply, analyze, synthesize, interpret, and evaluate information; makes recommendations to modify care plan	5	4	3	2	1
PSYCHOMOTOR DOMAIN					
4. Minimal errors, no critical errors; able to self-correct; performs all steps safely and accurately	5	4	3	2	1
5. Selects, assembles, and verifies proper function and cleanliness of equipment; assures operation and corrects malfunctions; provides adequate care and maintenance	5	4	3	2	1
6. Exhibits the required manual dexterity	5	4	3	2	1
7. Performs procedure in a reasonable time frame for clinical level	5	4	3	2	1
8. Applies and maintains aseptic technique and PPE as required	5	4	3	2	1
9. Maintains concise and accurate patient and clinical records	5	4	3	2	1
10. Reports promptly on patient status/needs to appropriate personnel	5	4	3	2	1
AFFECTIVE DOMAIN					
11. Exhibits courteous and pleasant demeanor; shows consideration and respect, honesty, and integrity	5	4	3	2	1
12. Communicates verbally and in writing clearly and concisely	5	4	3	2	1
13. Preserves confidentiality and adheres to all policies	5	4	3	2	1
14. Follows directions, exhibits sound judgment, and seeks help when required	5	4	3	2	1
15. Demonstrates initiative, self-direction, responsibility, and accountability	5	4	3	2	1

TOTAL POINTS =   /15 = AVERAGE GRADE =

ADDITIONAL COMMENTS: IDENTIFY AREAS OF EXCELLENCE; LIST ERRORS OF OMISSION OR COMMISSION, CRITICAL ERRORS

SUMMARY PERFORMANCE EVALUATION AND RECOMMENDATIONS

☐ PASS: Satisfactory Performance

  ☐ Minimal supervision needed, may progress to next level provided specific skills, clinical time completed

  ☐ Minimal supervision needed, able to progress to next level without remediation

☐ FAIL: Unsatisfactory Performance (check all that apply)

  ☐ Minor reevaluation only

  ☐ Needs additional clinical practice before reevaluation

  ☐ Needs additional laboratory practice before skills performed in clinical area

  ☐ Recommend clinical probation

SIGNATURES

Evaluator (print name):   Evaluator signature: Date:

Student Signature: Date:

Student Comments:

Procedural Competency Evaluation

STUDENT: _____   DATE: _____

CAPILLARY SAMPLING

				PERFORMANCE RATING	PERFORMANCE LEVEL
Evaluator: ☐ Peer ☐ Instructor		**Setting:** ☐ Lab	☐ Clinical Simulation		
Equipment Utilized:		**Conditions (Describe):**			

Performance Level:

S or ✓ = Satisfactory, no errors of omission or commission
U = Unsatisfactory Error of Omission or Commission
NA = Not applicable

Performance Rating:

5   **Independent:** Near flawless performance; minimal errors; able to perform without supervision; seeks out new learning; shows initiative; A = 4.7–5.0 average

4   **Minimally Supervised:** Few errors, able to self-correct; seeks guidance when appropriate; B = 3.7–4.65

3   **Competent:** Minimal required level; no critical errors; able to correct with coaching; meets expectations; safe; C = 3.0–3.65

2   **Marginal:** Below average; critical errors or problem areas noted; would benefit from remediation; D = 2.0–2.99

1   **Dependent:** Poor; unacceptable performance; unsafe; gross inaccuracies; potentially harmful; F = < 2.0

Two or more errors of commission or omission of mandatory or essential performance elements will terminate the procedure, and require additional practice and/or remediation and reevaluation. Student is responsible for obtaining additional evaluation forms as needed from the Director of Clinical Education (DCE).

EQUIPMENT AND PATIENT PREPARATION

1. Common Performance Elements Steps 1–8

ASSESSMENT AND IMPLEMENTATION

2. Common Performance Elements Steps 9 and 10
3. Warms the heel for 5–10 minutes
4. Evaluates effectiveness of warming before performing the puncture
5. Selects the appropriate puncture zone (lateral or medial to the calcaneus)
6. Disinfects the puncture site
7. Quickly punctures the appropriate site with the lancet, no deeper than 3 mm
8. Ensures the free flow of blood and does not squeeze the heel
9. Wipes away the first blood drop with a sterile gauze
10. Draws the sample into a heparinized capillary tube
11. Ensures no air bubbles are present
12. Compresses the puncture site and applies adhesive bandage if required
13. Seals one end of the capillary tube with a stopper
14. Inserts mixing flea and places circular magnet over the tube
15. Caps the other end
16. Mixes the sample by sliding the magnet up and down the tube
17. Labels sample according to facility policy
18. Transports the sample to the laboratory according to facility policy, icing if necessary
19. Removes the mixing flea prior to analysis

FOLLOW-UP

20. Common Performance Elements Steps 11–16

SIGNATURES   Student: _____   Evaluator: _____   Date: _____

Clinical Performance Evaluation

PERFORMANCE RATING:

5 **Independent:** Near flawless performance; minimal errors; able to perform without supervision; seeks out new learning; shows initiative; A = 4.7–5.0 average

4 **Minimally Supervised:** Few errors, able to self-correct; seeks guidance when appropriate; B = 3.7–4.65

3 **Competent:** Minimal required level; no critical errors; able to correct with coaching; meets expectations; safe; C = 3.0–3.65

2 **Marginal:** Below average; critical errors or problem areas noted; would benefit from remediation; D = 2.0–2.99

1 **Dependent:** Poor; unacceptable performance; unsafe; gross inaccuracies; potentially harmful; F = < 2.0

Circle the appropriate response below. Please be consistent, objective, and honest in your assessment of the student's clinical performance and ability.

PERFORMANCE CRITERIA

	SCORE				
COGNITIVE DOMAIN					
1. Consistently displays knowledge, comprehension, and command of essential concepts	5	4	3	2	1
2. Demonstrates the relationship between theory and clinical practice	5	4	3	2	1
3. Able to select, review, apply, analyze, synthesize, interpret, and evaluate information; makes recommendations to modify care plan	5	4	3	2	1
PSYCHOMOTOR DOMAIN					
4. Minimal errors, no critical errors; able to self-correct; performs all steps safely and accurately	5	4	3	2	1
5. Selects, assembles, and verifies proper function and cleanliness of equipment; assures operation and corrects malfunctions; provides adequate care and maintenance	5	4	3	2	1
6. Exhibits the required manual dexterity	5	4	3	2	1
7. Performs procedure in a reasonable time frame for clinical level	5	4	3	2	1
8. Applies and maintains aseptic technique and PPE as required	5	4	3	2	1
9. Maintains concise and accurate patient and clinical records	5	4	3	2	1
10. Reports promptly on patient status/needs to appropriate personnel	5	4	3	2	1
AFFECTIVE DOMAIN					
11. Exhibits courteous and pleasant demeanor; shows consideration and respect, honesty, and integrity	5	4	3	2	1
12. Communicates verbally and in writing clearly and concisely	5	4	3	2	1
13. Preserves confidentiality and adheres to all policies	5	4	3	2	1
14. Follows directions, exhibits sound judgment, and seeks help when required	5	4	3	2	1
15. Demonstrates initiative, self-direction, responsibility, and accountability	5	4	3	2	1

TOTAL POINTS =   /15 = AVERAGE GRADE =

ADDITIONAL COMMENTS: IDENTIFY AREAS OF EXCELLENCE; LIST ERRORS OF OMISSION OR COMMISSION, CRITICAL ERRORS

SUMMARY PERFORMANCE EVALUATION AND RECOMMENDATIONS

☐ PASS: Satisfactory Performance

    ☐ Minimal supervision needed, may progress to next level provided specific skills, clinical time completed

    ☐ Minimal supervision needed, able to progress to next level without remediation

☐ FAIL: Unsatisfactory Performance (check all that apply)

    ☐ Minor reevaluation only

    ☐ Needs additional clinical practice before reevaluation

    ☐ Needs additional laboratory practice before skills performed in clinical area

    ☐ Recommend clinical probation

SIGNATURES

Evaluator (print name):   Evaluator signature: Date:

Student Signature: Date:

Student Comments:

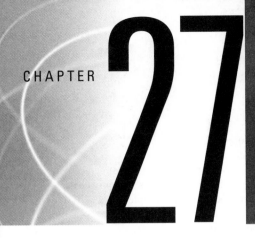

CHAPTER 27

Arterial Blood Gas Analysis and Maintenance

INTRODUCTION

Since very important clinical decisions are based on blood gas data, it is imperative that these values come from reliable and well-maintained blood gas equipment and laboratory. One of the most rapid and significant transformations in clinical practice that evolved from physiological research is the development of the modern, integrated blood gas analyzers. The current analyzers are incredibly sophisticated, stable, and fast.[1,2]

A total quality assurance program for a blood gas laboratory should include documented policies and procedures for the analysis of samples and machine maintenance, verifiable technician competence, scheduled preventive maintenance of the analyzers, performance of calibrations, quality control sampling, **proficiency** testing, and documentation of sample analysis results. Review of patient data would include the statistical analysis of sampling done and identifying whether procedures were indicated.

This chapter introduces students to the procedures involved in maintaining a blood gas laboratory. Because of the significant expense of equipment and **reagents** and the lack of real blood samples for programs that are not hospital-based, some of the procedures described may be performed only in the clinical setting.[3]

OBJECTIVES

Upon completion of this chapter, the student will be able to:

1. Apply infection control guidelines and standards associated with equipment and procedures, according to OSHA regulations and CDC guidelines.
2. Analyze an arterial blood gas sample for pH, $PaCO_2$, and PaO_2 via a standard blood gas analyzer.
3. Analyze an arterial blood gas sample for total hemoglobin and oxyhemoglobin saturation, and measure abnormal hemoglobins with a co-oximeter.
4. Perform one- and two-point calibrations of blood gas analyzers.
5. Perform daily and weekly maintenance according to manufacturer's specifications.
6. Re-membrane a pH, PCO_2, and PO_2 electrode.
7. Analyze quality control test samples and document the results.

KEY TERMS

diluent
proficiency

reagents
slope

Exercises

EQUIPMENT REQUIRED

- ☐ Blood gas analyzer
- ☐ Co-oximeter
- ☐ Reagents: pH buffers, PO_2 and PCO_2 electrolytes, flush solution, KCl solution, or KCl donuts
- ☐ Electrode cleaning solution
- ☐ Deproteinizing solution
- ☐ Calibration gases
- ☐ Barometer—mercury or anaeroid
- ☐ **Diluent**
- ☐ Zeroing solution
- ☐ Quality control test samples for analyzer and co-oximeter
- ☐ Blank blood gas report forms or equivalent
- ☐ Electrode membrane changing kits for pH, PCO_2, and PO_2
- ☐ Electrode membrane changing tools and holder

- ☐ 4×4 gauze
- ☐ Arterial blood gas syringes
- ☐ 3-mL syringes with 22- or 23-gauge needles
- ☐ Plastic specimen containers or equivalent
- ☐ Heparinized capillary sample tubes
- ☐ Magnet and metal rods ("fleas")
- ☐ Disposable waste containers
- ☐ Sharps containers
- ☐ 5.25% sodium hypochlorite (bleach) (1:10) solution
- ☐ Disposable latex and vinyl gloves, various sizes
- ☐ Goggles, disposable gowns (optional)
- ☐ Cotton swabs
- ☐ Stopwatch or watch with second hand
- ☐ Calculator (optional)

EXERCISE 27.1 BLOOD GAS ANALYSIS

EXERCISE 27.1.1 IDENTIFICATION OF COMPONENTS OF BLOOD GAS ANALYZERS

1. Identify the brand of blood gas analyzer being used for this exercise and **record it on your laboratory report.**
2. Identify the controls located on the control panel and **record them on your laboratory report. Draw a schematic representation of the location of these controls.** Be sure to include the location of the sampling ports and electrodes.
3. Locate the reagents and the waste receptacle. **Record the pH of the buffers for the analyzer on your laboratory report.**
4. Locate the calibration gases. Note the pressures on the gauges and **record them on your laboratory report.** Note the concentrations of gases in the tanks and **record them on your laboratory report.**
5. Locate the water bath (if applicable). **Record the temperature on your laboratory report.** Count the rate of gases bubbling through the water bath for 15 seconds and **record it on your laboratory report.**
6. Locate the barometer in your laboratory (Fig. 27.1).
7. Determine the barometric pressure in your laboratory and **record it on your laboratory report.**

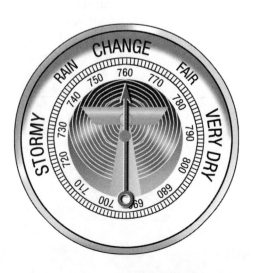

Figure 17.1. Barometer.

8. Calculate the calibration point for slope and balance based on your recorded barometric pressure using the following formula:

$$P = (\text{Barometric pressure} - 47 \text{ mm Hg}) \times F_I$$

where P is the partial pressure of calibration gas and F_I is the fractional decimal expression of the gas concentration. **Show your work and calculations on your laboratory report.**

EXERCISE 27.1.2 CALIBRATION OF BLOOD GAS ANALYZERS

Performance of this exercise and the specific sequence of steps will vary depending on the brand and level of automation of the analyzer used. Consult the operator's manual for the analyzer you are using.

Two-Point Calibration

Initiate the two-point calibration sequence for your analyzer. Using a stopwatch or a watch with a second hand, time how long the two-point calibration takes for your analyzer. **Record the time on your laboratory report.** Pay attention to the sequence in which the reagents and gases are introduced into the analyzer. **Record the sequence of reagents and gases on your laboratory report.**

The following steps are usually involved in a two-point calibration:

1. Flush the pH electrode.
2. Introduce the low-pH buffer into the pH electrode.
3. Allow sufficient time for the reading to stabilize.
4. Adjust the pH balance control.
5. Flush the pH electrode.
6. Introduce the high-pH buffer into the pH electrode.
7. Allow sufficient time for the reading to stabilize.
8. Adjust the pH slope control.
9. Calculate the balance and slope gas calibration points.
10. Introduce low-calibration gases into the PaO_2 and $PaCO_2$ electrodes.
11. Allow sufficient time for the readings to stabilize.
12. Adjust the PO_2 and PCO_2 balance controls.
13. Flush the electrodes.
14. Introduce high-calibration gases into the PO_2 and PCO_2 electrodes.
15. Allow sufficient time for the readings to stabilize.
16. Adjust the PO_2 and PCO_2 slope controls.
17. Flush the sampling chamber.
18. Determine from the analyzer manual or observation how often the machine performs a two-point calibration. **Record this information on your laboratory report.**

One-Point Calibration

Initiate the one-point calibration sequence for your analyzer. Using a stopwatch or a watch with a second hand, time how long the one-point calibration takes for your analyzer. **Record the time on your laboratory report.** Pay attention to the sequence in which the reagents and gases are introduced into the analyzer. **Record the sequence of reagents and gases on your laboratory report.**

The following steps are usually involved in a one-point calibration:

1. Flush the pH electrode.
2. Expose the pH electrode to the high-pH buffer.
3. Allow sufficient time for the readings to stabilize.
4. Adjust the balance control.
5. Flush the sampling chamber.
6. Introduce the low-calibration gases.
7. Allow sufficient time for the readings to stabilize.
8. Adjust the PCO_2 and PO_2 balance controls.
9. Determine how often the machine performs a one-point calibration. **Record the frequency on your laboratory report.**

EXERCISE 27.1.3 ANALYSIS OF QUALITY CONTROL TEST MEDIA

Three levels of controls must be analyzed every 8 hours and appropriately documented. Depending on the medium used, the medium may need to be anaerobically drawn up into sampling syringes before insertion into the blood gas analyzer. The following instructions are for media that come in small glass vials. If a different medium is used, follow the manufacturer's directions.

1. Apply latex or vinyl gloves and other standard precautions and transmission-based isolation procedures as applicable.
2. Perform a one-point calibration before analysis.
3. Verify the quality control medium expiration data and lot number.
4. Mix the quality control medium gently by swirling the vial. Break open the vial carefully, and draw up an anaerobic sample of the level I medium into a syringe using a 22- or 23-gauge needle, or aspirate directly into the analyzer's sampling tube. A glass ampule protection device may be used (Fig. 27.2).
5. Initiate the sampling sequence on your analyzer.
6. Insert the syringe into the sampling port (on some analyzers this may require inserting the analyzer sampling tube into the syringe).
7. Slowly inject the sample into the analyzer until a continuous line of the sample can be seen past the electrode block or until the machine indicates that enough blood has been introduced. Be certain that no air bubbles are introduced. In most modern machines less than 0.5 mL of sample is needed. In older machines 1 to 2 mL may be needed.
8. Allow sufficient time for the readings to stabilize.
9. **Record the results on your laboratory report.** Print out the results if a printer and blood gas recording slips are available.
10. Flush the sampling chamber (this will be done automatically on most machines).
11. Discard the syringe in a sharps container.
12. Repeat the preceding steps with level II and level III and **record the results on your laboratory report.**
13. If the control levels are out of range, take corrective actions. **Record the actions taken on your laboratory report.**
14. Remove your gloves and discard them in an infectious waste container. Wash your hands.

EXERCISE 27.1.4 TRENDING OF QUALITY CONTROL DATA: LEVY-JENNINGS PLOTS

For the following exercise, you will need to obtain quality control data for a period of time and do statistical analysis.

1. Determine what method or methods of recording and analyzing quality control data are performed at your clinical site (manual or computerized). **Record this information on your laboratory report.**
2. Collect at least 2 days worth of quality control data for all shifts and levels. **Attach this information to your laboratory report.**
3. Obtain the lot number of the quality control medium and the acceptable ranges for quality control data for each level. **Record this information on your laboratory report.**
4. Obtain a printout or copy of a Levy-Jennings plot, as shown in Figure 27.3, from your clinical site for the time period in which you collected your data. **Attach it to your laboratory report. Identify any values that indicate random error, trending, or out-of-control data.**

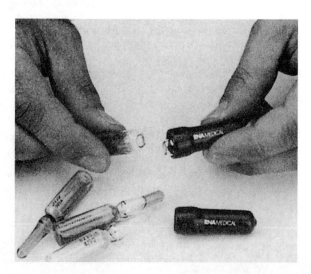

Figure 27.2. Glass ampule protection device. (Courtesy of RNA Medical, Division of Bionostics, Inc., Acton, MA.)

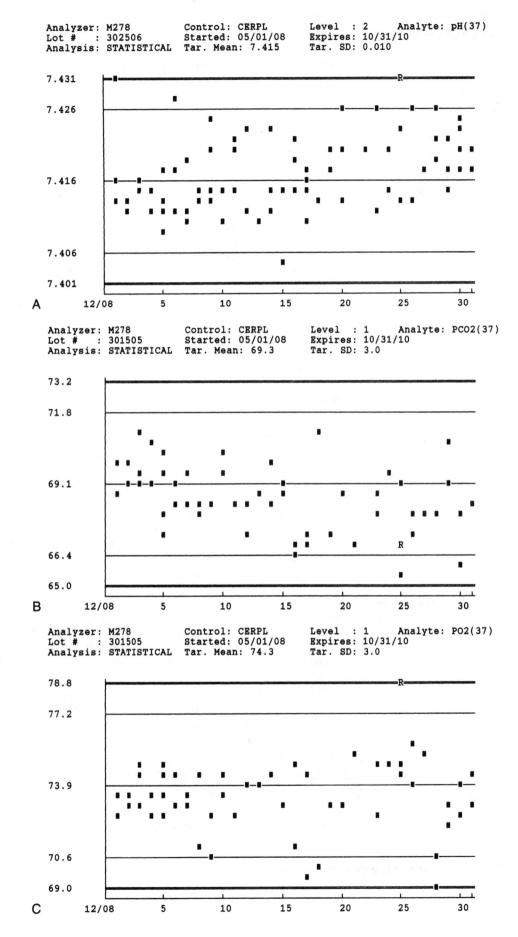

Figure 27.3. Sample Levy Jennings plot.

EXERCISE 27.1.5 BLOOD GAS ANALYSIS

Blood samples may not be readily available in a school laboratory setting. Do not introduce the red dye "blood" solution used in the arterial arm simulators into the blood gas analyzers. A saline or water solution or quality control medium may be used as a substitute for blood samples.

Record the type of specimen used on your lab report.

1. Apply latex or vinyl gloves and other standard precautions and transmission-based isolation procedures as applicable. Gowns and goggles may be worn when dealing with human blood samples.

2. Perform a one-point calibration before blood analysis.

3. Remove the sample from the ice bath and mix the blood sample by rolling it between your palms. Verify that it is an air-free sample.

4. Remove the cap from the sample syringe. Eject a small amount of blood into a gauze pad.

5. Initiate the sampling sequence on your analyzer. Analyzers interfaced with computers may require that patient data and other information be entered.

6. Insert the syringe into the sampling port (on some analyzers this may require inserting the analyzer sampling tube into the syringe).

7. Slowly inject the blood sample into the analyzer until a continuous line of blood can be seen past the electrode block or until the machine indicates that enough blood has been introduced. Be certain that no air bubbles or clots are introduced. In most modern machines less than 0.5 mL of blood is needed. In older machines 1 to 2 mL may be needed. In newer models, the blood sample is aspirated into the machine automatically.

8. Allow sufficient time for the readings to stabilize.

9. **Record the results on your laboratory report.** Print out the results if a printer and blood gas recording slips are available.

10. Flush the sampling chamber (this will be done automatically on most machines).

11. Discard the syringe in a sharps container.

12. Clean up any blood spills with a 1:10 solution of sodium hypochlorite (bleach) solution.

13. Remove your gloves and discard them in an infectious waste container. Wash your hands.

EXERCISE 27.1.6 MAINTENANCE OF A BLOOD GAS ANALYZER

The steps required for daily and weekly preventive maintenance will vary depending on the type of analyzer and the level of automation. Refer to the operator's manual for specific sequences. All activities should be performed with appropriate standard precautions, including gloves, gowns, and goggles if blood splashing may occur.

Daily Maintenance

1. Empty or change the waste container. Modern analyzers may have disposable waste bottles. Remove the container and replace it with a new one. If a disposable container is not available, discard the waste in an infectious waste container, followed by a small amount of bleach. Rinse the container with hot water, pour a small amount of bleach into the container, and place it back onto the analyzer.

2. Check the calibration gas tank pressures.

3. Check the fluid and reagent levels.

4. Check the barometric pressure. Zero the base of the manometer if needed.

5. Verify that the water bath temperature is 37°C.

6. Check the water level in the humidifier (if applicable). Refill it (if needed) with sterile water.

7. Clean the sample port with a cotton swab and bleach solution or alcohol.

8. Remove bubbles and dry the electrode chambers if disposable electrodes are not being used. Newer electrodes are maintenance-free.

Weekly or Biweekly Maintenance

1. Insert a syringe with cleaning solution once per week. Allow it to sit in sampling chamber. Flush when complete.

2. Insert a sample of deproteinizing solution. Allow it to sit in the sampling chamber. Flush when complete.

3. Change the membranes. Newer electrodes on some brands of analyzers are maintenance-free. The entire electrode block is replaced about once a year. Other brands have snap-on membrane kits that are easier to re-membrane. Figure 27.4 depicts a reference pH, PCO_2, and PO_2 electrode. The following steps are usually involved in membrane changing:

A. Remove the electrode from the machine.

B. Remove the old membrane, O-ring, and electrolyte solution.

C. Rinse with sterile water.

D. The PO_2 electrode tip may be polished with a small amount of pumice on a gauze pad and then rinsed with sterile water.

E. Soak the electrode in the appropriate solution.

F. Place a new O-ring on the appropriate membrane changing tool and insert it into the holder.

G. Place a new membrane over the tool, letters down.

H. Place a drop of electrolyte on the membrane.

I. For the CO_2 electrode, place a nylon spacer over the tip of the electrode.

J. Insert the tip of the electrode into the tool and push down until the O-ring snaps into place.

Reference Electrodes

pCO$_2$ Electrode

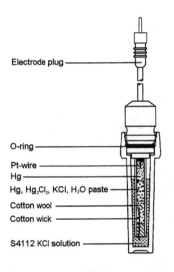

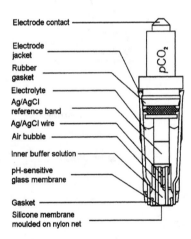

pH Electrode

pO$_2$ Electrode

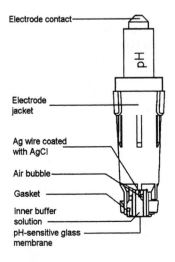

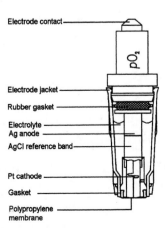

Figure 27.4. Schematic of pH, PCO_2, and PO_2 electrodes. (Courtesy of Radiometer America, Westlake, OH.)

A

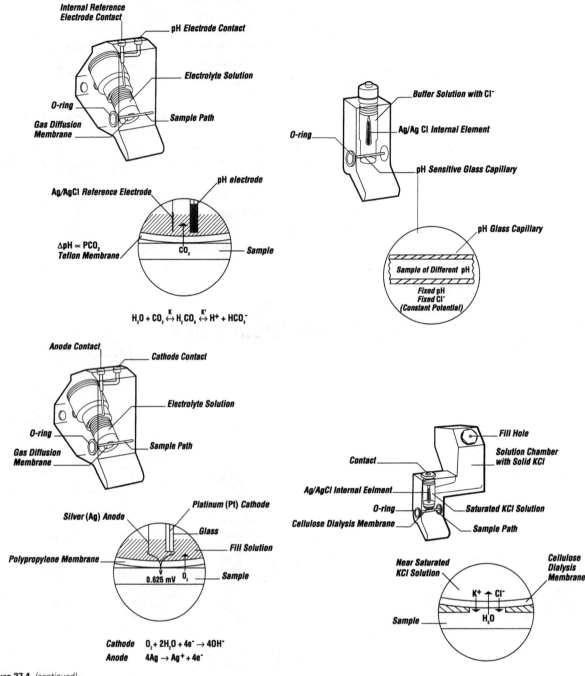

Figure 27.4. *(continued)*

K. Inspect the membrane and remove any wrinkles. Trim if necessary and remove the cardboard holder.

L. Fill the electrode with fresh electrolyte solution, leaving a 1-mm air bubble in the chamber.

M. Dry the outside of the electrode and check for leaks. Place the "boot" over the tip of the membrane.

EXERCISE 27.2 CO-OXIMETRY

EXERCISE 27.2.1 IDENTIFICATION OF CONTROLS FOR A CO-OXIMETER

1. Identify the brand of co-oximeter being used for this exercise, and **record it on your laboratory report.**

2. Identify the controls located on the control panel. **Record them on your laboratory report. Draw a schematic representation of the location of these controls.**

3. Locate the reagents and waste receptacle. **Record which reagents are used for the co-oximeter on your laboratory report.**

EXERCISE 27.2.2 CALIBRATION AND QUALITY CONTROLS FOR A CO-OXIMETER

The steps required for calibration and quality control media sampling will vary depending on the type of analyzer and the level of automation. Refer to the operator's manual for specific sequences. All activities should be performed with appropriate standard precautions and transmission-based isolation procedures, including gloves, gowns, and goggles if blood splashing may occur.

The following steps are usually involved for calibration and quality control for a co-oximeter:

1. Activate the flush.
2. Aspirate the sample chamber.
3. Alternate between flush and aspirate until all bubbles are removed from the fluidics.
4. Push the start button.
5. Insert the calibration sample into the sample port.
6. Once the readings stabilize, adjust the calibration value if necessary.
7. Repeat the procedure for the quality control media.

REFERENCES

1. Raff, H: The significance of the blood gas analyzer. APS 10:1152, 2004.
2. Severinghaus, JW, and Bradley, AF: Electrodes for blood PO_2 and PCO_2 determination. J Appl Physiol 13:515–520:1958.
3. American Association for Respiratory Care: AARC clinical practice guideline: In vitro pH and blood gas analysis and hemoximetry. Respir Care 46(5):498–505, 2001.

Laboratory Report

CHAPTER 27: ARTERIAL BLOOD GAS ANALYSIS AND MAINTENANCE

Name _____ Date _____

Course/Section _____ Instructor _____

Data Collection

EXERCISE 27.1 Blood Gas Analysis

EXERCISE 27.1.1 IDENTIFICATION OF COMPONENTS OF BLOOD GAS ANALYZERS

1. Analyzer brand: _____

2. Control panel:

_____   _____

_____   _____

_____   _____

_____   _____

_____   _____

_____   _____

_____   _____

_____   _____

_____   _____

Schematic:

3. pH of the buffers:

_____

_____

4. Calibration gas pressures: _____

Concentration of gases: _____

5. Water bath temperature: _____

Bubbling rate: _____/15 seconds

6. Type of barometer: _____

7. Barometric pressure: _____

8. Calculation of calibration points: **Show your work!**

$P_B =$ _____

Slope gases: $CO_2 =$ _____ $O_2 =$ _____

Balance gases: $CO_2 =$ _____ $O_2 =$ _____

EXERCISE 27.1.2 CALIBRATION OF BLOOD GAS ANALYZERS

Duration (time) of two-point calibration: _____

Sequence for reagents in two-point calibration: _____

_____

_____

Frequency (time) between two-point calibrations: _____

Duration of one-point calibration: _____

Sequence for reagents in one-point calibration: _____

_____

_____

Frequency of one-point calibration: _____

EXERCISE 27.1.3 ANALYSIS OF QUALITY CONTROL TEST MEDIA

Type of quality control media used: _____

Level I	Level II	Level III
EXPECTED RANGES	EXPECTED RANGES	EXPECTED RANGES
pH: _____	pH: _____	pH: _____
PCO_2: _____	PCO_2: _____	PCO_2: _____
PO_2: _____	PO_2: _____	PO_2: _____

ACTUAL RESULTS	ACTUAL RESULTS	ACTUAL RESULTS
pH: _____	pH: _____	pH: _____
PCO_2: _____	PCO_2: _____	PCO_2: _____
PO_2: _____	PO_2: _____	PO_2: _____

Describe corrective actions (if applicable) if out of range:

_____

_____

EXERCISE 27.1.4 TRENDING OF QUALITY CONTROL DATA: LEVY-JENNINGS PLOTS

1. Method(s) of recording and analyzing quality control data

Clinical site: _____

Method(s) used: _____

2. Quality control data: _____

3. Lot number: _____

Acceptable ranges for quality control data

Level I	Level II	Level III
pH: _____	pH: _____	pH: _____
PCO_2: _____	PCO_2: _____	PCO_2: _____
PO_2: _____	PO_2: _____	PO_2: _____

4. Attach the Levy-Jennings plot. Identify any values on the attached plot that indicate:

    A. Random error

    B. Trending

    C. Out-of-control

EXERCISE 27.1.5 BLOOD GAS ANALYSIS

Type of specimen used: _____ F_IO_2 _____

pH: _____

$PaCO_2$: _____

PaO_2: _____

HCO_3^-: _____

SaO_2: _____

EXERCISE 27.2 Co-oximetry

EXERCISE 27.2.1 IDENTIFICATION OF CONTROLS FOR A CO-OXIMETER

1. Brand of co-oximeter: _____

2. Control panel:

_____   _____

_____   _____

_____   _____

_____   _____

_____   _____

_____   _____

_____   _____

_____   _____

_____   _____

Schematic:

3. Reagents used for the co-oximeter: _____

Critical Thinking Questions

1. For each of the following, *identify* what it measures, *describe* the components of the device, and *explain* its principal of operation.

   A. Sanz electrode

   B. Severinghaus electrode

   C. Clark electrode

   D. Co-oximeter

2. What effect will a water bath temperature of less than 37°C have on the measured pH, $PaCO_2$, and PaO_2? What effect will a water bath temperature of greater than 37°C have on the measured pH, $PaCO_2$, and PaO_2? Whose gas law explains this?

3. Why is it important to eject a small amount of blood from the syringe sample onto a gauze pad before injecting the sample into the machine?

4. Under what circumstances and how often should a two-point calibration be performed on a blood gas analyzer? A one-point calibration?

5. Given a barometric pressure of 750 mm Hg, calculate the calibration points for the following (**show your work!**):

    A. 10% CO_2 and 0% oxygen

    B. 5% CO_2 and 12% oxygen

    C. 20% oxygen and 12% CO_2

6. List five common causes of inaccurate results obtained from blood gas sampling and analysis.

7. A patient is being treated for smoke inhalation and third-degree burns. Silvadene has been applied to large portions of the patient's body surface. How might the patient's condition affect the analysis of blood for co-oximetry?

8. Identify three factors that would make the reading of a co-oximeter unreliable.

Procedural Competency Evaluation

STUDENT: **DATE:**

ABG ANALYZER MAINTENANCE

	PERFORMANCE RATING	PERFORMANCE LEVEL
Evaluator: ☐ Peer ☐ Instructor **Setting:** ☐ Lab ☐ Clinical Simulation		
Equipment Utilized: **Conditions (Describe):**		
Performance Level:		
S or ✓ = Satisfactory, no errors of omission or commission U = Unsatisfactory Error of Omission or Commission NA = Not applicable		
Performance Rating:		
5 **Independent:** Near flawless performance; minimal errors; able to perform without supervision; seeks out new learning; shows initiative; A = 4.7–5.0 average		
4 **Minimally Supervised:** Few errors, able to self-correct; seeks guidance when appropriate; B = 3.7–4.65		
3 **Competent:** Minimal required level; no critical errors; able to correct with coaching; meets expectations; safe; C = 3.0–3.65		
2 **Marginal:** Below average; critical errors or problem areas noted; would benefit from remediation; D = 2.0–2.99		
1 **Dependent:** Poor; unacceptable performance; unsafe; gross inaccuracies; potentially harmful; F = < 2.0		
Two or more errors of commission or omission of mandatory or essential performance elements will terminate the procedure, and require additional practice and/or remediation and reevaluation. Student is responsible for obtaining additional evaluation forms as needed from the Director of Clinical Education (DCE).		
EQUIPMENT PREPARATION		
1. Performs daily maintenance:		
A. Checks fluid level of pH and flush		
B. Checks cal and slope tanks and gas flow		
C. Checks levels of humidifiers		
D. Empties waste bottle		
E. Inserts daily cleaner		
2. Calibrates blood gas analyzer:		
A. Obtains correct barometric pressure		
B. Performs a two point calibration going from low-high buffer (pH) then from low gas-high gas (PCO_2 and PO_2)		
C. Using the following formula, calculates correct gas values: $(PB - 47) \times \%$ gas in tank $=$ mm Hg to be calibrated		
3. Performs electrode maintenance (if applicable)		
A. Every 2 weeks the pH reference PCO_2 and PO_2 membranes should be replaced, if applicable		
1) Re-membranes according to procedure manual, if applicable; fills with electrolyte solution; cleans out chamber and places electrode back into machine		
2) PCO_2: removes from machine, empties solution, and removes membrane; cleans and re-membranes following procedure manual for the machine; fills with electrolyte solution; cleans out electrode chamber and places electrode back into machine		
3) PO_2 electrodes: removes from machine, empties solution, and removes membrane; cleans and re-membranes according to procedure manual for machine; fills with electrolyte solution		
4) Cleans out electrode chamber and places electrode back into machine		
B. On most analyzers, electrode block needs to be replaced annually		
4. Calibrates the machine prior to analyzing blood gas sample		
5. Performs quality controls:		
A. Verifies lot numbers and expected ranges		
B. Inserts three levels of quality control (acidosis, normal, alkalosis)		
C. Corrects any errors and reruns if necessary		
FOLLOW-UP		
6. Documents preventive maintenance procedures		
7. Produces Levy-Jennings plots		
A. Able to identify Levy-Jennings plots that are in control, random error, shift, trend, and out of control		

SIGNATURES   Student: Evaluator: Date:

Clinical Performance Evaluation

PERFORMANCE RATING:

5 **Independent:** Near flawless performance; minimal errors; able to perform without supervision; seeks out new learning; shows initiative; A = 4.7–5.0 average

4 **Minimally Supervised:** Few errors, able to self-correct; seeks guidance when appropriate; B = 3.7–4.65

3 **Competent:** Minimal required level; no critical errors; able to correct with coaching; meets expectations; safe; C = 3.0–3.65

2 **Marginal:** Below average; critical errors or problem areas noted; would benefit from remediation; D = 2.0–2.99

1 **Dependent:** Poor; unacceptable performance; unsafe; gross inaccuracies; potentially harmful; F = < 2.0

Circle the appropriate response below. Please be consistent, objective, and honest in your assessment of the student's clinical performance and ability.

PERFORMANCE CRITERIA	SCORE				
COGNITIVE DOMAIN					
1. Consistently displays knowledge, comprehension, and command of essential concepts	5	4	3	2	1
2. Demonstrates the relationship between theory and clinical practice	5	4	3	2	1
3. Able to select, review, apply, analyze, synthesize, interpret, and evaluate information; makes recommendations to modify care plan	5	4	3	2	1
PSYCHOMOTOR DOMAIN					
4. Minimal errors, no critical errors; able to self-correct; performs all steps safely and accurately	5	4	3	2	1
5. Selects, assembles, and verifies proper function and cleanliness of equipment; assures operation and corrects malfunctions; provides adequate care and maintenance	5	4	3	2	1
6. Exhibits the required manual dexterity	5	4	3	2	1
7. Performs procedure in a reasonable time frame for clinical level	5	4	3	2	1
8. Applies and maintains aseptic technique and PPE as required	5	4	3	2	1
9. Maintains concise and accurate patient and clinical records	5	4	3	2	1
10. Reports promptly on patient status/needs to appropriate personnel	5	4	3	2	1
AFFECTIVE DOMAIN					
11. Exhibits courteous and pleasant demeanor; shows consideration and respect, honesty, and integrity	5	4	3	2	1
12. Communicates verbally and in writing clearly and concisely	5	4	3	2	1
13. Preserves confidentiality and adheres to all policies	5	4	3	2	1
14. Follows directions, exhibits sound judgment, and seeks help when required	5	4	3	2	1
15. Demonstrates initiative, self-direction, responsibility, and accountability	5	4	3	2	1

TOTAL POINTS = _____ /15 = AVERAGE GRADE = _____

ADDITIONAL COMMENTS: IDENTIFY AREAS OF EXCELLENCE; LIST ERRORS OF OMISSION OR COMMISSION, CRITICAL ERRORS

SUMMARY PERFORMANCE EVALUATION AND RECOMMENDATIONS

☐ PASS: Satisfactory Performance

    ☐ Minimal supervision needed, may progress to next level provided specific skills, clinical time completed

    ☐ Minimal supervision needed, able to progress to next level without remediation

☐ FAIL: Unsatisfactory Performance (check all that apply)

    ☐ Minor reevaluation only

    ☐ Needs additional clinical practice before reevaluation

    ☐ Needs additional laboratory practice before skills performed in clinical area

    ☐ Recommend clinical probation

SIGNATURES

Evaluator (print name): _____ Evaluator signature: _____ Date: _____

Student Signature: _____ Date: _____

Student Comments:

28 Blood Gas Interpretation and Calculations

INTRODUCTION

The respiratory care practitioner must not only be proficient in obtaining blood gas samples but also must be able to interpret the results in order to make recommendations and modify therapeutic interventions related to acid–base, ventilation, and oxygenation status. Many calculations and formulas assist in estimating the adequacy of physiologic indexes or approximating needed changes in oxygen or ventilator parameters. Calculations also are helpful in verifying the accuracy of derived values from blood gas sampling measurements.[1,2]

OBJECTIVES

Upon completion of this chapter, the student will be able to:

1. Identify and correct **preanalytical** errors affecting blood gas results, including inadvertent venous sampling, air bubbles in sample, excess heparinization, and delayed sample analysis.
2. Interpret arterial blood gas analysis results and make recommendations for oxygen therapy based on the interpretations.
3. Calculate PaO_2, $P(A - a)DO_2$, arterial:alveolar oxygen tension (a:A) ratio, CaO_2, CvO_2, and $C(a - v)O_2$, VO_2, and cardiac output using the Fick equation, acid:base ratios, pH, HCO_3^-, and total carbon dioxide.
4. Estimate the F_IO_2 needed to obtain a desired PaO_2.
5. Using a graphic representation of the oxyhemoglobin dissociation curve, determine SaO_2, CaO_2, PaO_2, and P-50.

KEY TERMS

acidosis	exacerbation	logarithm	superimposed
alkalosis	hyperoxia	preanalytical	

Exercises

EQUIPMENT REQUIRED

- [ ] Arterial blood gas results
- [ ] Logs
- [ ] Computer runs
- [ ] Computer tutorials

- [ ] **Logarithm** table or calculator with log function
- [ ] Metric ruler

EXERCISE 28.1 INTERPRETATION OF ARTERIAL BLOOD GAS VALUES

Review normal arterial and venous values (Table 28.1). Perform the following steps to interpret arterial blood gas sample results:

1. Obtain blood gas analysis results to interpret. Your instructor will provide you with one or more of the following:

   Blood gas log records

   Computer runs of blood gas results

   Blood gas record slips

   Computerized practice and drill tutorials

2. Consider the following abnormalities:

   pH

   > <7.35: acidotic

   > >7.45: alkalotic

   PCO_2—Respiratory Component

   > >45 mm Hg: acidotic (hypoventilation)

   > <35 mm Hg: alkalotic (hyperventilation)

   HCO_3^- —Metabolic Component

   > <22 mEq/L: acidotic

   > >26 mEq/L: alkalotic

   BE—Metabolic Component

   > <−2: acidotic

   > >+2: alkalotic

   PO_2

   > <80 mm Hg mild hypoxemia

   > <60 mm Hg moderate hypoxemia

   > <40 mm Hg severe hypoxemia

   > >100 mm Hg **hyperoxia**

   A. Must consider correlation with oxygen therapy (uncorrected, corrected, or overcorrected).

   B. Must consider age of patient:

   i. Newborn normal PaO_2 is 40 to 70 mm Hg.

   ii. Over 60 years old, PaO_2 may decrease approximately 1 mm Hg per year.

   iii. Any PaO_2 below 60 mm Hg is abnormal.

Table 28.1 Normal Blood Gas Values

Arterial	Venous
pH: 7.40 (7.35–7.45)	pH: 7.34–7.36
$PaCO_2$: 40 (35–45) mm Hg	$PvCO_2$: 46–48 mm Hg
PaO_2: 100 (80–100) mm Hg	PvO_2: 40 (37–43) mm Hg
SaO_2: 97%	SvO_2: 70%–75%
HCO_3^-: 22–26 mEq/L	
BE: ±2	

3. Interpret acid:base status:
   A. Look at the pH and decide whether it is acidotic, alkalotic, or normal. If normal, is it on the acidotic or alkalotic side of 7.40? Mark your decision next to the pH value.
   B. Look at the $PaCO_2$ and determine whether it is normal, acidotic, or alkalotic.
   C. Look at HCO_3^-/BE. Determine whether it is normal, acidotic, or alkalotic.
   D. Determine whether the primary condition is respiratory or metabolic. See which component (CO_2 or base) matches the pH (same direction, alkalotic, or acidotic).
   E. Determine how much compensation is occurring:
      i. Look at the nonprimary component to see if it is normal. If normal, this is an *acute uncompensated* condition.
      ii. If the nonprimary component is abnormal, determine in which direction it is occurring. If it is in the opposite direction of the primary problem, *compensation* has begun. This is a *chronic, partially compensated* condition.
      iii. If the pH is normal, compensation is *complete*.
      iv. If the nonprimary component is abnormal in the same direction as the primary component, it is a *mixed* condition.

4. You *must* consider the patient history, diagnosis, and treatment, if known, to fully interpret. There may be an acute problem **superimposed** on a chronic problem—for example, a COPD patient with chronic hypercarbia placed on a mechanical ventilator or having an acute exacerbation. The following series of blood gases are given as an illustration:

	Normal State	On Admission	After Ventilation
pH	7.37	7.25	7.47
PCO_2	55	70	45
HCO_3^-	31	30	32
BE	+4	+5	+3

5. Oxygenation status:
   A. Look at the PO_2 and determine whether it is normal, hypoxemic, or hyperoxic.
   B. Look at the oxygen therapy being given, if any, and determine whether the PO_2 is uncorrected, corrected, or overcorrected.
   C. Remember to consider the age of the patient.
   D. Look at the hemoglobin, SO_2, oxygen content, and vital signs to determine whether there are any indications of tissue hypoxia.

6. Compare the results with the patient's previous results, if available, and the clinical condition.

7. Consider any possible sources of error, such as excess heparin, air bubbles, inadvertent venous sample, improperly iced sample or delayed analysis, or analyzer temperature not at 37°C.

   NOTE: There is a lack of a scientific basis for correction of blood gases for changes in patient body temperature. Appropriate clinical interpretation is better accomplished when temperature correction is avoided.[1]

EXERCISE 28.2 CALCULATION OF OXYGENATION PARAMETERS

EXERCISE 28.2.1 OXYGEN DISSOCIATION CURVE

The following problems should be answered using the oxygen dissociation curve in Figure 28.1. Do not "calculate" answers. Use your ruler to line up the y and x axes on the graph to determine the following parameters. **Record your answers on your laboratory report.**

1. With the curve in a normal position, for the following values of PO_2, determine the SaO_2.
   A. 60 mm Hg
   B. 50 mm Hg
   C. 90 mm Hg
   D. 40 mm Hg

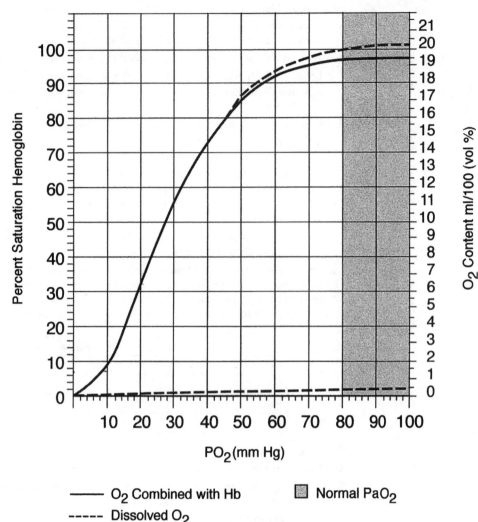

Figure 28.1. The oxyhemoglobin dissociation curve.

——— O₂ Combined with Hb   ▨ Normal PaO₂

----- Dissolved O₂

2. With the curve in the normal position, for the following values of PO_2, determine the CaO_2.
   A. 60 mm Hg
   B. 20 mm Hg
   C. 90 mm Hg
   D. 40 mm Hg

3. For the following P-50 values, determine whether the curve has shifted left or right.
   A. 20 mm Hg
   B. 30 mm Hg

4. For the shifted curves shown in Figure 28.2, determine the P-50 value by lining up your ruler with an SO_2 value of 50%, intersecting the curve, and then drawing a perpendicular line down to the corresponding PO_2 value. For the curves shifted to the left and to the right, **record your answers on your laboratory report.**

EXERCISE 28.2.2 CALCULATION OF ALVEOLAR AIR EQUATION, ALVEOLAR ARTERIAL OXYGEN GRADIENT, AND ARTERIAL:ALVEOLAR OXYGEN RATIO

The following equation can be used to determine the PaO_2. Because PaO_2 should approximate PaO_2, the formula is helpful in determining the maximum possible PaO_2 for a given F_IO_2. This is useful in evaluating possible preanalytical error from air bubble inclusion.

$$PaO_2 = [F_IO_2 (P_B - 47)] - (PaCO_2 \times 1.25)$$

From this calculation, the $P(A - a)DO_2$ can then be determined by using the following formula:

$$PaO_2 - PaO_2 = P(A - a)DO_2$$

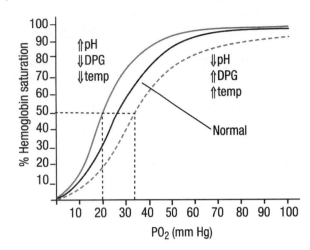

Figure 28.2. The shifted oxyhemoglobin dissociation curve.

This formula can be used to estimate the degree of hypoxemia or the degree of physiologic shunt.[2]

The arterial:alveolar oxygen ratio is an indicator of the efficiency of oxygen diffusion. A low a:A ratio reflects ventilation perfusion (V/Q) mismatches, diffusion defects, or shunts.[3] The a:A ratio is determined by the following formula:

$$PaO_2/PAO_2 = \text{a:A ratio}$$

For each of the following, calculate the PAO_2, the $P(A - a)DO_2$, and the a:A ratio. **Show your work and record your answers on your laboratory report.**

1. $F_IO_2 = 0.21$
   $P_B = 760$ mm Hg
   $PaCO_2 = 40$ mm Hg
   $PaO_2 = 100$ mm Hg
2. $F_IO_2 = 1.00$
   $P_B = 760$ mm Hg
   $PaCO_2 = 40$ mm Hg
   $PaO_2 = 650$ mm Hg
3. $F_IO_2 = 0.50$
   $P_B = 750$ mm Hg
   $PaCO_2 = 50$ mm Hg
   $PaO_2 = 60$ mm Hg
4. $F_IO_2 = 0.21$
   $P_B = 755$ mm Hg
   $PaCO_2 = 20$ mm Hg
   $PaO_2 = 110$ mm Hg
5. Calculate the highest possible values of PaO_2 for the following values of $PaCO_2$ for patients breathing room air at sea level.
   A. $PaCO_2 = 25$ mm Hg
   B. $PaCO_2 = 15$ mm Hg
   C. $PaCO_2 = 30$ mm Hg
   D. $PaCO_2 = 50$ mm Hg
   E. $PaCO_2 = 70$ mm Hg

EXERCISE 28.2.3 F_IO_2 NEEDED FOR A DESIRED PaO_2

This calculation is useful to estimate the F_IO_2 needed for a desired PaO_2 in a patient with hypoxemia caused by V/Q mismatch or hypoventilation. It is less reliable in severe intrapulmonary shunts.[4]

For the following blood gas examples, calculate the F_IO_2 needed. **Show your work and record your answers on your laboratory report.**

Step 1: Calculate the PAO_2 as in the preceding exercises.

Step 2: Calculate the a:A ratio as in the preceding exercises.

Step 3: Calculate the PAO_2 needed.

$$PAO_2 \text{ needed} = PaO_2 \text{ desired}/\text{a:A ratio}$$

Step 4: Calculate the F_IO_2 needed.

$$F_IO_2 \text{ needed} = PAO_2 \text{ needed} + (PaCO_2 \times 1.25)/PB - 47$$

1. $PaO_2 = 40$ mm Hg
   $PaCO_2 = 30$ mm Hg
   $F_IO_2 = 0.21$
   $PB = 760$ mm Hg
   Desired $PaO_2 = 80$ mm Hg
2. $PaO_2 = 50$ mm Hg
   $PaCO_2 = 60$ mm Hg
   $F_IO_2 = 0.25$
   $PB = 750$
   Desired $PaO_2 = 60$ mm Hg
3. $PaO_2 = 500$ mm Hg
   $PaCO_2 = 40$ mm Hg
   $F_IO_2 = 1.0$
   $PB = 765$
   Desired $PaO_2 = 90$ mm Hg

EXERCISE 28.2.4 ARTERIAL OXYGEN CONTENT, VENOUS OXYGEN CONTENT, ARTERIAL VENOUS OXYGEN DIFFERENCE, OXYGEN CONSUMPTION, AND CARDIAC OUTPUT USING THE FICK EQUATION

$$CaO_2 = (PaO_2 \times 0.003) + (Hb \times 1.39) SaO_2$$
$$CvO_2 = (PvO_2 \times 0.003) + (Hb \times 1.39) SvO_2$$
$$C(a - v)O_2 = CaO_2 - CvO_2$$
$$VO_2 = C(a - v)O_2 \times (\text{cardiac output}) \times 10$$

For each of the following, perform the above calculations. **Show your work and record your answers on your laboratory report.**

1.	Arterial	Mixed Venous
pH	7.25	7.22
PCO_2	55 mm Hg	62 mm Hg
PaO_2	60 mm Hg	30 mm Hg
SaO_2	88%	65%
Hb	18 g/100 mL	
Cardiac output	4.0 L/minute	
F_IO_2	0.21	

2.	Arterial	Mixed Venous
pH	7.35	7.32
PCO_2	65 mm Hg	72 mm Hg
PaO_2	50 mm Hg	20 mm Hg
SaO_2	85%	60%
Hb	18 g/100 mL	
VO_2	180 mL/minute	
F_IO_2	0.24	

EXERCISE 28.3 ACID–BASE CALCULATIONS

The following formulas are used to calculate acid–base parameters:

$$\text{Base:acid ratio} = \frac{HCO_3^-}{PaCO_2 \times 0.03}$$

$$pH = 6.1 + \log\left[\frac{HCO_3^-}{PaCO_2 \times 0.03}\right]$$

$$\text{Total } CO_2 \text{ mM/L} = (PaCO_2 \times 0.03) + HCO_3^-$$

For each of the following, calculate the base:acid ratio, pH, and total CO_2. **Show your work and record your answers on your laboratory report.**

1. HCO_3^- = 20 mEq/L
   PCO_2 = 37 mm Hg
2. HCO_3^- = 32 mEq/L
   PCO_2 = 42 mm Hg
3. HCO_3^- = 35 mEq/L
   PCO_2 = 55 mm Hg
4. HCO_3^- = 17 mEq/L
   PCO_2 = 28 mm Hg

For the following, calculate the HCO_3^-. **Show all work and record your answers on your laboratory report**

5. pH = 7.35
   PCO_2 = 60
6. pH = 7.45
   PCO_2 = 45
7. pH = 7.15
   PCO_2 = 20
8. pH = 7.55
   PCO_2 = 20

REFERENCES

1. Shapiro, BA, Peruzzi, WT, and Kozelowski-Templin, R: Clinical Application of Blood Gases. Mosby, St. Louis, 1994, p. 231.
2. American Association for Respiratory Care: AARC clinical practice guideline: In vitro pH and blood gas analysis and he-moximetry. Respir Care 46(5):498–505, 2001.
3. Chang, DW: Respiratory Care Calculations. Delmar, Albany, 1994, p. 14.
4. Chang, DW: Respiratory Care Calculations. Delmar, Albany, 1994, p. 48.

Laboratory Report

CHAPTER 28: BLOOD GAS INTERPRETATION AND CALCULATIONS

Name _____   Date _____

Course/Section _____   Instructor _____

Data Collection

EXERCISE 28.2 Calculation of Oxygen Parameters

EXERCISE 28.2.1 OXYGEN DISSOCIATION CURVE

1. A. 60 mm Hg = _____

   B. 50 mm Hg = _____

   C. 90 mm Hg = _____

   D. 40 mm Hg = _____

2. A. 60 mm Hg = _____

   B. 20 mm Hg = _____

   C. 90 mm Hg = _____

   D. 40 mm Hg = _____

3. For the following P-50 values, determine whether the curve has shifted left or right:

   A. 20 mm Hg _____

   B. 30 mm Hg _____

4. For the curve shifted to the left, P-50 = _____

   For the curve shifted to the right, P-50 = _____

EXERCISE 28.2.2 CALCULATION OF $P_{A}O_2$, $P(A - a)DO_2$, a:A RATIO

Show your work on the laboratory report.

1. $P_{A}O_2$ = _____

   $P(A - a)DO_2$ = _____

   a:A ratio = _____

2. $P_{A}O_2$ = _____

   $P(A - a)DO_2$ = _____

   a:A ratio = _____

3. P_AO_2 = _____

   $P(A - a)DO_2$ = _____

   a:A ratio = _____

4. P_AO_2 = _____

   $P(A - a)DO_2$ = _____

   a:A ratio = _____

5. Calculation of PaO_2 (see text):

   A. PaO_2 = _____

   B. PaO_2 = _____

   C. PaO_2 = _____

   D. PaO_2 = _____

   E. PaO_2 = _____

EXERCISE 28.2.3 F_IO_2 NEEDED FOR A DESIRED PaO_2

Show all work for all steps!

1. P_AO_2 = _____

   a:A ratio = _____

   P_AO_2 needed = _____

   F_IO_2 needed = _____

2. P_AO_2 = _____

   a:A ratio = _____

   P_AO_2 needed = _____

   F_IO_2 needed = _____

3. P_AO_2 = _____

   a:A ratio = _____

   P_AO_2 needed = _____

   F_IO_2 needed = _____

EXERCISE 28.2.4 CaO_2, CvO_2, $C(a - v)O_2$, VO_2, AND CARDIAC OUTPUT (C.O.) USING THE FICK EQUATION

Show all work for all steps!

1. CaO_2 = _____

   CvO_2 = _____

   $C(a - v)O_2$ = _____

   VO_2 = _____

2. CaO_2 = _____

   CvO_2 = _____

   $C(a - v)O_2$ = _____

   C.O. = _____

EXERCISE 28.3 Acid–Base Calculations

Show all work for all steps!

1. Base:acid ratio = _____

   pH = _____

   Total CO_2 = _____

2. Base:acid ratio = _____

   pH = _____

   Total CO_2 = _____

3. Base:acid ratio = _____

   pH = _____

   Total CO_2 = _____

4. Base:acid ratio = _____

   pH = _____

   Total CO_2 = _____

5. HCO_3^- = _____

6. HCO_3^- = _____

7. HCO_3^- = _____

8. HCO_3^- = _____

Critical Thinking Questions

Mr. Sample is a 33-year-old nonsmoking healthy man who has volunteered to serve as a control in a research study. An arterial blood gas sample is drawn on room air as part of the study. The blood gas kit used did not contain a preheparinized syringe. Liquid heparin was used to heparinize the syringe before sampling.

1. If the following blood gas result was obtained, what type of preanalytical error would you suspect, if any? What action would you take at this time, if any?

   pH = 7.35

   $PaCO_2$ = 46 mm Hg

   $PaCO_2$ = 45 mm Hg

   SaO_2 = 77%

   HCO_3^- = 23 mEq/L

2. If the following blood gas result was obtained, what type of preanalytical error would you suspect, if any? What action would you take at this time, if any?

   pH = 7.50

   $PaCO_2$ = 25 mm Hg

   $PaCO_2$ = 150 mm Hg

   SaO_2 = 100%

   HCO_3^- = 26 mEq/L

3. If excess heparin remained in the syringe during sampling, how would it affect the pH and $PaCO_2$ values obtained?

4. If analysis of the sample was delayed by 1 hour without icing the sample, how would the pH, $PaCO_2$, and PaO_2 be changed? Why?

Mr. Khan is a 65-year-old with a history of atrial fibrillation. He takes Coumadin. He complained of increasing shortness of breath and was transported to the ER by the paramedics with a nonrebreathing mask in place. The patient is lethargic. You are called to draw an arterial blood gas.

5. What factors might you consider while performing the puncture?

6. Interpret and explain the following results:

   pH = 7.30

   $PaCO_2$ = 68 mm Hg

   PaO_2 = 122 mm Hg

   HCO_3^- = 32 m Eq/L

7.   What recommendations would you make concerning an appropriate oxygen delivery device?

8.   After successful cardiopulmonary resuscitation, the following blood gas results were obtained while the patient was still being manually ventilated with an F_IO_2 of 0.50.

pH = 7.10

$PaCO_2$ = 50 mm Hg

PaO_2 = 55 mm Hg

HCO_3^- = 15 m Eq/L

   A.   Interpret the results.

   B.   Explain the cause(s) for these results.

   C.   What specific recommendations would you make at this time?

Procedural Competency Evaluation

STUDENT: **DATE:**

ARTERIAL BLOOD GAS INTERPRETATION

	PERFORMANCE RATING	PERFORMANCE LEVEL
Evaluator: ☐ Peer ☐ Instructor **Setting:** ☐ Lab ☐ Clinical Simulation		
Equipment Utilized: **Conditions (Describe):**		

Performance Level:

S or ✓ = Satisfactory, no errors of omission or commission
U = Unsatisfactory Error of Omission or Commission
NA = Not applicable

Performance Rating:

5   **Independent:** Near flawless performance; minimal errors; able to perform without supervision; seeks out new learning; shows initiative; A = 4.7–5.0 average

4   **Minimally Supervised:** Few errors, able to self-correct; seeks guidance when appropriate; B = 3.7–4.65

3   **Competent:** Minimal required level; no critical errors; able to correct with coaching; meets expectations; safe; C = 3.0–3.65

2   **Marginal:** Below average; critical errors or problem areas noted; would benefit from remediation; D = 2.0–2.99

1   **Dependent:** Poor; unacceptable performance; unsafe; gross inaccuracies; potentially harmful; F = < 2.0

Two or more errors of commission or omission of mandatory or essential performance elements will terminate the procedure, and require additional practice and/or remediation and reevaluation. Student is responsible for obtaining additional evaluation forms as needed from the Director of Clinical Education (DCE).

1. Obtains and analyzes an arterial blood gas sample		
2. Evaluates the pH		
3. Evaluates the $PaCO_2$		
4. Evaluates the HCO_3^-		
5. Evaluates the BE		
6. Interprets the acid-base status		
7. If the acid-base status is abnormal, correctly identifies if it is a metabolic or respiratory disturbance		
8. Determines if any compensation is present		
9. Evaluates the PaO_2		
10. Evaluates the SaO_2		
11. Interprets oxygenation status		
12. Uses P-50 to determine if there is a shift in the oxygen dissociation curve		
13. Determines CaO_2 using the oxygen dissociation curve		
14. Calculates $P(A - a)DO_2$		
15. Calculates the F_IO_2 needed for desired PaO_2		

SIGNATURES   Student: Evaluator: Date:

Clinical Performance Evaluation

PERFORMANCE RATING:

5   **Independent:** Near flawless performance; minimal errors; able to perform without supervision; seeks out new learning; shows initiative; A = 4.7–5.0 average

4   **Minimally Supervised:** Few errors, able to self-correct; seeks guidance when appropriate; B = 3.7–4.65

3   **Competent:** Minimal required level; no critical errors; able to correct with coaching; meets expectations; safe; C = 3.0–3.65

2   **Marginal:** Below average; critical errors or problem areas noted; would benefit from remediation; D = 2.0–2.99

1   **Dependent:** Poor; unacceptable performance; unsafe; gross inaccuracies; potentially harmful; F = < 2.0

Circle the appropriate response below. Please be consistent, objective, and honest in your assessment of the student's clinical performance and ability.

PERFORMANCE CRITERIA	SCORE				
COGNITIVE DOMAIN					
1. Consistently displays knowledge, comprehension, and command of essential concepts	5	4	3	2	1
2. Demonstrates the relationship between theory and clinical practice	5	4	3	2	1
3. Able to select, review, apply, analyze, synthesize, interpret, and evaluate information; makes recommendations to modify care plan	5	4	3	2	1
PSYCHOMOTOR DOMAIN					
4. Minimal errors, no critical errors; able to self-correct; performs all steps safely and accurately	5	4	3	2	1
5. Selects, assembles, and verifies proper function and cleanliness of equipment; assures operation and corrects malfunctions; provides adequate care and maintenance	5	4	3	2	1
6. Exhibits the required manual dexterity	5	4	3	2	1
7. Performs procedure in a reasonable time frame for clinical level	5	4	3	2	1
8. Applies and maintains aseptic technique and PPE as required	5	4	3	2	1
9. Maintains concise and accurate patient and clinical records	5	4	3	2	1
10. Reports promptly on patient status/needs to appropriate personnel	5	4	3	2	1
AFFECTIVE DOMAIN					
11. Exhibits courteous and pleasant demeanor; shows consideration and respect, honesty, and integrity	5	4	3	2	1
12. Communicates verbally and in writing clearly and concisely	5	4	3	2	1
13. Preserves confidentiality and adheres to all policies	5	4	3	2	1
14. Follows directions, exhibits sound judgment, and seeks help when required	5	4	3	2	1
15. Demonstrates initiative, self-direction, responsibility, and accountability	5	4	3	2	1

TOTAL POINTS =   /15 = AVERAGE GRADE =

ADDITIONAL COMMENTS: IDENTIFY AREAS OF EXCELLENCE; LIST ERRORS OF OMISSION OR COMMISSION, CRITICAL ERRORS

SUMMARY PERFORMANCE EVALUATION AND RECOMMENDATIONS

☐ PASS: Satisfactory Performance

    ☐ Minimal supervision needed, may progress to next level provided specific skills, clinical time completed

    ☐ Minimal supervision needed, able to progress to next level without remediation

☐ FAIL: Unsatisfactory Performance (check all that apply)

    ☐ Minor reevaluation only

    ☐ Needs additional clinical practice before reevaluation

    ☐ Needs additional laboratory practice before skills performed in clinical area

    ☐ Recommend clinical probation

SIGNATURES

Evaluator (print name):   Evaluator signature: Date:

Student Signature: Date:

Student Comments:

29 Phlebotomy

INTRODUCTION

Phlebotomy[1] is the act of drawing blood from a vein by incision or puncture to obtain a sample for analysis and diagnosis. It has also been known as **venesection** or **venipuncture**. Usually a 5- to 25-mL sample of blood is adequate, depending on what blood tests have been requested. In many circumstances it will be done by a **phlebotomist**, although nurses, doctors, and other medical staff (including respiratory therapists) are also trained to take blood. Phlebotomy is also the treatment of certain diseases such as **hemochromatosis** and primary and secondary **polycythemia**.

Properly performed, phlebotomy does not carry the risk of mortality. It may cause temporary pain and bleeding, but these are usually easily managed. On the other hand, of phlebotomy device injuries, 33% are sustained by phlebotomists and 7% by clinical lab workers; 11% occur while "disassembling" phlebotomy needles, and 22% during or after disposal.[2]

OBJECTIVES

Upon completion of this chapter, the student will be able to:

1. Demonstrate proper patient identification procedures.
2. Practice communication skills required for assessing the level of patient comprehension of the procedure.
3. Apply infection control guidelines and standards associated with equipment and procedures according to CDC guidelines.
4. Demonstrate proper selection and use of equipment necessary to perform a phlebotomy.
5. Demonstrate proper labeling procedures and completion of laboratory requisitions.
6. List preferred venous access sites and factors to consider in site selection.
7. Demonstrate ability to differentiate between the feel of a vein, tendon, and artery.
8. List six areas to be avoided when performing venipuncture and the reasons for the restrictions.
9. Demonstrate use of the different collection methods.
10. Demonstrate adequate preparation of patient.
11. Demonstrate adequate preparation of the venous access site.
12. Summarize the problems that may be encountered in accessing a vein, including the procedure to follow when a specimen is not obtained.
13. Demonstrate application of safety and infection control.

KEY TERMS

biohazard	phlebotomist	sharps container	venesection
hemochromatosis	phlebotomy	tourniquet	vacutainer
needle	polycythemia	venipuncture	

Exercises

EQUIPMENT REQUIRED

- [ ] Artificial phlebotomy practice arms and blocks
- [ ] Phlebotomy chairs with locking armrests
- [ ] **Vacutainer** assembly with shielded, retractable, or blunting needle
- [ ] Plastic vacuum blood-collecting tubes
- [ ] Disposable adapters and needles of differing gauges
- [ ] Dry, sterile sponges
- [ ] Holder/adapter
- [ ] **Tourniquet**
- [ ] Absorbent pad or towel
- [ ] Alcohol prep pads
- [ ] Povidone-iodine wipes/swabs
- [ ] Gauze sponges
- [ ] Adhesive bandages/tape
- [ ] **Biohazard** waste containers
- [ ] **Sharps container**
- [ ] Personal protective equipment—goggles, safety shields, lab coats, masks
- [ ] 5- or 10-mL safety syringes (may be used in place of the evacuated collection tube for special circumstances)
- [ ] Laboratory slip

EXERCISE 29.1 IDENTIFICATION OF VEINS

Identify the four veins illustrated in Figure 29.1 and **record the answers on your laboratory report.**

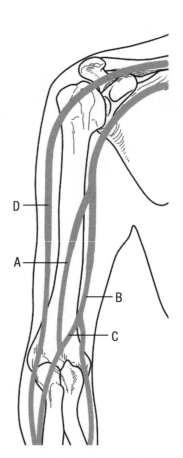

Figure 29.1. Identification of venipuncture sites.

EXERCISE 29.2 PREPARATION OF THE SUBJECT FOR PHLEBOTOMY

Scenario: *Charles Goldberg is a 55-year-old Caucasian male with a history of atrial fibrillation. A pacemaker was implanted 2 years ago and he is currently taking warfarin once a day.*

To perform this exercise, you will need a laboratory partner to simulate a patient and a phlebotomy training device or venipuncture arm.

1. Interview the "patient" and ask for the following:
   A. Use of medications and last therapeutic drug monitoring
   B. Last time exercise or physical activity took place
   C. Presence of stress or anxiety
   D. If pregnant
2. **Chart the answers on your laboratory report.**

EXERCISE 29.3 PREPARATION FOR PHLEBOTOMY

1. Check the requisition form for requested tests, patient information, and any special requirements or physician's orders for test to be obtained.
2. Wash your hands.
3. Gather equipment.
4. Open sterile packages.
5. **List the necessary equipment on your laboratory report.**

EXERCISE 29.4 PHLEBOTOMY PROCEDURE

1. Identify the "patient."
2. Introduce yourself and explain the procedure.
3. Don clean gloves.
4. Approach the "patient" in a friendly, calm manner. Provide for their comfort as much as possible and gain the "patient's" cooperation.
5. Position the "patient." The "patient" should sit in a chair, lie down, or sit up in bed. Hyperextend the "patient's" arm.
6. Place the arm in a straight and independent position, if possible.
7. Select a suitable site for venipuncture.
8. Palpate and trace the path of veins with the index finger. Arteries pulsate, are more elastic, and have thick walls.
9. Place an absorbent pad or towel under the arm to prevent soiling the linen with blood.
10. Place equipment close to work area.
11. Apply a tourniquet 3 to 4 inches above the selected puncture site. Tighten the tourniquet and tell the "patient" to open and close their fist to increase blood flow to arm. Do not leave the tourniquet on for more than 2 minutes.
12. Cleanse with antimicrobial wipe starting at the puncture site and moving in a circular fashion about 2 inches away from site.
13. Allow to air dry.
14. Hold skin taut with nondominant hand. Perform a venipuncture with bevel of needle pointed up at a 15- to 30-degree angle (Fig. 29.2).

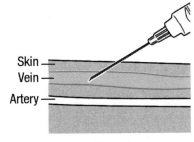

Skin
Vein
Artery

Figure 29.2. Proper bevel position for venipuncture.

15. Lower needle toward skin after needle has entered vein.

16. Thread needle along path of vein. Watch for backflow of blood in syringe.

17. If a syringe is used, pull plunger back gently and check for placement of the needle in the vein. If a vacutainer is used, insert blood collection tube into plastic holder while holding the plastic adapter steady. Press tube firmly into the short needle so that it pierces the top of the tube. Blood should begin to spurt quickly into the tube until filled.

18. If placement is correct, instruct the patient to relax their fist, release the tourniquet, wait a few seconds to allow fresh blood flow to flow into the vein, and then pull back gently on the plunger if the syringe is used.

19. Fill syringe to desired amount.

20. Remove needle from vein, cover the venipuncture site with a sterile sponge, and press firmly on the site for 2 to 3 minutes.

21. Do not remove the top from the laboratory tube. Place the needle straight through the top.

22. Gently eject blood drawn inside of the tube. Do not allow blood to foam or splash because red blood cells can be destroyed.

23. Rotate the tube gently to mix blood with tube contents.

24. Label tube promptly. Write "patient's" name, date, time, and initials of the phlebotomist. (Fig. 29.3).

25. Check "patient's" venipuncture site for oozing.

26. Dispose of shielded needle and syringe in biohazard receptacle.

    A. Do not bend, break, recap, or resheath needles to avoid accidental needle puncture or splashing of contents.

27. Remove gloves, wash hands.

28. Take blood specimens to a designated station or laboratory according to hospital procedure. If you stick yourself with a contaminated needle:

    A. Remove your gloves and dispose of them properly.

    B. Squeeze the puncture site to promote bleeding.

    C. Wash the area well with soap and water.

    D. Record the "patient's" name and ID number.

    E. Follow the institution's guidelines regarding treatment and follow-up.

    NOTE: The use of prophylactic zidovudine following blood exposure to HIV has shown effectiveness (about 79%) in preventing seroconversion.

29. **Summarize the procedure on your laboratory report.**

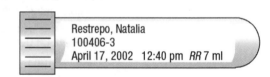

Figure 29.3. Proper labeling of a blood tube.

Restrepo, Natalia
100406-3
April 17, 2002 12:40 pm *RR* 7 ml

EXERCISE 29.5 PHLEBOTOMY TROUBLESHOOTING

If an incomplete collection or no blood is obtained:

1. Change the position of the needle. Move it forward (it may not be in the lumen) (Fig. 29.4) or move it backward (it may have penetrated too far) (Fig. 29.5).

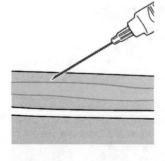

Figure 29.4. Needle not advanced into the vein.

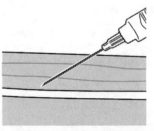

Figure 29.5. Needle advanced through the vein.

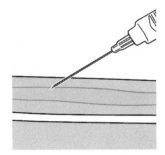

Figure 29.6. Needle positioned against the vein wall.

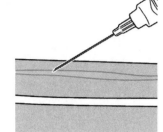

Figure 29.7. Vein collapse.

2. Adjust the angle (the bevel may be against the vein wall) (Fig. 29.6).
3. Loosen the tourniquet (it may be obstructing blood flow).
4. Try another tube (there may be no vacuum in the one being used).
5. Re-anchor the vein (veins sometimes roll away from the point of the needle and puncture site).

If blood stops flowing into the tube or syringe:

1. The vein may have collapsed; resecure the tourniquet to increase venous filling. If this is not successful, remove the needle, take care of the puncture site, and redraw (Fig. 29.7).
2. The needle may have pulled out of the vein when switching tubes. Hold equipment firmly and place fingers against patient's arm, using the flange for leverage when withdrawing and inserting tubes.

Problems Other Than an Incomplete Collection

1. *A hematoma forms under the skin adjacent to the puncture site.* Release the tourniquet immediately and withdraw the needle. Apply firm pressure (Fig. 29.8).
2. *The blood is bright red (arterial) rather than venous.* Apply firm pressure for more than 5 minutes (Fig. 29.9).

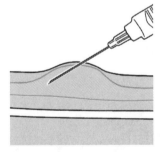

Figure 29.8. Hematoma formation.

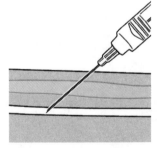

Figure 29.9. Arterial puncture.

REFERENCES
1. Ernst, DJ: Applied Phlebotomy, ed 1. Lippincott Williams & Wilkins, Philadelphia, 2005.
2. EPINet Multihospital Needlestick and Sharp-Object Injury Data Report, 1993–2001; International Health Care Worker Safety Center, University of Virginia Health System (90 healthcare facilities contributing data). (Report provided 5/22/03.)

Laboratory Report

CHAPTER 29: PHLEBOTOMY

Name _____   Date _____

Course/Section _____   Instructor _____

Data Collection

EXERCISE 29.1 Identification of Veins

Label all veins in Figure 29.1.

A. _____

B. _____

C. _____

D. _____

EXERCISE 29.2 Preparation of the Subject for Phlebotomy

Scenario: Charles Goldberg

Document relevant patient history and explain impact on the procedure:

_____

_____

_____

_____

_____

_____

_____

_____

EXERCISE 29.3 Preparation for Phlebotomy

List the necessary equipment for venipuncture:

_____

_____

_____

_____

EXERCISE 29.4 Phlebotomy Procedure

Summarize in chronological order the most important steps in performing a venipuncture.

_____

_____

_____

_____

_____

_____

_____

EXERCISE 29.5 Phlebotomy Troubleshooting

Identify the situations illustrated in Figure 29.10 and describe the corrective action for each.

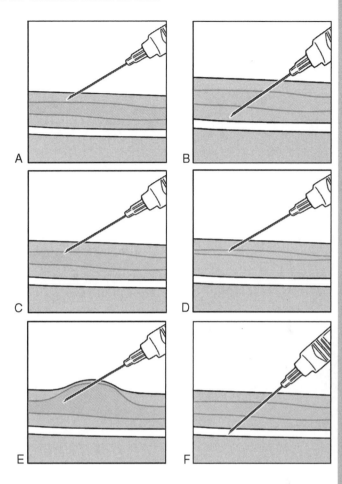

Figure 29.10. Troubleshooting and correcting common phlebotomy problems.

A. _____

B. _____

C. _____

D. _____

E. _____

F. _____

Procedural Competency Evaluation

STUDENT: **DATE:**

VENIPUNCTURE

	PERFORMANCE RATING	PERFORMANCE LEVEL

Evaluator: ☐ Peer   ☐ Instructor   **Setting:** ☐ Lab   ☐ Clinical Simulation

Equipment Utilized: **Conditions (Describe):**

Performance Level:

S or ✓ = Satisfactory, no errors of omission or commission
U = Unsatisfactory Error of Omission or Commission
NA = Not applicable

Performance Rating:

5   **Independent:** Near flawless performance; minimal errors; able to perform without supervision; seeks out new learning; shows initiative; A = 4.7–5.0 average

4   **Minimally Supervised:** Few errors, able to self-correct; seeks guidance when appropriate; B = 3.7–4.65

3   **Competent:** Minimal required level; no critical errors; able to correct with coaching; meets expectations; safe; C = 3.0–3.65

2   **Marginal:** Below average; critical errors or problem areas noted; would benefit from remediation; D = 2.0–2.99

1   **Dependent:** Poor; unacceptable performance; unsafe; gross inaccuracies; potentially harmful; F = < 2.0

Two or more errors of commission or omission of mandatory or essential performance elements will terminate the procedure, and require additional practice and/or remediation and reevaluation. Student is responsible for obtaining additional evaluation forms as needed from the Director of Clinical Education (DCE).

EQUIPMENT AND PATIENT PREPARATION

1. Common Performance Elements Steps 1–8

ASSESSMENT AND IMPLEMENTATION

2. Common Performance Elements Steps 9 and 10

3. Selects the proper blood tubes based on laboratory policy and procedure

4. Hyperextends the arm in a straight and independent position

5. Selects a suitable site for puncture by palpating and tracing veins

6. Applies the tourniquet 3–4 inches above puncture site

7. Tightens tourniquet and asks the patient to make a fist

8. Cleanses puncture site with antimicrobial swab in a circular fashion moving 2 inches away from the puncture site

9. Holds skin taut with the non-dominant hand

10. Inserts needle at a 15- to 30-degree angle with the bevel up

11. Threads needle into vein and observes for a backflow of blood into the needle or syringe

12. If a syringe is used, pulls back on plunger and fills to the proper amount

13. If a vacutainer is used, puts blood tube into the plastic holder and fills to proper amount

14. If blood is not obtained, withdraws needle to below the surface of the skin and repositions needle

15. Removes needle after blood sample is obtained and compresses puncture site for at least 2–3 minutes with sterile gauze

16. Transfers blood from syringe to blood tube

17. Gently mixes blood in the tube

18. Assesses puncture site for active bleeding or oozing

19. Applies adhesive bandage

20. Labels blood tube properly with patient name and ID number

21. Disposes of all sharps properly

22. Delivers sample to designated station or laboratory

FOLLOW-UP

23. Common Performance Elements Steps 11–16

SIGNATURES   Student: Evaluator: Date:

Clinical Performance Evaluation

PERFORMANCE RATING:

5   **Independent:** Near flawless performance; minimal errors; able to perform without supervision; seeks out new learning; shows initiative; A = 4.7–5.0 average

4   **Minimally Supervised:** Few errors, able to self-correct; seeks guidance when appropriate; B = 3.7–4.65

3   **Competent:** Minimal required level; no critical errors; able to correct with coaching; meets expectations; safe; C = 3.0–3.65

2   **Marginal:** Below average; critical errors or problem areas noted; would benefit from remediation; D = 2.0–2.99

1   **Dependent:** Poor; unacceptable performance; unsafe; gross inaccuracies; potentially harmful; F = < 2.0

Circle the appropriate response below. Please be consistent, objective, and honest in your assessment of the student's clinical performance and ability.

PERFORMANCE CRITERIA	SCORE				
COGNITIVE DOMAIN					
1. Consistently displays knowledge, comprehension, and command of essential concepts	5	4	3	2	1
2. Demonstrates the relationship between theory and clinical practice	5	4	3	2	1
3. Able to select, review, apply, analyze, synthesize, interpret, and evaluate information; makes recommendations to modify care plan	5	4	3	2	1
PSYCHOMOTOR DOMAIN					
4. Minimal errors, no critical errors; able to self-correct; performs all steps safely and accurately	5	4	3	2	1
5. Selects, assembles, and verifies proper function and cleanliness of equipment; assures operation and corrects malfunctions; provides adequate care and maintenance	5	4	3	2	1
6. Exhibits the required manual dexterity	5	4	3	2	1
7. Performs procedure in a reasonable time frame for clinical level	5	4	3	2	1
8. Applies and maintains aseptic technique and PPE as required	5	4	3	2	1
9. Maintains concise and accurate patient and clinical records	5	4	3	2	1
10. Reports promptly on patient status/needs to appropriate personnel	5	4	3	2	1
AFFECTIVE DOMAIN					
11. Exhibits courteous and pleasant demeanor; shows consideration and respect, honesty, and integrity	5	4	3	2	1
12. Communicates verbally and in writing clearly and concisely	5	4	3	2	1
13. Preserves confidentiality and adheres to all policies	5	4	3	2	1
14. Follows directions, exhibits sound judgment, and seeks help when required	5	4	3	2	1
15. Demonstrates initiative, self-direction, responsibility, and accountability	5	4	3	2	1

TOTAL POINTS =   /15 = AVERAGE GRADE =

ADDITIONAL COMMENTS: IDENTIFY AREAS OF EXCELLENCE; LIST ERRORS OF OMISSION OR COMMISSION, CRITICAL ERRORS

SUMMARY PERFORMANCE EVALUATION AND RECOMMENDATIONS

☐ PASS: Satisfactory Performance

    ☐ Minimal supervision needed, may progress to next level provided specific skills, clinical time completed

    ☐ Minimal supervision needed, able to progress to next level without remediation

☐ FAIL: Unsatisfactory Performance (check all that apply)

    ☐ Minor reevaluation only

    ☐ Needs additional clinical practice before reevaluation

    ☐ Needs additional laboratory practice before skills performed in clinical area

    ☐ Recommend clinical probation

SIGNATURES

Evaluator (print name):   Evaluator signature: Date:

Student Signature: Date:

Student Comments:

30 Intravenous Insertion and Maintenance

INTRODUCTION

An intravenous insertion site is where a **catheter** is introduced through the skin into a vein for the administration of drugs or fluids. **Intravenous (IV) catheters** are indispensable in modern-day medical practice. Although such catheters provide necessary vascular access, proper insertion and maintenance are critical to reduce the risk for local and systemic infectious complications. Organisms may enter the circulatory system via the intravenous insertion site, directly from the catheter, administration set or IV fluids, or from another site in the body via the bloodstream.[1-6] It is essential for respiratory therapists to be proficient in obtaining intravenous access and assisting with the maintenance of the catheters since their help is becoming more necessary in transport teams.

OBJECTIVES

Upon completion of this chapter, the student will be able to:

1. Demonstrate proper patient identification procedures.
2. Practice communication skills required for assessing the level of patient comprehension of the procedure.
3. Apply infection control guidelines and standards associated with equipment and procedures according to CDC guidelines.
4. Demonstrate proper selection and use of equipment necessary for insertion and maintenance of an intravenous catheter.
5. List preferred venous access sites, and identify factors to consider in site selection.
6. Demonstrate ability to differentiate between the feel of a vein, tendon, and artery.
7. Demonstrate adequate preparation of patient.
8. Demonstrate adequate preparation of the venous access site.
9. Demonstrate proper connection of the intravenous fluids to the catheter.
10. Demonstrate adequate maintenance of the insertion site.
11. Demonstrate removal of the intravenous catheter.
12. Demonstrate application of proper safety and infection control measures.

KEY TERMS

angiocath
biohazard containers

dressing
intravenous catheter

intravenous solution
intravenous tubing

sharps container
tourniquet

Exercises

EQUIPMENT REQUIRED

- [ ] Artificial phlebotomy practice arms and blocks
- [ ] Phlebotomy chairs with locking armrests
- [ ] Intravenous catheters or angiocaths of different gauges
- [ ] Intravenous fluids
- [ ] IV tubing and IV poles
- [ ] Infusion pump
- [ ] Dry, sterile sponges
- [ ] Holder/adapter
- [ ] **Tourniquet**

- [ ] Absorbent pad or towel
- [ ] Alcohol prep pads
- [ ] Povidone-iodine wipes/swabs
- [ ] Semitransparent occlusive dressings
- [ ] Gauze sponges
- [ ] Securing devices/tape
- [ ] **Biohazard** waste containers
- [ ] **Sharps container**
- [ ] Personal protective equipment: gloves, goggles, safety shields, lab coats, masks

EXERCISE 30.1 IDENTIFICATION OF VEINS AND CATHETER PARTS

Review the procedure in Exercise 29.1. Avoid hand veins because of the risk of nerve injuries. Identify the parts of an intravenous catheter as shown in Figure 30.1 and **record them on your lab report.**

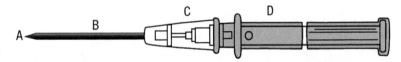

Figure 30.1. Components of an IV catheter.

EXERCISE 30.2 PREPARATION OF THE SUBJECT FOR INTRAVENOUS INSERTION

Scenario 1: Valentina Forgy is a 23-year-old Caucasian woman admitted to the emergency room after a motor vehicle accident. She appeared to suffer a splenic injury and tomography reveals fluid in the abdomen consistent with bleeding. An IV catheter needs to be inserted in the right arm, so IV fluids can be initiated to replace her blood loss. To perform this exercise, you will need a laboratory partner to simulate a patient and a phlebotomy training device or venipuncture arm plus an IV fluid setup.

1. Identify the relevant patient history **and record it on your laboratory report.**

EXERCISE 30.3 INTRAVENOUS INSERTION PROCEDURE

1. Identify the "patient."
2. Wash your hands.
3. Gather equipment and check sterility and expiration dates on the IV fluids.
4. Prepare IV infusion and prime tubing.
5. Introduce yourself and explain the procedure.
6. Don clean gloves.
7. Approach the "patient" in a friendly, calm manner. Provide for their comfort as much as possible and gain the "patient's" cooperation.

8. Position the patient. Hyperextend the patient's arm.

9. Place the arm in a straight and independent position, if possible.

10. Select appropriate venipuncture site. Avoid shaving but trim hair with scissors or clippers.

11. Palpate and trace the path of veins with the index finger. Arteries pulsate, are most elastic, and have thick walls.

12. Place an absorbent pad or towel under the arm to prevent soiling the linen with blood.

13. Place equipment close to work area.

14. Apply a tourniquet 3 to 4 inches above the selected puncture site.

15. Clean the insertion site with an antiseptic solution starting at the insertion site and moving in a circular fashion about 2 inches away from site.

16. Allow to air dry. Do not palpate site after applying antiseptics if wearing nonsterile gloves.

17. Select the smallest-gauge catheter possible. For routine hydration, 22- to 27-gauge is appropriate.

18. Inspect the catheter before insertion to ensure that the needle is fully inserted into the plastic cannula. Prior to venipuncture, hold the catheter hub and rotate the barrel 360 degrees to lose connection.

19. Hold the skin taut with nondominant hand. Perform the venous insertion with bevel of the needle inside the catheter pointed up at a 15- to 30-degree angle.

20. Thread the catheter along path of vein. Observe flashback along the catheter.

21. Upon flashback visualization, lower the catheter almost parallel to the skin.

22. Advance the entire unit slightly before threading the catheter.

23. Thread the catheter into the vein while maintaining skin traction.

24. Release the tourniquet.

25. Apply digital pressure beyond the catheter tip.

26. Gently stabilize the catheter hub.

27. Remove the needle.

28. Flush the cannula with normal saline.

29. Connect primed IV administration to the catheter hub. Handle sterile connections with sterile gloves. Use sterile scissors to anchor the catheter.

30. Initiate flow of IV fluid and assess for signs of extravasation or infiltration.

31. Secure the catheter with tape.

32. Cover with transparent, semipermeable polyurethane dressings where possible to allow visual inspection of the insertion site. Use sterile gauze dressings if the "patient" is perspiring profusely or if the insertion site is bleeding or oozing (Fig. 30.2).

33. Set the fluid infusion rate manually or by using an IV pump (Fig. 30.3).

34. Label dressing with date, time, catheter gauge, and initials (Fig. 30.4).

35. Reconfirm flow after securing the IV catheter.

36. Discard supplies in a biohazard container.

    a. Do not bend, break, recap, or resheath needles to avoid accidental needle puncture or splashing of contents.

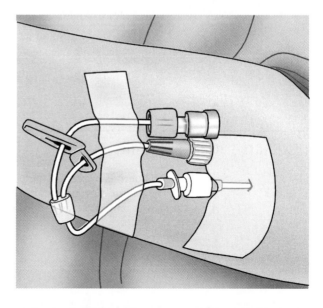

Figure 30.2. IV site dressing.

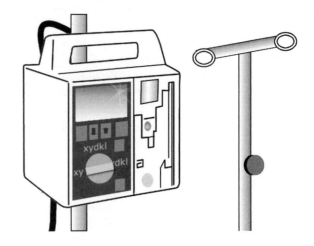

Figure 30.3. IV pump.

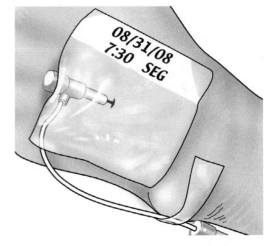

Figure 30.4. Labeling of an IV dressing.

37. Summarize the steps of the procedure and **record them on your laboratory report.**
38. Remove gloves, wash hands.
39. **Record the type of solution, the amount, and the rate of flow on your laboratory report.**

EXERCISE 30.4 INTRAVENOUS RATE INFUSION CALCULATION

The goal of this exercise is to be able to quickly formulate and calculate IV drip rates.

$$\frac{[\text{No. of mL to be infused}] \times [\text{No. of drops in a mL (drop factor)}]}{\text{No. of minutes to infuse the above amount}} = \text{drops/minute}$$

or

$$\frac{\text{IV fluid ordered} \times \text{drop factor}}{\text{Time frame ordered}} = \text{drip rate}$$

EXERCISE 30.4.1 SCENARIO 2

Dr. Cohen has ordered your patient to receive 125 mL of D5W per hour for the next 24 hours. The patient care unit uses tubing with a drop factor of 10. Calculate the drip rate and **record your answer on your laboratory report.**

EXERCISE 30.4.2 SCENARIO 3

Dr. Usuga has ordered a liter of D5W to run this 8-hour shift. If the drop factor is 15, what will be the rate of infusion in drops/minute? **Calculate and record your answer on your laboratory report.**

EXERCISE 30.5 INTRAVENOUS CATHETER MAINTENANCE

1. Check insertion site at least daily and check that the line is patent before each use.
2. Remove the peripheral catheter, and resite if necessary, at least every 72 to 96 hours. If infusing blood, blood products, or lipid emulsions, repeat this step every 24 hours.
3. Change the dressing when soiled or if no longer intact.
4. Assess the external length of the catheter to determine whether migration of the catheter has occurred.
5. For intermittent use, use saline flush once each week or after each use.
6. If the lumen will either not flush or not aspirate and is occluded with blood, a declotting procedure may be necessary per institution protocol.
7. **"Chart" insertion, manipulations, and initial insertion site care on your laboratory report.**

EXERCISE 30.6 INTRAVENOUS CATHETER REMOVAL

1. Remove dressing.
2. Grasp the catheter near the insertion site.
3. Remove it slowly without using excessive force.
4. If resistance is felt, stop removal. Apply warm compress and wait 20 to 30 minutes.
5. Resume removal procedure until the catheter is completely out the insertion site.
6. Gently apply pressure until bleeding, if any, has stopped.
7. Apply a Band-Aid® over the insertion site and follow up a few minutes later to confirm that no bleeding or oozing is present.
8. **"Chart" the IV catheter removal on your laboratory report.**

REFERENCES

1. O'Grady, NO, Alexander, M, Dellinger, EP, et al.: Guidelines for the prevention of intravascular catheter-related infections. MMWR 51(RR10):1–26, 2003.
2. Maki, DG and Ringer, M: Risk factors for infusion-related phlebitis with small peripheral venous catheters: A randomized controlled trial. Ann Intern Med 114:845–854, 1991.
3. Rosenthal, K: Tailor your I.V. insertion techniques for special populations. Nursing 35(5):36–41, 2005.
4. Hadaway, L: Anatomy and physiology related to IV therapy. Intravenous Therapy: Clinical Principles and Practice. WB Saunders, Philadelphia, 1995, pp. 81–110.
5. Royal College of Nursing: Competencies: An education and training competency framework for administering medicines intravenously to children and young people. RCN, London, Publication Code 003 005, 2005.
6. Scales, K: Vascular access: A guide to peripheral venous cannulation. Nursing Standard 19(49):48–52, 2005.

Laboratory Report

CHAPTER 30: INTRAVENOUS INSERTION AND MAINTENANCE

Name _____   Date _____

Course/Section _____   Instructor _____

Data Collection

EXERCISE 30.1 Identification of Veins and Catheter Parts

Please refer to Exercise 29.1 to identify the veins.

Label all parts of the catheter in Figure 30.1

A. _____

B. _____

C. _____

D. _____

EXERCISE 30.2 Preparation of the Subject for Intravenous Insertion

Scenario1: Document relevant patient history and explain impact on the procedure:

_____

_____

_____

_____

_____

EXERCISE 30.3 Intravenous Insertion Procedure

Summarize the most important steps to insert an intravenous catheter in chronological order: _____

_____

_____

_____

_____

_____

_____

_____

_____

_____

_____

_____

_____

_____

EXERCISE 30.4 Intravenous Rate Infusion Calculation

Calculate the rate of infusion for Scenarios 2 and 3. **Show your work!**

Scenario 2 =

Scenario 3 =

EXERCISE 30.5 Intravenous Catheter Maintenance

"Chart" the maintenance of an intravenous catheter:

_____

_____

_____

_____

_____

_____

_____

EXERCISE 30.6 Intravenous Catheter Removal

"Chart" the removal of an intravenous catheter:

_____

_____

_____

_____

Critical Thinking Questions

1.   What is the corrective action if resistance is felt while removing an IV catheter?

2.   If routine hydration is ordered, what type of IV catheter should you use?

3.   What is the purpose of using transparent dressings?

Procedural Competency Evaluation

STUDENT: _____ **DATE:** _____

IV INSERTION		PERFORMANCE RATING	PERFORMANCE LEVEL
Evaluator: ☐ Peer ☐ Instructor **Setting:** ☐ Lab ☐ Clinical Simulation			
Equipment Utilized: **Conditions (Describe):**			
Performance Level: S or ✓ = Satisfactory, no errors of omission or commission U = Unsatisfactory Error of Omission or Commission NA = Not applicable			
Performance Rating: **5** **Independent:** Near flawless performance; minimal errors; able to perform without supervision; seeks out new learning; shows initiative; A = 4.7–5.0 average **4** **Minimally Supervised:** Few errors, able to self-correct; seeks guidance when appropriate; B = 3.7–4.65 **3** **Competent:** Minimal required level; no critical errors; able to correct with coaching; meets expectations; safe; C = 3.0–3.65 **2** **Marginal:** Below average; critical errors or problem areas noted; would benefit from remediation; D = 2.0–2.99 **1** **Dependent:** Poor; unacceptable performance; unsafe; gross inaccuracies; potentially harmful; F = < 2.0 *Two or more errors of commission or omission of mandatory or essential performance elements will terminate the procedure, and require additional practice and/or remediation and reevaluation. Student is responsible for obtaining additional evaluation forms as needed from the Director of Clinical Education (DCE).*			

	PERFORMANCE RATING	PERFORMANCE LEVEL
EQUIPMENT AND PATIENT PREPARATION		
1. Common Performance Elements Steps 1–8		
ASSESSMENT AND IMPLEMENTATION		
2. Common Performance Elements Steps 9 and 10		
3. Selects the proper IV fluid per MD order		
4. Assembles the IV administration set and primes the tubing		
5. Selects the proper gauge IV catheter		
6. Selects a suitable site for IV insertion by palpating and tracing veins		
7. Applies the tourniquet 3–4 inches above puncture site		
8. Tightens tourniquet and asks the patient to make a fist		
9. Cleanses puncture site with antimicrobial swab in a circular fashion moving 2 inches away from the puncture site		
10. Holds skin taut with the nondominant hand		
11. Inserts needle at a 15- to 30-degree angle with the bevel up		
12. Threads needle into vein and observes for a backflow of blood into the needle or syringe		
13. Loosens the tourniquet		
14. Removes the needle while holding the catheter stable		
15. Connects primed IV tubing		
16. Initiates flow of IV fluid		
17. Assesses for infiltration or extravasation		
18. Secures catheter with tape		
19. Covers site with transparent, semi-permeable dressing, allowing for visualization of puncture site		
20. Labels dressing with date, time, catheter size and initials		
21. Initiates fluid infusion rate manually or by IV pump per MD order		
22. Reconfirms flow of IV fluid		
23. Discards all used supplies in biohazard container		
FOLLOW-UP		
24. Common Performance Elements Steps 11–16		

SIGNATURES Student: _____ Evaluator: _____ Date: _____

Clinical Performance Evaluation

PERFORMANCE RATING:

5 **Independent:** Near flawless performance; minimal errors; able to perform without supervision; seeks out new learning; shows initiative; A = 4.7–5.0 average

4 **Minimally Supervised:** Few errors, able to self-correct; seeks guidance when appropriate; B = 3.7–4.65

3 **Competent:** Minimal required level; no critical errors; able to correct with coaching; meets expectations; safe; C = 3.0–3.65

2 **Marginal:** Below average; critical errors or problem areas noted; would benefit from remediation; D = 2.0–2.99

1 **Dependent:** Poor; unacceptable performance; unsafe; gross inaccuracies; potentially harmful; F = < 2.0

Circle the appropriate response below. Please be consistent, objective, and honest in your assessment of the student's clinical performance and ability.

PERFORMANCE CRITERIA	SCORE				
COGNITIVE DOMAIN					
1. Consistently displays knowledge, comprehension, and command of essential concepts	5	4	3	2	1
2. Demonstrates the relationship between theory and clinical practice	5	4	3	2	1
3. Able to select, review, apply, analyze, synthesize, interpret, and evaluate information; makes recommendations to modify care plan	5	4	3	2	1
PSYCHOMOTOR DOMAIN					
4. Minimal errors, no critical errors; able to self-correct; performs all steps safely and accurately	5	4	3	2	1
5. Selects, assembles, and verifies proper function and cleanliness of equipment; assures operation and corrects malfunctions; provides adequate care and maintenance	5	4	3	2	1
6. Exhibits the required manual dexterity	5	4	3	2	1
7. Performs procedure in a reasonable time frame for clinical level	5	4	3	2	1
8. Applies and maintains aseptic technique and PPE as required	5	4	3	2	1
9. Maintains concise and accurate patient and clinical records	5	4	3	2	1
10. Reports promptly on patient status/needs to appropriate personnel	5	4	3	2	1
AFFECTIVE DOMAIN					
11. Exhibits courteous and pleasant demeanor; shows consideration and respect, honesty, and integrity	5	4	3	2	1
12. Communicates verbally and in writing clearly and concisely	5	4	3	2	1
13. Preserves confidentiality and adheres to all policies	5	4	3	2	1
14. Follows directions, exhibits sound judgment, and seeks help when required	5	4	3	2	1
15. Demonstrates initiative, self-direction, responsibility, and accountability	5	4	3	2	1

TOTAL POINTS =   /15 = AVERAGE GRADE =

ADDITIONAL COMMENTS: IDENTIFY AREAS OF EXCELLENCE; LIST ERRORS OF OMISSION OR COMMISSION, CRITICAL ERRORS

SUMMARY PERFORMANCE EVALUATION AND RECOMMENDATIONS

☐ PASS: Satisfactory Performance

  ☐ Minimal supervision needed, may progress to next level provided specific skills, clinical time completed

  ☐ Minimal supervision needed, able to progress to next level without remediation

☐ FAIL: Unsatisfactory Performance (check all that apply)

  ☐ Minor reevaluation only

  ☐ Needs additional clinical practice before reevaluation

  ☐ Needs additional laboratory practice before skills performed in clinical area

  ☐ Recommend clinical probation

SIGNATURES

Evaluator (print name):   Evaluator signature: Date:

Student Signature: Date:

Student Comments:

31 Pulmonary Function Testing

INTRODUCTION

The development and use of advanced medical techniques have allowed people to live longer, particularly patients with lung disease and victims of major trauma. Because of these medical advances, more people with severe respiratory disease and other diseases with respiratory complications are accessing medical care. It therefore became necessary to develop sophisticated methods to objectively measure the function of the respiratory system in order to better evaluate these individuals.

Many lung diseases develop insidiously over time. The pulmonary system has a significant amount of functional reserve so that a large degree of dysfunction can occur through illness or injury[1] before outward signs and symptoms are noted. Detection of lung dysfunction is important for the diagnosis, prevention, treatment, and rehabilitation of patients with lung disease.

Pulmonary function testing (PFT) is a series of diagnostic tests devised to evaluate all aspects of respiratory system function, including,[1] but not limited to, the following:

1. Ventilatory volumes and capacities
2. Airway integrity through measurement of flows and resistance
3. Respiratory muscle strength
4. Mechanical properties of lungs and thoracic cage
5. Efficiency of gas exchange and function of alveolar-capillary membrane
6. Exercise response
7. Response to irritants and bronchoactive drugs

The goals of pulmonary function testing include the following[1]:

1. Determine absence or presence of pulmonary disease abnormalities.
2. Allow for earlier detection and intervention.
3. Measure the severity of the disorder (degree of impairment and extent of disability—how it affects daily activities).
4. Characterize the type of pathophysiology.
5. Follow the course of disease and progression.

6. Measure response to therapy regimens and rehabilitation efforts.

7. Preoperative evaluation—determine surgical risk for postoperative pulmonary complications.

Pulmonary function testing has some limitations. One cannot identify specific diseases entirely without other correlating information, such as the patient's history and physical examination and other diagnostic tests. The variable sensitivity of pulmonary function tests and the large **variability** of what is considered normal make early detection difficult.

Four factors that play an important role in determining the **validity** and **reliability** of pulmonary function testing are equipment use, technician competence, level of patient cooperation and effort, and **reproducibility** of the results. Standards for equipment and test performance help minimize variability and improve the reliability and validity of the test results.

Many different testing protocols, including bedside assessment, screening, complete testing, and specialized testing, are performed for various indications. This chapter focuses on simple spirometry, screening, protocols, flow–volume loops, and postbronchodilator studies.

OBJECTIVES

Upon completion of this chapter, the student will be able to:

1. Practice communication skills needed for the active forceful coaching instruction of subjects performing a forced vital capacity (FVC) maneuver.
2. Practice medical charting for maintaining legal records of pulmonary function results.
3. Apply infection control guidelines and standards associated with equipment and procedures, according to OSHA regulations and CDC guidelines.
4. Calibrate and maintain volume displacement and flow-sensing spirometry equipment.
5. Perform valid and reliable pulmonary function testing of a slow vital capacity (SVC) and FVC maneuver, postbronchodilator study, and maximum voluntary ventilation (MVV) according to American Thoracic Society (ATS) guidelines for spirometry.
6. Interpret graphic representations of volume–time and flow–volume tracings of FVC maneuvers.
7. Manually calculate the FVC, FEV_1, $FEF_{25\%-75\%}$, predicted values, and percent predicted values for a valid spirogram.
8. Interpret pulmonary function testing results.
9. Define the four lung volumes and four lung capacities and analyze their interrelationships.

KEY TERMS

accuracy	intersection	pneumotachometer	validity
calibration	kymograph	reliability	variability
displacement	nomogram	reproducibility	
extrapolation	plateau	sensitivity	

Exercises

EQUIPMENT REQUIRED

- ☐ Volume **displacement** spirometers
- ☐ Disposable mouthpieces
- ☐ Main large-bore tubing
- ☐ Flow-sensing spirometers
- ☐ Disposable flow sensors or in-line filters
- ☐ Disposable noseclips
- ☐ Calibrated graph paper
- ☐ Marking pens
- ☐ Chair
- ☐ Centigrade thermometer
- ☐ 3-liter calibration syringe and adaptors

- ☐ Unit-dose bronchodilators
- ☐ Small-volume nebulizer, connecting tubing, and gas source
- ☐ Metric rulers
- ☐ Tissues
- ☐ Medical waste receptacles
- ☐ Pencils
- ☐ Calculators
- ☐ Stopwatch
- ☐ BTPS conversion charts
- ☐ Predicted values tables or **nomograms**

EXERCISE 31.1 EQUIPMENT IDENTIFICATION

EXERCISE 31.1.1 IDENTIFICATION OF VOLUME DISPLACEMENT SPIROMETERS

Identify the types of volume displacement spirometers shown in Figure 31.1 and **record them on your laboratory report.**

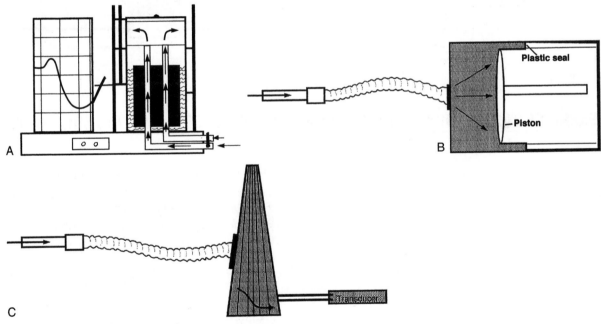

Figure 31.1. Types of volume displacement spirometers.

EXERCISE 31.1.2 IDENTIFICATION OF FLOW-SENSING SPIROMETERS (PNEUMOTACHOMETERS)

Identify the types of flow-sensing spirometers (**pneumotachometers**) shown in Figure 31.2 and record them on your laboratory report.

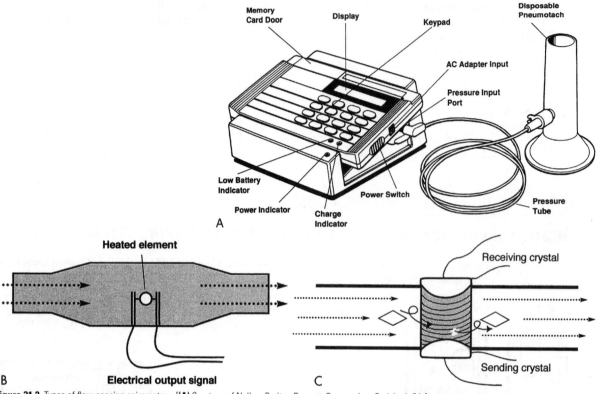

Figure 31.2. Types of flow-sensing spirometers. [(**A**) Courtesy of Nellcor Puritan Bennett Corporation, Carlsbad, CA.]

EXERCISE 31.2 CALIBRATION AND MAINTENANCE OF SPIROMETRIC EQUIPMENT

1. Identify the type of spirometer and brand used and **record it on your laboratory report.**
2. Check to make sure you have an adequate paper supply. Note the paper speed of the machine used (**calibration** in mm/second), and **record it on your laboratory report.**
3. Check to make sure the recording pen (if applicable) is functional and that spares are available.
4. Plug the unit in, if applicable. If a computerized device is used, follow the manufacturer's instructions to enter the date and time.
5. If a volume displacement spirometer is used, check the unit for leaks by occluding the main inlet and attempting to move the piston/bell/bellows connection where the recording pen attaches. No movement should be observed if no leaks are present.
6. Attach the main tubing and repeat step 5. If a leak is detected, check the tubing for holes or tears and replace as necessary.
7. If possible, turn on the recording device and make sure the pen is recording on the baseline.
8. Check the room temperature. Enter it into your computerized spirometer as applicable. **Record the temperature in both Fahrenheit and Celsius on your laboratory report.**
9. Using a 3-liter calibration syringe, check the spirometer for accuracy.
   A. Turn the machine on and enter the calibration mode, if applicable, on a computerized machine.
   B. Pull back the plunger to set the syringe to the 3-liter volume.
   C. Attach the syringe (an adaptor may be required) securely to the main tubing or flow sensing device.
   D. Start the recording device or activate the machine according to manufacturer's directions, and push the entire 3-liter volume into the device. The calibration tracing will appear as shown in Figure 31.3.

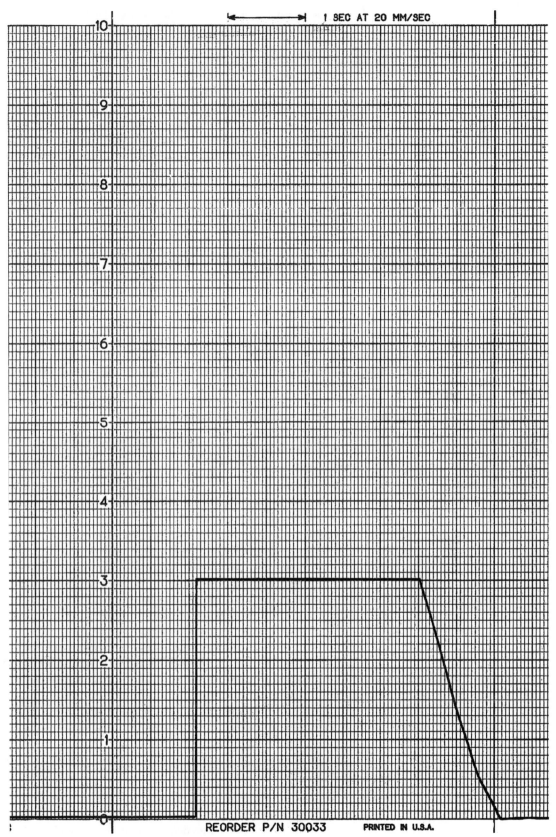

Figure 31.3. Calibration tracing.

E. **Record the measured volume on your laboratory report.** According to ATS standards, the spirometer must be accurate to 3% of the calibrating volume or ±50 mL, whichever is greater.[2]

F. Calculate the percent accuracy of your measurement by the following formula, and **record it on your laboratory report:**

Measured volume: 3 L / 3 L × 100 = Percent accuracy

G. Repeat the calibration while varying the speed at which the calibration volume is injected. **Record your observations of how fast or slow the volume is injected and the effects on the calibration volume on your laboratory report.**

H. For volume displacement spirometers using a kymograph recording device, verify the time calibration by checking the paper speed using a stopwatch. Make a mark on your recording paper. Simultaneously start the recording device and activate the stopwatch. At exactly 10 seconds, simultaneously stop the recording and the stopwatch. Verify that 10 seconds of recording paper have been used.

EXERCISE 31.3 RESPIRATORY HISTORY

Using your lab partner as the patient, obtain a baseline spirometry screening test. This involves obtaining three valid, reproducible FVC maneuvers that meet all ATS standards for spirometry. A screening should not be performed on anyone with an acute illness.

1. Introduce yourself and your department to your subject.

2. Briefly explain the purpose of the test and confirm your subject's understanding by having the subject repeat the instructions back to you.

3. **Have your subject record his or her information on his or her own laboratory report. Record your information on your laboratory report.** Although you will be performing testing on your laboratory partner, for purposes of student confidentiality, **use only your own information and test results for your laboratory report.**

    A. Name and identification number

    B. Age on day of testing

    C. Height in stocking feet

    D. Gender

    E. Race (indicate white or nonwhite for purposes of race correction according to NIOSH and OSHA regulations for spirometry)

4. Determine whether previous testing has ever been done and whether it was done sitting or standing. **Record the information on your laboratory report.**

5. Elicit a respiratory history by asking your subject the following questions. **Record the information on your laboratory report.**

    A. Do you usually have a cough first thing in the morning? Do you cough up any secretions? If so, how much and what color is it usually?

    B. Do you cough for as much as 3 months a year?

    C. Do you ever experience chest tightness, wheezing, shortness of breath on exertion or at rest, or chest pain? Describe quality and location. Are you having any chest pain now?

    D. Have you ever had or been told you have asthma, allergies, pneumonia, chronic bronchitis, emphysema, or tuberculosis?

    E. Do you have a heart condition for which you are under a doctor's care?

    F. Do you take or have you ever taken prescription medicine for a respiratory or cardiac illness? If so, what medications?

    G. Do you take nonprescription medicine for a respiratory illness?

    H. Smoking history:

        i.   Have you ever smoked?

        ii. Do you smoke now?

        iii. How many packs of cigarettes do/did you smoke per day?

        iv. How old were you when you started smoking?

        v.   How long ago did you quit smoking?

        vi. How many years/months have you been smoking?

        vii. Calculate the subject's pack/year history: [(Age now − Age started smoking) − years since stopped smoking] × packs per day = packs/years. **Show your work and answer on your laboratory report.**

I.   Occupational history:
    i.   What type of work do you presently do?
    ii.   What other types of work have you done in the past?
    iii. Have you ever worked in mining, construction, or with insulation? Have you ever been exposed to dusts, fumes, or mists at work?
J.   Family history: List ages, state of health, age at death, and cause of death for mother, father, and siblings.

EXERCISE 31.4 SPIROMETRY SCREENING

NOTE: The following exercises should be done with a volume displacement spirometer if available so that hand calculation of the results can be practiced as part of the laboratory exercises. It should be repeated with a flow-sensing spirometer as well so students gain experience with both types of equipment. Also, each student must practice being both tester and subject in order to have appropriate data to complete the laboratory report.

EXERCISE 31.4.1 IDENTIFICATION OF LUNG VOLUMES AND CAPACITIES

Identify the lung volumes and capacities labeled in Figure 31.4. **Record them on your laboratory report.**

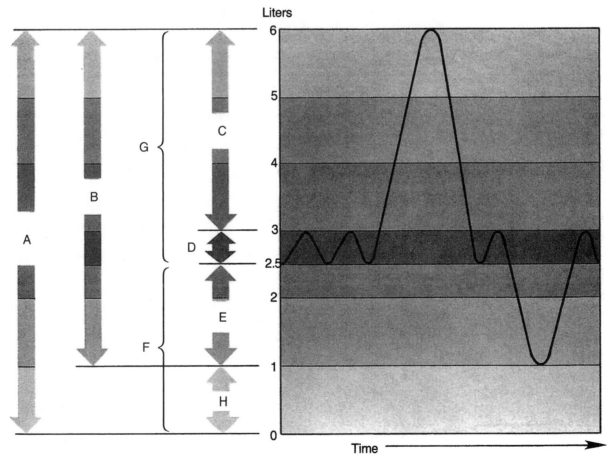

Figure 31.4. Lung volumes and capacities. (From Scanlon, VC and Sanders, T: Essentials of Anatomy and Physiology, ed 2. FA Davis, Philadelphia, 1991, p. 349, with permission.)

EXERCISE 31.4.2 MEASURING SPIROMETRIC LUNG VOLUMES AND CAPACITIES

1. Wash your hands and apply standard precautions and transmission-based isolation procedures as applicable.

2. Aseptically take a clean disposable mouthpiece or flow-sensing device and attach it to the main tubing. If disposable pneumotachometers are used, each one should be calibrated before use in testing.

3. Instruct the subject in the performance of a simple spirogram. Instruct the subject, when indicated, to place the mouthpiece tightly between the teeth with the lips sealed, without the tongue blocking the opening and without biting down, and to relax and breathe normally in and out for five or six breaths. Observe for consistency of tidal volume and breathing pattern. Instruct the subject to take the deepest breath possible and then blow it out *slowly* until you say to stop. Confirm your subject's understanding by having the subject repeat the instructions back to you.

4. Place the noseclips on the subject and verify that there are no leaks. If the subject refuses to use the noseclips, have the subject hold his or her nose if possible.

5. Have the subject sit or stand straight, chin slightly elevated. If the subject is obese, pregnant, or a child, the test should be performed standing. A chair without wheels should be placed behind the subject under these circumstances for safety.

6. Have the subject begin tidal breathing until a relaxed pattern is noted, and then activate the machine and the recording device. Reinforce instructions throughout the test. Record five or six tidal breaths.

7. Actively coach the subject throughout inspiration and expiration to perform the SVC maneuver. At the end of a normal exhalation, instruct the subject to take a maximal inspiration until the lungs are completely full and then exhale slowly until the lungs are completely empty. Remind the subject to continue exhaling until instructed to stop.

8. Observe the subject for adequate effort and proper performance during the maneuver. Reinstruct as necessary.

9. Remove the noseclips and allow the subject to be seated if needed between tests.

10. **Have the subject sign the tracing. Record the room temperature on your laboratory report. Attach the spirogram tracing to the subject's laboratory report. From the spirogram, calculate the values listed on the laboratory report.**

EXERCISE 31.4.3 PERFORMANCE OF SLOW VITAL CAPACITY AND FORCED VITAL CAPACITY MANEUVERS

1. Determine whether there are any contraindications to the performance of a baseline spirometry screening at this time by asking the subject the following questions (the following mnemonic "FRED'S SAFE" may help you remember them):

   "F" Have you had upper respiratory tract illness, inFluenza, or bronchitis within the last 3 weeks?

   "R" Are you wearing any tight or Restrictive clothing that may interfere with the performance of the test?

   "E" Have you Eaten a heavy meal within the last 2 hours?

   "D" Do you have any Dental appliances, loose teeth, caps, gum, or candy in your mouth? Note that dentures should usually be left in place to allow for an adequate seal around the mouthpiece unless they are so loose that they may come out during the test.

   "S" Have you Smoked within the last hour?

   "S" Have you had any recent Surgeries?

   "A" Have you used an Aerosolized bronchodilator within the last 4 to 6 hours?

   "F" How are you Feeling today? Do you have any acute illness at the present time?

   "E" Have you had any Ear infections in the last 3 weeks?

2. If a positive response is obtained to any of the preceding questions, the problem should be corrected or screening spirometry should be postponed for the appropriate length of time. The subject must be free from any acute illness for at least 3 weeks before screening.[3]

3. Wash your hands and apply standard precautions and transmission-based isolation procedures as applicable.

4. Aseptically take a clean disposable mouthpiece or flow-sensing device and attach it to the main tubing. If disposable pneumotachometers are used, each one should be calibrated before use in testing.

5. Instruct the subject in the performance of the SVC maneuver. Explain (and demonstrate, if necessary) the following:

   A. When you indicate, the subject should take as deep a breath as possible, completely filling his or her lungs.

   B. The subject should place the mouthpiece tightly between the teeth with the lips sealed, without the tongue blocking the opening and without biting down.

   C. Without hesitation, the subject should then *slowly* blow the air out until the lungs are as completely empty as possible, until you say to stop.

6. Confirm your subject's understanding by having the subject repeat the instructions back to you.

7. Place the noseclips on the subject and verify that there are no leaks. If the subject refuses to use the noseclips, have the subject hold his or her nose if possible.

8. Have the subject sit or stand straight, chin slightly elevated. If the subject is obese, pregnant, or a child, the test should be performed standing. A chair without wheels should be placed behind the subject under these circumstances for safety.

9. Activate the machine and the recording device. Actively coach the subject throughout inspiration and expiration, and perform the SVC.

10. Observe the subject for adequate effort and proper performance during the maneuver. Reinstruct as necessary.

11. Note the volume obtained and **record it on your laboratory report.**

12. Allow for adequate recovery of the subject. Remove the noseclips and allow the subject to be seated if needed between tests.

13. Replace the noseclips, reinstruct the subject, and repeat the SVC maneuver with active, forceful coaching until three tracings of consistent volume are observed. The two best volumes should be within 200 mL or 5%.

14. Instruct the subject in the performance of the FVC maneuver. Explain (and demonstrate, if necessary) the following:

   A. When you indicate, the subject should take as deep a breath as possible, completely filling his or her lungs.

   B. The subject should place the mouthpiece tightly between the teeth with the lips sealed, without the tongue blocking the opening and without biting down.

   C. Without hesitation, the subject should then blow the air out as hard, fast, and completely as possible, until you say to stop.

15. Confirm your subject's understanding by having the subject repeat the instructions back to you.

16. Place the noseclips on the subject and verify that there are no leaks. If the subject refuses to use the noseclips, have the subject hold his or her nose if possible.

17. Have the subject sit or stand straight, chin slightly elevated. If the subject is obese, pregnant, or a child, the test should be performed standing. A chair without wheels should be placed behind the subject under these circumstances for safety.

18. Activate the machine and the recording device. Actively coach the subject throughout inspiration and expiration, and perform the FVC.

19. Observe the subject for adequate effort and proper performance during the maneuver. Reinstruct as necessary.

20. Note the volume obtained, the shape, and the appearance of the graphic representation, if available.

21. Allow for adequate recovery of the subject. Remove the noseclips and allow the subject to be seated if needed between tests.

22. Verify that the results meet ATS standards for acceptability. The FVC tracings should be free from the following[3]:

   A. Cough or glottic closure (Fig. 31.5).

   B. Variable effort (Fig. 31.6).

   C. Early termination (Fig. 31.7). A plateau should be achieved and is defined as no change in volume in the last 1 second of the tracing. The test should be at least 6 seconds in duration. In subjects with severe chronic obstructive lung disease, the spirometer should be capable of recording for at least 15 seconds. Failure to plateau is shown in Figure 31.8.

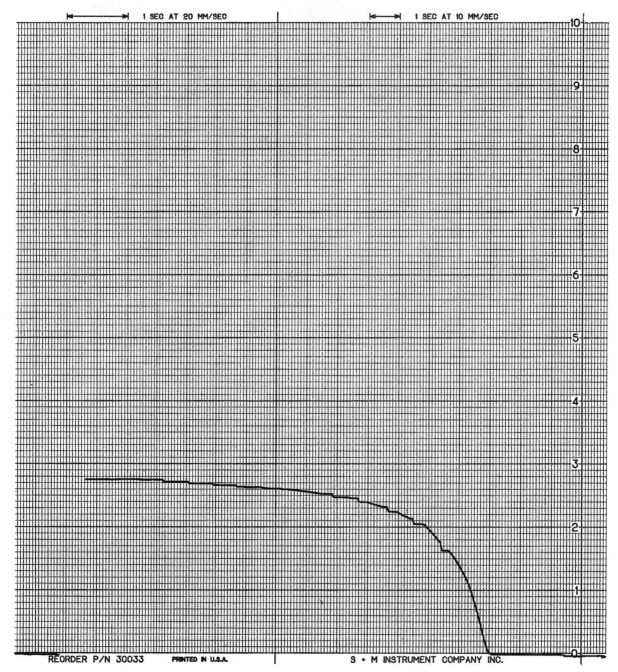

Figure 31.5. Cough or glottic closure on a volume–time tracing. Shown at reduced size.

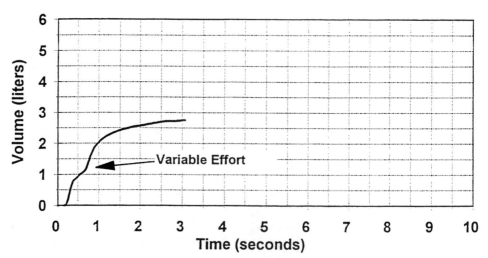

Figure 31.6. Variable effort on a volume–time tracing.

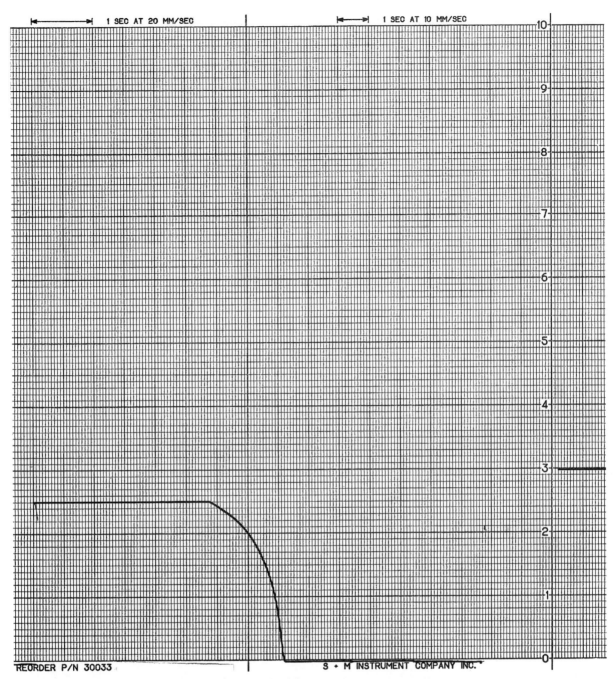

Figure 31.7. Early termination on a volume–time tracing. Shown at reduced size.

  D. Hesitation at the start of the test (Fig. 31.9). Extrapolated volume must be less than 5% of the FVC if the FVC is >3.00 liters or 150 mL if the FVC is <3.00 liters.
  E. Baseline error or leaks.
  F. Excessive variability. There should be less than 5% or 200-mL difference between the two best FVC and FEV$_1$ results. The 1994 ATS standards require less than 200 mL; however, this variability may be excessive with smaller lung volumes.[2,3]

23. It is advisable to have the subject sign and date the spirometric tracing, due to the often litigious nature of pulmonary disability or workers' compensation cases. **Attach it to his or her laboratory report.**

24. Repeat spirometry with a flow-sensing computerized spirometer. **Attach the subject's results to his or her laboratory report for comparison.**

25. Discard any disposable noseclips, mouthpieces, or flow sensors in an infectious waste container when testing is completed. Disinfect any nondisposable mouthpieces and tubings when finished with the laboratory.

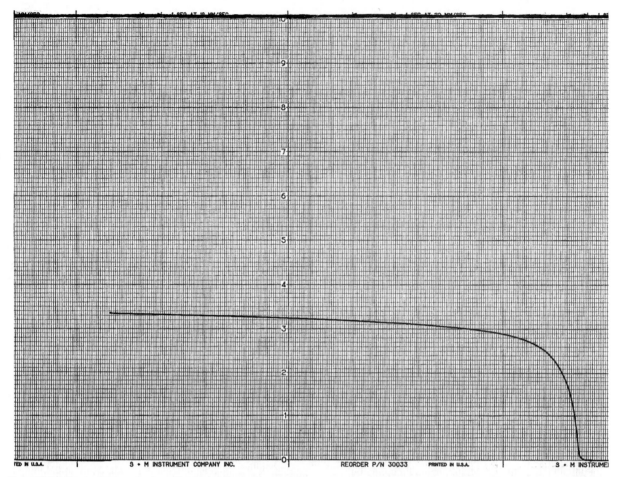

Figure 31.8. Failure to plateau on a volume–time tracing. Shown at reduced size.

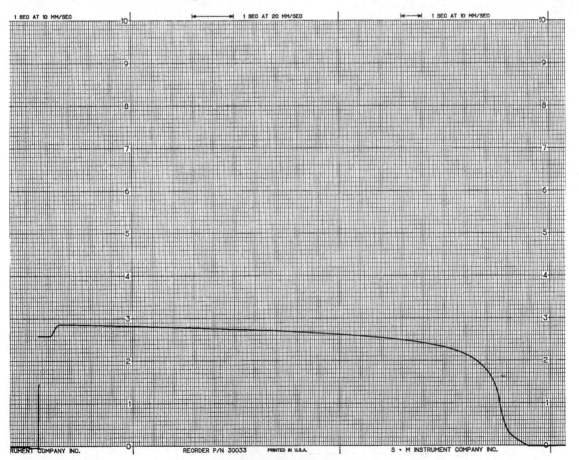

Figure 31.9. Hesitation at the start of the test on a volume–time tracing. Shown at reduced size.

EXERCISE 31.5 CALCULATION OF SPIROMETRIC RESULTS

Using your own graph obtained from a volume displacement spirometer, calculate the following. **Show your work and record the results on your laboratory report.**

1. Determine validity as indicated by three acceptable FVC tracings free from the following:

   Cough or glottic closure

   Early termination of expiration

   Variable effort

   Baseline error

   Excessive hesitation at start of test

2. Measure the SVC at the highest point of the plateau.

3. Measure the FVC in each tracing at the highest point of the plateau.

   A. No excessive variability: two best curves within 5% or 100 mL, whichever is greater.

   Volume A (largest) − Volume B / Volume A (largest) × 100 = Percent

   B. Select the largest FVC.

4. Calculate the variability between the SVC and FVC:

   SVC − FVC / SVC × 100 = Percent

5. Using a metric ruler placed on the volume–time tracing, draw back-extrapolation lines on all FVC tracings on the steepest portion of the curve, as shown in Figure 31.10.

   A. The tracing is valid if the extrapolation volume is less than 5% or 150 mL of the FVC on that curve (volume inside triangle as shown in Fig. 31.11).

   B. Use the point at which the back-extrapolation line intersects the baseline (x axis) as the zero point determination.

6. Measure the FEV_1 on all three tracings by measuring the 1-second distance from the zero point determined in step 3 (Fig. 31.12). Choose the best FEV_1 regardless of which curve it is from, even if it is not the same curve as the best FVC.

7. Calculate the $FEV_1/FVC\%$ ratio.

   $FEV_1/FVC \times 100 = FEV_1/FVC\%$ ($FEV_1\%$)

8. Determine the BTPS correction factor from Table 31.1 using ambient temperature. Correct all volumes and flow rates to BTPS. *Do not* correct the FEV1/FVC% ratio.

   SVC × BTPS correction factor = SVC actual BTPS corrected

   FVC × BTPS correction factor = FVC actual BTPS corrected

   FEV_1 × BTPS correction factor = FEV_1 actual BTPS corrected

   $FEF_{25\%-75\%}$ × BTPS correction factor = $FEF_{25\%-75\%}$ actual BTPS corrected

9. Determine predicted values from tables or nomograms. Correct for race if necessary (NOTE: If NHANES III predicted tables are used, then use the appropriate table for race and do not race-correct).

   Predicted value × 0.85 = Race-corrected value

10. Calculate the percent predicted.

    Actual (BTPS)/Predicted (race-corrected if necessary) × 100 = Percent predicted

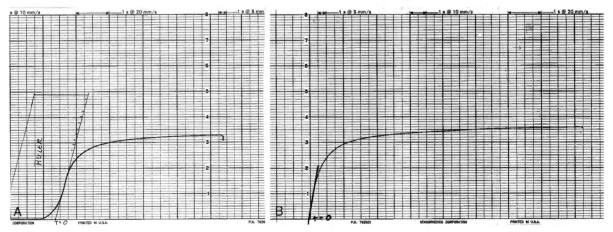

Figure 31.10. Measuring the extrapolation volumes under the curve. Shown at reduced size.

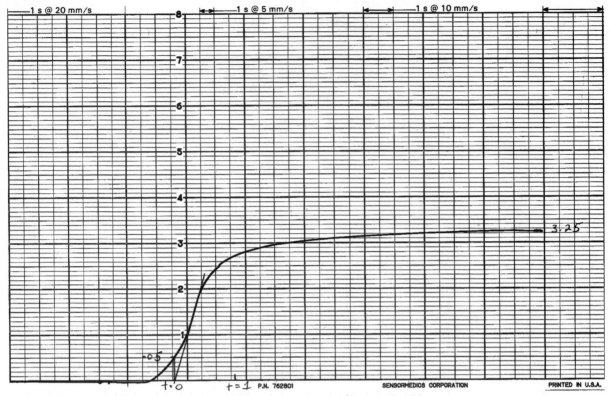

Figure 31.11. Measuring the FEV$_1$ by measuring the 1 second distance from the zero point. Shown at reduced size.

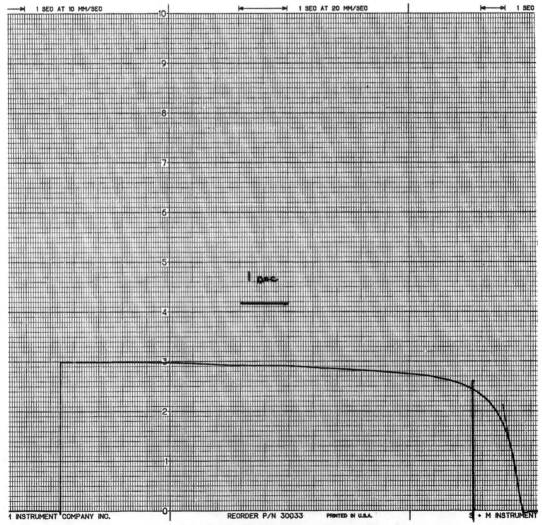

Figure 31.12. Drawing the back extrapolation lines on all FVC tracings along the steepest portion of the curve. Shown at reduced size.

Table 31.1 BTPS Conversion
Factors

Gas Temperature °C (ATPS)	Conversion Factor
18	1.114
19	1.111
20	1.102
21	1.096
22	1.091
23	1.085
24	1.080
25	1.075
26	1.068
27	1.063
28	1.057
29	1.051
30	1.045
31	1.039
32	1.032
33	1.026
34	1.020
35	1.014
36	1.007
37	1.000

$°C = 5 (°F - 32)/9$

NOTE: Round all volumes to two decimal places and all percentages to one decimal place. Label all results correctly.

11. $FEF_{25\%-75\%}$ (Fig. 31.13):
    A. Choose the "best" curve (i.e., the one with best sum of FEV_1 and FVC).
    B. Calculate 25% of FVC. Calculate 75% of FVC. Mark 25% and 75% points on the curve.
    C. Draw a line connecting the 25% and 75% points.
    D. Find any two points *A* and *B* that are 1 second apart on the FEF line.
    E. Measure the volumes at points *A* and *B* (note that these are *not* the 25% and 75% points).
    F. Subtract the difference in volume (point *B* − *A*).
    G. Correct for BTPS. Answer in liters per second.
    H. Obtain a predicted value for the $FEF_{25\%-75\%}$.

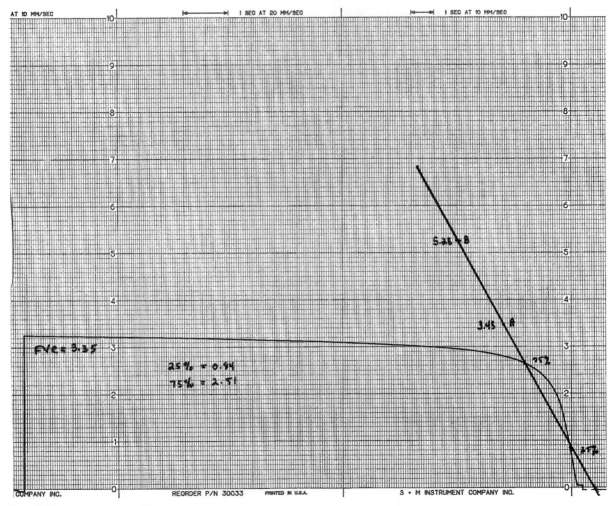

Figure 31.13. FEF$_{25\%-75\%}$ calculation. Shown at reduced size.

EXERCISE 31.6 POSTBRONCHODILATOR STUDY

If any students presently have a prescription for bronchodilators, a prebronchodilator–postbronchodilator comparison may be done with the student's consent.

1. Have the subject administer the bronchodilator via MDI or SVN as previously instructed (Chapter 15).
2. Repeat Exercise 31.4.3.
3. Calculate the percent change in FEV_1 as follows, and **record on your laboratory report:**

   FEV_1 postbronchodilator − FEV_1 prebronchodilator/FEV_1 prebronchodilator × 100
4. Calculate the percent change in FEV_1/FVC ratio ($FEV_1\%$) as follows, and **record on your laboratory report:**

   $FEV_1\%$ pre − $FEV_1\%$ post = Percent change

EXERCISE 31.7 MAXIMUM VOLUNTARY VENTILATION

1. Introduce yourself and your department to your subject.
2. Briefly explain the purpose of the test. Confirm your subject's understanding by having the subject repeat the instructions back to you.
3. Wash your hands and apply standard precautions and transmission-based isolation procedures as applicable.
4. Aseptically attach the mouthpiece to the main tubing.
5. Instruct the subject in the performance of the test. Explain that he or she will be breathing as rapidly and deeply as possible for 12 to 15 seconds (depending on the device used).

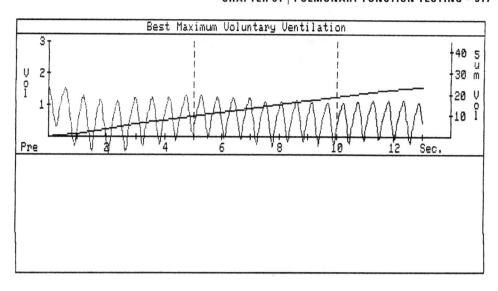

Figure 31.14. MVV tracing.

6. With the subject seated, actively coach him or her to begin breathing as rapidly and deeply as possible. Activate the machine and obtain a tracing (Fig. 31.14). **Record the result on your laboratory report and attach the tracing.**

7. Multiply the volume achieved by 5 (for a 12-second observation) or 4 (for a 15-second observation) to obtain the volume per minute. **Record the duration of the test on your laboratory report. Record the result on your laboratory report.**

EXERCISE 31.8 FLOW–VOLUME LOOPS

If the spirometer you are using is capable of performing a flow–volume loop, follow the manufacturer's directions and complete the following:

1. Introduce yourself and your department to the subject.
2. Explain the purpose of the test. Confirm understanding by having the subject repeat the instructions back to you.
3. Obtain subject information (age, gender, height, weight, and race) and enter the data into the spirometer.
4. Wash your hands and apply standard precautions and transmission-based isolation procedures as applicable.
5. Aseptically take a clean disposable mouthpiece or flow-sensing device and attach it to the main tubing. If disposable pneumotachometers are used, each one should be calibrated before use in testing.
6. Instruct the subject in the performance of the flow–volume loop maneuver. Explain (and demonstrate, if necessary) the following:
   A. The subject should place the mouthpiece tightly between the teeth with the lips sealed, without the tongue blocking the opening and without biting down.
   B. When you indicate, the subject should take as deep a breath as possible, completely filling the lungs.
   C. Without hesitation, the subject should then blow the air out as hard, fast, and completely as possible, until you say to stop. As soon as the subject's lungs are empty, the subject should take a maximum deep breath without removing the mouthpiece.
7. Confirm your subject's understanding by having the subject repeat the instructions back to you.
8. Place the noseclips on the subject and verify that there are no leaks. If the subject refuses to use the noseclips, have the subject hold his or her nose if possible.
9. Have the subject sit or stand straight, chin slightly elevated. If the subject is obese, pregnant, or a child, the test should be performed standing. A chair without wheels should be placed behind the subject under these circumstances for safety.
10. Activate the machine and the recording device. Actively coach the subject throughout inspiration and expiration, and perform the flow–volume loop.
11. Observe the subject for adequate effort and proper performance during the maneuver. Reinstruct as necessary.

12. Note the volume obtained on the first effort and the shape and appearance of the graphic representation if available.

13. Allow for adequate recovery of the subject. Remove the noseclips and allow the subject to be seated if needed between tests.

14. Replace the noseclips, reinstruct the subject, and repeat the maneuver with active, forceful coaching until three acceptable tracings are obtained according to ATS standards. The three tracings should be free from the following:

> Cough or glottic closure (Fig. 31.15)
>
> Variable effort (Fig. 31.16)
>
> Early termination (Fig. 31.17)
>
> Hesitation at the start of the test (Fig. 31.18). The extrapolated volume must be less than 5% of the FVC or 150 mL , whichever is greater.
>
> Baseline error
>
> Excessive variability. There should be no more than a 5% or 200-mL difference between the two best FVC and FEV_1 results.

15. Have the subject sign and date the spirometric tracing. **Attach it to his or her laboratory report.**

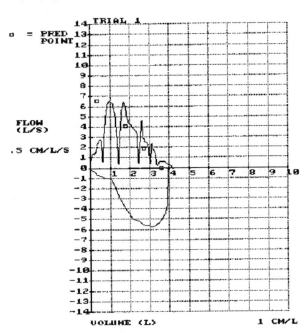

Figure 31.15. Flow–volume loop with cough or glottic closure.

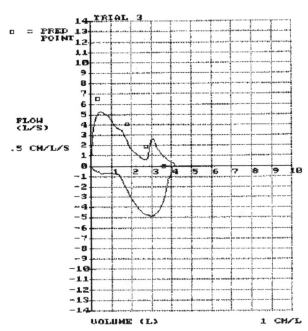

Figure 31.16. Flow–volume loop with variable effort.

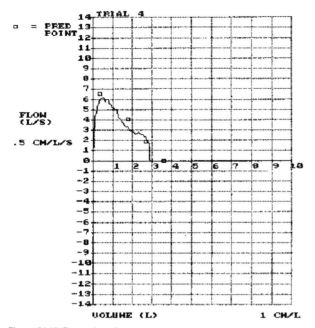

Figure 31.17. Flow–volume loop with early termination.

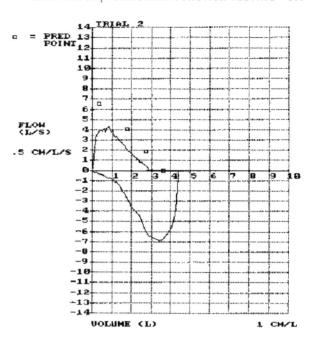

Figure 31.18. Flow–volume loop with hesitation at the start of the test.

REFERENCES

1. American Association for Respiratory Care: AARC clinical practice guideline: Spirometry. Respir Care 36:1414–1417, 1991.
2. NIOSH Spirometry Training Guide. Universities Occupational Safety and Health Educational Resource Center, Continuing Education and Outreach Program; and Centers for Disease Control and Prevention, National Institute for Occupational Safety and Health, Morgantown, WV, 1997.
3. American Thoracic Society: Standardization of spirometry: 1994 update. Am J Respir Crit Care Med 152:1107–1136, 1995.

Laboratory Report

CHAPTER 31: PULMONARY FUNCTION TESTING

Name _____ Date _____

Course/Section _____ Instructor _____

Data Collection

EXERCISE 31.1 Equipment Identification

EXERCISE 31.1.1 IDENTIFICATION OF VOLUME DISPLACEMENT SPIROMETERS

A. _____

B. _____

C. _____

EXERCISE 31.1.2 IDENTIFICATION OF FLOW-SENSING SPIROMETERS (PNEUMOTACHOMETERS)

A. _____

B. _____

C. _____

EXERCISE 31.2 Calibration and Maintenance of Spirometric Equipment

1. Type: _____

Brand: _____

2. Paper speed (calibration mm/sec): _____

3. Room temperature: _____ °F (_____°C)

4. Calibration volume: _____

Percent accuracy: _____ (**show your work!**)

Calibration injection speed observations: _____

_____

_____

EXERCISE 31.3 Respiratory History

1. Name and identification number: _____

2. Age on day of testing: _____

3. Height in stocking feet: _____

4. Gender: _____

5. Race: _____

6. Previous testing: _____

7. Sitting or standing: _____

8. Respiratory history

   A. Do you usually have a cough first thing in the morning? _____

   B. Do you cough up any secretions? If so, how much and what color is it usually? _____

   C. Do you cough for as much as 3 months a year? _____

   D. Do you ever experience chest tightness, wheezing, shortness of breath (on exertion or at rest), or chest pain (quality and duration)? _____

   E. Have you ever had or been told you have asthma, allergies, pneumonia, chronic bronchitis, emphysema, or tuberculosis? _____

   F. Do you have a heart condition for which you are under a doctor's care? Do you have any chest pain now?

       _____

   G. Do you take or have you ever taken prescription medicine for a respiratory or cardiac illness? If so, what medications? _____

   H. Do you take nonprescription medicine for a respiratory illness? _____

9. Smoking history

   A. Have you ever smoked? _____

   B. Do you smoke now? _____

   C. How many packs of cigarettes do/did you smoke per day? _____

   D. How old were you when you started smoking? _____

   E. How long ago did you quit smoking? _____

   F. How many years/months have you been smoking? _____

   G. Calculate the subject's pack/year history

       (Show your work): _____

       _____

       _____

10. Occupational history

    A. What type of work do you presently do? _____

    B. What other types of work have you done in the past? _____

    C. Have you ever worked in mining, in construction, or with insulation? Have you ever been exposed to dusts, fumes, or mists at work? _____

11. Family history

    A. Mother: _____

    B. Father: _____

    C. Siblings: _____

EXERCISE 31.4 Spirometry Screening

EXERCISE 31.4.1 IDENTIFICATION OF LUNG VOLUMES AND CAPACITIES

A. _____

B. _____

C. _____

D. _____

E. _____

F. _____

G. _____

H. _____

EXERCISE 31.4.2 MEASURING SPIROMETRIC LUNG VOLUMES AND CAPACITIES

From the attached spirogram, calculate the following:

Room temperature: _____

Measure all tidal breaths recorded: _____

Average the V_T (**show your work**): _____

_____

Correct for BTPS: $V_T \times$ BTPS correction factor: _____

Measure the following from the spirometric tracing:

IC (BTPS) = _____

IRV (BTPS) = _____

VC (BTPS) = _____

ERV (BTPS) = _____

EXERCISE 31.4.3 PERFORMANCE OF SLOW VITAL CAPACITY AND FORCED VITAL CAPACITY MANEUVERS

Recorded SVC: _____

Attach results from volume displacement and flow-sensing spirometer.

EXERCISE 31.5 Calculation of Spirometric Results

Attach the spirometric volume–time tracing obtained with your measurements and calculate the following (show your work):

Date: _____

Time: _____

Temperature: _____

FVC results

A: _____

B: _____

C: _____

Percent variability for FVC: _____

SVC results: _____

Percent variability between SVC and FVC: _____

FEV_1 results

A: _____

B: _____

C: _____

Whose predicted values used: _____

Best FEV_1 (BTPS): _____

FEV_1 predicted: _____

FEV_1 percent predicted: _____

Best FVC (BTPS): _____

FVC predicted: _____

FVC percent predicted: _____

FEV_1/FVC%: _____

$FEF_{25\%-75\%}$: _____

Compare your hand-calculated results with the computerized spirometric results: _____

_____

_____

EXERCISE 31.6 Postbronchodilator Study

Attach results of postbronchodilator study, if applicable. Compare prebronchodilator and postbronchodilator results:

Percent change FEV_1: _____

Percent change FEV_1/FVC%: _____

EXERCISE 31.7 Maximum Voluntary Ventilation

Duration (seconds) of test: _____

MVV: _____ L/min

EXERCISE 31.8 Flow–Volume Loops

Attach the results of the flow–volume loop, if available.

Critical Thinking Questions

1. What lung volumes and capacities cannot be measured directly by spirometry?

2. Identify three methods to measure the volumes and capacities listed in Critical Thinking Question 1.

3. What is considered a significant change in preshift to postshift, or prebronchodilator to postbronchodilator spirometric results? What factors might account for a change in spirometric values from preshift to postshift workers?

4. What is considered a significant change in annual spirometric results? What factors might account for changes in annual spirometry?

5. Calculate the following (**show all work**):

    V_T = 500 mL

    IRV = 3,000 mL

    ERV = 1,000 mL

    RV = 1,500 mL

    A. TLC = _____

    B. VC = _____

    C. IC = _____

    D. FRC = _____

6. Calculate the following (**show all work**):

    V_T = 400 mL

    IC = 1,000 mL

    FRC = 3,000 mL

    ERV = 600 mL

    A. VC = _____

    B. TLC = _____

    C. RV = _____

    D. IRV: _____

7. Calculate the following (**show all work**):

    TLC = 6,000 mL

    FRC = 3,500 mL

    ERV = 1,500 mL

    V_T = 500 mL

    A. VC = _____

    B. IC = _____

8. For the flow–volume loop shown in Figure 31.19, calculate the FVC, FIVC, PEF_{max} (peak expiratory flow), PIF_{max} (peak inspiratory flow), and ratio of $PEF_{50\%}/PIF_{50\%}$.

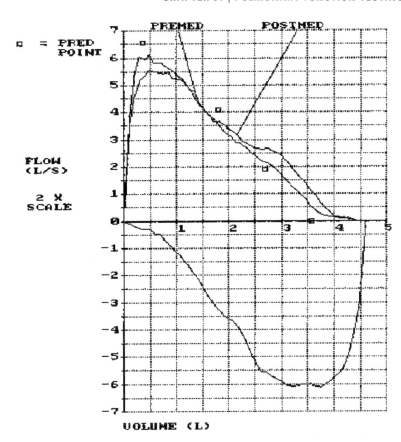

Figure 31.19. Flow–volume loop for calculation.

9. What would sawtoothing on the inspiratory loop of a flow–volume tracing most likely represent?

10. Interpret the following pulmonary function tests:

    A. A 39-year-old man has a chief complaint of shortness of breath on exertion. Results of the spirometry screening are as follows:

Prebronchodilator	Predicted	Percent predicted	Postbronchodilator	Percent predicted
FVC 4.09 L	4.64 L	88.1%	4.00 L	86.2%
FEV$_1$ 1.94 L	3.73 L	52.0%	1.98 L	53.1%
FEV$_1$/FVC%	47.4%	80.4%	—	49.5%

B. A slightly dyspneic coal miner who is a heavy smoker has a respiratory rate of 25/minute with the following ABG and PFT results:

pH   7.43
$PaCO_2$ 50 mm Hg
HCO_3^- 32 mm Hg
PaO_2 55 mm Hg (drawn breathing room air)

	Predicted	Actual
VC	4.4 L	3.0 L
FEV_1	3.4	1.8 L
$FEF_{25\%-75\%}$	3.8 L/sec	2.0 L/sec
D_LCO	26	24
MVV	150 Lpm	85 Lpm
FRC	6.0 L	4.0 L

C. John Bart, 40 years of age, 72 inches tall, and 165 pounds, had been working in the steel mill since he was 17 years old. During the past 6 months he has been experiencing worsening of his shortness of breath. He is now not able to work. He quit smoking 1 week ago. He had been smoking one pack a day since he was 16. Results are as follows:

Spirometry	Prebronchodilator	Predicted	Percent predicted	Postbronchodilator	Percent predicted
FVC	3.25 L	5.42	60.0%	3.22 L	59.4%
FEV_1	2.30 L	4.08 L	56.4%	2.35 L	57.6%
FEV_1/FVC %	70.8	75.3	—	73.0	—
$FEF_{25\%-75\%}$	1.59 L/sec	4.55 L/sec	35.0%	1.77 L/sec	38.9%
MVV	88 Lpm	147 Lpm	60.0%	95 Lpm	64.6%
FRC	2.98 L	4.20 L	71.0%		
RV	1.52 L	2.20 L	69.0%		
TLC	4.77 L	7.62 L	63.0%		
RV/TLC%	31.9%	28.9%			
D_LCO	8.4	30.9	27.2%		

Procedural Competency Evaluation

STUDENT: **DATE:**

SCREENING SPIROMETRY CASE

Evaluator:	☐ Peer	☐ Instructor		**Setting:**	☐ Lab		☐ Clinical Simulation

Equipment Utilized: **Conditions (Describe):**

Performance Level:

S or ✓ = Satisfactory, no errors of omission or commission
U = Unsatisfactory Error of Omission or Commission
NA = Not applicable

Performance Rating:

5   **Independent:** Near flawless performance; minimal errors; able to perform without supervision; seeks out new learning; shows initiative; A = 4.7–5.0 average

4   **Minimally Supervised:** Few errors, able to self-correct; seeks guidance when appropriate; B = 3.7–4.65

3   **Competent:** Minimal required level; no critical errors; able to correct with coaching; meets expectations; safe; C = 3.0–3.65

2   **Marginal:** Below average; critical errors or problem areas noted; would benefit from remediation; D = 2.0–2.99

1   **Dependent:** Poor; unacceptable performance; unsafe; gross inaccuracies; potentially harmful; F = < 2.0

Two or more errors of commission or omission of mandatory or essential performance elements will terminate the procedure, and require additional practice and/or remediation and reevaluation. Student is responsible for obtaining additional evaluation forms as needed from the Director of Clinical Education (DCE).

(Columns at right: PERFORMANCE RATING | PERFORMANCE LEVEL)

PATIENT AND EQUIPMENT PREPARATION

1. Common Performance Elements Steps 1–8

2. Plugs the unit in if applicable; enters the date and time and patient information; confirms correct normal values are being utilized

3. If a volume displacement spirometer is used, checks the unit for leaks

4. Turns on the recording device and makes sure the pen is recording on the baseline, if applicable

5. Checks and enters the room temperature

6. Using a 3-liter calibration syringe, checks the spirometer for accuracy; calculates and records the percent accuracy

    A. Repeats the calibration while varying the speed of volume injection; ensures within 3% or 50 mL

ASSESSMENT AND IMPLEMENTATION

7. Common Performance Elements Steps 9 and 10

8. Assesses subject by obtaining the following information:
    A. Name and identification number
    B. Age on day of testing
    C. Height in stocking feet (or arm span, if subject unable to stand)
    D. Gender
    E. Race; indicate as white or non-white for purposes of race correction according to NIOSH and OSHA regulations for spirometry

9. Determines if previous testing has ever been done and whether it was done sitting or standing

10. Elicits a respiratory history including cough/sputum production, smoking history, dyspnea at rest and on exertion, medications, employment history, and previous illnesses

11. Determines if there are any contraindications to the performance of a baseline spirometry screening at this time by asking the subject the following questions: (acronym FREDS SAFE)
    A. (F) Upper respiratory tract illness, influenza, or bronchitis within the last 3 weeks?
    B. (R) Wearing any tight or restrictive clothing that may interfere with the performance of the test?
    C. (E) Eaten a heavy meal within the last 2 hours?
    D. (D) Any dental appliances, loose teeth, caps, gum or candy in your mouth? Remove as appropriate.
    E. (S) Have you smoked within the last hour?
    F. (S) Recent surgeries?
    G. (A) Used an aerosolized bronchodilator within the last 4 to 6 hours?
    H. (F) How are you feeling today? Do you have any acute illness at the present time?
    I. (E) Ear infections in the last 3 weeks?
    J. If a positive response is obtained to any of the above questions, corrects problems or postpones test for the appropriate time period.

12. Aseptically attaches clean disposable mouthpiece or flow sensing device to the main tubing; calibrates as needed

13. Instructs the subject in the performance of the SVC maneuver and confirms subject's understanding

14. Places the noseclips on the subject and verifies that there are no leaks

15. Positions the subject by instructing him or her to sit or stand straight as appropriate, with chin slightly elevated; places a chair without wheels behind the subject if standing

16. Activates the machine and recording device; actively coaches the subject throughout inspiration and expiration and performs the SVC

17. Observes the subject for adequate effort and proper performance during the maneuver; reinstructs as necessary

Procedural Competency Evaluation

STUDENT: _____ DATE: _____

SCREENING SPIROMETRY CASE *(continued)*

	PERFORMANCE RATING	PERFORMANCE LEVEL
18. Notes the volume obtained		
19. Allows for adequate recovery of the subject		
20. Repeats the SVC maneuver with active, forceful coaching until three tracings within 5% or 200 mL of each other are obtained		
21. Instructs the subject in the performance of the FVC maneuver and confirms subject's understanding		
22. Places the noseclips on the subject and verifies that there are no leaks; repositions subject		
23. Activates machine and performs FVC with active, forceful coaching throughout		
24. Observes the subject for adequate effort and proper performance during the maneuver; reinstructs as necessary		
25. Notes the volume obtained and the shape and the appearance of the graphic representation if available		
26. Allows for adequate recovery of the subject		
27. Determines validity of the test:		
A. Three acceptable tracings free from:		
1) Cough or glottic closure		
2) Early termination of expiration		
3) Variable effort		
4) Baseline error		
5) Excessive hesitation at start of test		
B. Extrapolated volume must be less than 5% of the FVC or 150 mL, whichever is greater		
C. Plateau is defined as no change in volume in the last 1 second of the tracing		
D. The test should be at least 6 seconds in duration		
E. Excessive variability: There should be less than 5% or 200 mL difference between the two best FVC and FEV_1 results		
28. Compares the SVC and FVC volumes and explains any discrepancies		
29. If a post-bronchodilator test is ordered, administers the medication, waits an appropriate length of time, and repeats the FVC		
A. Calculates the percent change in FEV_1		
B. Calculate the percent change in FEV_1/FVC ratio (FEV_1%)		
30. Instructs the subject in the MVV maneuver, if appropriate, and confirms understanding		
A. With the subject seated, has subject begin breathing as rapidly and deeply as possible		
B. Activates the machine and actively coaches test performance for 12 to 15 seconds		
C. Allows for adequate recovery of subject		
D. Multiplies the volume achieved by 6 or 4 to obtain the volume/minute; records the results		
E. Repeats the test; assures variability no greater than 10%		
FOLLOW-UP		
31. Common Performance Elements Steps 11–16		
32. Has the subject sign and date the spirometric tracing		

SIGNATURES   Student: _____   Evaluator: _____   Date: _____

Clinical Performance Evaluation

SCREENING SPIROMETRY CASE

PERFORMANCE RATING:

5 **Independent:** Near flawless performance; minimal errors; able to perform without supervision; seeks out new learning; shows initiative; A = 4.7–5.0 average

4 **Minimally Supervised:** Few errors, able to self-correct; seeks guidance when appropriate; B = 3.7–4.65

3 **Competent:** Minimal required level; no critical errors; able to correct with coaching; meets expectations; safe; C = 3.0–3.65

2 **Marginal:** Below average; critical errors or problem areas noted; would benefit from remediation; D = 2.0–2.99

1 **Dependent:** Poor; unacceptable performance; unsafe; gross inaccuracies; potentially harmful; F = < 2.0

Circle the appropriate response below. Please be consistent, objective, and honest in your assessment of the student's clinical performance and ability.

PERFORMANCE CRITERIA	SCORE				
COGNITIVE DOMAIN					
1. Consistently displays knowledge, comprehension, and command of essential concepts	5	4	3	2	1
2. Demonstrates the relationship between theory and clinical practice	5	4	3	2	1
3. Able to select, review, apply, analyze, synthesize, interpret, and evaluate information; makes recommendations to modify care plan	5	4	3	2	1
PSYCHOMOTOR DOMAIN					
4. Minimal errors, no critical errors; able to self-correct; performs all steps safely and accurately	5	4	3	2	1
5. Selects, assembles, and verifies proper function and cleanliness of equipment; assures operation and corrects malfunctions; provides adequate care and maintenance	5	4	3	2	1
6. Exhibits the required manual dexterity	5	4	3	2	1
7. Performs procedure in a reasonable time frame for clinical level	5	4	3	2	1
8. Applies and maintains aseptic technique and PPE as required	5	4	3	2	1
9. Maintains concise and accurate patient and clinical records	5	4	3	2	1
10. Reports promptly on patient status/needs to appropriate personnel	5	4	3	2	1
AFFECTIVE DOMAIN					
11. Exhibits courteous and pleasant demeanor; shows consideration and respect, honesty, and integrity	5	4	3	2	1
12. Communicates verbally and in writing clearly and concisely	5	4	3	2	1
13. Preserves confidentiality and adheres to all policies	5	4	3	2	1
14. Follows directions, exhibits sound judgment, and seeks help when required	5	4	3	2	1
15. Demonstrates initiative, self-direction, responsibility, and accountability	5	4	3	2	1

TOTAL POINTS =   /15 = AVERAGE GRADE =

ADDITIONAL COMMENTS: IDENTIFY AREAS OF EXCELLENCE; LIST ERRORS OF OMISSION OR COMMISSION, CRITICAL ERRORS

SUMMARY PERFORMANCE EVALUATION AND RECOMMENDATIONS

☐ PASS: Satisfactory Performance

☐ Minimal supervision needed, may progress to next level provided specific skills, clinical time completed

☐ Minimal supervision needed, able to progress to next level without remediation

☐ FAIL: Unsatisfactory Performance (check all that apply)

☐ Minor reevaluation only

☐ Needs additional clinical practice before reevaluation

☐ Needs additional laboratory practice before skills performed in clinical area

☐ Recommend clinical probation

SIGNATURES

Evaluator (print name):   Evaluator signature: Date:

Student Signature: Date:

Student Comments:

Procedural Competency Evaluation

STUDENT: **DATE:**

FLOW–VOLUME LOOP (FVL)

Evaluator: ☐ Peer ☐ Instructor   **Setting:** ☐ Lab   ☐ Clinical Simulation

Equipment Utilized: **Conditions (Describe):**

Performance Level:

S or ✓ = Satisfactory, no errors of omission or commission
U = Unsatisfactory Error of Omission or Commission
NA = Not applicable

Performance Rating:

5   **Independent:** Near flawless performance; minimal errors; able to perform without supervision; seeks out new learning; shows initiative; A = 4.7–5.0 average

4   **Minimally Supervised:** Few errors, able to self-correct; seeks guidance when appropriate; B = 3.7–4.65

3   **Competent:** Minimal required level; no critical errors; able to correct with coaching; meets expectations; safe; C = 3.0–3.65

2   **Marginal:** Below average; critical errors or problem areas noted; would benefit from remediation; D = 2.0–2.99

1   **Dependent:** Poor; unacceptable performance; unsafe; gross inaccuracies; potentially harmful; F = < 2.0

Two or more errors of commission or omission of mandatory or essential performance elements will terminate the procedure, and require additional practice and/or remediation and reevaluation. Student is responsible for obtaining additional evaluation forms as needed from the Director of Clinical Education (DCE).

	PERFORMANCE RATING	PERFORMANCE LEVEL
EQUIPMENT AND PATIENT PREPARATION		
1. Common Performance Elements Steps 1–8		
ASSESSMENT AND IMPLEMENTATION		
2. Common Performance Elements Steps 9 and 10		
3. Properly calibrates equipment with a 3.00 liter calibration syringe		
4. Properly sets-up equipment for the FVL maneuver		
5. Gathers necessary patient demographic information		
6. Instructs the patient in the proper performance of the maneuver		
7. Demonstrates the performance of the FVL maneuver correctly		
8. Uses noseclips according to facility policy		
9. Instructs patient in proper placement of the mouthpiece		
10. Forcefully coaches patient in the expiratory maneuver		
11. Forcefully coaches patient in the inspiratory maneuver		
12. Determines validity according to ATS Guidelines		
13. Repeats maneuver as necessary		
14. Allows patient to rest sufficiently in between tests		
15. Performs post-bronchodilator FVL if ordered		
16. Analyzes results for accuracy		
FOLLOW-UP		
17. Common Performance Elements Steps 11–16		

SIGNATURES   Student: Evaluator: Date:

Clinical Performance Evaluation

PERFORMANCE RATING:

5   **Independent:** Near flawless performance; minimal errors; able to perform without supervision; seeks out new learning; shows initiative; A = 4.7–5.0 average

4   **Minimally Supervised:** Few errors, able to self-correct; seeks guidance when appropriate; B = 3.7–4.65

3   **Competent:** Minimal required level; no critical errors; able to correct with coaching; meets expectations; safe; C = 3.0–3.65

2   **Marginal:** Below average; critical errors or problem areas noted; would benefit from remediation; D = 2.0–2.99

1   **Dependent:** Poor; unacceptable performance; unsafe; gross inaccuracies; potentially harmful; F = < 2.0

Circle the appropriate response below. Please be consistent, objective, and honest in your assessment of the student's clinical performance and ability.

PERFORMANCE CRITERIA	SCORE				
COGNITIVE DOMAIN					
1. Consistently displays knowledge, comprehension, and command of essential concepts	5	4	3	2	1
2. Demonstrates the relationship between theory and clinical practice	5	4	3	2	1
3. Able to select, review, apply, analyze, synthesize, interpret, and evaluate information; makes recommendations to modify care plan	5	4	3	2	1
PSYCHOMOTOR DOMAIN					
4. Minimal errors, no critical errors; able to self-correct; performs all steps safely and accurately	5	4	3	2	1
5. Selects, assembles, and verifies proper function and cleanliness of equipment; assures operation and corrects malfunctions; provides adequate care and maintenance	5	4	3	2	1
6. Exhibits the required manual dexterity	5	4	3	2	1
7. Performs procedure in a reasonable time frame for clinical level	5	4	3	2	1
8. Applies and maintains aseptic technique and PPE as required	5	4	3	2	1
9. Maintains concise and accurate patient and clinical records	5	4	3	2	1
10. Reports promptly on patient status/needs to appropriate personnel	5	4	3	2	1
AFFECTIVE DOMAIN					
11. Exhibits courteous and pleasant demeanor; shows consideration and respect, honesty, and integrity	5	4	3	2	1
12. Communicates verbally and in writing clearly and concisely	5	4	3	2	1
13. Preserves confidentiality and adheres to all policies	5	4	3	2	1
14. Follows directions, exhibits sound judgment, and seeks help when required	5	4	3	2	1
15. Demonstrates initiative, self-direction, responsibility, and accountability	5	4	3	2	1

TOTAL POINTS =   /15 = AVERAGE GRADE =

ADDITIONAL COMMENTS: IDENTIFY AREAS OF EXCELLENCE; LIST ERRORS OF OMISSION OR COMMISSION, CRITICAL ERRORS

SUMMARY PERFORMANCE EVALUATION AND RECOMMENDATIONS

☐ PASS: Satisfactory Performance

    ☐ Minimal supervision needed, may progress to next level provided specific skills, clinical time completed

    ☐ Minimal supervision needed, able to progress to next level without remediation

☐ FAIL: Unsatisfactory Performance (check all that apply)

    ☐ Minor reevaluation only

    ☐ Needs additional clinical practice before reevaluation

    ☐ Needs additional laboratory practice before skills performed in clinical area

    ☐ Recommend clinical probation

SIGNATURES

Evaluator (print name):   Evaluator signature: Date:

Student Signature: Date:

Student Comments:

Procedural Competency Evaluation

STUDENT: **DATE:**

MAXIMUM VOLUNTARY VENTILATION (MVV)

Evaluator: ☐ Peer   ☐ Instructor   **Setting:** ☐ Lab   ☐ Clinical Simulation

Equipment Utilized: **Conditions (Describe):**

Performance Level:

S or ✓ = Satisfactory, no errors of omission or commission
U = Unsatisfactory Error of Omission or Commission
NA = Not applicable

Performance Rating:

5   **Independent:** Near flawless performance; minimal errors; able to perform without supervision; seeks out new learning; shows initiative; A = 4.7–5.0 average

4   **Minimally Supervised:** Few errors, able to self-correct; seeks guidance when appropriate; B = 3.7–4.65

3   **Competent:** Minimal required level; no critical errors; able to correct with coaching; meets expectations; safe; C = 3.0–3.65

2   **Marginal:** Below average; critical errors or problem areas noted; would benefit from remediation; D = 2.0–2.99

1   **Dependent:** Poor; unacceptable performance; unsafe; gross inaccuracies; potentially harmful; F = < 2.0

Two or more errors of commission or omission of mandatory or essential performance elements will terminate the procedure, and require additional practice and/or remediation and reevaluation. Student is responsible for obtaining additional evaluation forms as needed from the Director of Clinical Education (DCE).

	PERFORMANCE RATING	PERFORMANCE LEVEL
EQUIPMENT AND PATIENT PREPARATION		
1. Common Performance Elements Steps 1–8		
ASSESSMENT AND IMPLEMENTATION		
2. Common Performance Elements Steps 9 and 10		
3. Properly calibrates equipment with a 3.00 liter calibration syringe		
4. Properly sets-up equipment for the MVV maneuver		
5. Gathers necessary patient demographic information		
6. Instructs the patient in the proper performance of the maneuver		
7. Demonstrates the performance of the MVV maneuver correctly		
8. Uses noseclips according to facility policy		
9. Instructs patient in proper placement of the mouthpiece		
10. Forcefully coaches patient to breath as rapidly and as deeply as possible for 10–12 seconds		
11. Forcefully coaches patient during the entire maneuver		
12. Allows patient to rest sufficiently		
13. Analyzes results for accuracy		
FOLLOW-UP		
14. Common Performance Elements Steps 11–16		

SIGNATURES   Student: Evaluator: Date:

Clinical Performance Evaluation

PERFORMANCE RATING:

5 **Independent:** Near flawless performance; minimal errors; able to perform without supervision; seeks out new learning; shows initiative; A = 4.7–5.0 average

4 **Minimally Supervised:** Few errors, able to self-correct; seeks guidance when appropriate; B = 3.7–4.65

3 **Competent:** Minimal required level; no critical errors; able to correct with coaching; meets expectations; safe; C = 3.0–3.65

2 **Marginal:** Below average; critical errors or problem areas noted; would benefit from remediation; D = 2.0–2.99

1 **Dependent:** Poor; unacceptable performance; unsafe; gross inaccuracies; potentially harmful; F = < 2.0

Circle the appropriate response below. Please be consistent, objective, and honest in your assessment of the student's clinical performance and ability.

PERFORMANCE CRITERIA	SCORE				
COGNITIVE DOMAIN					
1. Consistently displays knowledge, comprehension, and command of essential concepts	5	4	3	2	1
2. Demonstrates the relationship between theory and clinical practice	5	4	3	2	1
3. Able to select, review, apply, analyze, synthesize, interpret, and evaluate information; makes recommendations to modify care plan	5	4	3	2	1
PSYCHOMOTOR DOMAIN					
4. Minimal errors, no critical errors; able to self-correct; performs all steps safely and accurately	5	4	3	2	1
5. Selects, assembles, and verifies proper function and cleanliness of equipment; assures operation and corrects malfunctions; provides adequate care and maintenance	5	4	3	2	1
6. Exhibits the required manual dexterity	5	4	3	2	1
7. Performs procedure in a reasonable time frame for clinical level	5	4	3	2	1
8. Applies and maintains aseptic technique and PPE as required	5	4	3	2	1
9. Maintains concise and accurate patient and clinical records	5	4	3	2	1
10. Reports promptly on patient status/needs to appropriate personnel	5	4	3	2	1
AFFECTIVE DOMAIN					
11. Exhibits courteous and pleasant demeanor; shows consideration and respect, honesty, and integrity	5	4	3	2	1
12. Communicates verbally and in writing clearly and concisely	5	4	3	2	1
13. Preserves confidentiality and adheres to all policies	5	4	3	2	1
14. Follows directions, exhibits sound judgment, and seeks help when required	5	4	3	2	1
15. Demonstrates initiative, self-direction, responsibility, and accountability	5	4	3	2	1

TOTAL POINTS = /15 = AVERAGE GRADE =

ADDITIONAL COMMENTS: IDENTIFY AREAS OF EXCELLENCE; LIST ERRORS OF OMISSION OR COMMISSION, CRITICAL ERRORS

SUMMARY PERFORMANCE EVALUATION AND RECOMMENDATIONS

☐ PASS: Satisfactory Performance

    ☐ Minimal supervision needed, may progress to next level provided specific skills, clinical time completed

    ☐ Minimal supervision needed, able to progress to next level without remediation

☐ FAIL: Unsatisfactory Performance (check all that apply)

    ☐ Minor reevaluation only

    ☐ Needs additional clinical practice before reevaluation

    ☐ Needs additional laboratory practice before skills performed in clinical area

    ☐ Recommend clinical probation

SIGNATURES

Evaluator (print name):   Evaluator signature: Date:

Student Signature: Date:

Student Comments:

Procedural Competency Evaluation

STUDENT: **DATE:**

SPIROMETRY SCREENING INTERPRETATION

	PERFORMANCE RATING	PERFORMANCE LEVEL
Evaluator: ☐ Peer ☐ Instructor **Setting:** ☐ Lab ☐ Clinical Simulation		
Equipment Utilized: **Conditions (Describe):**		
Performance Level:		
S or ✓ = Satisfactory, no errors of omission or commission U = Unsatisfactory Error of Omission or Commission NA = Not applicable		
Performance Rating:		
5 **Independent:** Near flawless performance; minimal errors; able to perform without supervision; seeks out new learning; shows initiative; A = 4.7–5.0 average		
4 **Minimally Supervised:** Few errors, able to self-correct; seeks guidance when appropriate; B = 3.7–4.65		
3 **Competent:** Minimal required level; no critical errors; able to correct with coaching; meets expectations; safe; C = 3.0–3.65		
2 **Marginal:** Below average; critical errors or problem areas noted; would benefit from remediation; D = 2.0–2.99		
1 **Dependent:** Poor; unacceptable performance; unsafe; gross inaccuracies; potentially harmful; F = < 2.0		
Two or more errors of commission or omission of mandatory or essential performance elements will terminate the procedure, and require additional practice and/or remediation and reevaluation. Student is responsible for obtaining additional evaluation forms as needed from the Director of Clinical Education (DCE).		

EQUIPMENT AND PATIENT PREPARATION

1. Common Performance Elements Steps 1–8		

ASSESSMENT AND IMPLEMENTATION

2. Common Performance Elements Steps 9 and 10		
3. Performs spirometry as ordered by the physician		
4. Interprets the following values by comparing actual values to predicted values:		
FVC		
FEV$_1$		
FEV$_1$/FVC%		
5. Analyzes the shape of the volume–time tracing and flow–volume loop		
6. Determines if the results are within normal limits or abnormal		
7. Accurately determines if the results are obstructive, restrictive, or mixed pattern of disease		
8. Accurately determines if results are mild, moderate, or severe		
9. Determines the degree of effectiveness of bronchodilator administration		

FOLLOW-UP

10. Common Performance Elements Steps 11–16		

SIGNATURES   Student: Evaluator: Date:

Clinical Performance Evaluation

PERFORMANCE RATING:

5 **Independent:** Near flawless performance; minimal errors; able to perform without supervision; seeks out new learning; shows initiative; A = 4.7–5.0 average

4 **Minimally Supervised:** Few errors, able to self-correct; seeks guidance when appropriate; B = 3.7–4.65

3 **Competent:** Minimal required level; no critical errors; able to correct with coaching; meets expectations; safe; C = 3.0–3.65

2 **Marginal:** Below average; critical errors or problem areas noted; would benefit from remediation; D = 2.0–2.99

1 **Dependent:** Poor; unacceptable performance; unsafe; gross inaccuracies; potentially harmful; F = < 2.0

Circle the appropriate response below. Please be consistent, objective, and honest in your assessment of the student's clinical performance and ability.

PERFORMANCE CRITERIA	SCORE				
COGNITIVE DOMAIN					
1. Consistently displays knowledge, comprehension, and command of essential concepts	5	4	3	2	1
2. Demonstrates the relationship between theory and clinical practice	5	4	3	2	1
3. Able to select, review, apply, analyze, synthesize, interpret, and evaluate information; makes recommendations to modify care plan	5	4	3	2	1
PSYCHOMOTOR DOMAIN					
4. Minimal errors, no critical errors; able to self-correct; performs all steps safely and accurately	5	4	3	2	1
5. Selects, assembles, and verifies proper function and cleanliness of equipment; assures operation and corrects malfunctions; provides adequate care and maintenance	5	4	3	2	1
6. Exhibits the required manual dexterity	5	4	3	2	1
7. Performs procedure in a reasonable time frame for clinical level	5	4	3	2	1
8. Applies and maintains aseptic technique and PPE as required	5	4	3	2	1
9. Maintains concise and accurate patient and clinical records	5	4	3	2	1
10. Reports promptly on patient status/needs to appropriate personnel	5	4	3	2	1
AFFECTIVE DOMAIN					
11. Exhibits courteous and pleasant demeanor; shows consideration and respect, honesty, and integrity	5	4	3	2	1
12. Communicates verbally and in writing clearly and concisely	5	4	3	2	1
13. Preserves confidentiality and adheres to all policies	5	4	3	2	1
14. Follows directions, exhibits sound judgment, and seeks help when required	5	4	3	2	1
15. Demonstrates initiative, self-direction, responsibility, and accountability	5	4	3	2	1

TOTAL POINTS = _____ /15 = AVERAGE GRADE = _____

ADDITIONAL COMMENTS: IDENTIFY AREAS OF EXCELLENCE; LIST ERRORS OF OMISSION OR COMMISSION, CRITICAL ERRORS

SUMMARY PERFORMANCE EVALUATION AND RECOMMENDATIONS

☐ PASS: Satisfactory Performance

　☐ Minimal supervision needed, may progress to next level provided specific skills, clinical time completed

　☐ Minimal supervision needed, able to progress to next level without remediation

☐ FAIL: Unsatisfactory Performance (check all that apply)

　☐ Minor reevaluation only

　☐ Needs additional clinical practice before reevaluation

　☐ Needs additional laboratory practice before skills performed in clinical area

　☐ Recommend clinical probation

SIGNATURES

Evaluator (print name): _____　　Evaluator signature: _____　　Date: _____

Student Signature: _____　　Date: _____

Student Comments: _____

32

Chest Tube Drainage Systems

INTRODUCTION

Excess air or fluid may accumulate in the **pleural space** due to **pneumothorax**, **pleural effusion**, **hemothorax**, **chylothorax**, **empyema**, or following thoracic surgery. As a result, the negative pressure normally found in the pleural cavity is disrupted and the patient will develop shortness of breath and an increase in work of breathing. Over time, small volumes of air and/or fluid can be absorbed by the body, but lung expansion will be limited by large volumes.[1-6]

The purpose of the chest tube is to remove air and/or fluid from the pleural cavity to help re-establish normal intrathoracic pressures. This aids in the re-expansion of the lung and restoration of normal breathing dynamics. Once the chest tube is in place, it is connected to a chest drainage system. The purpose of the chest drainage system is to collect fluid as it drains from the pleural cavity, allow air to exit the pleural cavity, and provide suction for enhanced pleural drainage.[1-6]

OBJECTIVES

Upon completion of this chapter, the student will be able to:

1. Identify the parts of a chest drainage system.
2. Discuss the function of each of the three chambers of a chest drainage system.
3. Demonstrate the proper setup of a chest drainage system.
4. Compare and contrast a water-seal system to a dry suction chest drainage system.
5. Discuss maintenance and troubleshooting of the chest drainage system.

KEY TERMS

chylothorax
collection chamber
empyema

hemothorax
pleural effusion
pleural space

pneumothorax
suction control chamber

tidaling
water-seal chamber

Exercises

EQUIPMENT REQUIRED

☐ Chest tube
☐ Wet chest drainage system
☐ Dry chest drainage system
☐ Human patient simulator (if available)

☐ Nonsterile disposable nonlatex gloves, various sizes
☐ Sterile water
☐ Suction tubing
☐ Suction source

EXERCISE 32.1 WET CHEST DRAINAGE SYSTEMS

EXERCISE 32.1.1 WET CHEST DRAINAGE SYSTEM COMPONENT IDENTIFICATION

Compare the equipment provided in the laboratory with Figure 32.1. **Identify each item and record them on your laboratory report.**

Calibrated **water-seal chamber**

Carrying handle

Collection chamber

High-negativity float valve and relief chamber

High-negativity relief valve

Patient air leak meter

Positive-pressure relief valve

Self-sealing diaphragm

Suction control chamber

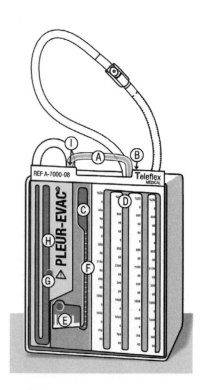

Figure 32.1. Pleur-evac® wet chest drainage system.

EXERCISE 32.1.2 ASSEMBLING A WET CHEST TUBE DRAINAGE SYSTEM

1. Wash or sanitize your hands and apply standard precautions and transmission-based isolation procedures as appropriate.
2. Put on nonsterile gloves.
3. Remove the chest drainage system from its packaging. **Record the brand used on your laboratory report.**
4. Lock the floor stand into place.
5. Instill sterile water into the water-seal chamber.
   A. Attach a funnel to the short suction chamber tubing.
   B. Kink the tubing by holding the funnel below the top of the chest drainage unit.
   C. Fill the funnel with sterile water to the 2 cm level.
   D. Raise the funnel above the chest drainage unit to fill the water-seal chamber.
6. Connect the "patient's" chest tube to the collection chamber tube.
7. Pour sterile water directly into the suction control chamber through the atmospheric vent to the prescribed level (usually 20 cm).
8. Connect the suction tubing to the suction source if suction is required.
   A. Gradually increase wall suction until gentle bubbling is seen in the suction control chamber.
9. Position the chest drainage system so that it is hanging from the bed or standing on the floor. The unit should be at least 1 foot below the level of the "patient's" chest.
10. Assess the "patient" for signs of respiratory distress.
11. Assess the chest tube entry site for drainage and subcutaneous emphysema.
12. Assess all the tubing and ensure that there are no kinks or dependent loops and all connections are tightly connected.
13. Assess the chest drainage unit:
    A. Assess the suction control chamber:
       i. Ensure that the suction level in the suction control chamber is set at the ordered level.
       ii. Assess the suction control chamber for gentle, continuous bubbling.
       iii. If the "patient" is not on suction, ensure that the air vent is open.
    B. Assess the water-seal chamber:
       i. Ensure that the water-seal chamber is filled to the appropriate level.
       ii. Assess the water-seal chamber for bubbling and tidaling.
    C. Assess the collection chamber:
       i. Assess the volume, type, and rate of drainage.
14. Remove your gloves and wash or sanitize your hands.
15. Dispose of all infectious waste in the proper receptacles.

EXERCISE 32.2 DRY CHEST DRAINAGE SYSTEMS

EXERCISE 32.2.1 DRY CHEST DRAINAGE SYSTEM COMPONENT IDENTIFICATION

Compare the equipment provided in the laboratory with Figure 32.2. **Identify each item and record them on your laboratory report.**

Calibrated water seal
Carrying handle
Collection chamber
High-negativity float valve and relief chamber
High-negativity relief valve
Patient air leak meter
Positive-pressure relief valve
Self-sealing diaphragm
Suction control dial
Suction control indicator window

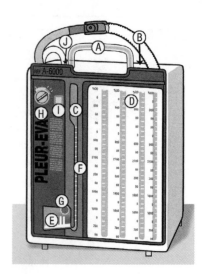

Figure 32.2. Pleur-evac® dry chest drainage system.

EXERCISE 32.2.2 ASSEMBLING A DRY CHEST TUBE DRAINAGE SYSTEM

1. Wash or sanitize your hands and apply standard precautions and transmission-based isolation procedures as appropriate.
2. Put on nonsterile gloves.
3. Remove the chest drainage system from its packaging. **Record the brand used on your laboratory report.**
4. Lock the floor stand into place.
5. Connect the "patient's" chest tube to the collection chamber tube.
6. Add sterile water to the water-seal chamber through the needleless injection site on the back of the unit if applicable.
7. Connect the suction tubing to the suction source if suction is required.
   A. Set the dry suction control dial to the desired suction setting.
   B. Gradually increase wall suction until the desired suction level appears in the suction control indicator.
8. Position the chest drainage system so that it is hanging from the bed or standing on the floor. The unit should be at least 1 foot below the level of the "patient's" chest.
9. Assess the "patient" for signs of respiratory distress.
10. Assess the chest tube entry site for drainage and subcutaneous emphysema.
11. Assess all the tubing and ensure that there are no kinks or dependent loops and all connections are tightly connected.
12. Assess the chest drainage unit:
    A. Assess the suction control chamber:
       i. Ensure that the suction level in the suction control indicator is set at the ordered level.
       ii. Ensure that the suction source indicator is visible.
       iii. If the "patient" is not on suction, ensure that the air vent is open.
    B. Assess the water-seal chamber:
       i. Ensure that the water-seal chamber is filled to the appropriate level.
       ii. Assess the water-seal chamber for bubbling and tidaling.
    C. Assess the collection chamber:
       i. Assess the volume, type, and rate of drainage.
13. Remove your gloves and wash or sanitize your hands.
14. Dispose of all infectious waste in the proper receptacles.

EXERCISE 32.3 MAINTAINING AND TROUBLESHOOTING CHEST DRAINAGE SYSTEMS

Using outside sources, complete Table 32.1 and **record your answers on your laboratory report.**

Table 32.1 Maintaining and Troubleshooting Chest Drainage Systems

Location	Assessment	Indication/ Action
Collection Chamber	Drainage has *suddenly* stopped.	
	The collection chamber is full.	
Water-Seal Chamber	The water level is not at 2 cm.	
		This is a normal finding called *tidaling*.
	Tidaling is *not* seen.	
	Continuous bubbling is seen.	
		This indicates that the patient has an air leak in the pleural space. This is expected during expiration in a patient with a pneumothorax. Notify the physician if this is a new leak.
		This indicates that the lung has re-expanded and air is no longer leaking into the pleural space. Verify full lung expansion on chest x-ray.
Wet Suction Control	There is too much water in this chamber.	
	Aggressive bubbling is seen.	
	Continuous gentle bubbling is seen.	
	No bubbling is seen.	
Dry Suction Control	The suction control indicator is not visible.	

REFERENCES
1. Carroll, P: Exploring chest drain options. RN 63(10):50–58, 2000.
2. Coughlin, A and Parchinsky, C: Go with the flow of chest tube therapy. Nursing 36(3):36–41, 2006.
3. Erickson, R: Mastering the ins and outs of chest drainage. Part 2. Nursing 19(6):46–49, 1989.
4. O'Hanlon-Nichols, T: Commonly asked questions about chest tubes. Am J Nursing 96(5):60–64, 1996.
5. Pettinicchi, T: Troubleshooting chest tubes. Nursing 28(3):58–59, 1998.
6. Roman, M and Mercado, D: Review of chest tube use. Nursing 15(1):41–43, 2006.

Laboratory Report

CHAPTER 32: CHEST TUBE DRAINAGE SYSTEMS

Name _____ Date _____

Course/Section _____ Instructor _____

Data Collection

EXERCISE 32.1 Wet Chest Drainage Systems

EXERCISE 32.1.1 WET CHEST DRAINAGE SYSTEM COMPONENT IDENTIFICATION

A. _____

B. _____

C. _____

D. _____

E. _____

F. _____

G. _____

H. _____

I. _____

EXERCISE 32.1.2 ASSEMBLING A WET CHEST TUBE DRAINAGE SYSTEM

Brand used: _____

EXERCISE 32.2. Dry Chest Drainage Systems

EXERCISE 32.2.1 DRY CHEST DRAINAGE SYSTEM COMPONENT IDENTIFICATION

A. _____

B. _____

C. _____

D. _____

E. _____

F. _____

G. _____

H. _____

I. _____

J. _____

EXERCISE 32.2.2 ASSEMBLING A DRY CHEST TUBE DRAINAGE SYSTEM

Brand used: _____

EXERCISE 32.3 Maintaining and Troubleshooting Chest Drainage Systems

Table 32.1 Maintaining and Troubleshooting Chest Drainage Systems

Location	Assessment	Indication/ Action
Collection Chamber	Drainage has *suddenly* stopped.	
	The collection chamber is full.	
Water-Seal Chamber	The water level is not at 2 cm.	
		This is a normal finding called *tidaling*.
	Tidaling is *not* seen.	
	Continuous bubbling is seen.	
		This indicates that the patient has an air leak in the pleural space. This is expected during expiration in a patient with a pneumothorax. Notify the physician if this is a new leak.
		This indicates that the lung has re-expanded and air is no longer leaking into the pleural space. Verify full lung expansion on chest x-ray.
Wet Suction Control	There is too much water in this chamber.	
	Aggressive bubbling is seen.	
	Continuous gentle bubbling is seen.	
	No bubbling is seen.	
Dry Suction Control	The suction control indicator is not visible.	

Critical Thinking Questions

1. Describe the function of the three chambers of a chest drainage unit.

2. Your patient has a chest tube in place and is showing signs of respiratory distress. What is the most likely cause of these findings and what would you recommend the respiratory therapist do at this time?

3. If your patient with a chest tube develops swelling of chest tissue and you hear a crackling sound upon palpation of the area, what would you suspect?

4. Describe tidaling in the following patients:

    A. Spontaneously breathing

    B. Mechanically ventilated

5. State three conditions that are indicated by the absence of tidaling in the water-seal chamber and how to troubleshoot each situation, if necessary.

6. The respiratory therapist caring for a patient with a treated pneumothorax receiving mechanical ventilation with positive end-expiratory pressure should expect to see what type of bubbling in the water-seal chamber?

Procedural Competency Evaluation

STUDENT: **DATE:**

CHEST DRAINAGE SYSTEM ASSEMBLY

					PERFORMANCE RATING	PERFORMANCE LEVEL
Evaluator: ☐ Peer ☐ Instructor			**Setting:** ☐ Lab	☐ Clinical Simulation		

Equipment Utilized: **Conditions (Describe):**

Performance Level:

    S or ✓ = Satisfactory, no errors of omission or commission
    U = Unsatisfactory Error of Omission or Commission
    NA = Not applicable

Performance Rating:

    5   **Independent:** Near flawless performance; minimal errors; able to perform without supervision; seeks out new learning; shows initiative; A = 4.7–5.0 average

    4   **Minimally Supervised:** Few errors, able to self-correct; seeks guidance when appropriate; B = 3.7–4.65

    3   **Competent:** Minimal required level; no critical errors; able to correct with coaching; meets expectations; safe; C = 3.0–3.65

    2   **Marginal:** Below average; critical errors or problem areas noted; would benefit from remediation; D = 2.0–2.99

    1   **Dependent:** Poor; unacceptable performance; unsafe; gross inaccuracies; potentially harmful; F = < 2.0

    Two or more errors of commission or omission of mandatory or essential performance elements will terminate the procedure, and require additional practice and/or remediation and reevaluation. Student is responsible for obtaining additional evaluation forms as needed from the Director of Clinical Education (DCE).

	PERFORMANCE RATING	PERFORMANCE LEVEL
EQUIPMENT AND PATIENT PREPARATION		
1. Common Performance Elements Steps 1–8		
2. Locks floor stand into place		
3. Instills sterile water into the water-seal chamber		
4. Connects the patient's chest tube to the collection chamber tube		
5. Instills sterile water into the suction control chamber to the prescribed level (wet system)		
6. Connects the suction tubing to the suction source if required		
7. Set the dry suction control dial to the desired suction setting (dry system)		
8. Adjusts vacuum pressure to appropriate level		
9. Positions the chest drainage system appropriately		
ASSESSMENT AND IMPLEMENTATION		
10. Common Performance Elements Steps 9 and 10		
11. Assesses the chest tube entry site		
12. Assesses all tubing		
13. Assesses the suction control chamber		
14. Assesses the water-seal chamber		
15. Assesses the collection chamber		
FOLLOW-UP		
16. Common Performance Elements Steps 11–16		

SIGNATURES   Student: Evaluator: Date:

Clinical Performance Evaluation

PERFORMANCE RATING:

5   **Independent:** Near flawless performance; minimal errors; able to perform without supervision; seeks out new learning; shows initiative; A = 4.7–5.0 average

4   **Minimally Supervised:** Few errors, able to self-correct; seeks guidance when appropriate; B = 3.7–4.65

3   **Competent:** Minimal required level; no critical errors; able to correct with coaching; meets expectations; safe; C = 3.0–3.65

2   **Marginal:** Below average; critical errors or problem areas noted; would benefit from remediation; D = 2.0–2.99

1   **Dependent:** Poor; unacceptable performance; unsafe; gross inaccuracies; potentially harmful; F = < 2.0

Circle the appropriate response below. Please be consistent, objective, and honest in your assessment of the student's clinical performance and ability.

PERFORMANCE CRITERIA	SCORE				
COGNITIVE DOMAIN					
1. Consistently displays knowledge, comprehension, and command of essential concepts	5	4	3	2	1
2. Demonstrates the relationship between theory and clinical practice	5	4	3	2	1
3. Able to select, review, apply, analyze, synthesize, interpret, and evaluate information; makes recommendations to modify care plan	5	4	3	2	1
PSYCHOMOTOR DOMAIN					
4. Minimal errors, no critical errors; able to self-correct; performs all steps safely and accurately	5	4	3	2	1
5. Selects, assembles, and verifies proper function and cleanliness of equipment; assures operation and corrects malfunctions; provides adequate care and maintenance	5	4	3	2	1
6. Exhibits the required manual dexterity	5	4	3	2	1
7. Performs procedure in a reasonable time frame for clinical level	5	4	3	2	1
8. Applies and maintains aseptic technique and PPE as required	5	4	3	2	1
9. Maintains concise and accurate patient and clinical records	5	4	3	2	1
10. Reports promptly on patient status/needs to appropriate personnel	5	4	3	2	1
AFFECTIVE DOMAIN					
11. Exhibits courteous and pleasant demeanor; shows consideration and respect, honesty, and integrity	5	4	3	2	1
12. Communicates verbally and in writing clearly and concisely	5	4	3	2	1
13. Preserves confidentiality and adheres to all policies	5	4	3	2	1
14. Follows directions, exhibits sound judgment, and seeks help when required	5	4	3	2	1
15. Demonstrates initiative, self-direction, responsibility, and accountability	5	4	3	2	1

TOTAL POINTS =   /15 = AVERAGE GRADE =

ADDITIONAL COMMENTS: IDENTIFY AREAS OF EXCELLENCE; LIST ERRORS OF OMISSION OR COMMISSION, CRITICAL ERRORS

SUMMARY PERFORMANCE EVALUATION AND RECOMMENDATIONS

☐ PASS: Satisfactory Performance

    ☐ Minimal supervision needed, may progress to next level provided specific skills, clinical time completed

    ☐ Minimal supervision needed, able to progress to next level without remediation

☐ FAIL: Unsatisfactory Performance (check all that apply)

    ☐ Minor reevaluation only

    ☐ Needs additional clinical practice before reevaluation

    ☐ Needs additional laboratory practice before skills performed in clinical area

    ☐ Recommend clinical probation

SIGNATURES

Evaluator (print name):   Evaluator signature: Date:

Student Signature: Date:

Student Comments:

33 Basic Chest X-ray Interpretation

INTRODUCTION

Radiologists and pulmonologists develop x-ray interpretation skills over the course of several years and hundreds of films. Although respiratory care practitioners are not expected to achieve this level of expertise, the ability to identify a normal chest x-ray and common cardiopulmonary abnormalities should be a part of the basic skills an advanced-level practitioner can perform. In a critical situation, knowledge of x-ray interpretation can be crucial to patient care. In conjunction with other patient assessment techniques, atelectasis, pneumothorax, or endotracheal tube placement can be confirmed by radiography. Recognition of frequently encountered findings such as hyperinflation, infiltrates, pulmonary edema, and pneumonia is an asset to the practitioner and improves patient care.

The x-ray film is similar to a photographic negative. The x-ray precipitates silver and an image is created. A cassette is used to enhance this process. It contains a fluorescent screen that, when stimulated by the x-ray, helps darken the film and enhance the image. Thus objects that are the densest absorb the x-rays and the film is not altered photographically. These objects are called radiopaque, or **radiodense**, and appear white to gray depending on the density. Objects that absorb fewer rays are called **radiolucent**. Air, which allows the rays to pass through, appears black.[1]

One must remember that the image created is two-dimensional and the position and distance of the patient relative to the x-ray machine are important. Chest x-rays can be taken in several positions and describe the path or direction in which the ray passes through the patient onto the cassette. The most common view is the postero-anterior (PA) in an ambulatory patient. The anteroposterior (AP) is the usual view of a portable film in a more critically ill patient. The lateral, **lordotic** (used to expose the upper lobes), and decubitus projections are also used.[2]

The proficient interpretation of x-rays by respiratory therapists takes much practice. The learning process can be aided when a systematic approach is used.

Other techniques may also be used to determine lung abnormalities. **Transillumination** of an infant chest may help identify pneumothorax. Ventilation perfusion scans may assist in the diagnosis of pulmonary emboli. The chest x-ray is limited by its two-dimensional nature. Patient complaints and symptomatology sometimes do not correlate with the chest x-ray findings. Advanced techniques such as computerized **tomography** (CT) scans or magnetic resonance imaging (MRI) are then used to define a pulmonary abnormality that might or might not be identifiable on routine chest x-ray. The interpretation of these techniques is well beyond the scope of the respiratory care practitioner.

OBJECTIVES

Upon completion of this chapter, the student will be able to:

1. Differentiate between radiopaque and radiolucent structures.
2. Given a chest x-ray, verify the patient identity, film projection, position, and quality of the film.
3. Identify the major organs and anatomic landmarks on adult and infant chest x-ray films, including the aortic knob and heart shadow, costophrenic angles, hemi-diaphragms, spinal column, ribs and rib angles, sternum, clavicles, hila, trachea and bifurcation (carina), air bronchogram, stomach bubble, and breast shadows.
4. Confirm the position of an endotracheal tube.
5. Identify the placement of chest tubes and pulmonary artery catheters.
6. Locate the following abnormalities on a chest x-ray: atelectasis, pneumothorax, hyperinflation, pleural effusion, large masses, infiltrates, pneumonia, hilar adenopathy, cavitary lesions, respiratory distress syndrome (RDS), epiglottitis, croup, and bronchopulmonary dysplasia (BPD).
7. Differentiate chest deformities from normal chest structure.

KEY TERMS

adenopathy	cardiomegaly	infiltrates	radiodense
air bronchogram	costophrenic	lordotic	radiolucent
bifurcation	dysplasia	mass	tomography
blunted	hyperlucent	nodule	transillumination

Exercises

EQUIPMENT REQUIRED

- ☐ Grease pencil
- ☐ Measuring tape
- ☐ X-ray view boxes
- ☐ Spare fluorescent bulbs
- ☐ Chest x-rays of the following:
  - ☐ Normal PA and lateral views
  - ☐ AP view
  - ☐ Lateral decubitus view
  - ☐ Lordotic view
  - ☐ Kyphoscoliosis
  - ☐ Pectus carinatum
  - ☐ Adult respiratory distress syndrome
  - ☐ Atelectasis
  - ☐ Asthma
  - ☐ Cardiomegaly
  - ☐ Congestive heart failure
  - ☐ COPD
    - ☐ Hyperinflation
  - ☐ Intubated patient
    - ☐ Endotracheal tube in proper placement
    - ☐ Improperly placed endotracheal tube
- ☐ Pulmonary artery catheter placement
- ☐ Bronchiectasis
- ☐ Flail chest
- ☐ Lung cancer
- ☐ Pleural effusion
- ☐ Pneumonia—lobar and diffuse
- ☐ Pneumothorax
  - ☐ Chest tube placement
- ☐ Pulmonary edema
- ☐ Pulmonary fibrosis
- ☐ Sarcoidosis
- ☐ Subcutaneous emphysema
- ☐ Trached patient
- ☐ Tuberculosis
- ☐ Pediatric chest films
  - ☐ Normal infant chest film
  - ☐ Bronchopulmonary dysplasia
  - ☐ Croup
  - ☐ Epiglottitis
  - ☐ Respiratory distress syndrome

EXERCISE 33.1 IDENTIFICATION OF POSITIONS

Identify the position of the film in Figures 33.1 through 33.4 and label each one. **Record the answers on your laboratory report.**

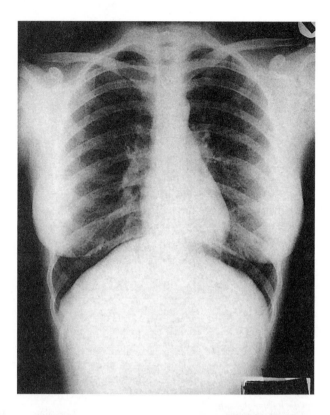

Figure 33.1. Film A.

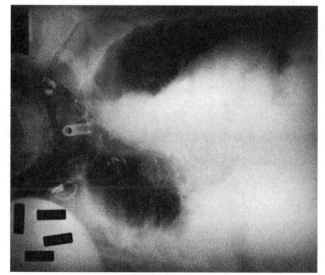

Figure 33.2. Film B.

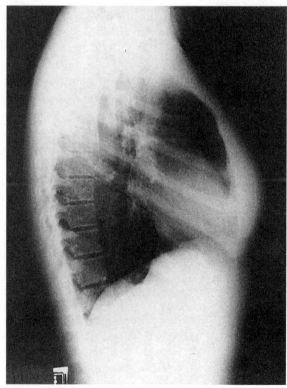

Figure 33.3. Film C.

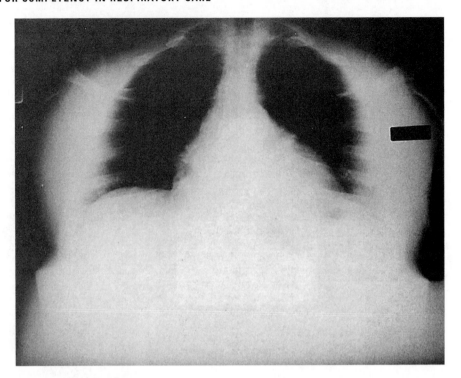

Figure 33.4. Film D.

EXERCISE 33.2 IDENTIFICATION OF MAJOR ORGANS AND LANDMARKS

A systematic approach is needed when viewing a chest film. The following method can be used as a guide. It is helpful to use your index finger to trace along the structure that you are viewing. This helps identify and delineate the object you are viewing.

1. Obtain a normal PA chest x-ray, insert it onto the view box, and turn on the view box.
2. Verify that you have the correct patient's film.
   NOTE: In the laboratory setting, for reasons of patient confidentiality, the patient name should be removed or masked.
3. The film should be placed so that it seems as if the patient is facing you. This is the standard method of viewing.[3] Look for the lead marker.
4. Observe the entire film for symmetry:
   A. Identify the clavicles, scapulae, and ribs.
   B. Identify the spinal column. Is it midline?
   C. Identify the lungs, right and left.
   D. Are there breast shadows?
   E. Locate the gastric air bubble.
   F. Observe the film to ensure that none of the peripheral structures were "clipped," or incompletely shown, because of patient positioning.
5. Observe the film for the quality of the exposure. Is the overall quality too dark or too white? The thoracic spine should be just visible on a routine chest x-ray.[4]
6. Starting in the upper left side, trace your finger along the edge of the lungs down to the edge where the lung meets the diaphragm. This is the costophrenic angle. Is it sharp or blurred (possible fluid), or is it less sharp (blunted)?
7. Note the rib level of the hemi-diaphragms. Chest x-rays are taken at the peak of inspiration, and the diaphragms should be at the level of rib 8 or rib 9. This helps the radiologist determine whether the film is of good or poor inspiratory quality.
8. Trace the outline of each rib, starting from the sternum and moving outward. Do they go to the edge of the film? Are they continuous or interrupted (indicating a fracture)? Note the angle of the ribs anteriorly. Are they horizontal? Estimate the angle.
9. Observing the center of the film, observe the trachea's position. The trachea appears as a column of air. Is it midline? Follow the trachea to the point of bifurcation.
10. Identify the carina and the mainstem bronchi (the air bronchogram). Count the level of vertebrae and intercostal spaces corresponding to the carina. The carina should be at approximately T5 and between the second and third intercostal space.

11. Examine the hila for size and position. Because of anatomy, the left hilum normally appears higher than the right. The radiopaque image represents the pulmonary vasculature. Trace the lines out. These are the "lung markings" and also represent blood vessels, not airways.

12. In the center of the film, identify the aortic knob and the heart shadow. The cardiothoracic ratio is used to express heart size. If the shadow occupies more than 50% it is considered abnormally enlarged.[5] Approximate how much of the film is occupied by the heart shadow, as shown in Figure 33.5, and **record it on your laboratory report.**

    NOTE: On AP films the heart will appear larger than its actual size. Therefore, this projection should not be used to measure heart size.

13. Label the following structures on Figure 33.6 and **record them on your laboratory report.**

    Rib
    Carina
    Clavicle
    Scapula
    Lung field
    Left heart border (apex)
    Right heart border
    Hila
    Larynx
    Trachea
    Carina (tracheal bifurcation)
    Left hemi-diaphragm
    Right hemi-diaphragm
    Costophrenic angles
    Aortic knob
    Gastric bubble

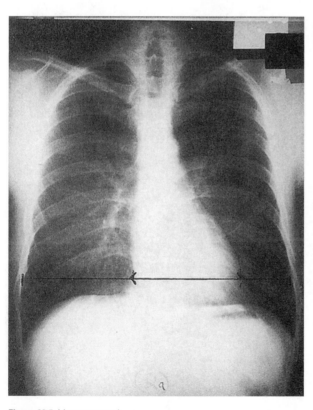

Figure 33.5. Measurement of heart size.

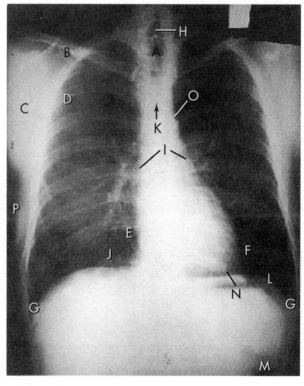

Figure 33.6. Label the x-ray, naming the anatomic landmarks and other characteristics.

EXERCISE 33.3 HYPERINFLATION

1. Obtain an x-ray film already interpreted as hyperinflation, as shown in Figure 33.7, and compare it with the normal film used in Exercise 33.2.

2. Using the technique practiced in the previous exercise, observe and identify the following. **Record them on your laboratory report.**

   Projection used

   Patient position

   Flattening of the hemi-diaphragms. Note the level of the ribs. Location of the diaphragms at the level of rib 11 is an indicator of hyperinflation.

   Horizontal rib margins

   Increased intercostal spaces

   Areas of hyperlucency with decreased lung markings

   Lung size: compare the size of the lungs.

   Increased AP diameter on a lateral film.

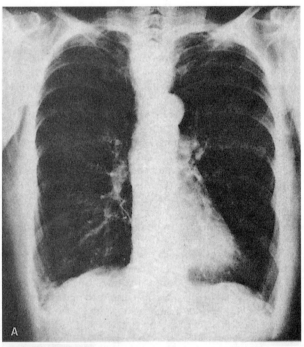

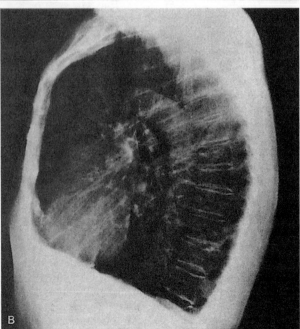

Figure 33.7. X-ray typical of emphysema. (From Wilkins, RF and Dexter, JR: Respiratory Disease: Principles of Patient Care. FA Davis, Philadelphia, 1993, p. 48, with permission.)

EXERCISE 33.4 PNEUMOTHORAX

1. Obtain a film with a confirmed pneumothorax, as shown in Figure 33.8, and compare it with the normal film used in Exercise 33.2.
2. Using the technique practiced in the previous exercise, observe and identify the following. **Record them on your laboratory report.**

   Film ID, patient demographics (if available)

   Projection used

   Tracheal or mediastinal shift indicating a tension pneumothorax. Note that not all films display a shift.

   Area of darker region without lung markings

   Line of demarcation indicating the edge of the collapsed lung

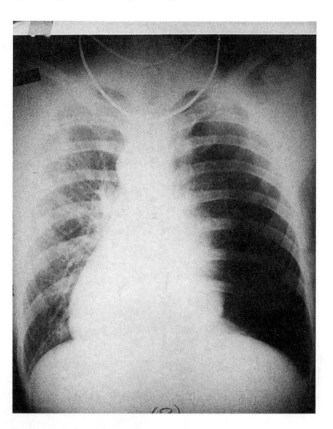

Figure 33.8. Pneumothorax.

EXERCISE 33.5 ATELECTASIS OR CONSOLIDATION

1. Obtain a film with a confirmed atelectasis or consolidated lung, as shown in Figure 33.9, and compare it with the normal film used in Exercise 33.2.
2. Using the technique practiced in Exercise 33.2, observe and identify the following. **Record them on your laboratory report.**

   Film ID, patient demographics (if available)

   Projection used

   Hemi-diaphragm positions (relative to normal and relative to each other)

   Area of radiopaque image in an area where it should be radiolucent

   Mediastinal shift (if any)

   Decreased lung volumes

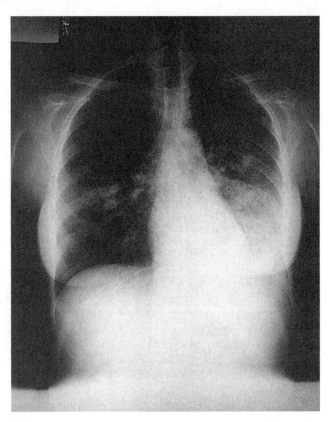

Figure 33.9. Atelectasis or consolidation.

EXERCISE 33.6 ENDOTRACHEAL TUBE POSITION

1. Obtain a film with a confirmed endotracheal tube, as shown in Figure 33.10, and compare it with the normal film used in Exercise 33.2.
2. Using the technique practiced in Exercise 33.2, observe and identify the following. **Record them on your laboratory report.**

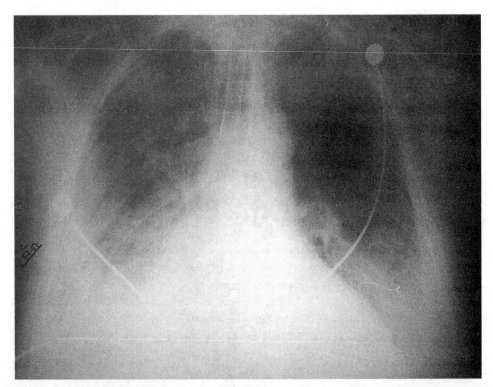

Figure 33.10. Endotracheal tube in position.

Film ID, patient demographics (if available)
Projection used
The radiopaque line of the endotracheal tube
Aortic knob
The carina (at approximately T5)
Tip of the endotracheal tube (at what level?). State three identifying landmarks.

3. Once you have identified the structures, identify the following. **Record the answers on your laboratory report.**
    A. Count the ribs. At the level of what rib or intercostal space anteriorly is the tube?
    B. Count the vertebrae. At the level of what vertebra is the tube?
    C. Approximately how far is the tip of the endotracheal tube above the carina?

EXERCISE 33.7 CHEST DEFORMITIES

1. Obtain a film of kyphoscoliosis (Fig. 33.11).
2. Using the technique practiced in the previous exercises, compare the abnormalities to a normal chest film. **Record them on your laboratory report.**

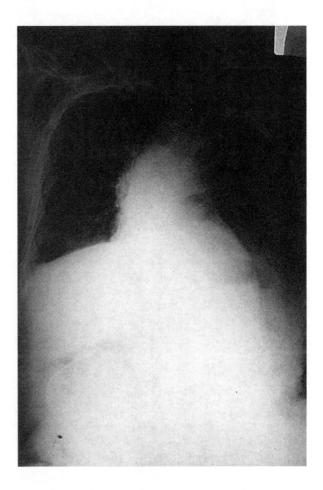

Figure 33.11. Kyphoscoliosis.

EXERCISE 33.8 INFANT AND PEDIATRIC FILMS

1. Obtain a normal infant film (Fig. 33.12). Using the technique practiced in the previous exercises, observe the film and compare it with a normal adult chest x-ray. **Record your findings on your laboratory report.**

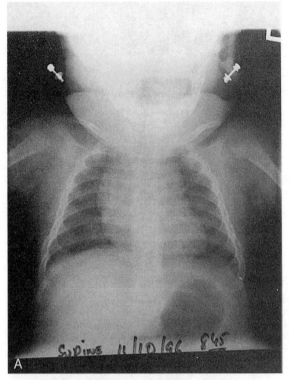
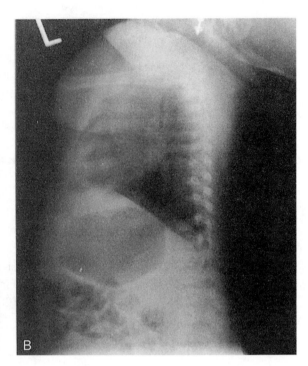

Figure 33.12. (A) and **(B)**: Normal infant chest films.

2. Obtain films of the following:

   Steeple sign in croup (Fig. 33.13)
   Thumb sign in epiglottitis (Fig. 33.14)
   Respiratory distress syndrome (RDS) (Fig. 33.15)
   Bronchopulmonary dysplasia (BPD) (Fig. 33.16)

3. Using the technique practiced in the previous exercises, compare the abnormalities to a normal chest film. **Record them on your laboratory report.**

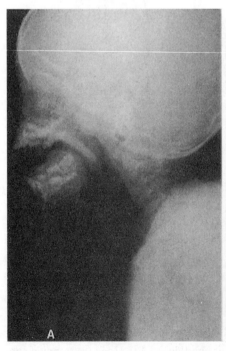
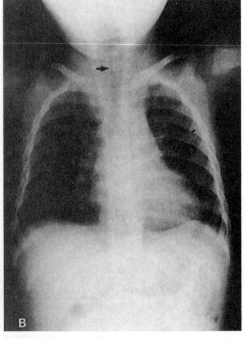

Figure 33.13. Steeple sign in croup. (From Wilkins, RF and Dexter, JR: Respiratory Disease: Principles of Patient Care. FA Davis, Philadelphia, 1993, p. 335, with permission.)

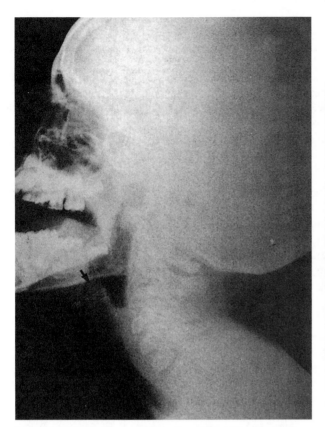

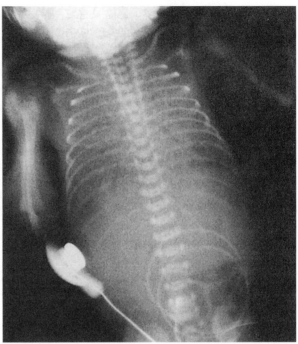

Figure 33.14. Thumb signs in epiglottitis. (From Wilkins, RF and Dexter, JR: Respiratory Disease: Principles of Patient Care. FA Davis, Philadelphia, 1993, p. 332, with permission.)

Figure 33.15. Infant respiratory distress syndrome. (From Wilkins, RF and Dexter, JR: Respiratory Disease: Principles of Patient Care. FA Davis, Philadelphia, 1993, p. 359, with permission.)

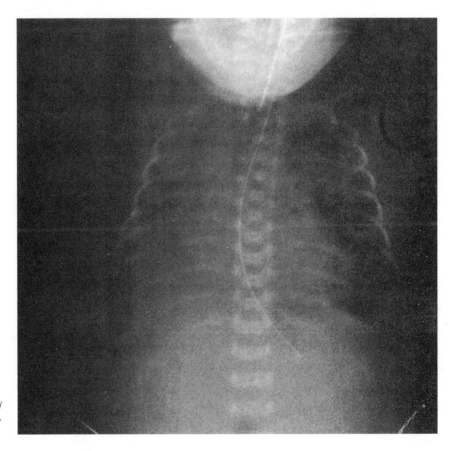

Figure 33.16. Bronchopulmonary dysplasia. (From Wilkins, RF and Dexter, JR: Respiratory Disease: Principles of Patient Care. FA Davis, Philadelphia, 1993, p. 373, with permission.)

EXERCISE 33.9 OTHER ABNORMAL PATTERNS

1. Obtain films from your instructor that are consistent with pulmonary edema, cavitary lesion, hilar adenopathy, chest tube, pulmonary artery catheter, and pleural effusion. Compare them with the normal adult film used in Exercise 33.2.

2. Using the technique practiced in the previous exercises, observe and identify the differences in each film. **Record them on your laboratory report.**

REFERENCES

1. Squire, LF and Novelline, RA: Fundamentals of Radiology, ed 4. Harvard University Press, Cambridge, 1988, p. 3.
2. Squire, LF and Novelline, RA: Fundamentals of Radiology, ed 4. Harvard University Press, Cambridge, 1988, p. 4.
3. Squire, LF and Novelline, RA: Fundamentals of Radiology, ed 4. Harvard University Press, Cambridge, 1988, p. 13.
4. Squire, LF and Novelline, RA: Fundamentals of Radiology, ed 4. Harvard University Press, Cambridge, 1988, p. 40–41.
5. Squire, LF and Novelline, RA: Fundamentals of Radiology, ed 4. Harvard University Press, Cambridge, 1988, p. 129

Laboratory Report

CHAPTER 33: BASIC CHEST X-RAY INTERPRETATION

Name _____   Date _____

Course/Section _____   Instructor _____

Data Collection

EXERCISE 33.1 Identification of Positions

A. _____   B. _____

C. _____   D. _____

EXERCISE 33.2 Identification of Major Organs and Landmarks

Cardiothoracic ratio = Heart size / Lung width

Label the chest film on Figure 33.6.

- Aortic knob
- Carina
- Clavicle
- Costophrenic angle
- Gastric bubble
- Hila
- Larynx
- Left heart border (apex)
- Left hemi-diaphragm
- Lung field
- Pleural edge
- Rib
- Right heart border
- Right hemi-diaphragm
- Scapula
- Trachea

A.	B.
C.	D.
E.	F.
G.	H.
I.	J.
K.	L.
M.	N.
O.	P.

EXERCISE 33.3 Hyperinflation

Film ID: _____ Patient demographics if known: _____

Projection used: _____

Flattening of the hemi-diaphragms: _____

Lung expansion to level of rib no.: _____

Horizontal rib margins present: _____

Increased intercostal spaces: _____

Areas of hyperlucency with decreased lung markings: _____

Comparison of lung size: _____

EXERCISE 33.4 Pneumothorax

Film ID: _____ Patient demographics if known: _____

Projection used: _____

Mediastinal shift: _____

Area of darker region without lung markings: _____

Edge of the collapsed lung: _____

EXERCISE 33.5 Atelectasis or Consolidation

Film ID: _____ Patient demographics if known: _____

Patient position: _____

Projection used: _____

Hemi-diaphragm positions: _____

Area of radiopaque image in an area where it should be radiolucent: _____

Mediastinal shift: _____

Decreased lung volumes: _____

EXERCISE 33.6 Endotracheal Tube Position

Film ID: _____ Patient demographics if known: _____

Projection used: _____

Tip of the endotracheal tube at: _____

Level of carina: _____

Lung expansion to rib level: _____

Distance above the carina: _____

EXERCISE 33.7 Chest Deformities

Film ID: _____ Patient demographics if known: _____

Kyphoscoliosis: _____

Differences observed: _____

EXERCISE 33.8 Infant and Pediatric Films

Film ID: _____ Patient demographics if known: _____

Comparison of normal infant chest x-ray with a normal adult chest x-ray: _____

Film ID: _____ Patient demographics if known: _____

Differences observed: _____

Steeple sign in croup_____

Film ID: _____ Patient demographics if known: _____

Differences observed: _____

Thumb sign in epiglottitis _____

Film ID: _____ Patient demographics if known: _____

Differences observed: _____

Respiratory distress syndrome_____

Film ID: _____ Patient demographics if known: _____

Differences observed: _____

Bronchopulmonary dysplasia _____

EXERCISE 33.9 Other Abnormal Patterns

Film ID: _____ Patient demographics if known: _____

Differences observed: _____

Abnormality: _____

_____

Film ID: _____ Patient demographics if known: _____

Differences observed: _____

Abnormality: _____

_____

Film ID: _____ Patient demographics if known: _____

Differences observed: _____

Abnormality: _____

_____

Film ID: _____ Patient demographics if known: _____

Differences observed: _____

Location of the chest tube: _____

Film ID: _____ Patient demographics if known: _____

Differences observed: _____

Location of the pulmonary artery catheter: _____

Differences observed: _____

Abnormality: _____

_____

Critical Thinking Questions

1. Why would the patient be asked to remove all necklaces, charms, and medals before a chest x-ray?

2. The physician requires a yearly chest x-ray for his or her patient with COPD. Of what benefit is the previous film?

3. Where is the carina normally found on the chest x-ray?

4. Can the chest x-ray determine if the tube is in the esophagus? Why or why not?

5. What factors might make the interpretation of a film difficult?

6.   Given the chest x-rays shown in Figures 33.17 through 33.21, what might the interpretation be?

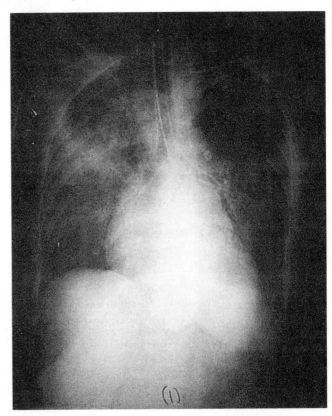

Figure 33.17. Unknown film A.

Figure 33.17 _____

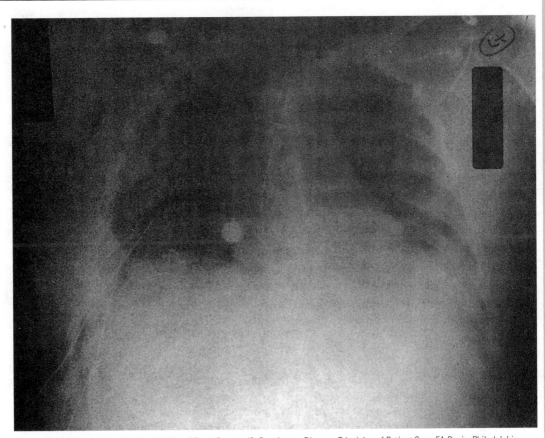

Figure 33.18. Unknown film B. (From Wilkins, RF and Dexter, JR: Respiratory Disease: Principles of Patient Care. FA Davis, Philadelphia, 1993, p. 207, with permission.)

Figure 33.18 _____

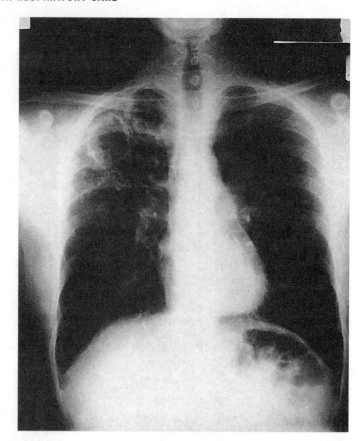

Figure 33.19. Unknown film C.

Figure 33.19 _____

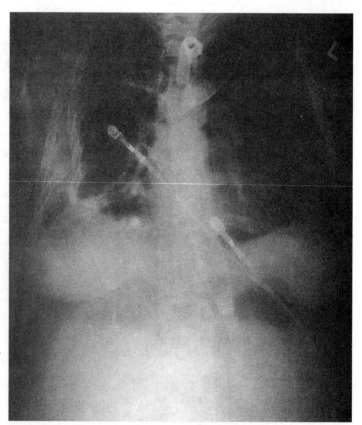

Figure 33.20. Unknown film D. (From Wilkins, RF and Dexter, JR: Respiratory Disease: Principles of Patient Care. FA Davis, Philadelphia, 1993, p. 212, with permission.)

Figure 33.20 _____

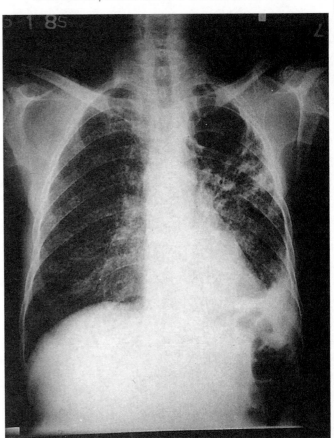

Figure 33.21. Unknown film E.

Figure 33.21 _____

Procedural Competency Evaluation

STUDENT: _____ DATE: _____

CHEST X-RAY INTERPRETATION

		PERFORMANCE RATING	PERFORMANCE LEVEL
Evaluator: ☐ Peer ☐ Instructor **Setting:** ☐ Lab ☐ Clinical Simulation			
Equipment Utilized: _____ **Conditions (Describe):** _____			
Performance Level:			
S or ✓ = Satisfactory, no errors of omission or commission U = Unsatisfactory Error of Omission or Commission NA = Not applicable			
Performance Rating:			
5 **Independent:** Near flawless performance; minimal errors; able to perform without supervision; seeks out new learning; shows initiative; A = 4.7–5.0 average			
4 **Minimally Supervised:** Few errors, able to self-correct; seeks guidance when appropriate; B = 3.7–4.65			
3 **Competent:** Minimal required level; no critical errors; able to correct with coaching; meets expectations; safe; C = 3.0–3.65			
2 **Marginal:** Below average; critical errors or problem areas noted; would benefit from remediation; D = 2.0–2.99			
1 **Dependent:** Poor; unacceptable performance; unsafe; gross inaccuracies; potentially harmful; F = < 2.0			
Two or more errors of commission or omission of mandatory or essential performance elements will terminate the procedure, and require additional practice and/or remediation and reevaluation. Student is responsible for obtaining additional evaluation forms as needed from the Director of Clinical Education (DCE).			

EQUIPMENT AND PATIENT PREPARATION

1. Common Performance Elements Steps 1–8		

ASSESSMENT AND IMPLEMENTATION

2. Common Performance Elements Steps 9 and 10		
3. Obtains the chest x-ray film; verifies film identification		
4. Inserts film onto the view box with correct orientation and turns on view box light		
5. Identifies projection view of the film and patient position		
6. Observes the entire film for symmetry and quality and identifies:		
A. Clavicles, scapulae, and ribs		
B. Spinal column and thoracic vertebrae; midline visible?		
C. Lungs, right and left		
D. Costophrenic angles; notes if they are sharp, blurred (possible fluid), or less sharp (blunted)		
E. Level of diaphragms; notes the rib level to determine if the film is of good or poor inspiratory quality		
F. Stomach air bubble		
G. Breast shadows		
H. Traces the outline of each rib noting the angle and any fractures or other abnormalities		
I. Tracheal position		
J. Identifies the carina and the mainstem bronchi		
K. Examines hila for size and position		
L. Presence or absence of lung markings		
M. Aortic knob and the heart shadow		
N. Examines for silhouette sign		
O. Measures and estimates the cardiothoracic ratio		
P. Notes the presence and position of any artificial airways or catheters		
7. States an overall impression of the film		
8. Correlates the film with the clinical findings and interprets results		

FOLLOW-UP

9. Common Performance Elements Steps 11–16		

SIGNATURES Student: _____ Evaluator: _____ Date: _____

Clinical Performance Evaluation

PERFORMANCE RATING:

5 **Independent:** Near flawless performance; minimal errors; able to perform without supervision; seeks out new learning; shows initiative; A = 4.7–5.0 average

4 **Minimally Supervised:** Few errors, able to self-correct; seeks guidance when appropriate; B = 3.7–4.65

3 **Competent:** Minimal required level; no critical errors; able to correct with coaching; meets expectations; safe; C = 3.0–3.65

2 **Marginal:** Below average; critical errors or problem areas noted; would benefit from remediation; D = 2.0–2.99

1 **Dependent:** Poor; unacceptable performance; unsafe; gross inaccuracies; potentially harmful; F = < 2.0

Circle the appropriate response below. Please be consistent, objective, and honest in your assessment of the student's clinical performance and ability.

PERFORMANCE CRITERIA	SCORE				
COGNITIVE DOMAIN					
1. Consistently displays knowledge, comprehension, and command of essential concepts	5	4	3	2	1
2. Demonstrates the relationship between theory and clinical practice	5	4	3	2	1
3. Able to select, review, apply, analyze, synthesize, interpret, and evaluate information; makes recommendations to modify care plan	5	4	3	2	1
PSYCHOMOTOR DOMAIN					
4. Minimal errors, no critical errors; able to self-correct; performs all steps safely and accurately	5	4	3	2	1
5. Selects, assembles, and verifies proper function and cleanliness of equipment; assures operation and corrects malfunctions; provides adequate care and maintenance	5	4	3	2	1
6. Exhibits the required manual dexterity	5	4	3	2	1
7. Performs procedure in a reasonable time frame for clinical level	5	4	3	2	1
8. Applies and maintains aseptic technique and PPE as required	5	4	3	2	1
9. Maintains concise and accurate patient and clinical records	5	4	3	2	1
10. Reports promptly on patient status/needs to appropriate personnel	5	4	3	2	1
AFFECTIVE DOMAIN					
11. Exhibits courteous and pleasant demeanor; shows consideration and respect, honesty, and integrity	5	4	3	2	1
12. Communicates verbally and in writing clearly and concisely	5	4	3	2	1
13. Preserves confidentiality and adheres to all policies	5	4	3	2	1
14. Follows directions, exhibits sound judgment, and seeks help when required	5	4	3	2	1
15. Demonstrates initiative, self-direction, responsibility, and accountability	5	4	3	2	1

TOTAL POINTS = _____ /15 = AVERAGE GRADE = _____

ADDITIONAL COMMENTS: IDENTIFY AREAS OF EXCELLENCE; LIST ERRORS OF OMISSION OR COMMISSION, CRITICAL ERRORS

SUMMARY PERFORMANCE EVALUATION AND RECOMMENDATIONS

☐ PASS: Satisfactory Performance

    ☐ Minimal supervision needed, may progress to next level provided specific skills, clinical time completed

    ☐ Minimal supervision needed, able to progress to next level without remediation

☐ FAIL: Unsatisfactory Performance (check all that apply)

    ☐ Minor reevaluation only

    ☐ Needs additional clinical practice before reevaluation

    ☐ Needs additional laboratory practice before skills performed in clinical area

    ☐ Recommend clinical probation

SIGNATURES

Evaluator (print name): _____ Evaluator signature: _____ Date: _____

Student Signature: _____ Date: _____

Student Comments:

34 Bronchoscopy Assisting

INTRODUCTION

Bronchoscopy is the general term used to describe the insertion of a visualization instrument (endoscope) into the bronchi. It has become an increasingly important diagnostic and therapeutic tool for the management of patients with pulmonary disease. Although this chapter will emphasize **flexible bronchoscopy**, respiratory therapists should gain some basic knowledge of **rigid bronchoscopy**.

The rigid **bronchoscope** is an open metal tube with a distal light source and a port for attaching oxygen or ventilating equipment. The rigid bronchoscope is used most often by otorhinolaryngologists or thoracic surgeons. It requires the use of general anesthesia and, therefore, the use of an operating suite and the services of an anesthesiologist. Rigid bronchoscopy cannot access the smaller airways. Some of the indications for rigid bronchoscopy include massive **hemoptysis**, laser therapy, foreign body retrieval, and placement of airway stents.

Flexible bronchoscopy has progressively replaced rigid bronchoscopy. The main indications for performing a flexible bronchoscopy are: inspection of the airway, remotion of objects from the airway, collection of samples from the airway, and the placement of devices into the airway.[1] Additionally, in the intensive care setting bronchoscopy may be used in the placement or change of an endotracheal tube, evaluation of chemical/thermal injuries, and evaluation of the upper airway after extubation.

Respiratory care practitioners can be utilized to prepare all the required equipment and assist the physician with the procedure.[2,3]

OBJECTIVES

Upon completion of this chapter, the student will be able to:

1. Practice communication skills required for assessing the level of patient comprehension of the procedure.
2. Practice medical charting for the bronchoscopy procedure.
3. Apply infection control guidelines and standards associated with equipment and procedures according to CDC guidelines.
4. Identify indications for rigid and flexible bronchoscopy.
5. Select the proper equipment necessary to assist during a bronchoscopy.
6. Assemble and verify equipment function.
7. Demonstrate use of the different ports of the bronchoscope.
8. Demonstrate adequate preparation of patient.
9. Demonstrate adequate preparation of the airway.
10. Demonstrate the setup of monitoring devices required during bronchoscopy.

11. Relate the complications that may be encountered during the insertion and manipulation of a bronchoscope.

12. Discuss the criteria for discharging the patient from the bronchoscopy suite.

KEY TERMS

atomizer	bronchoscope	hemoptysis	thumb control
bite block	flexible bronchoscopy	rigid bronchoscopy	

Exercises

EQUIPMENT REQUIRED

☐ Masks
☐ Gloves
☐ Gown
☐ Endotracheal tubes
☐ Fiberoptic bronchoscope adapter
☐ Yankauer-type suction catheters
☐ Suction pump
☐ Suction tubing
☐ **Bite block**
☐ Adhesive tape
☐ Water-soluble lubricant
☐ 10- and 20-mL syringes, Luer-Lok™
☐ 10- and 20-mL syringes, non-Luer-Lok™
☐ Needles, sharp tip
☐ Needles, blunt tip
☐ Saline
☐ Nonbacteriostatic saline
☐ Bronchoscope accessories
☐ Specimen cups
☐ Sputum traps
☐ Bronchoscope light source
☐ Denture cups
☐ Emesis basins
☐ Medicine cups
☐ Cotton 4×4 and 2×2 pads

☐ Pulse oximeter
☐ Oxygen cannula
☐ ECG leads
☐ Cardiac monitor
☐ Jackson forceps
☐ Cotton balls
☐ Heparin locks or caps
☐ Intravenous catheters or "butterflies"
☐ Alcohol wipes
☐ Band-Aids®
☐ Sterile swabs
☐ **Atomizer** and accessories
☐ Epinephrine 1:1000
☐ Heparin lock flush solution
☐ Sedatives (e.g., meperidine, codeine, morphine, diazepam, midazolam)
☐ Topical anesthetics [e.g., lidocaine (1%, 2%, and 4%), cocaine (4% or 10%), Cetacaine]
☐ Consent forms
☐ Specimen labels
☐ Laboratory specimen forms
☐ Radiology requisitions
☐ Bronchoscopy charge slips
☐ Physician order forms

EXERCISE 34.1 IDENTIFICATION OF COMPONENTS

Identify the components of a typical fiberoptic bronchoscope, as shown in Figure 34.1, and **record them on your laboratory report:**

Connection to light and video source

Brush/forceps/instillation port

Suction/oxygen port

Camera attachment/eyepiece

Thumb control

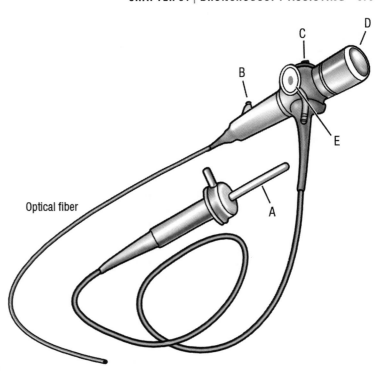

Figure 34.1. Components of a flexible fiberoptic bronchoscope.

EXERCISE 34.2 PREPARATION OF THE SUBJECT FOR BRONCHOSCOPY

Scenario 1

Paula Swanson is a 43-year-old Hispanic woman with a history of hemoptysis. A chest radiograph showed a mass in the right middle lobe and she has been scheduled for a bronchoscopy and possibly a biopsy.

To perform this exercise, you will need a mannequin and a laboratory partner to simulate a clinical situation. Before the initiation of the bronchoscopic procedure:

1. Ask the patient whether food or drink has been ingested in the last 8 hours.
2. Explain the need for premedication with benzodiazepines prior to the procedure to decrease anxiety.
3. Obtain vascular access.
4. **Record the relevant patient history on your laboratory report.**

EXERCISE 34.3 EQUIPMENT PREPARATION FOR BRONCHOSCOPY

1. Check the orders to confirm the request for bronchoscopy, patient information, and any special requirements or physician's orders prior to the procedure.
2. Wash your hands.
3: Gather equipment and check for proper function, tight connections, and integrity of the following.
   A. Light
   B. Thumb control
   C. Eyepiece focus
   D. Patency of suction and biopsy channel
4. **Record verification of proper function on your laboratory report.**

EXERCISE 34.4 BRONCHOSCOPY PROCEDURE

For this exercise, you will need a laboratory partner and a mannequin to simulate a patient undergoing bronchoscopy.

1. Identify the "patient."
2. Introduce yourself and explain the procedure.
3. Don clean gloves.
4. Approach the "patient" in a friendly, calm manner. Provide for his/her comfort as much as possible, and gain the "patient's" cooperation. Create a calm and soothing environment.
5. Position the "patient" in a semirecumbent position.
6. Place equipment close to work area.
7. Prepare the airway on the mannequin:
   A. Apply topical vasoconstrictors to prevent bleeding through nasal passage if indicated by the physician.
   B. Apply topical anesthetic to the nose using an atomizer, by mouthwash to the oropharynx, and by nebulizer or direct instillation in the bronchoscope.
8. Set up monitoring devices on your laboratory partner:
   A. Connect pulse oximetry. Provide supplemental oxygen if necessary.
   B. Attach leads to continuous electrocardiogram monitor.
   C. Place blood pressure cuff around "patient's" arm. **Record patient assessment data on your laboratory report.**
9. During mechanical ventilation (you need an intubated mannequin for this exercise):
   A. Increase F_IO_2 to 1.0.
   B. Maintain PEEP at preset levels.
   C. Attach a fiberoptic bronchoscope adapter, as shown in Figure 34.2, to the endotracheal tube adapter to introduce the bronchoscope.
   D. Adjust high-pressure alarm on the ventilator if necessary. **Record the adjustments made to the ventilator on your laboratory report.**
10. Insert a bite block.
11. Insert the bronchoscope (physician).
12. Introduce forceps and brushes.
13. Introduce syringes filled with anesthetic, vasoconstrictor, mucolytic agents, or lavage solution as available in your lab.
14. Apply suction to simulate sputum or tissue sampling.
15. Remove the bronchoscope.
16. Clean bronchoscope using a gluteraldehyde disinfecting solution.

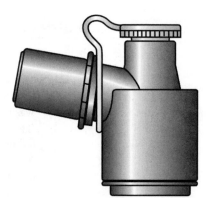

Figure 34.2. Fiberoptic bronchoscope adapter. (Courtesy of Smiths Medical, Rockland, MA.)

EXERCISE 34.5 BRONCHOSCOPY RECOVERY

To perform this exercise, you will need a partner to simulate a patient after the bronchoscopic procedure. Before discharge you will:

1. Confirm adequate oxygenation by measuring pulse oximetry on your "patient."
2. Keep "patient" in sitting position until fully awake and alert.
3. Instruct "patient" to refrain from eating or drinking until sensation is fully recovered.
4. Assess for presence of stridor and/or bronchospasm.
5. **"Chart" the post-bronchoscopy assessment on your laboratory report.**

EXERCISE 34.6 BRONCHOSCOPY COMPLICATIONS

Using your textbooks and other sources, prepare a list of common complications associated with bronchoscopy. List them in increasing order of severity. **Record the list on your laboratory report.**

REFERENCES
1. Leibler, JM and Markin, CJ: Fiberoptic bronchoscopy for diagnosis and treatment. Crit Care Clin 16:83, 2000.
2. Wilkins, RL, Stoller, JK, and Scanlan CL (eds): Egan's Fundamentals of Respiratory Care, ed 8. Mosby, St. Louis, 2003, p. 700.
3. Treanor, S, Benitez, WD, and Raffin, TA: Respiratory therapists as fiberoptic bronchoscopy assistants. Respir Care 30(38):321, 1985.

Laboratory Report

CHAPTER 34: BRONCHOSCOPY ASSIST

Name _____   Date _____

Course/Section _____   Instructor _____

Data Collection

EXERCISE 34.1 Identification of Components

Label all of the parts of the bronchoscope in Figure 34.1:

A. _____

B. _____

C. _____

D. _____

E. _____

EXERCISE 34.2 Preparation of the Subject for Bronchoscopy

Scenario 1

Relevant patient history and its impact on the procedure:

_____

_____

_____

_____

_____

EXERCISE 34.3 Equipment Preparation for Bronchoscopy

Verification of equipment function:

_____

_____

_____

EXERCISE 34.4 Bronchoscopy Procedure

Patient assessment data:

_____

_____

_____

Adjustments made to the mechanical ventilator:

_____

_____

_____

_____

EXERCISE 34.5 Bronchoscopy Recovery

Post-bronchoscopy assessment:

_____

_____

_____

_____

EXERCISE 34.6 Bronchoscopy Complications

Name four common complications during bronchoscopy:

_____

_____

_____

_____

Critical Thinking Questions

1. For Mrs. Swanson in Exercise 34.2, would you have recommended rigid bronchoscopy? YES ____ NO _____. Explain your answer.

2. While a bronchoscopy is being performed on a mechanically ventilated patient, you notice that the high-pressure alarm is sounding. What are the possible causes and corrective actions?

3. If the physician informs you that the light on the scope is no longer visible, what would you suggest to correct the problem?

4. A pulmonary fellow is performing her first bronchoscopy and informs you that the entire airway is blurry and suggests instillation of saline to clear the scope. You proceed with the instillation of saline and suction but the field fails to clear. What would you suggest in order to clear the field?

5. A patient with documented hypertension has been scheduled for a flexible bronchoscopy. Which of the commonly administered medications during bronchoscopy might cause an adverse reaction? Explain your answer in detail.

Procedural Competency Evaluation

STUDENT: **DATE:**

BRONCHOSCOPY ASSISTING

				PERFORMANCE RATING	PERFORMANCE LEVEL
Evaluator: ☐ Peer ☐ Instructor		**Setting:** ☐ Lab	☐ Clinical Simulation		
Equipment Utilized:		**Conditions (Describe):**			

Performance Level:

S or ✓ = Satisfactory, no errors of omission or commission
U = Unsatisfactory Error of Omission or Commission
NA = Not applicable

Performance Rating:

5   **Independent:** Near flawless performance; minimal errors; able to perform without supervision; seeks out new learning; shows initiative; A = 4.7–5.0 average

4   **Minimally Supervised:** Few errors, able to self-correct; seeks guidance when appropriate; B = 3.7–4.65

3   **Competent:** Minimal required level; no critical errors; able to correct with coaching; meets expectations; safe; C = 3.0–3.65

2   **Marginal:** Below average; critical errors or problem areas noted; would benefit from remediation; D = 2.0–2.99

1   **Dependent:** Poor; unacceptable performance; unsafe; gross inaccuracies; potentially harmful; F = < 2.0

Two or more errors of commission or omission of mandatory or essential performance elements will terminate the procedure, and require additional practice and/or remediation and reevaluation. Student is responsible for obtaining additional evaluation forms as needed from the Director of Clinical Education (DCE).

EQUIPMENT AND PATIENT PREPARATION		
1. Common Performance Elements Steps 1–8		
ASSESSMENT AND IMPLEMENTATION		
2. Common Performance Elements Steps 9 and 10		
3. Observes/assists with preparation of the bronchoscope		
4. Reviews indications, contraindications, hazards, and precautions of the procedure		
5. Assists with procedure as instructed by the physician		
6. Administers any anesthetic or medication as instructed		
7. Communicates effectively with the patient during the procedure		
8. Communicates effectively with the physician during the procedure		
9. Labels any specimens according to facility policy		
FOLLOW-UP		
10. Common Performance Elements Steps 11–16		

SIGNATURES   Student: Evaluator: Date:

Clinical Performance Evaluation

PERFORMANCE RATING:

5 **Independent:** Near flawless performance; minimal errors; able to perform without supervision; seeks out new learning; shows initiative; A = 4.7–5.0 average

4 **Minimally Supervised:** Few errors, able to self-correct; seeks guidance when appropriate; B = 3.7–4.65

3 **Competent:** Minimal required level; no critical errors; able to correct with coaching; meets expectations; safe; C = 3.0–3.65

2 **Marginal:** Below average; critical errors or problem areas noted; would benefit from remediation; D = 2.0–2.99

1 **Dependent:** Poor; unacceptable performance; unsafe; gross inaccuracies; potentially harmful; F = < 2.0

Circle the appropriate response below. Please be consistent, objective, and honest in your assessment of the student's clinical performance and ability.

PERFORMANCE CRITERIA	SCORE				
COGNITIVE DOMAIN					
1. Consistently displays knowledge, comprehension, and command of essential concepts	5	4	3	2	1
2. Demonstrates the relationship between theory and clinical practice	5	4	3	2	1
3. Able to select, review, apply, analyze, synthesize, interpret, and evaluate information; makes recommendations to modify care plan	5	4	3	2	1
PSYCHOMOTOR DOMAIN					
4. Minimal errors, no critical errors; able to self-correct; performs all steps safely and accurately	5	4	3	2	1
5. Selects, assembles, and verifies proper function and cleanliness of equipment; assures operation and corrects malfunctions; provides adequate care and maintenance	5	4	3	2	1
6. Exhibits the required manual dexterity	5	4	3	2	1
7. Performs procedure in a reasonable time frame for clinical level	5	4	3	2	1
8. Applies and maintains aseptic technique and PPE as required	5	4	3	2	1
9. Maintains concise and accurate patient and clinical records	5	4	3	2	1
10. Reports promptly on patient status/needs to appropriate personnel	5	4	3	2	1
AFFECTIVE DOMAIN					
11. Exhibits courteous and pleasant demeanor; shows consideration and respect, honesty, and integrity	5	4	3	2	1
12. Communicates verbally and in writing clearly and concisely	5	4	3	2	1
13. Preserves confidentiality and adheres to all policies	5	4	3	2	1
14. Follows directions, exhibits sound judgment, and seeks help when required	5	4	3	2	1
15. Demonstrates initiative, self-direction, responsibility, and accountability	5	4	3	2	1

TOTAL POINTS = _____ /15 = AVERAGE GRADE = _____

ADDITIONAL COMMENTS: IDENTIFY AREAS OF EXCELLENCE; LIST ERRORS OF OMISSION OR COMMISSION, CRITICAL ERRORS

SUMMARY PERFORMANCE EVALUATION AND RECOMMENDATIONS

☐ PASS: Satisfactory Performance

    ☐ Minimal supervision needed, may progress to next level provided specific skills, clinical time completed

    ☐ Minimal supervision needed, able to progress to next level without remediation

☐ FAIL: Unsatisfactory Performance (check all that apply)

    ☐ Minor reevaluation only

    ☐ Needs additional clinical practice before reevaluation

    ☐ Needs additional laboratory practice before skills performed in clinical area

    ☐ Recommend clinical probation

SIGNATURES

Evaluator (print name): _____ Evaluator signature: _____ Date: _____

Student Signature: _____ Date: _____

Student Comments:

35

Electrocardiography

INTRODUCTION

Electrocardiography (ECG) is commonly used for both diagnostic and monitoring purposes. The ECG recording is an integral part of patient assessment for any patient with chest pain or symptoms that suggest myocardial infarction or other cardiac dysfunction. Many procedures performed by respiratory care practitioners (RCPs) can affect cardiac function and electrical conduction. Whether to perform routine ECG recording, to monitor changes in heart rate and rhythm during therapeutic procedures, or to rapidly respond to changes in ECG during emergency procedures, RCPs are frequently called on to perform or identify and interpret common abnormalities in electrocardiogram tracings.

OBJECTIVES

Upon completion of this chapter, the student will be able to:

1. Identify normal anatomy of the heart and electrical conduction system.
2. Perform a 12-lead ECG recording.
3. Identify and correct common causes of artifacts that may interfere with the ECG.
4. Analyze and interpret ECG tracings for rate and rhythm, including normal sinus rhythm and common dysrhythmias.
5. Relate the pharmacological treatments of choice according to American Heart Association (AHA) advanced cardiac life support (ACLS) standards for common life-threatening dysrhythmias.

KEY TERMS

artifact   atrium   ventricle

Exercises

EQUIPMENT REQUIRED

- ☐ 4×4 nonsterile gauze
- ☐ Anatomical heart model
- ☐ Alcohol prep pads
- ☐ Bed linens
- ☐ Bed or table
- ☐ Clean towels or washcloths
- ☐ Disposable ECG electrode pads
- ☐ ECG calipers
- ☐ ECG monitor or Holter monitoring system, if available

- ☐ ECG recording paper
- ☐ Electrical outlets
- ☐ Electrocardiograph (ECG) machine
- ☐ Electrode gel
- ☐ Infectious waste container
- ☐ Limb and chest leads
- ☐ Privacy screen
- ☐ Ventilator, compressor, or any other large piece of electrical equipment

EXERCISE 35.1 CARDIAC ANATOMY

Obtain an anatomical model of the heart. Identify the vessels, coronary circulation chambers, and valves in comparison with Figure 35.1.

Label Figure 35.2, anatomy of the heart, label Figure 35.3, cardiac conduction system, **and record on your laboratory report.**

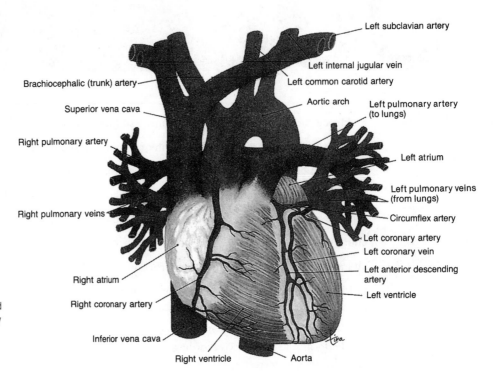

Figure 35.1. Anatomy of the heart: vessels and coronary circulation. (From Scanlon, VC and Sanders, T: Essentials of Anatomy and Physiology, ed 2. FA Davis, Philadelphia, 1991, p. 266, with permission.)

Left subclavian artery
Left internal jugular vein
Left common carotid artery
Aortic arch
Left pulmonary artery (to lungs)
Left atrium
Left pulmonary veins (from lungs)
Circumflex artery
Left coronary artery
Left coronary vein
Left anterior descending artery
Left ventricle

Brachiocephalic (trunk) artery
Superior vena cava
Right pulmonary artery
Right pulmonary veins
Right atrium
Right coronary artery
Inferior vena cava
Right ventricle
Aorta

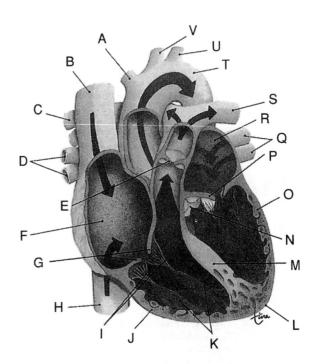

Figure 35.2. Label the anatomy of the heart: vessels, valves, and chambers. (From Scanlon, VC and Sanders, T: Essentials of Anatomy and Physiology, ed 2. FA Davis, Philadelphia, 1991, p. 266, with permission.)

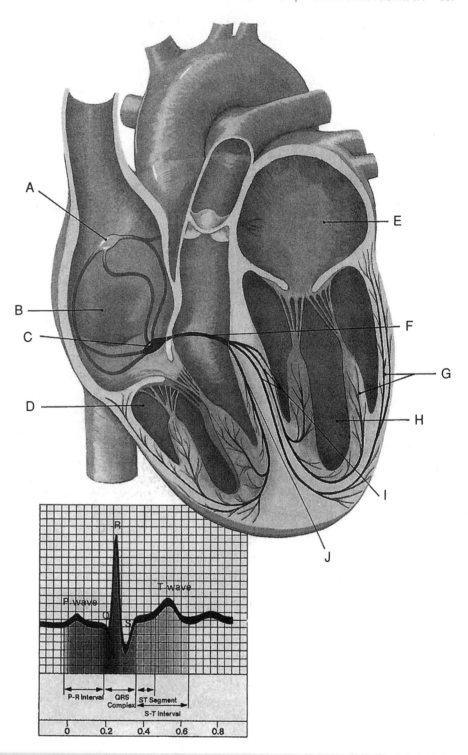

Figure 35.3. Cardiac conduction system. (From Scanlon, VC and Sanders, T: Essentials of Anatomy and Physiology, ed 2. FA Davis, Philadelphia, 1991, p. 271, with permission.)

EXERCISE 35.2 IDENTIFICATION OF ELECTROCARDIOGRAPH MACHINE CONTROLS

Depending on laboratory resources, your instructor will provide you with either a single-channel or a multichannel ECG machine. In either case, certain features are common to all ECG machines.

Identify the following controls on the ECG machine provided:

On/off switch

Stylus position

Lead marker

Calibration standard

Lead selector

Sensitivity

Paper speed

Identify the type of machine used and the specific controls found on this machine. **Record on your laboratory report.**

EXERCISE 35.3 PREPARATION AND ATTACHMENT OF LIMB LEADS

The following exercises will be performed on your laboratory partner or instructor.

1. Gather the necessary equipment:
   ECG machine
   Limb leads
   Disposable electrodes or reusable electrodes and gel
   Alcohol prep pads
2. Wash or sanitize your hands and apply standard precautions and transmission-based isolation procedures as appropriate.
3. Introduce yourself to the subject, verify the subject's identification, and explain the procedure.
4. Have the subject remove all jewelry or metal.
5. Place the subject in a supine position on the bed or table.
6. Plug in the ECG machine. Ensure that there is an adequate paper supply.
7. Apply clean electrodes (Fig. 35.4) to the muscular areas of the arms and legs, as shown in Figure 35.5. The placement should be in a similar location on both arms and legs. Avoid placing the electrodes on any bony prominences. NOTE: In the case of limb deformities or amputation, the electrode should be placed on the torso as close to the point of limb attachment as possible.

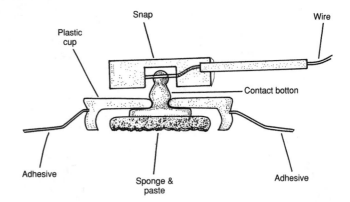

Figure 35.4. Cross-section of a disposable self-adhesive electrode.

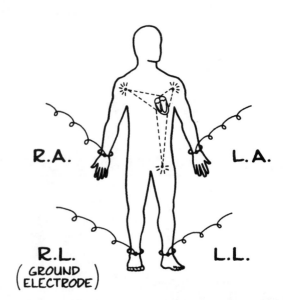

Figure 35.5. Limb leads. (From Lipman, BC and Cascio, T: ECG Assessment and Interpretation. FA Davis, Philadelphia, 1994, p. 15, with permission.)

It may be necessary to prepare the skin by rubbing it with an alcohol prep pad before electrode application. Excess body hair may interfere with the contact of an individual electrode; consequently, in a clinical situation, the area may need to be shaved before electrode application. For the purposes of this lab, shaving will not be performed.

If disposable electrode pads are used, peel off the backing and stick securely to the subject's skin. If nondisposable electrodes are used, an alcohol prep pad or electrode gel should be applied to the skin first. NOTE: The limb leads may be color-coded or alphabetically coded as follows:

Electrode location	Color
Right arm (RA)	White
Left arm (LA)	Black
Left leg (LL)	Red
Chest	Brown

8. Instruct the subject to attempt to relax completely.
9. If the machine is capable of recording single-channel leads, record the tracings for limb leads I, II, III, AVR, AVL, and AVF at this time.
10. Turn the machine on.
11. Turn to the record position. Check that the stylus is centered on the paper.
12. Make sure the paper speed is set at 25 mm/second.
13. Press the calibration standard mark at the beginning of each tracing (if it is not done automatically). Adjust the sensitivity as necessary so that the size of the complex is not too large or too small.
14. Run each lead for at least 6 seconds (approximately 6 inches). Use the lead marker to identify each lead recorded (if it is not done automatically).
15. Document the subject's name, date, and time of the recording on the ECG tracing when finished.

Attach the ECG tracing to your laboratory report. If only one subject is used to demonstrate to the class, have the instructor make copies of lead II for each student in the class and **attach the copy to your laboratory report.** Alternatively, you may run a long strip so that a minimum of a 6-second strip is available for each student in the laboratory.

You may continue with your partner for Exercise 35.4. However, if you are not performing Exercise 35.4 at this time, you should disconnect and remove the leads from your subject and clean up now. See Exercise 35.6 for directions.

EXERCISE 35.4 PREPARATION AND ATTACHMENT OF PRECORDIAL (CHEST) LEADS

EXERCISE 35.4.1 STANDARD CHEST LEADS

Because the chest leads must be attached to bare skin, it is preferable that a volunteer be used for this exercise. A student should not perform a 12-lead ECG on a female student without the permission of the female student and the instructor. Adequate privacy should be ensured. The chest, or precordial, leads are recorded with either a single electrode or multiple electrodes. If a single chest electrode is used, it must be repositioned before recording each precordial lead.

1. Place a small amount of ECG electrode gel on the skin over the correct position before electrode placement.
2. Place the chest electrodes in the following locations, as shown in Figure 35.6:
   V1: Fourth intercostal space, right sternal margin
   V2: Fourth intercostal space, left sternal margin
   V3: Midway between V2 and V4
   V4: Fifth intercostal space, left midclavicular line (MCL)
   V5: Fifth intercostal space, left anterior axillary line (AAL)
   V6: Sixth intercostal space, left midaxillary line (MAL)
3. Record the ECG tracing for each precordial lead, making sure to mark the calibration standard and lead marker for each lead.
4. If a multichannel 12-lead ECG machine is being used, record the entire 12-lead ECG at this time.
5. Document the subject's name, the date, and the time of the procedure on the ECG tracing. **Attach the tracing to your laboratory report.** If only one subject is used to demonstrate to the class, have the instructor make copies of V5 for each student, and **attach the copy to your laboratory report.**

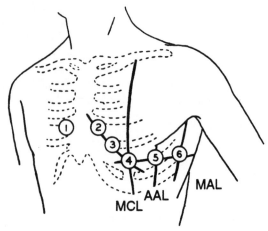

Figure 35.6. Precordial chest leads in relation to ribs. (From Lipman, BC and Cascio, T: ECG Assessment and Interpretation. FA Davis, Philadelphia, 1994, p. 16, with permission.)

EXERCISE 35.4.2 MODIFIED CHEST LEADS

The accompanying figures show modified leads used for continuous ECG monitoring (Fig. 35.7) and for ambulatory or Holter monitoring (Fig. 35.8). If an ECG monitor or Holter monitor is available, students should place electrodes on the chest as shown and run a strip.

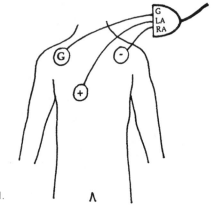

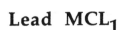

Figure 35.7. Modified chest lead MCL1. (From Lipman, BC and Cascio, T: ECG Assessment and Interpretation. FA Davis, Philadelphia, 1994, p. 20, with permission.)

Lead MCL₁

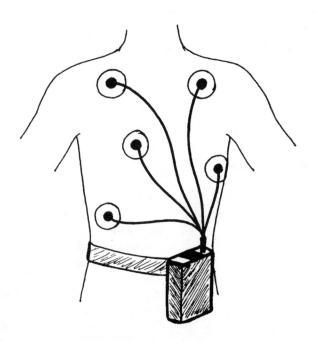

Figure 35.9. Ambulatory or Holter monitoring. (From Lipman, BC and Cascio, T: ECG Assessment and Interpretation. FA Davis, Philadelphia, 1994, p. 243, with permission.)

EXERCISE 35.5 ELECTROCARDIOGRAPH ARTIFACT

EXERCISE 35.5.1 IDENTIFICATION OF ARTIFACT

Match the ECG rhythm strips in Figures 35.9 through 35.12 with the following **artifacts and record them on your laboratory report:**

- Wandering baseline
- Muscle tremor
- 60-cycle interference
- Intermittent loss of signal

Figure 35.9. Tracing A. (From Frew, MA, Lane, K, and Frew, DR: Comprehensive Medical Assisting, ed 3. FA Davis, Philadelphia, 1995, p. 844, with permission.)

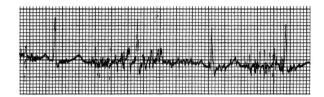

Figure 35.10. Tracing B. (From Frew, MA, Lane, K, and Frew, DR: Comprehensive Medical Assisting, ed 3. FA Davis, Philadelphia, 1995, p. 844, with permission.)

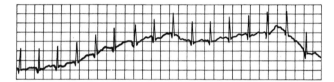

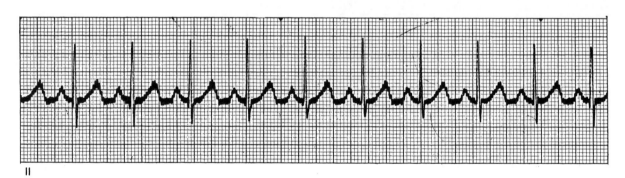

II

Figure 35.11. Tracing C. (From Brown, KR and Jacobson, S: Mastering Dysrhythmia: A Problem-Solving Guide. FA Davis, Philadelphia, 1988, p. 164, with permission.)

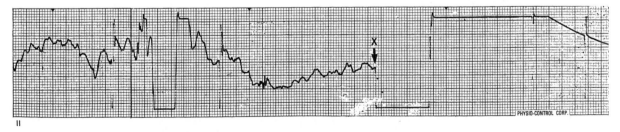

II

Figure 35.12. Tracing D. (From Brown, KR and Jacobson, S: Mastering Dysrhythmia: A Problem-Solving Guide. FA Davis, Philadelphia, 1988, p. 173, with permission.)

EXERCISE 35.5.2 SIMULATION OF ARTIFACT

1. Prepare your patient as instructed in Exercise 35.3.
2. Set the ECG machine to record lead II. Have the subject perform the following maneuvers to simulate ECG artifacts while recording the ECG tracing.
   A. Have the subject take deep breaths for several seconds. **Record your observations on, or attach the ECG tracing to, your laboratory report.**
   B. Have the subject tense his or her muscles for several seconds. **Record your observations on, or attach the ECG tracing to, your laboratory report.**
   C. Have the subject move his or her limbs. **Record your observations on, or attach the ECG tracing to, your laboratory report.**
   D. Have the subject touch the metal bed rails or ECG machine while recording. Alternatively, you may plug in another electrical device into the same electrical outlet while recording the ECG. **Record your observations on, or attach the ECG tracing to, the laboratory report.**
3. Loosen the right electrode lead. **Record your observations on, or attach the ECG tracing to, the laboratory report.**
4. Loosen the left electrode lead. **Record your observations on, or attach the ECG tracing to, the laboratory report.**
5. Reverse the right and left electrode leads. **Record your observations on, or attach the ECG tracing to, the laboratory report.**
6. If nondisposable electrodes are used, replace one without using electrode gel or alcohol prep pad. **Record your observations on, or attach the ECG tracing to, the laboratory report.**

EXERCISE 35.6 CLEANUP PROCEDURES

1. Remove the electrodes gently, especially if disposable electrodes are being used over body hair.
2. Clean off the skin using a washcloth or towel.
3. Discard the disposable electrodes in an infectious waste container.
4. Nondisposable electrodes must be thoroughly cleaned and disinfected before storage. Follow manufacturer's recommendations.
5. Neatly store limb leads and other supplies.

EXERCISE 35.7 RATE AND RHYTHM INTERPRETATION

1. To calculate the heart rate, one of three methods may be used:
   A. An estimation may be determined by counting the number of QRS complexes on a 6-second strip and multiplying by 10 (Fig. 35.13).

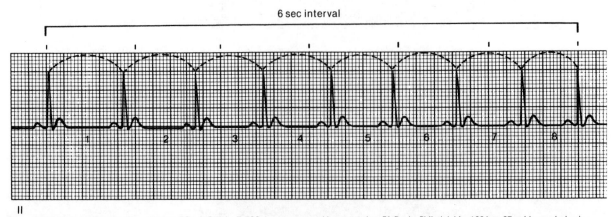

Figure 35.13. A 6-second strip. (From Lipman, BC and Cascio, T: ECG Assessment and Interpretation. FA Davis, Philadelphia, 1994, p. 67, with permission.)

B. The RR method. First find an R wave in which the peak of the QRS falls on a heavy, dark line. Then find the next QRS. For each dark line between the R waves, count backward (300, 150, 100, and so on) until you reach the second QRS, as shown in Figure 35.14.

C. Use the calipers to count the number of small boxes between two R waves, and divide that number into 1,500 (Fig. 35.15). This is the most accurate method.

2. Each small box is equal to 0.04 second. Each large box contains five small boxes across for duration of 0.20 second (see Fig. 35.3). Examine the PR intervals and the QRS widths on the rhythm strips obtained from previous exercises. Measure duration of each in seconds, and **record the results on your laboratory report.**

3. To interpret the rhythm, the following systematic approach is recommended:

A. Perform a general inspection of the rhythm strip. Look for possible artifacts.

B. Identify specific waves and intervals.

C. Is the rhythm regular or irregular? Using calipers, check the distance between R waves. A regular rhythm should have the same distance (within two small boxes) between all R waves. The conduction ratio is the number of P waves for each QRS complex.

D. Calculate the rate.

E. P waves: Are they present? What is their shape? Are they all alike? Is each followed by a QRS? What is the PR interval?

F. QRS: Are they present? What is their shape? Are they all alike? What is the QRS width?

G. ST segment: Is it baseline? Is it elevated or depressed?

H. T wave: Is it normal? Is it inverted?

I. Identify the rhythm.

Given practice tracings by your instructor, use the above method to interpret the rate and rhythm for each. **Attach the strips and results to your laboratory report.**

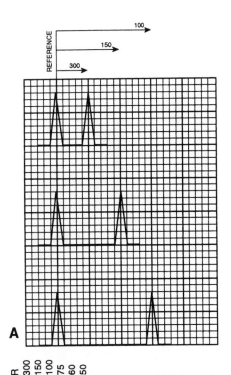

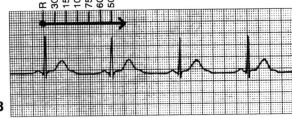

Figure 35.14. R-R method of calculating rate on an ECG. (From Lipman, BC and Cascio, T: ECG Assessment and Interpretation. FA Davis, Philadelphia, 1994, p. 66, with permission.)

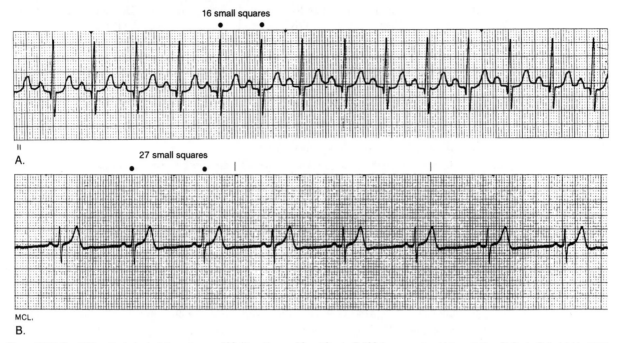

Figure 35.15. The 1500 method of calculating rate on an ECG. (From Lipman, BC and Cascio, T: ECG Assessment and Interpretation. FA Davis, Philadelphia, 1994, p. 63, with permission.)

Laboratory Report

CHAPTER 35: ELECTROCARDIOGRAPHY

Name _____ Date _____

Course/Section _____ Instructor _____

Data Collection

EXERCISE 35.1 Cardiac Anatomy

Label the heart diagram in Figure 35.2:

A._____   B._____

C._____   D._____

E._____   F._____

G._____   H._____

I._____   J._____

K._____   L._____

M._____   N._____

O._____   P._____

Q._____   R._____

S._____   T._____

U._____   V._____

Label the conduction system in Figure 35.3:

A._____   B._____

C._____   D._____

E._____   F._____

G._____   H._____

I._____   J._____

EXERCISE 35.2 Identification of Electrocardiograph Machine Controls

Type of machine used: _____

Controls identified: _____

_____

_____

_____

EXERCISE 35.3 Preparation and Attachment of Limb Leads

Attach the ECG tracing or copy to the laboratory report.

EXERCISE 35.4 Preparation and Attachment of Precordial (Chest) Leads

EXERCISE 35.4.1 STANDARD CHEST LEADS

Attach the ECG tracing or copy to the laboratory report.

EXERCISE 35.5 Electrocardiograph Artifact

EXERCISE 35.5.1 IDENTIFICATION OF ARTIFACT

Figure 35.9: _____

Figure 35.10: _____

Figure 35.11: _____

Figure 35.12: _____

EXERCISE 35.5.2 SIMULATION OF ARTIFACT

Tracings or observations: _____

Deep breathing: _____

Tensing of muscles: _____

Limb movement: _____

Touching metal bed rails or ECG machine or plugging in electrical device (record method used): _____

Loosening the right electrode lead: _____

Loosening the left electrode lead: _____

Reversal of the right and left electrode leads: _____

Replacement of electrode without gel or alcohol swab: _____

EXERCISE 35.7 Rate and Rhythm Interpretation

Using the tracings obtained from Exercise 35.3 or 35.4, perform the following:

1. General inspection: _____

2. Are all the P waves upright? Are they alike? _____

3. Is there a P wave for every QRS? _____

    A. Measure the PR interval: _____

    B. Number of small boxes: _____

    C. PR interval duration in seconds: _____

    D. Normal PR interval: _____

4. Look at the QRSs. Are they all alike? _____

    A. Is there a QRS for every P? _____

    B. Measure the QRS width: _____

C. Number of small boxes: _____

D. QRS width in seconds: _____

E. Normal QRS width: _____

F. Are all the RR intervals the same? _____

5. Is the ST segment baseline, elevated, or depressed? _____

6. Is the T wave normal? Is it inverted? _____

7. Is the rhythm regular or irregular? _____

8. Calculate the heart rate by all three methods. Show your work for each!

A. 6-second strip: _____

B. RR method: _____

C. 1500 method: _____

9. Interpretation: _____

_____

Critical Thinking Questions

Interpret the following ECG rhythm tracings:

1. A patient was found unconscious at home (Fig. 35.16). Paramedics sent the strip via telemetry.

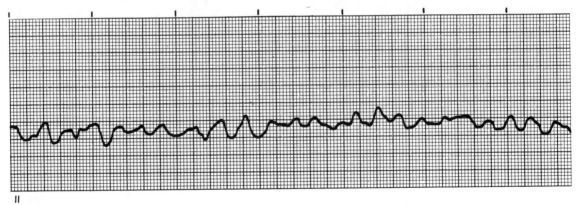

II

Figure 35.16. Rhythm strip #1. (From Brown, KR and Jacobson, S: Mastering Dysrhythmias: A Problem-Solving Guide. FA Davis, Philadelphia, 1988, p. 25, with permission.)

A. Rate:

B. Rhythm: regular or irregular?

C. P waves: present, shape, all alike, followed by normal QRS?

D. PR interval:

E.   QRS: present, shape, all alike?

F.   QRS width:

G.   ST segment: baseline, elevated, or depressed?

H.   T wave: normal or inverted?

I.   Identification of rhythm:

J.   Pharmacological treatment of choice or other treatment (if applicable):

2.   An 84-year-old man was seen in the doctor's office complaining of dizziness and light-headedness (Fig. 35.17).

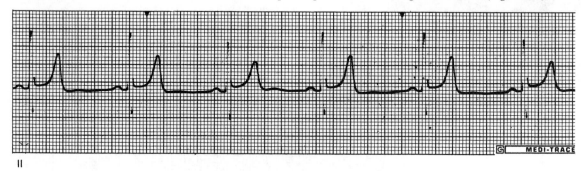

Figure 35.17. Rhythm strip #2. (From Brown, KR and Jacobson, S: Mastering Dysrhythmias: A Problem-Solving Guide. FA Davis, Philadelphia, 1988, p. 39, with permission.)

A.   Rate:

B.   Rhythm: regular or irregular?

C.   P waves: present, shape, all alike, followed by normal QRS?

D.   PR interval:

E.   QRS: present, shape, all alike?

F.   QRS width:

G.   ST segment: baseline, elevated, or depressed?

H.   T wave: normal or inverted?

I.   Identification of rhythm:

J.   Pharmacological treatment of choice (if applicable):

3.   A patient with a history of COPD being treated for an acute exacerbation began complaining of palpitations (Fig. 35.18).

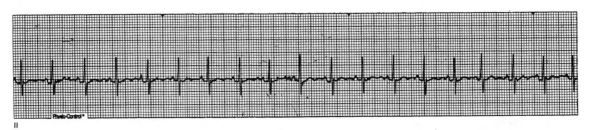

Figure 35.18. Rhythm strip #3. (From Brown, KR and Jacobson, S: Mastering Dysrhythmias: A Problem-Solving Guide. FA Davis, Philadelphia, 1988, p. 238, with permission.)

A.   Rate:

B.   Rhythm: regular or irregular?

C.   P waves: present, shape, all alike, followed by normal QRS?

D.   PR interval:

E.   QRS: present, shape, all alike?

F.   QRS width:

G.   ST segment: baseline, elevated, or depressed?

H.   T wave: normal or inverted?

I.   Identification of rhythm:

J.   Pharmacological treatment of choice (if applicable):

4.   A 64-year-old woman was brought to the ER with a chief complaint of heaviness in the chest and tightness in the back and left shoulder (Fig. 35.19).

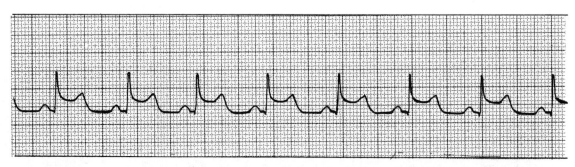

Figure 35.19. Rhythm strip #4. (Courtesy of Laerdal Medical Corporation, Wappingers Falls, NY.)

A.   Rate:

B.   Rhythm: regular or irregular?

C.   P waves: present, shape, all alike, followed by normal QRS?

D.   PR interval:

E.   QRS: present, shape, all alike?

F. QRS width:

G. ST segment: baseline, elevated, or depressed?

H. T wave: normal or inverted?

I. Identification of rhythm:

J. Pharmacological treatment of choice (if applicable):

5. Figure 35.20 was obtained several days later on the patient in Critical Thinking Question 4.

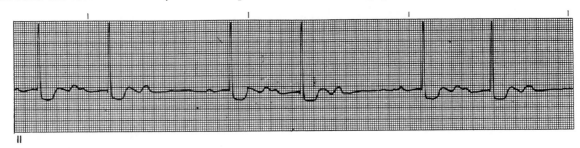

Figure 35.20. Rhythm strip #5. (From Brown, KR and Jacobson, S: Mastering Dysrhythmias: A Problem-Solving Guide. FA Davis, Philadelphia, 1988, p. 90, with permission.)

A. Rate:

B. P waves: present, shape, all alike, followed by normal QRS?

C. PR interval:

D. QRS: present, shape, all alike?

E. QRS width:

F. ST segment: baseline, elevated, or depressed?

G. T wave: normal or inverted?

H.   Rhythm: regular or irregular?

I.   Identification of rhythm:

J.   Pharmacological treatment of choice (if applicable):

You enter a patient's room to perform an arterial blood gas. During preparation for the procedure, you notice the rhythm shown in Figure 35.21 on the ECG monitor.

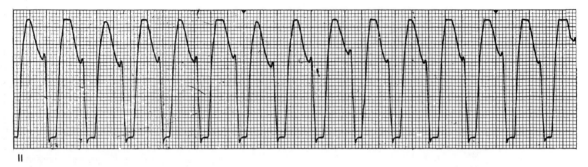

II

Figure 35.21. Rhythm strip #6 (From Brown, KR and Jacobson, S: Mastering Dysrhythmias: A Problem-Solving Guide. FA Davis, Philadelphia, 1988, p. 125, with permission.)

K.   What should you do first?

L.   You have determined that the patient has no respirations or pulse. What would your next action(s) be?

M.   Once advanced life support emergency equipment is available, what should be done first to treat this rhythm?

N.   The patient's pulse and blood pressure have returned and the rhythm shown in Figure 35.22 is noted on the ECG monitor. What is the most indicated pharmacological treatment for this rhythm?

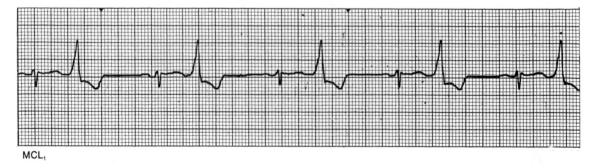

MCL₁

Figure 35.22. Rhythm strip #7. (From Brown, KR and Jacobson, S: Mastering Dysrhythmias: A Problem-Solving Guide. FA Davis, Philadelphia, 1988, p. 117, with permission.)

Procedural Competency Evaluation

STUDENT: **DATE:**

ELECTROCARDIOGRAPHY

		PERFORMANCE RATING	PERFORMANCE LEVEL
Evaluator: ☐ Peer ☐ Instructor **Setting:** ☐ Lab ☐ Clinical Simulation			
Equipment Utilized: **Conditions (Describe):**			

Performance Level:
 	
    S or ✓ = Satisfactory, no errors of omission or commission
    U = Unsatisfactory Error of Omission or Commission
    NA = Not applicable			

Performance Rating:
 	
  5 **Independent:** Near flawless performance; minimal errors; able to perform without supervision; seeks out new learning; shows initiative; A = 4.7–5.0 average
  4 **Minimally Supervised:** Few errors, able to self-correct; seeks guidance when appropriate; B = 3.7–4.65
  3 **Competent:** Minimal required level; no critical errors; able to correct with coaching; meets expectations; safe; C = 3.0–3.65
  2 **Marginal:** Below average; critical errors or problem areas noted; would benefit from remediation; D = 2.0–2.99
  1 **Dependent:** Poor; unacceptable performance; unsafe; gross inaccuracies; potentially harmful; F = < 2.0
 	
  Two or more errors of commission or omission of mandatory or essential performance elements will terminate the procedure, and require additional practice and/or remediation and reevaluation. Student is responsible for obtaining additional evaluation forms as needed from the Director of Clinical Education (DCE).			

EQUIPMENT AND PATIENT PREPARATION			
1. Common Performance Elements Steps 1–8			
2. Obtains ECG machine, electrodes, gel, gauze, and paper; ensures that the machine has sufficient paper and supplies available			
ASSESSMENT AND IMPLEMENTATION			
3. Common Performance Elements Steps 9 and 10			
4. Assures patient comfort and respects patient privacy and modesty			
5. Places patient appropriately in supine or semi-Fowler's position; instructs patient to relax completely			
6. Has patient remove all jewelry or metal			
7. Applies clean limb electrodes to muscular areas of arms and legs; placement should be in a similar location on both arms and legs			

8. Places chest leads in proper location:
  A. V1: 4th intercostal space right sternal margin   D. V4: Fifth intercostal space, left midclavicular line
  B. V2: 4th intercostal space left sternal margin   E. V5: Fifth intercostal space, left anterior axillary line
  C. V3: Midway between V2 and V4 F. V6: Sixth intercostal space, left midaxillary line			

9. Calibrates machine; runs test strip			

10. Inspects rhythm strip for:
  A. Wandering baseline   D. Disconnected lead or intermittent loss of signal
  B. 60-cycle artifact   E. Poor prep (contact) artifact
  C. Muscle tremor artifact			

11. Runs complete 12-lead ECG			
12. Scans cardiogram for any major dysrhythmias			

13. Measures, analyzes, or interprets:
  A. Rhythm   F. ST segment
  B. Rate   G. T wave
  C. P wave appearance   H. QT interval
  D. PR interval   I. Interprets ECG results
  E. QRS complex appearance and width			

FOLLOW-UP			
14. Maintains patient's privacy			
15. Common Performance Elements Steps 11–16			
16. Removes electrodes and cleans electrode sites			
17. Cleans electrodes and machine			

SIGNATURES   Student: Evaluator: Date:

Clinical Performance Evaluation

PERFORMANCE RATING:

5 **Independent:** Near flawless performance; minimal errors; able to perform without supervision; seeks out new learning; shows initiative; A = 4.7–5.0 average

4 **Minimally Supervised:** Few errors, able to self-correct; seeks guidance when appropriate; B = 3.7–4.65

3 **Competent:** Minimal required level; no critical errors; able to correct with coaching; meets expectations; safe; C = 3.0–3.65

2 **Marginal:** Below average; critical errors or problem areas noted; would benefit from remediation; D = 2.0–2.99

1 **Dependent:** Poor; unacceptable performance; unsafe; gross inaccuracies; potentially harmful; F = < 2.0

Circle the appropriate response below. Please be consistent, objective, and honest in your assessment of the student's clinical performance and ability.

PERFORMANCE CRITERIA	SCORE				
COGNITIVE DOMAIN					
1. Consistently displays knowledge, comprehension, and command of essential concepts	5	4	3	2	1
2. Demonstrates the relationship between theory and clinical practice	5	4	3	2	1
3. Able to select, review, apply, analyze, synthesize, interpret, and evaluate information; makes recommendations to modify care plan	5	4	3	2	1
PSYCHOMOTOR DOMAIN					
4. Minimal errors, no critical errors; able to self-correct; performs all steps safely and accurately	5	4	3	2	1
5. Selects, assembles, and verifies proper function and cleanliness of equipment; assures operation and corrects malfunctions; provides adequate care and maintenance	5	4	3	2	1
6. Exhibits the required manual dexterity	5	4	3	2	1
7. Performs procedure in a reasonable time frame for clinical level	5	4	3	2	1
8. Applies and maintains aseptic technique and PPE as required	5	4	3	2	1
9. Maintains concise and accurate patient and clinical records	5	4	3	2	1
10. Reports promptly on patient status/needs to appropriate personnel	5	4	3	2	1
AFFECTIVE DOMAIN					
11. Exhibits courteous and pleasant demeanor; shows consideration and respect, honesty, and integrity	5	4	3	2	1
12. Communicates verbally and in writing clearly and concisely	5	4	3	2	1
13. Preserves confidentiality and adheres to all policies	5	4	3	2	1
14. Follows directions, exhibits sound judgment, and seeks help when required	5	4	3	2	1
15. Demonstrates initiative, self-direction, responsibility, and accountability	5	4	3	2	1

TOTAL POINTS = _____ /15 = AVERAGE GRADE = _____

ADDITIONAL COMMENTS: IDENTIFY AREAS OF EXCELLENCE; LIST ERRORS OF OMISSION OR COMMISSION, CRITICAL ERRORS

SUMMARY PERFORMANCE EVALUATION AND RECOMMENDATIONS

☐ PASS: Satisfactory Performance

    ☐ Minimal supervision needed, may progress to next level provided specific skills, clinical time completed

    ☐ Minimal supervision needed, able to progress to next level without remediation

☐ FAIL: Unsatisfactory Performance (check all that apply)

    ☐ Minor reevaluation only

    ☐ Needs additional clinical practice before reevaluation

    ☐ Needs additional laboratory practice before skills performed in clinical area

    ☐ Recommend clinical probation

SIGNATURES

Evaluator (print name): _____ Evaluator signature: _____ Date: _____

Student Signature: _____ Date: _____

Student Comments:

Procedural Competency Evaluation

STUDENT: _____ DATE: _____

ECG INTERPRETATION

Evaluator: ☐ Peer ☐ Instructor	**Setting:** ☐ Lab ☐ Clinical Simulation
Equipment Utilized:	**Conditions (Describe):**

Performance Level:

S or ✓ = Satisfactory, no errors of omission or commission
U = Unsatisfactory Error of Omission or Commission
NA = Not applicable

Performance Rating:

5   **Independent:** Near flawless performance; minimal errors; able to perform without supervision; seeks out new learning; shows initiative; A = 4.7–5.0 average

4   **Minimally Supervised:** Few errors, able to self-correct; seeks guidance when appropriate; B = 3.7–4.65

3   **Competent:** Minimal required level; no critical errors; able to correct with coaching; meets expectations; safe; C = 3.0–3.65

2   **Marginal:** Below average; critical errors or problem areas noted; would benefit from remediation; D = 2.0–2.99

1   **Dependent:** Poor; unacceptable performance; unsafe; gross inaccuracies; potentially harmful; F = < 2.0

Two or more errors of commission or omission of mandatory or essential performance elements will terminate the procedure, and require additional practice and/or remediation and reevaluation. Student is responsible for obtaining additional evaluation forms as needed from the Director of Clinical Education (DCE).

	PERFORMANCE RATING	PERFORMANCE LEVEL
1. Obtains an ECG rhythm strip		
2. Analyzes strip for the presence of artifact		
3. Differentiates artifact from actual ECG tracing		
4. Calculates heart rate by 6-second, RR, or box counting method		
5. Determines regularity by analyzing R wave distance with calipers		
6. Evaluates presence and shape of P waves		
7. Calculates PR interval		
8. Evaluates QRS width		
9. Evaluates ST segment for elevation or depression		
10. Evaluates T wave for inversion		
11. Identifies any ectopic beats		
12. Correctly interprets rate and rhythm		

SIGNATURES   Student: _____   Evaluator: _____   Date: _____

Clinical Performance Evaluation

PERFORMANCE RATING:

5 **Independent:** Near flawless performance; minimal errors; able to perform without supervision; seeks out new learning; shows initiative; A = 4.7–5.0 average

4 **Minimally Supervised:** Few errors, able to self-correct; seeks guidance when appropriate; B = 3.7–4.65

3 **Competent:** Minimal required level; no critical errors; able to correct with coaching; meets expectations; safe; C = 3.0–3.65

2 **Marginal:** Below average; critical errors or problem areas noted; would benefit from remediation; D = 2.0–2.99

1 **Dependent:** Poor; unacceptable performance; unsafe; gross inaccuracies; potentially harmful; F = < 2.0

Circle the appropriate response below. Please be consistent, objective, and honest in your assessment of the student's clinical performance and ability.

PERFORMANCE CRITERIA | SCORE

PERFORMANCE CRITERIA					
COGNITIVE DOMAIN					
1. Consistently displays knowledge, comprehension, and command of essential concepts	5	4	3	2	1
2. Demonstrates the relationship between theory and clinical practice	5	4	3	2	1
3. Able to select, review, apply, analyze, synthesize, interpret, and evaluate information; makes recommendations to modify care plan	5	4	3	2	1
PSYCHOMOTOR DOMAIN					
4. Minimal errors, no critical errors; able to self-correct; performs all steps safely and accurately	5	4	3	2	1
5. Selects, assembles, and verifies proper function and cleanliness of equipment; assures operation and corrects malfunctions; provides adequate care and maintenance	5	4	3	2	1
6. Exhibits the required manual dexterity	5	4	3	2	1
7. Performs procedure in a reasonable time frame for clinical level	5	4	3	2	1
8. Applies and maintains aseptic technique and PPE as required	5	4	3	2	1
9. Maintains concise and accurate patient and clinical records	5	4	3	2	1
10. Reports promptly on patient status/needs to appropriate personnel	5	4	3	2	1
AFFECTIVE DOMAIN					
11. Exhibits courteous and pleasant demeanor; shows consideration and respect, honesty, and integrity	5	4	3	2	1
12. Communicates verbally and in writing clearly and concisely	5	4	3	2	1
13. Preserves confidentiality and adheres to all policies	5	4	3	2	1
14. Follows directions, exhibits sound judgment, and seeks help when required	5	4	3	2	1
15. Demonstrates initiative, self-direction, responsibility, and accountability	5	4	3	2	1

TOTAL POINTS = _____ /15 = AVERAGE GRADE = _____

ADDITIONAL COMMENTS: IDENTIFY AREAS OF EXCELLENCE; LIST ERRORS OF OMISSION OR COMMISSION, CRITICAL ERRORS

SUMMARY PERFORMANCE EVALUATION AND RECOMMENDATIONS

☐ PASS: Satisfactory Performance

☐ Minimal supervision needed, may progress to next level provided specific skills, clinical time completed

☐ Minimal supervision needed, able to progress to next level without remediation

☐ FAIL: Unsatisfactory Performance (check all that apply)

☐ Minor reevaluation only

☐ Needs additional clinical practice before reevaluation

☐ Needs additional laboratory practice before skills performed in clinical area

☐ Recommend clinical probation

SIGNATURES

Evaluator (print name): _____ Evaluator signature: _____ Date: _____

Student Signature: _____ Date: _____

Student Comments:

36 Hemodynamic Monitoring

INTRODUCTION

The role of the respiratory therapist has evolved greatly over the past several decades. Respiratory therapists have progressed from being transporters of oxygen cylinders to the experts in a variety of sophisticated invasive therapeutic and patient-monitoring techniques. Likewise, diagnostic capabilities and expectations have progressed from obtaining basic vital signs to the performance of technologically advanced hemodynamic and laboratory techniques. In particular, major advancements have been made in the evaluation of the cardiovascular system and the efficiency of oxygen delivery in the care of the critically ill.[1] Application of physiologic principles and the interpretation of the data obtained from hemodynamic monitoring aid in the care of the critically ill, enhance patient-ventilator management, and improve clinical outcomes.[2] Although the involvement of the respiratory therapist with hemodynamic monitoring varies from facility to facility, mastering the use of this equipment—including setup, troubleshooting, and interpretation of results—helps make the respiratory therapist an indispensable member of the patient care team. In addition, the National Board for Respiratory Care recognizes, particularly for those seeking the advanced (RRT) level credential, that practitioners must demonstrate a basic competency in this area.

It should be noted that although there are noninvasive methods that are used for hemodynamic monitoring, this chapter focuses on invasive techniques that the respiratory therapist is most likely to encounter.[3]

OBJECTIVES

Upon completion of this chapter, the student will be able to:

1. Practice communication skills needed for the instruction of patients during hemodynamic monitoring.
2. Identify the components of a pulmonary artery catheter.
3. Identify the proper port for mixed venous blood sampling on a pulmonary artery catheter.
4. Select, assemble, and calibrate the equipment required for a fluid-filled monitoring system.
5. Calibrate a pressure transducer.
6. Simulate the procedure for obtaining a **cardiac output** using the thermodilution method.
7. Identify central venous, right ventricle, pulmonary artery, and pulmonary capillary wedge waveforms.
8. Identify and correct problems with a fluid-filled monitoring system.
9. Practice the calculations to obtain derived hemodynamic data: **body surface area,** Fick equation, mean arterial pressure, **cardiac index,** various shunt equations, **systemic vascular resistance,** and **pulmonary vascular resistance.**
10. Practice documentation and reporting of hemodynamic data collected.

11. Apply infection control guidelines and standards associated with equipment and procedures, according to OSHA regulations and CDC guidelines.

KEY TERMS

body surface area
cardiac index
cardiac output

central venous pressure
pulmonary capillary
  wedge pressure

pulmonary vascular
  resistance
systemic vascular
  resistance

Exercises

EQUIPMENT REQUIRED

☐ Quadruple-lumen or triple-lumen pulmonary
  artery catheter
☐ IV pole
☐ IV tubing (high-pressure)
☐ Microdrip chamber
☐ IV saline solution (1-L bag)
☐ Heparin
☐ Medication label
☐ Alcohol prep pads
☐ Ice
☐ Basin
☐ Sterile normal saline
☐ Pressure and cardiac output monitor
☐ Equipment manual

☐ Pressure transducer
☐ Inflatable pressure bag or pressure infuser
☐ Female caps
☐ Intraflow or flush device
☐ Three-way stopcocks
☐ T-connectors
☐ Tuberculin syringe
☐ 10-mL syringes (five)
☐ Mercury manometer with inflation bulb
☐ Hemodynamic simulator (if available)
☐ DuBois body surface area chart
☐ Medical scale

EXERCISE 36.1 IDENTIFICATION OF THE COMPONENTS OF A FLOW-DIRECTED PULMONARY ARTERY CATHETER

1. Select a pulmonary artery catheter as shown in Figure 36.1. **Identify the components on your laboratory report.**

   Thermistor connection

   Balloon inflation port

   Proximal port

   Distal port

   Thermistor opening

   Balloon

   Distal opening

   Centimeter markings

   Proximal opening

   Extra injection port

2. Using a tuberculin syringe, inflate the balloon with 0.5 mL of air. *Overinflation of the balloon will cause it to rupture. This is expensive in the laboratory setting and dangerous in the clinical setting.*

3. Feel the balloon.

4. Deflate the balloon.

5. Identify the port used for mixed venous blood sampling and **record it on your laboratory report.**

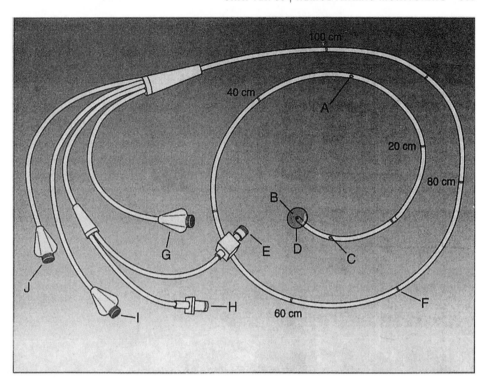

Figure 36.1. The components of a flow-directed pulmonary artery catheter. (From Persing, G: Advanced Practitioner Respiratory Care Review. WB Saunders, Philadelphia, 1994, p. 109, with permission.)

EXERCISE 36.2 ASSEMBLY AND CALIBRATION OF A FLUID-FILLED MONITORING SYSTEM[1]

1. Gather the necessary equipment and assemble it as shown in Figure 36.2. Make sure your handling of the equipment maintains the sterility of all ports. All ports should be capped with female caps to avoid inadvertent contamination.

2. Simulate heparinizing the IV solution and label the bag. Use 10 mg of a 1% solution of heparin per 500 mL. **Record on your laboratory report how much heparin is needed for the size IV solution bag used in your setup.**

3. Insert the microdrip chamber spike and IV tubing into the bag.

4. Squeeze all the air out of the IV bag.

5. Gravity-fill the tubing and transducer assembly.

6. Inspect for the presence of air bubbles. Remove any air bubbles found.

7. Place the IV bag into the inflatable pressure bag or pressure infuser.

8. Inflate the pressure bag or infuser to 300 mm Hg.

9. Turn on the pressure monitor and allow 5 to 10 minutes for warm-up.

10. Zero the monitor and transducer according to the manufacturer's instructions, as shown in Figure 36.3.

11. Close the system by closing the stopcock to all ports.

12. Connect the proximal port of the catheter to the IV tubing.

13. The completed setup is shown in Figure 36.4.

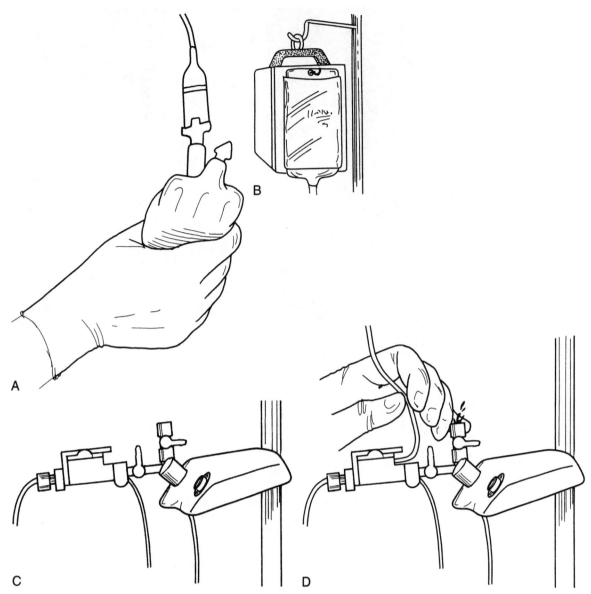

Figure 36.2. The components of a fluid-filled monitoring system.

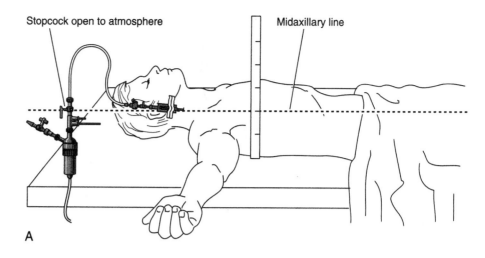

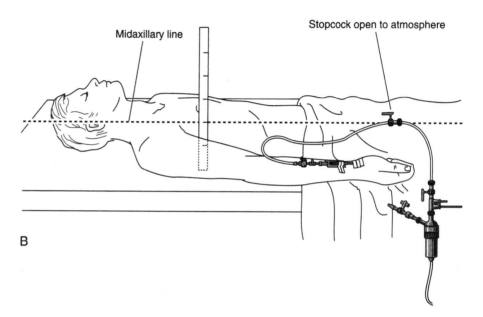

Figure 36.3. Zeroing the pressure transducer. (From Gardner, RM and Hollingsworth, KW: Optimizing the electrocardiogram and pressure monitoring. Crit Care Med 14:651, 1986, with permission.)

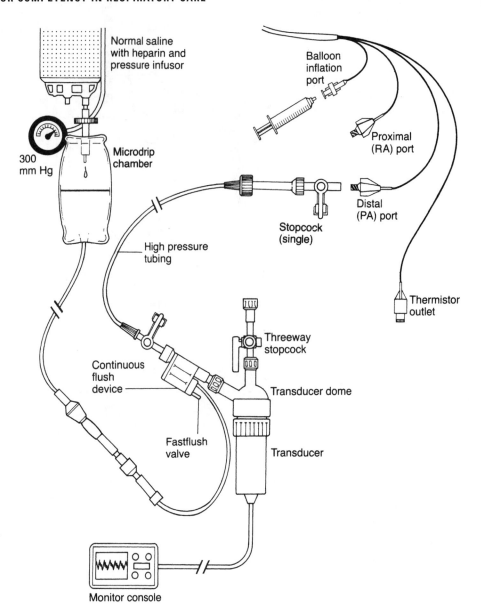

Normal saline
with heparin and
pressure infusor

Balloon
inflation
port

300
mm Hg

Microdrip
chamber

Proximal
(RA) port

Distal
(PA) port

Stopcock
(single)

High pressure
tubing

Thermistor
outlet

Threeway
stopcock

Continuous
flush
device

Transducer dome

Fastflush
valve

Transducer

Monitor console

Figure 36.4. Completed assembly of a fluid-filled monitoring system. (From Darovic, GO: Hemodynamic Monitoring: Invasive and Noninvasive Clinical Application, ed 2. WB Saunders, Philadelphia, 1995, p. 266, with permission.)

EXERCISE 36.3 TRANSDUCER CALIBRATION

1. Select and assemble the equipment as shown in Figure 36.5.
2. Open the stopcock to ensure communication between the manometer and the pressure monitor.
3. Inflate the manometer to 90 mm Hg by squeezing the bulb.
4. Observe the pressure monitor and **record the pressure reading on your laboratory report.**
5. Disassemble the equipment.

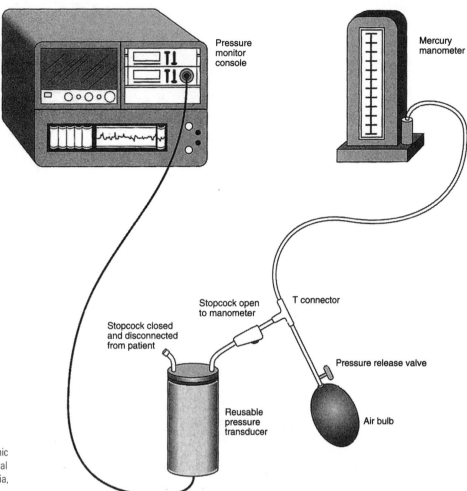

Figure 36.5. Assembly of a pressure transducer and manometer for transducer calibration. (From Darovic, GO: Hemodynamic Monitoring: Invasive and Noninvasive Clinical Application, ed 2. WB Saunders, Philadelphia, 1995, p. 171, with permission.)

EXERCISE 36.4 IDENTIFICATION OF PRESSURE WAVEFORMS

1. **Identify the pressure waveforms in Figures 36.6, 36.7, 36.8, and 36.9 on your laboratory report.**
2. Using a simulator (if available), generate and identify the following problem waveforms. **Print out (if possible) the waveforms associated with these problems and attach them to your laboratory report, or draw them on a separate sheet.** Common problems associated with a fluid-filled monitoring system are shown in Figure 36.10.

    Overdamped system
    Underdamped system
    Flush
    Catheter whip

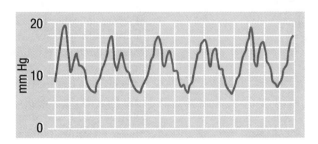

Figure 36.6. Waveform A.

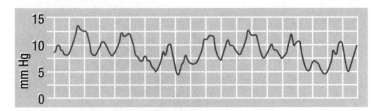

Figure 36.7. Waveform B.

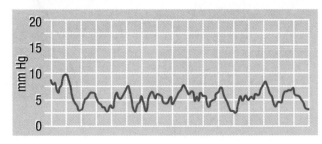

Figure 36.8. Waveform C.

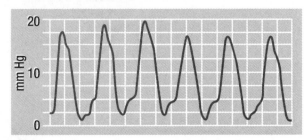

Figure 36.9. Waveform D.

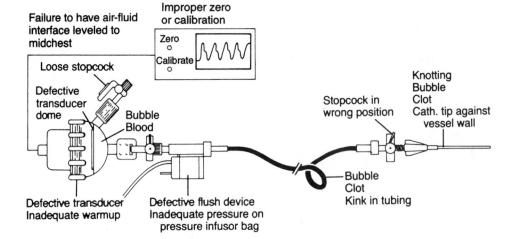

Figure 36.10. Step-by-step approach to problem identification. (From Darovic, GO: Hemodynamic Monitoring: Invasive and Noninvasive Clinical Application, ed 2. WB Saunders, Philadelphia, 1995, p. 312, with permission.)

EXERCISE 36.5 THERMODILUTION CARDIAC OUTPUT DETERMINATION

This exercise simulates the preparation of materials necessary to obtain a cardiac output.

1. Wash your hands and apply standard precautions and transmission-based isolation procedures as appropriate.

2. Explain the purpose of the procedure to the "patient."

3. Prepare an ice/slush solution on the basin. Be sure to maintain the sterility of all solutions, ports, and connectors.

4. Make sure that the cardiac output pressure monitor is turned on and properly calibrated and zeroed according to the instructions in the manual.

5. Connect the temperature probe to the monitor.

6. Fill four 10-mL syringes with sterile normal saline. Be sure to maintain sterility. Inspect the syringes and ensure that they are free from any air bubbles.

7. Insert the probe into one of the syringes to verify injectate temperature.

8. Place the syringes in the ice/slush bath.

9. Ensure that the thermistor port of the catheter is connected to the monitor. The system should be similar to Figure 36.11.

10. Position the "patient" in the supine position (not elevated more than 30 degrees).

11. Verify catheter position by identification of the proper pressure waveform for the pulmonary artery.

12. Record the temperature of the injectate solution by pressing the appropriate key on the face of the monitor. The temperature should be between 0 and 4 °C.

13. Take one of the injectate syringes and connect it to the proximal port of the catheter. A three-way stopcock may be used.

14. Press the "Start" key on the monitor.

15. Steadily and rapidly inject the 10-mL solution. The injection should take no longer than 4 seconds. Observe the waveform produced.

16. Observe the cardiac output reading.

17. Repeat the procedure at intervals of 90 seconds until three readings have been obtained. The readings should be within 10%. If they are not, a technical error may have occurred. Using the fourth syringe, obtain another cardiac output. **Record all readings on your laboratory report.**

18. Average the three readings to report the cardiac output and **record the results on your laboratory report.**

19. Ensure the "patient's" comfort after the procedure.

20. Clean the area and discard any medical waste in the appropriate containers.

21. Remove and properly dispose of any PPE. Wash your hands.

22. **Record any data and your observations on your laboratory report.**

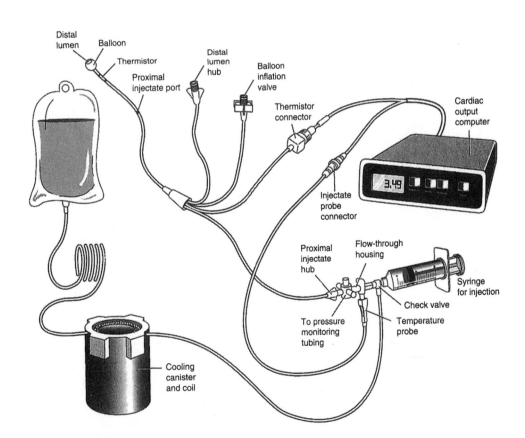

Figure 36.11. System for obtaining a thermodilution cardiac output. (From Baxter Healthcare Corporation, Edwards Critical Care Division, Santa Ana, CA, with permission.)

EXERCISE 36.6   HEMODYNAMIC CALCULATIONS

Normal hemodynamic data are shown in Table 36.1.

Table 36.1 Normal Adult Hemodynamic Data*

Cardiac output	4–8 Lpm
Cardiac index	2.5–4.2 Lpm/m²
Arterial blood pressure	100–140/60–90 mm Hg
Central venous pressure	2–6 mm Hg
Right ventricular pressure	15–25/0–8 mm Hg
Pulmonary artery pressure	15–25/6–12 mm Hg
Pulmonary wedge pressure	4–12 mm Hg
Percent shunt	3–5%
Systemic vascular resistance	770–1500 dyne·sec/cm⁵
Pulmonary vascular resistance	150–250 dyne·sec/cm⁵

It should be noted that normal values may vary somewhat from text to text or from institution to institution.

EXERCISE 36.6.1 MEAN ARTERIAL PRESSURE

Calculate the mean arterial pressure (MAP) using the following formula:

$$MAP = systolic + 2(diastolic) / 3$$

1. Systolic = 120 mm Hg, diastolic = 80 mm Hg
2. Systolic = 170 mm Hg, diastolic = 100 mm Hg
3. Systolic = 90 mm Hg, diastolic = 40 mm Hg

EXERCISE 36.6.2 CARDIAC OUTPUT USING THE FICK EQUATION

Calculate the cardiac output using the Fick equation for the following data.

$$Cardiac\ output = Oxygen\ consumption / C(a - v)O_2$$

Record the cardiac output on your laboratory report.

PaO_2 = 85 mm Hg
$PaCO_2$ = 40 mm Hg
SaO_2 = 93%
Hb = 14 g/dL
PvO_2 = 38 mm Hg
$PvCO_2$ = 44 mm Hg
SvO_2 = 68%
F_IO_2 = 0.50
Oxygen consumption = 260 mL/min

EXERCISE 36.6.3 CARDIAC INDEX

1. Using your laboratory partner as the patient, obtain your partner's height and weight. **Record them on your laboratory report.**
2. Using the DuBois body surface area (BSA) chart in Figure 36.12, obtain your partner's body surface area. **Record it on your laboratory report.**
3. Calculate BSA using the following formula. **Record the BSA on your laboratory report.**
   BSA 5 (4 3 weight in kg) 1 7 / Weight in kg 1 90
4. Assuming a cardiac output of 5.0 L, calculate the cardiac index using the following formula. **Record it on your laboratory report.**
   Cardiac index 5 Cardiac output / Body surface area

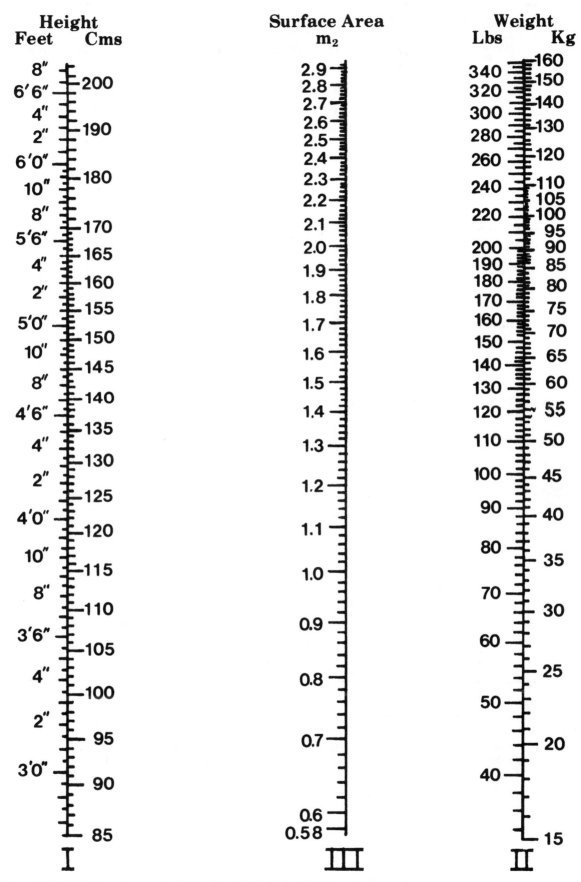

Figure 36.12. DuBois body surface area chart. (Adapted from DuBois, EF: Basal Metabolism in Health and Disease. Philadelphia, Lea & Febiger, 1936.)

EXERCISE 36.6.4 SYSTEMIC AND PULMONARY VASCULAR RESISTANCE

Using the following data and formulas, calculate systemic vascular resistance (SVR) and pulmonary vascular resistance (PVR). **Record them in your laboratory report.**

$$\text{SVR dyne·sec/cm}^5 = \text{Mean arterial pressure} - \text{CVP / cardiac output} \times 80$$
$$\text{PVR dyne·sec/cm}^5 = \text{Mean PAP} - \text{PWP / cardiac output} \times 80$$

Blood pressure = 108/60 mm Hg
PAP = 24/12 mm Hg
PWP = 8 mm Hg
CVP = 0 mm Hg
Cardiac output (CO): Use answer from Exercise 36.6.2.

EXERCISE 36.6.5 SHUNT CALCULATION

Using the following data, calculate the percent shunt using all three formulas. **Record and compare the results on your laboratory report.**

Classic Shunt Formula

$$\text{Percent shunt} = CcO_2 - CaO_2/CcO_2 - CvO_2 \times 100/$$
$$CcO_2 = 1.0 \,(1.34 \times Hb) + (0.003 \times P_AO_2)$$

Modified Estimated Shunt Equation: QS/QT

$$(P_AO_2 - PaO_2) \times 0.003/(CaO_2 - CvO_2) + [(P_AO_2 - PaO_2) \times 0.003]$$

Can use 5 for $C(a-v)O_2$ in stable individuals or 3.5 in critically ill.

Estimated Shunt

$AaDO_2/5$ on room air
PaO_2 = 485 mm Hg
$PaCO_2$ = 35 mm Hg
SaO_2 = 99%
Hb = 12 g/dL
PvO_2 = 380 mm Hg
Pv = 47 mm Hg
SvO_2 = 99%
F_IO_2 = 1.0

REFERENCES

1. Darovic, GO: Hemodynamic Monitoring: Invasive and Noninvasive Clinical Application, ed 3. Elsevier, St. Louis, 2002.
2. Hadian, M and Pinsky, MR: Functional hemodynamic monitoring. Curr Opin Crit Care 13:318–323, 2007.
3. Chan, JS, Segara, D, and Nair, P: Measurement of cardiac output with a non-invasive continuous wave Doppler device versus the pulmonary artery catheter: A comparative study. Crit Care Resusc 8:309–314, 2006.

Laboratory Report

CHAPTER 36: HEMODYNAMIC MONITORING

Name _____ Date _____

Course/Section _____ Instructor _____

Data Collection

EXERCISE 36.1 Identification of the Components of a Flow-Directed Pulmonary Artery Catheter

A: _____

B: _____

C: _____

D: _____

E: _____

F: _____

G: _____

H: _____

I: _____

J: _____

Blood sampling port: _____

EXERCISE 36.2 Assembly and Calibration of a Fluid-Filled Monitoring System

Amount of heparin used (**show your work!**): _____

_____

EXERCISE 36.3 Transducer Calibration

Pressure reading: _____

EXERCISE 36.4 Identification of Pressure Waveforms

Figure 36.6: _____

Figure 36.7: _____

Figure 36.8: _____

Figure 36.9: _____

Overdamped system: _____

Underdamped system: _____

Flush: _____

Catheter whip: _____

EXERCISE 36.5 Thermodilution Cardiac Output (CO) Determination

CO 1: _____

CO 2: _____

CO 3: _____

CO 4: _____

Average CO (**show your work!**): _____

Observations: _____

_____

_____

_____

_____

EXERCISE 36.6 Hemodynamic Calculations

Show all your work!

EXERCISE 36.6.1 MEAN ARTERIAL PRESSURE

1. MAP = _____

2. MAP = _____

3. MAP = _____

EXERCISE 36.6.2 CARDIAC OUTPUT USING THE FICK EQUATION

Cardiac output: _____

EXERCISE 36.6.3 CARDIAC INDEX

Partner's height: _____

Partner's weight: _____

DuBois BSA: _____

Calculated BSA: _____

Cardiac index: _____

EXERCISE 36.6.4 SYSTEMIC AND PULMONARY VASCULAR RESISTANCE

Mean arterial pressure: _____

SVR dyne·sec/cm^5: _____

PVR dyne·sec/cm^5: _____

EXERCISE 36.6.5 SHUNT CALCULATION

CcO_2: _____

CaO_2: _____

CvO_2: _____

Percent shunt (classic): _____

Percent shunt (modified): _____

Percent shunt (estimated): _____

Critical Thinking Questions

For each of the pressure tracings shown in Figures 36.13 through 36.16, identify and interpret the waveforms for channels 1 (ECG tracing) and 2 (hemodynamic tracing). Identify what is being monitored in channel 3. If the tracing indicates a malfunction, state what corrective action(s) would be needed. Correlate the tracings with possible clinical findings, and recommend any necessary therapeutic interventions, if possible.

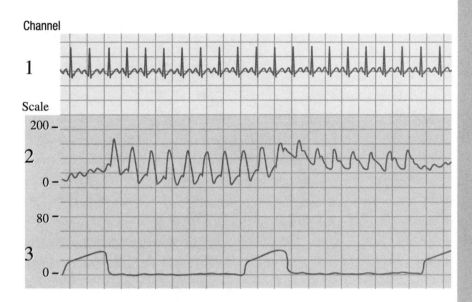

Figure 36.13. Unknown A.

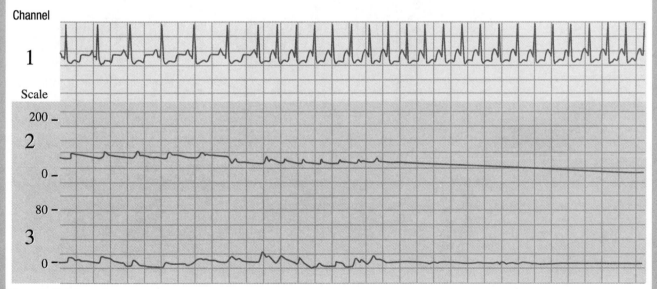

Figure 36.14. Unknown B.

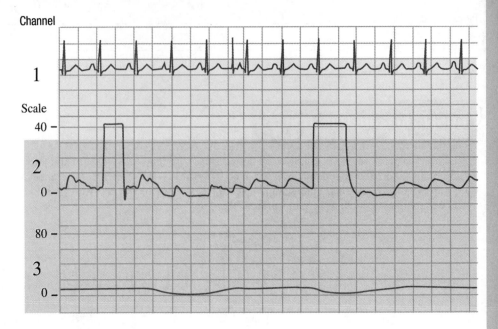

Figure 36.15. Unknown C.

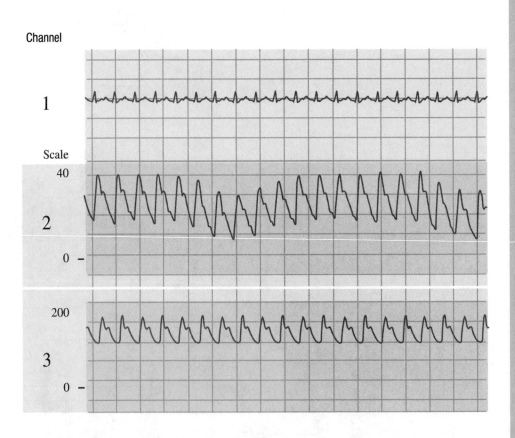

Figure 36.16. Unknown D.

Procedural Competency Evaluation

STUDENT: _____   DATE: _____

HEMODYNAMIC MEASUREMENTS

			PERFORMANCE RATING	PERFORMANCE LEVEL
Evaluator: ☐ Peer ☐ Instructor	**Setting:** ☐ Lab	☐ Clinical Simulation		
Equipment Utilized:	**Conditions (Describe):**			

Performance Level:

S or ✓ = Satisfactory, no errors of omission or commission
U = Unsatisfactory Error of Omission or Commission
NA = Not applicable

Performance Rating:

5 **Independent:** Near flawless performance; minimal errors; able to perform without supervision; seeks out new learning; shows initiative; A = 4.7–5.0 average

4 **Minimally Supervised:** Few errors, able to self-correct; seeks guidance when appropriate; B = 3.7–4.65

3 **Competent:** Minimal required level; no critical errors; able to correct with coaching; meets expectations; safe; C = 3.0–3.65

2 **Marginal:** Below average; critical errors or problem areas noted; would benefit from remediation; D = 2.0–2.99

1 **Dependent:** Poor; unacceptable performance; unsafe; gross inaccuracies; potentially harmful; F = < 2.0

Two or more errors of commission or omission of mandatory or essential performance elements will terminate the procedure, and require additional practice and/or remediation and reevaluation. Student is responsible for obtaining additional evaluation forms as needed from the Director of Clinical Education (DCE).

	PERFORMANCE RATING	PERFORMANCE LEVEL
PATIENT AND EQUIPMENT PREPARATION		
1. Common Performance Elements Steps 1–8		
ASSESSMENT AND IMPLEMENTATION		
2. Common Performance Elements Steps 9 and 10		
3. Identifies components of Swan-Ganz catheter:		
A. Inflation lumen port		
B. Distal lumen port		
C. Proximal lumen port		
D. Thermistor connection		
E. Proximal lumen orifice		
F. Balloon		
G. Distal orifice		
4. Identifies proper injectate site (proximal port)		
5. Identifies pressure waves; states the normal pressure ranges for each:		
A. CVP		
B. RA		
C. RV systolic		
D. RV diastolic		
E. PA systolic		
F. PA diastolic		
G. PAP mean		
H. PWP		
6. Corrects any malfunctions of pressure measuring system		
7. Records cardiac output from monitor for a minimum of three injections within 10%		
8. Averages three measurements		
9. Interprets all data obtained		
FOLLOW-UP		
10. Common Performance Elements Steps 11–16		

SIGNATURES   Student: _____   Evaluator: _____   Date: _____

Clinical Performance Evaluation

PERFORMANCE RATING:

5 **Independent:** Near flawless performance; minimal errors; able to perform without supervision; seeks out new learning; shows initiative; A = 4.7–5.0 average

4 **Minimally Supervised:** Few errors, able to self-correct; seeks guidance when appropriate; B = 3.7–4.65

3 **Competent:** Minimal required level; no critical errors; able to correct with coaching; meets expectations; safe; C = 3.0–3.65

2 **Marginal:** Below average; critical errors or problem areas noted; would benefit from remediation; D = 2.0–2.99

1 **Dependent:** Poor; unacceptable performance; unsafe; gross inaccuracies; potentially harmful; F = < 2.0

Circle the appropriate response below. Please be consistent, objective, and honest in your assessment of the student's clinical performance and ability.

PERFORMANCE CRITERIA	SCORE				
COGNITIVE DOMAIN					
1. Consistently displays knowledge, comprehension, and command of essential concepts	5	4	3	2	1
2. Demonstrates the relationship between theory and clinical practice	5	4	3	2	1
3. Able to select, review, apply, analyze, synthesize, interpret, and evaluate information; makes recommendations to modify care plan	5	4	3	2	1
PSYCHOMOTOR DOMAIN					
4. Minimal errors, no critical errors; able to self-correct; performs all steps safely and accurately	5	4	3	2	1
5. Selects, assembles, and verifies proper function and cleanliness of equipment; assures operation and corrects malfunctions; provides adequate care and maintenance	5	4	3	2	1
6. Exhibits the required manual dexterity	5	4	3	2	1
7. Performs procedure in a reasonable time frame for clinical level	5	4	3	2	1
8. Applies and maintains aseptic technique and PPE as required	5	4	3	2	1
9. Maintains concise and accurate patient and clinical records	5	4	3	2	1
10. Reports promptly on patient status/needs to appropriate personnel	5	4	3	2	1
AFFECTIVE DOMAIN					
11. Exhibits courteous and pleasant demeanor; shows consideration and respect, honesty, and integrity	5	4	3	2	1
12. Communicates verbally and in writing clearly and concisely	5	4	3	2	1
13. Preserves confidentiality and adheres to all policies	5	4	3	2	1
14. Follows directions, exhibits sound judgment, and seeks help when required	5	4	3	2	1
15. Demonstrates initiative, self-direction, responsibility, and accountability	5	4	3	2	1

TOTAL POINTS = _____ /15 = AVERAGE GRADE = _____

ADDITIONAL COMMENTS: IDENTIFY AREAS OF EXCELLENCE; LIST ERRORS OF OMISSION OR COMMISSION, CRITICAL ERRORS

SUMMARY PERFORMANCE EVALUATION AND RECOMMENDATIONS

☐ PASS: Satisfactory Performance

    ☐ Minimal supervision needed, may progress to next level provided specific skills, clinical time completed

    ☐ Minimal supervision needed, able to progress to next level without remediation

☐ FAIL: Unsatisfactory Performance (check all that apply)

    ☐ Minor reevaluation only

    ☐ Needs additional clinical practice before reevaluation

    ☐ Needs additional laboratory practice before skills performed in clinical area

    ☐ Recommend clinical probation

SIGNATURES

Evaluator (print name): _____ Evaluator signature: _____ Date: _____

Student Signature: _____ Date: _____

Student Comments:

Procedural Competency Evaluation

STUDENT: DATE:

SHUNT STUDIES

			PERFORMANCE RATING	PERFORMANCE LEVEL
Evaluator: ☐ Peer ☐ Instructor **Setting:** ☐ Lab ☐ Clinical Simulation				
Equipment Utilized: **Conditions (Describe):**				

Performance Level:

S or ✓ = Satisfactory, no errors of omission or commission
U = Unsatisfactory Error of Omission or Commission
NA = Not applicable

Performance Rating:

5   **Independent:** Near flawless performance; minimal errors; able to perform without supervision; seeks out new learning; shows initiative; A = 4.7–5.0 average

4   **Minimally Supervised:** Few errors, able to self-correct; seeks guidance when appropriate; B = 3.7–4.65

3   **Competent:** Minimal required level; no critical errors; able to correct with coaching; meets expectations; safe; C = 3.0–3.65

2   **Marginal:** Below average; critical errors or problem areas noted; would benefit from remediation; D = 2.0–2.99

1   **Dependent:** Poor; unacceptable performance; unsafe; gross inaccuracies; potentially harmful; F = < 2.0

Two or more errors of commission or omission of mandatory or essential performance elements will terminate the procedure, and require additional practice and/or remediation and reevaluation. Student is responsible for obtaining additional evaluation forms as needed from the Director of Clinical Education (DCE).

	Performance Rating	Performance Level
PATIENT AND EQUIPMENT PREPARATION		
1. Common Performance Elements Steps 1–8		
ASSESSMENT AND IMPLEMENTATION		
2. Common Performance Elements Steps 9 and 10		
3. Draws a mixed venous sample from proximal port of pulmonary artery catheter		
4. Draws an arterial blood gas sample		
5. Analyzes and records the results of both samples		
6. Calculates the following values:		
PAO_2		
$PAaDO_2$		
a/A ratio		
Oxygenation ratio		
CaO_2		
CvO_2		
Cardiac output		
Percent shunt		
MAP		
SVR		
F_IO_2 needed for a desired PaO_2		
7. Interprets results		
FOLLOW-UP		
8. Common Performance Elements Steps 11–16		

SIGNATURES   Student: Evaluator: Date:

Clinical Performance Evaluation

PERFORMANCE RATING:

5 **Independent:** Near flawless performance; minimal errors; able to perform without supervision; seeks out new learning; shows initiative; A = 4.7–5.0 average

4 **Minimally Supervised:** Few errors, able to self-correct; seeks guidance when appropriate; B = 3.7–4.65

3 **Competent:** Minimal required level; no critical errors; able to correct with coaching; meets expectations; safe; C = 3.0–3.65

2 **Marginal:** Below average; critical errors or problem areas noted; would benefit from remediation; D = 2.0–2.99

1 **Dependent:** Poor; unacceptable performance; unsafe; gross inaccuracies; potentially harmful; F = < 2.0

Circle the appropriate response below. Please be consistent, objective, and honest in your assessment of the student's clinical performance and ability.

PERFORMANCE CRITERIA	SCORE				
COGNITIVE DOMAIN					
1. Consistently displays knowledge, comprehension, and command of essential concepts	5	4	3	2	1
2. Demonstrates the relationship between theory and clinical practice	5	4	3	2	1
3. Able to select, review, apply, analyze, synthesize, interpret, and evaluate information; makes recommendations to modify care plan	5	4	3	2	1
PSYCHOMOTOR DOMAIN					
4. Minimal errors, no critical errors; able to self-correct; performs all steps safely and accurately	5	4	3	2	1
5. Selects, assembles, and verifies proper function and cleanliness of equipment; assures operation and corrects malfunctions; provides adequate care and maintenance	5	4	3	2	1
6. Exhibits the required manual dexterity	5	4	3	2	1
7. Performs procedure in a reasonable time frame for clinical level	5	4	3	2	1
8. Applies and maintains aseptic technique and PPE as required	5	4	3	2	1
9. Maintains concise and accurate patient and clinical records	5	4	3	2	1
10. Reports promptly on patient status/needs to appropriate personnel	5	4	3	2	1
AFFECTIVE DOMAIN					
11. Exhibits courteous and pleasant demeanor; shows consideration and respect, honesty, and integrity	5	4	3	2	1
12. Communicates verbally and in writing clearly and concisely	5	4	3	2	1
13. Preserves confidentiality and adheres to all policies	5	4	3	2	1
14. Follows directions, exhibits sound judgment, and seeks help when required	5	4	3	2	1
15. Demonstrates initiative, self-direction, responsibility, and accountability	5	4	3	2	1

TOTAL POINTS = _____ /15 = AVERAGE GRADE = _____

ADDITIONAL COMMENTS: IDENTIFY AREAS OF EXCELLENCE; LIST ERRORS OF OMISSION OR COMMISSION, CRITICAL ERRORS

SUMMARY PERFORMANCE EVALUATION AND RECOMMENDATIONS

☐ PASS: Satisfactory Performance

　☐ Minimal supervision needed, may progress to next level provided specific skills, clinical time completed

　☐ Minimal supervision needed, able to progress to next level without remediation

☐ FAIL: Unsatisfactory Performance (check all that apply)

　☐ Minor reevaluation only

　☐ Needs additional clinical practice before reevaluation

　☐ Needs additional laboratory practice before skills performed in clinical area

　☐ Recommend clinical probation

SIGNATURES

Evaluator (print name): _____　　Evaluator signature: _____　　Date: _____

Student Signature: _____　　Date: _____

Student Comments:

37 Noninvasive Ventilation

Some of the most common complications associated with mechanical ventilation arise from the use of artificial airways. Besides trauma to the airway and the potential for obstruction, endotracheal tubes and tracheostomy tubes provide a route for infection and serve as a barrier to communication. During the polio epidemic in the 1900s in the United States, negative pressure ventilators were designed to provide long-term ventilatory assistance to patients with this neuromuscular disease. Although more physiologic than positive pressure ventilation, they proved awkward and made routine care difficult. Today, the **cuirass** and the **poncho** types provide an alternative to positive-pressure ventilation.[1]

Other alternative methods to positive pressure ventilation have been employed with varying degrees of success. Rocking beds, pneumobelts, and phrenic nerve stimulators (diaphragmatic pacemakers) are used primarily for a select group of quadriplegic patients in rehabilitation facilities. However, hands-on practice with these devices is beyond the scope of the laboratory setting.[2]

Microprocessor-controlled positive pressure devices are now capable of providing another noninvasive alternative in the forms of continuous positive airway pressure (CPAP), bilevel positive airway pressure (BiPAP™), and, more recently, demand positive airway pressure (DPAP).[3] When coupled with the appropriate mask, mouthpiece, or other interface, these devices help patients maintain adequate ventilation in acute care and alternative sites such as long-term facilities and home care. The respiratory care practitioner must be familiar with the capabilities and limitations of these devices.[4]

This lab exercise will review the equipment required for and proper setup of **noninvasive positive pressure ventilation (NPPV)** therapy.

OBJECTIVES

Upon completion of this chapter, the student will be able to:

1. Practice communication skills needed for the instruction of patients or their families in noninvasive ventilator initiation.
2. Identify the components of negative pressure (cuirass shell or poncho) CPAP, BiPAP™, and DPAP units.
3. Assess patient for indications requiring noninvasive ventilation.
4. Apply infection control guidelines and standards associated with noninvasive ventilation equipment and procedures, according to OSHA regulations and CDC guidelines.

5. Select the equipment needed
6. Select and properly fit appropriate mask, mouthpiece, or other interface, as appropriate.
7. Initiate noninvasive ventilation.
8. Troubleshoot and solve common problems associated with noninvasive ventilators.
9. Assess the patient for tolerance and response to noninvasive ventilation.
10. Titrate oxygen in conjunction with noninvasive ventilators to vary F_IO_2.
11. Make recommendations or modifications to ventilation techniques or equipment as needed.
12. Practice medical charting for application of noninvasive ventilation procedures.

KEY TERMS

BiPAP™ unit	EPAP	noninvasive positive
CPAP unit	nasal mask	pressure ventilation
cuirass	nasal pillows	(NPPV)
IPAP		poncho

Exercises

EQUIPMENT REQUIRED[5]

- ☐ Negative pressure ventilators
- ☐ Cuirass shells or ponchos, various sizes if available
- ☐ CPAP unit
- ☐ BiPAP™ unit
- ☐ DPAP unit
- ☐ Mask sizing gauge
- ☐ **Nasal masks, nasal pillows,** or mouthpiece
- ☐ Head gear
- ☐ Spacers

- ☐ Oxygen supply tubing
- ☐ Oxygen analyzer
- ☐ Adaptors
- ☐ Oxygen enrichment adaptor
- ☐ Oxygen source or concentrator
- ☐ Watch with second hand
- ☐ Respirometer
- ☐ One-way valves
- ☐ Blood pressure cuffs and sphygmomanometer
- ☐ Pulse oximeter

EXERCISE 37.1 NEGATIVE PRESSURE VENTILATOR

1. Select a negative pressure ventilator as shown in Figure 37.1. **Record the type used on your laboratory report.**
2. Identify the controls. **Record the available controls on your laboratory report.**
3. Use your laboratory partner as the patient.
4. Wash your hands and apply standard precautions and transmission-based isolation procedures as appropriate.
5. Identify your "patient." Introduce yourself and your department. Explain to your partner in nonmedical terms that you are going to place the "patient" in the noninvasive ventilator device and what is involved. Confirm your partner's understanding and answer any questions or concerns. The partner should simulate a patient's concern and fears about having this procedure performed. You should respond appropriately.
6. Assess the "patient" for vital signs, SpO_2, breath sounds, and ventilatory status. **Record your findings on your laboratory report.**
7. Prepare the "patient" for noninvasive ventilation. Select the correct size cuirass shell or poncho.
8. Place the cuirass or poncho on the "patient" and check for proper fit and "patient" comfort.
9. Adjust the negative pressure to -10 cm H_2O.
10. Adjust the rate to 12/minute. Have your partner count from 1 to 10 as the ventilator cycles. **Record your observations on your laboratory report.**

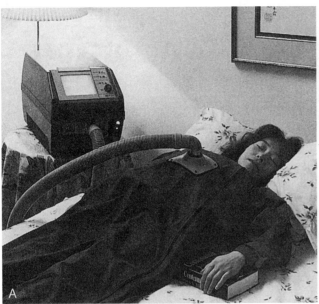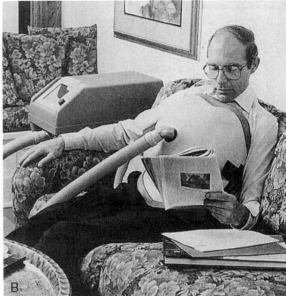

Figure 37.1. Negative pressure ventilators. (Courtesy of LIFECARE International, Inc., Westminster, CO.)

11. Using the spirometer and one-way valve, measure the exhaled tidal volume and compare it to desired tidal volume. **Record the volume on your laboratory report.**

12. Reassess your "patient's" vital signs, SpO$_2$, breath sounds, and ventilatory status. **Record your findings on your laboratory report.**

13. Based on "patient" assessment and measured exhaled tidal volume, recommend any appropriate settings changes to the physician.

14. **"Chart" the application of noninvasive ventilation on your laboratory report.**

15. Loosen the cuirass or the poncho.

16. Measure the exhaled tidal volume and note any difference from that measured in step 11 above. **Record the volume on your laboratory report.**

EXERCISE 37.2 CONTINUOUS POSITIVE AIRWAY PRESSURE SETUP

1. Select a **CPAP** unit and identify the controls. **Record the type of unit used and the available controls on your laboratory report.** If a commercial CPAP unit is not available, a system can be assembled as shown in Figure 37.2.

2. Wash your hands and apply standard precautions and transmission-based isolation procedures as appropriate.

3. Use your laboratory partner as the patient. Identify your "patient." Introduce yourself and your department. Explain to your partner in nonmedical terms that you are going to apply a mask CPAP device and what is involved. Confirm your partner's understanding and answer any questions or concerns. The partner should simulate a patient's concern and fears about having this procedure performed. You should respond appropriately.

4. Assess the "patient's" vital signs, SpO$_2$, breath sounds, and ventilatory status. **Record your findings on your laboratory report.**

5. Assess your lab partner for the appropriate interface. This may be done by using the mask sizing gauge to measure your lab partner. Select the smallest mask possible that will come close to, but not contact, the nasal bone, external nares, and upper lip, as shown in Figure 37.3. In any case, a mask or other interface that maximizes comfort and minimizes leaks should be selected. **Record the mask size on your laboratory report.** Remember to explain everything to your partner.

6. Use spacers to fill any gaps, as shown in Figure 37.4.

7. Attach the mask to the hose, ensuring the presence of an exhalation port such as a Whisper Swivel®, as shown in Figure 37.5.

8. Turn the CPAP unit or system on.

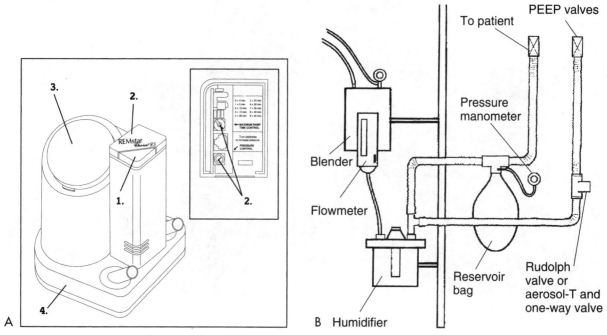

Figure 37.2. Continuous positive airway pressure (CPAP) systems: **(A)** Commercial CPAP system; **(B)** Assembly of a CPAP system from component parts.

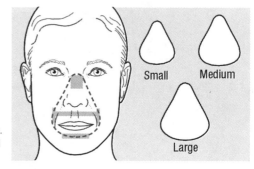

Figure 37.3. Fitting a CPAP mask. (Courtesy of Respironics, Inc. and its affiliates.)

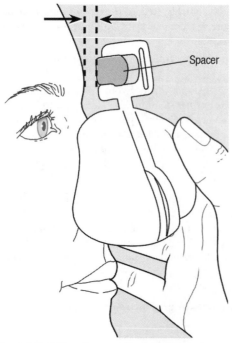

Figure 37.4. CPAP mask spacers. (Courtesy of Respironics, Inc. and its affiliates.)

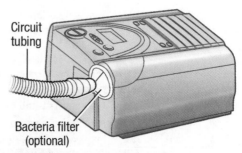

Figure 37.5. Hose attachment. (Courtesy of Respironics, Inc. and its affiliates.)

9. Attach the headgear or straps to your partner's head, as shown in Figure 37.6. Confirm proper fit and comfort.

10. Adjust the CPAP pressure to 5 cm H_2O.

11. Reassess vital signs, SpO_2, breath sounds, and ventilatory status. **Record your findings on your laboratory report.**

12. Based on "patient" assessment, recommend any appropriate settings changes to the physician.

13. Ask your partner how he or she is tolerating the pressure. Have your partner try to mouth-breathe and talk. **Record your observations on your laboratory report.**

14. **"Chart" the initiation of CPAP on your laboratory report.**

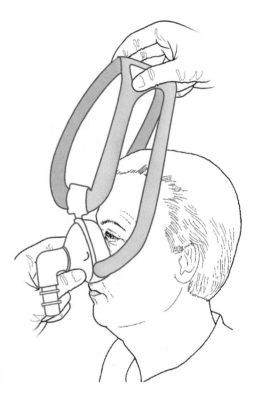

Figure 37.6. Head strap attachment. (Courtesy of Respironics, Inc. and its affiliates.)

EXERCISE 37.3 BIPAP™ SETUP

1. Select a **BiPAP™ unit,** as shown in Figure 37.7. Note the various connections and air filter locations and identify the controls. **Record the type of unit and the available controls on your laboratory report.**

2. Wash your hands and apply standard precautions and transmission-based isolation procedures as appropriate.

3. Use your laboratory partner as the patient. Identify your "patient." Introduce yourself and your department. Explain to your partner in nonmedical terms that you are going to apply a mask BiPAP™ device and what is involved. Confirm your partner's understanding and answer any questions or concerns.

4. Assess the "patient's" vital signs, SpO_2, breath sounds, and ventilatory status. **Record your findings on your laboratory report.**

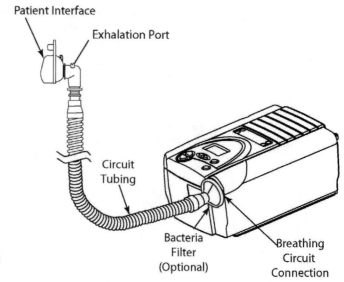

Figure 37.7. BiPAP™ S/T ventilatory support system. (Courtesy of Respironics, Inc. and its affiliates.)

5. Using the same steps as in the CPAP exercise, determine the appropriate interface, measure your partner for the correct size mask, and attach your partner to the unit using the following settings:

   Mode: Spontaneous

   IPAP: 10 cm H_2O

   EPAP: 6 cm H_2O

   Percent IPAP: 20%

   Low-pressure alarm: 4 cm H_2O

   High-pressure alarm: 15 cm H_2O

   F_IO_2: 21% (room air)

6. Observe the pressure manometer for several breathing cycles. Determine the I:E ratio. Ask your partner whether they feel any differences between breathing on a CPAP unit versus BiPAP™. **Record your observations on your laboratory report.**

7. Adjust the low-pressure alarm to 8 cm H_2O. Note any pressure changes and other occurrences. **Record your observations on your laboratory report.** Correct any malfunctions or alarms. **Record what adjustments were made on your laboratory report.**

8. Loosen the mask from your lab partner. Note any pressure changes and other occurrences. **Record your observations on your laboratory report.** Resecure the mask in place.

9. Change the mode to spontaneous/timed and set the rate to 14/minute.

10. Ask your partner if any appreciable difference is felt. **Record your observations on your laboratory report.**

11. Obtain an oxygen enrichment adaptor and oxygen analyzer. Place in-line as shown in Figure 37.8.

12. Titrate low-flow oxygen until an F_IO_2 of 0.28 is achieved. **Record the liter flow required on your laboratory report.** NOTE: Supplemental oxygen may also be directly titrated into the mask via the oxygen bleed-in port.

13. Adjust the unit to the following settings:

    Mode: spontaneous

    IPAP: 2 cm H_2O

    EPAP: 10 cm H_2O

    Percent IPAP: 20%

    Low-pressure alarm: 0 cm H_2O

14. Ask your partner whether any appreciable difference is felt. Note any pressure changes and other occurrences. **Record your observations on your laboratory report.**

15. Adjust the settings to correct any malfunctions or alarms. **Record what adjustments were made on your laboratory report.**

16. Reassess the "patient's" vital signs, SpO_2, breath sounds, and ventilatory status. **Record your findings on your laboratory report.**

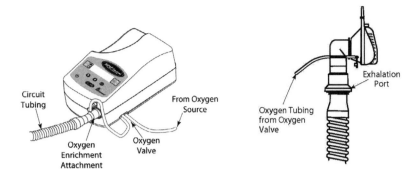

Figure 37.8. Titrating oxygen with BiPAP™. (Courtesy of Respironics, Inc. and its affiliates.)

17. Based on "patient" assessment, recommend any appropriate setting changes to the physician.

18. Obtain a DPAP unit. Set it up according to the manufacturer's instructions and apply it to your laboratory partner.

19. Ask your partner whether any appreciable difference is felt between DPAP and BiPAP™. Note any pressure changes and other occurrences. **Record your observations on your laboratory report.**

REFERENCES

1. Kacmarek, RM, Mack, CW, and Dimas, S: The Essentials of Respiratory Care, ed 4. Mosby, St. Louis, 2005.
2. Hess, DR: Noninvasive ventilation in neuromuscular disease: Equipment and application. Respir Care 51:896–911, 2006.
3. Aloia, MS, Stanchina, M, Arnedt, JT et al.: Treatment adherence and outcomes in flexible vs standard continuous positive airway pressure therapy. Chest 127:2085–2087, 2005.
4. Hess, DR: The evidence for noninvasive positive-pressure ventilation in the care of patients in acute respiratory failure: A systematic review of the literature. Respir Care 49:810–829, 2004.
5. Hill, NS and Bach, JR: Noninvasive mechanical ventilation. Respir Care Clin N Am 2:161–352, 1996.

Laboratory Report

CHAPTER 37: NONINVASIVE VENTILATION

Name _____   Date _____

Course/Section _____   Instructor _____

Data Collection

EXERCISE 37.1 Negative Pressure Ventilator

Type of ventilator used: _____

Controls available: _____

_____

_____

"Patient" assessment: _____

_____

Observations: _____

_____

_____

_____

Exhaled tidal volume: _____

"Patient" assessment: _____

_____

Chart the initiation of noninvasive ventilation as you would on a legal medical record:

_____

_____

_____

_____

_____

_____

_____

_____

Exhaled tidal volume with loosened cuirass: _____

EXERCISE 37.2 Continuous Positive Airway Pressure Setup

Type of ventilator used: _____

Controls available: _____

Mask size: _____

"Patient" assessment: _____

_____

Observation: _____

_____

_____

_____

_____

_____

Chart the initiation of CPAP as you would on a legal medical record:

_____

_____

_____

_____

_____

_____

_____

_____

_____

_____

EXERCISE 37.3 BiPAP™ Setup

Type of ventilator used: _____

Controls available: _____

_____

"Patient" assessment: _____

_____

I:E ratio: _____

(Show your work for any calculations!)

IPAP = 10 cm H_2O; EPAP = 6 cm H_2O; pressure alarm = 4 cm H_2O.

Observations: _____

_____

_____

_____

Pressure alarm = 8 cm H_2O.

Observations: _____

_____

_____

_____

Adjustments made: _____

Observation with loose mask: _____

_____

_____

Observations in the timed mode: _____

_____

_____

Liter flow: _____

Observations with IPAP = 2, EPAP = 10: _____

_____

_____

_____

Adjustments made: _____

DPAP observations: _____

_____

_____

_____

Critical Thinking Questions

1. What settings change would you recommend to a physician to increase the tidal volume for a patient on a negative pressure ventilator?

2. What types of patients would not be candidates for noninvasive ventilation?

3. Based on the exercises, what limitations of noninvasive ventilation did you observe?

Mr. Pickwick has obstructive sleep apnea, and the doctor has ordered him placed on BiPAP™ at the following settings: mode, S/T; rate, 12/minute; IPAP = 12 cm H_2O; EPAP = 6 cm H_2O. You enter his room, identify yourself, and explain everything to him. You also perform a complete assessment. After applying BiPAP™ you note a drop in blood pressure and oxygen saturation.

4. What are possible causes of the drop in blood pressure and SpO_2 and what changes or modifications would you recommend?

5. What would you recommend to Mr. Pickwick for infection control in the home?

You are a newly employed home care therapist and are visiting Mr. Pickwick for the first time. While checking his BiPAP™ setup you observe that 2 Lpm of oxygen from an oxygen concentrator is being titrated directly into the mask.

6. How would you determine the F_IO_2 being delivered? Explain your answer.

7. How can you assess the adequacy of the oxygen therapy being provided?

Procedural Competency Evaluation

STUDENT: _____ **DATE:** _____

CPAP/BIPAP™ INITIATION (NON-INVASIVE VENTILATION)

Evaluator: ☐ Peer ☐ Instructor	**Setting:** ☐ Lab ☐ Clinical Simulation
Equipment Utilized:	**Conditions (Describe):**

Performance Level:

S or ✓ = Satisfactory, no errors of omission or commission
U = Unsatisfactory Error of Omission or Commission
NA = Not applicable

Performance Rating:

5 **Independent:** Near flawless performance; minimal errors; able to perform without supervision; seeks out new learning; shows initiative; A = 4.7–5.0 average

4 **Minimally Supervised:** Few errors, able to self-correct; seeks guidance when appropriate; B = 3.7–4.65

3 **Competent:** Minimal required level; no critical errors; able to correct with coaching; meets expectations; safe; C = 3.0–3.65

2 **Marginal:** Below average; critical errors or problem areas noted; would benefit from remediation; D = 2.0–2.99

1 **Dependent:** Poor; unacceptable performance; unsafe; gross inaccuracies; potentially harmful; F = < 2.0

Two or more errors of commission or omission of mandatory or essential performance elements will terminate the procedure, and require additional practice and/or remediation and reevaluation. Student is responsible for obtaining additional evaluation forms as needed from the Director of Clinical Education (DCE).

	PERFORMANCE RATING	PERFORMANCE LEVEL
PATIENT AND EQUIPMENT PREPARATION		
1. Common Performance Elements Steps 1–8		
2. Identifies the circuit components of a continuous flow noninvasive circuit and assembles:		
A. 6-foot smooth bore tubing		
B. Exhalation port or mask with integrated exhalation port		
C. Proximal pressure tubing		
D. Interface		
E. Bacteria filter to machine outlet		
3. Performs required leak test (if applicable)		
ASSESSMENT AND IMPLEMENTATION		
4. Common Performance Elements Steps 9 and 10		
5. Differentiates between CPAP and BiPAP modes		
6. Turns the unit or system on and selects proper mode, pressures, ramp or rise time, F_1O_2, and timed inspiration		
7. Checks alarm function and sets alarms		
8. Positions patient and measures the patient for the appropriate mask size		
9. Uses spacers to fill any gaps		
10. Attaches the mask to the hose		
11. Attaches the head straps to the patient's head; confirms proper fit and comfort		
12. Evaluates waveforms to identify tidal volume, rate, pressures and flow, and air trapping or auto-PEEP		
13. Adjusts the pressure(s) (CPAP, IPAP, EPAP) to conform with the physician's order		
14. Reassesses vital signs, SpO_2, breath sounds, and ventilatory status		
15. Determines how patient is tolerating the pressure; readjusts mask if necessary		
16. Evaluates for alternative interface if patient is not tolerating the mask		
FOLLOW-UP		
17. Common Performance Elements Steps 11–16		

SIGNATURES Student: _____ Evaluator: _____ Date: _____

Clinical Performance Evaluation

PERFORMANCE RATING:

5 **Independent:** Near flawless performance; minimal errors; able to perform without supervision; seeks out new learning; shows initiative; A = 4.7–5.0 average

4 **Minimally Supervised:** Few errors, able to self-correct; seeks guidance when appropriate; B = 3.7–4.65

3 **Competent:** Minimal required level; no critical errors; able to correct with coaching; meets expectations; safe; C = 3.0–3.65

2 **Marginal:** Below average; critical errors or problem areas noted; would benefit from remediation; D = 2.0–2.99

1 **Dependent:** Poor; unacceptable performance; unsafe; gross inaccuracies; potentially harmful; F = < 2.0

Circle the appropriate response below. Please be consistent, objective, and honest in your assessment of the student's clinical performance and ability.

PERFORMANCE CRITERIA — SCORE

PERFORMANCE CRITERIA					
COGNITIVE DOMAIN					
1. Consistently displays knowledge, comprehension, and command of essential concepts	5	4	3	2	1
2. Demonstrates the relationship between theory and clinical practice	5	4	3	2	1
3. Able to select, review, apply, analyze, synthesize, interpret, and evaluate information; makes recommendations to modify care plan	5	4	3	2	1
PSYCHOMOTOR DOMAIN					
4. Minimal errors, no critical errors; able to self-correct; performs all steps safely and accurately	5	4	3	2	1
5. Selects, assembles, and verifies proper function and cleanliness of equipment; assures operation and corrects malfunctions; provides adequate care and maintenance	5	4	3	2	1
6. Exhibits the required manual dexterity	5	4	3	2	1
7. Performs procedure in a reasonable time frame for clinical level	5	4	3	2	1
8. Applies and maintains aseptic technique and PPE as required	5	4	3	2	1
9. Maintains concise and accurate patient and clinical records	5	4	3	2	1
10. Reports promptly on patient status/needs to appropriate personnel	5	4	3	2	1
AFFECTIVE DOMAIN					
11. Exhibits courteous and pleasant demeanor; shows consideration and respect, honesty, and integrity	5	4	3	2	1
12. Communicates verbally and in writing clearly and concisely	5	4	3	2	1
13. Preserves confidentiality and adheres to all policies	5	4	3	2	1
14. Follows directions, exhibits sound judgment, and seeks help when required	5	4	3	2	1
15. Demonstrates initiative, self-direction, responsibility, and accountability	5	4	3	2	1

TOTAL POINTS =   /15 = AVERAGE GRADE =

ADDITIONAL COMMENTS: IDENTIFY AREAS OF EXCELLENCE; LIST ERRORS OF OMISSION OR COMMISSION, CRITICAL ERRORS

SUMMARY PERFORMANCE EVALUATION AND RECOMMENDATIONS

☐ PASS: Satisfactory Performance

    ☐ Minimal supervision needed, may progress to next level provided specific skills, clinical time completed

    ☐ Minimal supervision needed, able to progress to next level without remediation

☐ FAIL: Unsatisfactory Performance (check all that apply)

    ☐ Minor reevaluation only

    ☐ Needs additional clinical practice before reevaluation

    ☐ Needs additional laboratory practice before skills performed in clinical area

    ☐ Recommend clinical probation

SIGNATURES

Evaluator (print name):   Evaluator signature: Date:

Student Signature: Date:

Student Comments:

CHAPTER

38 Pressure Ventilators

INTRODUCTION

With **pressure-limited/volume-variable ventilators**, the breath generally continues until a preset pressure is reached. Hence, the amount of volume for each breath depends on the set pressure as well as the patient's compliance and airway resistance.[1]

In general, pressure-limited/volume-variable ventilation is not used as a long-term ventilatory mode in the adult intensive care setting. However, it may be used as an alternative short-term modality for patients with ventilatory insufficiency. Beyond this and perhaps more importantly, this chapter examines the relationships between pressure, flow, volume, and time. In this sense, it will help the reader grasp the complexities of mechanical ventilation. By understanding the concepts covered in this chapter, the reader will be better prepared to initiate ventilation and monitor patients using the more advanced modes available on more highly sophisticated equipment.

This chapter is intended to introduce the relationships between pressure, flow, volume, and time. In this sense, this material will help prepare for a more in-depth exploration of mechanical ventilation in later chapters. In preparation for these exercises, the IPPB exercises in Chapter 16 should be reviewed.[2]

OBJECTIVES

Upon completion of this chapter, the student will be able to:

1. Identify the components of an adult breathing circuit.
2. Test the circuit for leaks.
3. Identify and operate the controls of a pressure-limited ventilator.
4. Initiate and monitor pressure-limited ventilation.
5. Compare the interrelationships between pressure, volume, flow, and time.
6. Relate the changes that might occur in the parameters of pressure, volume, flow, and time with changes in compliance and resistance.
7. Chart data related to pressure-limited ventilation in the medical record.

KEY TERMS

airway resistance
compliance
I:E ratio

pressure-limited/
volume-variable
ventilator

pressure ventilator

Exercises

EQUIPMENT REQUIRED

- ☐ Pressure ventilator (Bird series, Bennett PR II, or AP-5)
- ☐ Respirometer and adaptor
- ☐ Lung simulator or test lungs
- ☐ Adult breathing circuits
- ☐ Corrugated tubing
- ☐ Watch with second hand
- ☐ 50-psi gas source
- ☐ High-pressure hose

EXERCISE 38.1 IDENTIFICATION OF AN ADULT BREATHING CIRCUIT AND LEAK TESTING

1. Select an adult breathing circuit for a pressure-limited ventilator.
2. Examine the components shown in Figure 38.1.
3. Connect the circuit to the unit as practiced in Chapter 16.
4. Using the same technique as in Chapter 16, Exercise 16.3, step 3, test the circuit for leaks. Observe for leaks and correct if necessary. **Record the ventilator used, your observations, and any corrective actions on your laboratory report.**

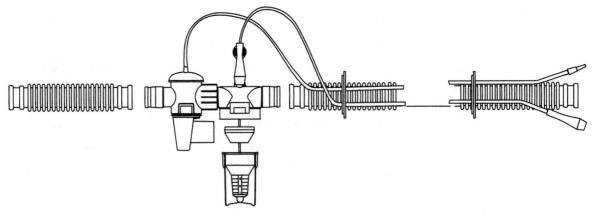

Figure 38.1. Adult breathing circuit for pressure ventilators. (Courtesy of Cardinal Health, Dublin, OH.)

EXERCISE 38.2 CONTROLS

1. Attach the ventilator circuit to a lung simulator or test lung as shown in Figure 38.2. Adjust the lung simulator to normal compliance and resistance values.
2. Adjust the pressure to 10 cm H_2O.
3. Adjust the flow rate to 15 if using a Bird.
4. If using a PR II, turn the peak flow to the minimum setting and the terminal flow to maximum.
5. Adjust the apnea control or rate control to achieve a breath rate of 12.
6. Attach a respirometer to the exhalation port. **Record the tidal volume achieved on your laboratory report.**
7. Measure the inspiratory and expiratory times and **record them on your laboratory report.** Calculate the I:E ratio and **record it on your laboratory report.**
8. Increase the pressure to 15 cm H_2O. **Record the tidal volume achieved on your laboratory report.**

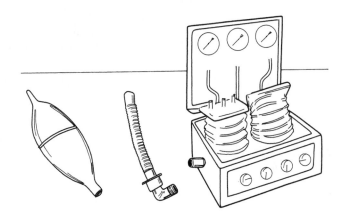

Figure 38.2. Attaching the circuit to a test lung.

9. Measure the inspiratory and expiratory times and **record them on your laboratory report.** Calculate the I:E ratio and **record it on your laboratory report.**

10. Return the pressure to 10 cm H_2O.

11. Increase the flow rate to 20 (Bird) or maximum peak flow (PR II). **Record the tidal volume achieved on your laboratory report.**

12. Measure the inspiratory and expiratory times and **record them on your laboratory report.** Calculate the I:E ratio and **record it on your laboratory report.**

13. Decrease the flow rate to 10 (Bird). **Record the volume achieved on your laboratory report.**

14. Measure the inspiratory and expiratory times and **record them on your laboratory report.** Calculate the I:E ratio **on your laboratory report.**

15. Increase the pressure to 20 cm H_2O and the flow to 20. **Record the tidal volume achieved on your laboratory report.**

16. Measure the inspiratory and expiratory times and **record them on your laboratory report.** Calculate the I:E ratio and **record it on your laboratory report.**

EXERCISE 38.3 INITIATION AND MONITORING

*Given the following information, complete the exercise as directed. Use the lung simulator as your patient. Your instructor will show you how to operate the simulator. Depending on the brand of simulator, you might have to change adaptors or settings in order to vary **compliance** and **airway resistance**. Use the settings on your simulator that correspond to the compliance and resistance settings in the exercises. Initially use the R5 resistance adaptors (normal resistance) and set the compliance of both lungs at 0.10 L/cm H_2O (normal resistance and compliance settings).*

Mrs. Gandhi is a 45-year-old nonsmoker with a history of asthma. She is in the recovery room following a colon resection. She is not yet reactive and is not breathing spontaneously. She weighs 150 lb. You have been called to place her on a pressure ventilator until she becomes reactive.

1. Using the formula of 10 to 15 mL/kg, set the ventilator to give the patient an appropriate tidal volume and respiratory rate of 12/minute. **Record your settings for pressure and flow on your laboratory report.**

2. Measure the tidal volume, inspiratory time, and expiratory time, and **record them on your laboratory report. Calculate the I:E ratio on your laboratory report.**

3. Simulate an increase in resistance perhaps by switching to an R20 adapter. Measure the tidal volume, and observe any changes in volume and I:E ratio. **Record them on your laboratory report.**

4. Increase the pressure until you have achieved the tidal volume in step 1. **Record it on your laboratory report.**

5. Using the flow control, adjust the inspiratory time until the I:E ratio returns to original value. **Record the settings and your observations on your laboratory report.**

6. Return to normal resistance, perhaps by switching back to an R5 adapter. Reduce the compliance on the right lung to 0.08 L/cm H_2O (low compliance). Measure the tidal volume, inspiratory time, and expiratory time, and **record them on your laboratory report. Calculate the I:E ratio on your laboratory report.**

7. Set the left lung to the same compliance setting as in step 6. Measure the tidal volume, inspiratory time, and expiratory time, and **record them on your laboratory report. Calculate the I:E ratio on your laboratory report.**

8. Increase the pressure until you have achieved the tidal volume in step 1. **Record it on your laboratory report.**

9. Using the flow control, set an appropriate I:E ratio. **Record the settings and your observations on your laboratory report.**

10. Finally, reduce the compliance to 0.01 L/cm H_2O and increase the resistance to R20. Measure the tidal volume, inspiratory time, and expiratory time, and **record them on your laboratory report. Calculate the I:E ratio on your laboratory report.**

11. Note how changes in compliance and resistance affect tidal volume, inspiratory time, expiratory time, and I:E ratio, and **discuss what changes occurred.**

REFERENCES

1. Denehy, L and Berney, S: The use of positive pressure devices by physiotherapists. Eur Respir J 17:821–829, 2001.
2. American Association for Respiratory Care: The AARC clinical practice guideline: Intermittent positive pressure breathing: 2003 revision and update. Respir Care 48(5):540–546, 2003.

Laboratory Report

CHAPTER 38: PRESSURE VENTILATORS

Name _____   Date _____

Course/Section _____   Instructor _____

Data Collection

EXERCISE 38.1 Identification of an Adult Breathing Circuit and Leak Testing

Ventilator used: _____

Observations: _____

_____

_____

_____

_____

EXERCISE 38.2 Controls

NORMAL RESISTANCE AND COMPLIANCE

PRESSURE = 10 cm H_2O, FLOW = 15

Tidal volume: _____

Inspiratory time: _____

Expiratory time: _____

I:E ratio (show your work!): _____

PRESSURE = 15 cm H_2O, FLOW = 15

Tidal volume: _____

Inspiratory time: _____

Expiratory time: _____

I:E ratio (show your work!): _____

PRESSURE = 10 cm H_2O, FLOW = 20

Tidal volume: _____

Inspiratory time: _____

Expiratory time: _____

I:E ratio (show your work!) _____

PRESSURE = 10 cm H_2O, FLOW = 10

Tidal volume: _____

Inspiratory time: _____

Expiratory time: _____

I:E ratio (**show your work!**) _____

PRESSURE = 20 cm H_2O, FLOW = 20

Tidal volume: _____

Inspiratory time: _____

Expiratory time: _____

I:E ratio (**show your work!**) _____

EXERCISE 38.3 Initiation and Monitoring

Peak pressure: _____

Respiratory rate: _____

Peak flow: _____

Tidal volume: _____

Inspiratory time: _____

Expiratory time: _____

I:E ratio: _____

Tidal volume with high resistance (R20): _____

Inspiratory time: _____

Expiratory time: _____

I:E ratio: _____

Pressure setting: _____

Flow setting: _____

Tidal volume with decreased compliance right lung (C_L 0.08 L/cm H_2O): _____

Inspiratory time: _____

Expiratory time: _____

I:E ratio: _____

Pressure setting: _____

Flow setting: _____

Tidal volume with decreased compliance both lungs (C_L 0.08 L/cm H_2O): _____

Inspiratory time: _____

Expiratory time: _____

I:E ratio: _____

Pressure setting: _____

Flow setting: _____

Tidal volume with low compliance and high resistance (C_L 0.01 and R20): _____

Inspiratory time: _____

Expiratory time: _____

I:E ratio: _____

Pressure setting: _____

Flow setting: _____

Critical Thinking Questions

1. Given the scenario with Mrs. Gandhi, answer the following:

   A. What clinical situations were simulated by increasing the airway resistance?

   B. What clinical situations were simulated by decreasing the compliance in the right lung? In both lungs?

2. What patient assessment techniques would you use to evaluate the ventilatory status of Mrs. Gandhi?

3. Construct a sample charting note using the initial settings and data obtained in Exercise 38.3. Be sure to include all assessment information.

4. Based on your observations and measurements:

   A. What effect did increasing resistance have on the exhaled tidal volume and I:E ratio?

   B. What parameter(s) would you change to maintain adequate ventilation and I:E ratio?

   C. What effect did decreasing compliance have on the exhaled tidal volume and I:E ratio?

   D. What parameter(s) would you change to maintain adequate ventilation and I:E ratio?

39 Continuous Mechanical Ventilation

INTRODUCTION

During volume-limited/pressure-variable ventilation, the breath continues until a preset volume is reached. The amount of pressure required to deliver the tidal volume preset will depend on the patient's compliance and resistance. Although pressure-limited and volume-limited ventilation have been the most common modes used in critical care, combinations of volume and pressure ventilation, or dual modes, are increasingly used as an alternative modality.

This chapter is intended to introduce the student to the initiation of volume ventilation. In subsequent chapters the relationships between pressure, flow, volume, and time during volume ventilation will be explored. The student must be able to apply these concepts to initiate ventilation and monitor patients using the more advanced modes available on current highly sophisticated equipment.[1]

OBJECTIVES

Upon completion of this chapter, the student will be able to:

1. Initiate and monitor volume-limited ventilation.
2. Compare the interrelationships between pressure, volume, flow, and time.
3. Relate the changes that might occur in the parameters of pressure, volume, flow, and time with changes in compliance and resistance.
4. Chart data related to volume-limited ventilation in the medical record.

KEY TERMS

flow	time	volume-limited/	volume ventilator
pressure	volume	pressure-variable	

Exercises

EQUIPMENT REQUIRED

- ☐ Volume ventilator
- ☐ Manufacturer's operation and maintenance manuals (videos if available)
- ☐ 50-psi oxygen source
- ☐ 50-psig regulator
- ☐ High-pressure hoses
- ☐ Air compressor
- ☐ Blender
- ☐ Wrench
- ☐ Test lung or lung simulator

- ☐ Water traps
- ☐ Humidifiers (HME, cascade, and wick)
- ☐ Sterile water
- ☐ Respirometer and adaptor
- ☐ Adult breathing circuits with and without exhalation valve
- ☐ Corrugated tubing
- ☐ Watch with second hand
- ☐ 50-psi gas source
- ☐ HEPA bacteria filter

EXERCISE 39.1 VENTILATOR ASSEMBLY

1. Select a volume ventilator, water traps, bacteria filters, humidifier, and test lung. **Record the ventilator brand and model on your laboratory report.**

2. Obtain the maintenance manual for the ventilator selected. In the manual, find the manufacturer's recommendations for changing and cleaning of bacteria filters and fan filters, sterilization or disinfection instructions for internal and external parts and surfaces, and requirements for routine maintenance. **Record this information on your laboratory report.**

3. Locate the **chronometer,** if available, and **record the number of hours of use on your laboratory report.**

4. Assemble the ventilator as shown in Figure 39.1 (with humidifier) and Figure 39.2 (with HME). Note any difficulties encountered while assembling the ventilator and **record them on your laboratory report.**

5. Repeat this exercise for each ventilator provided.

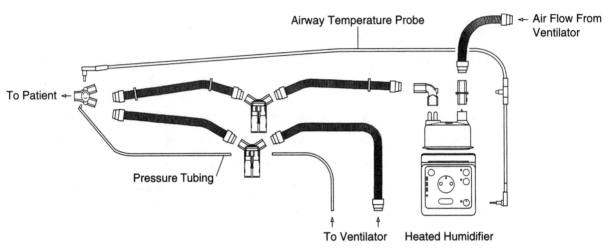

Figure 39.1. Ventilator circuit assembly with humidifier and water traps. (Courtesy of Fisher & Paykel Healthcare, Auckland, New Zealand.)

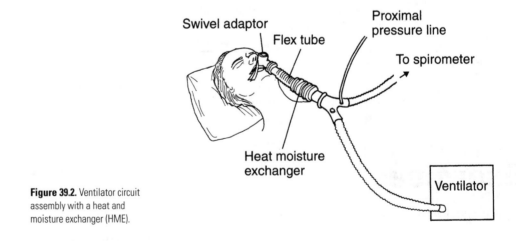

Figure 39.2. Ventilator circuit assembly with a heat and moisture exchanger (HME).

EXERCISE 39.2 IDENTIFICATION OF CONTROLS

1. On the volume ventilator selected, identify the following controls. It is important to note that not all ventilators have the same controls, but they have several controls in common. **Record the ventilator used and the controls identified on your laboratory report.**

   Tidal volume or minute volume

   Rate

   F_IO_2

   Flow or percent inspiratory time

   Sigh volume

   Sigh rate

   High-pressure limit

   Low-pressure limit

   F_IO_2 alarms

   Low-exhaled volume alarm

2. Repeat this exercise for each ventilator provided.

EXERCISE 39.3 LEAK TESTING

Using the same equipment from the previous exercises,

1. Turn all settings to the minimum or off setting.
2. Increase the tidal volume to 400 mL.
3. Increase the high-pressure limit to 80 cm H_2O or to the maximum setting.
4. Occlude the patient adaptor at the wye.
5. Cycle the ventilator. **Record your observations and the pressure achieved on your laboratory report.**

EXERCISE 39.4 DETERMINATION OF TUBING COMPLIANCE FACTOR AND CALCULATION OF LOST VOLUME

Utilizing the same volume ventilator, attach it to the test lung as in Figure 39.1 and perform the following:

1. Set the flow to the minimum setting.
2. Set the tidal volume to 300 mL.
3. Ensure that the high-pressure limit is set at the maximum.
4. Occlude the patient adaptor at the wye.
5. Cycle the ventilator. **Record your observations and the pressure achieved on your laboratory report.**
6. Determine the **compressibility factor** (CF) using the following formula:

   Set V_T − Observed exhaled V_T / Pressure = Compressibility factor
7. **Record the compressibility factor on your laboratory report.**

REFERENCES
1. McPherson, S: Respiratory Care Equipment, ed 7. Mosby, St. Louis, 2004.

Laboratory Report

CHAPTER 39: CONTINUOUS MECHANICAL VENTILATION

Name _____ Date _____

Course/Section _____ Instructor _____

Data Collection

EXERCISE 39.1 Ventilator Assembly

Ventilator brand and model: _____

Ventilator brand and model: _____

Ventilator brand and model: _____

Hours of use: _____

Difficulties encountered: _____

_____

_____

EXERCISE 39.2 Identification of Controls

(Attach separate sheet for additional ventilators used)

Ventilator brand and model: _____

Controls identified: _____

_____

_____

_____

EXERCISE 39.3 Leak Testing

Observations and pressure achieved: _____

_____

_____

EXERCISE 39.4 Determination of Tubing Compliance Factor and Calculation of Lost Volume

Set tidal volume: _____

Observed exhaled tidal volume: _____

Pressure reading : _____

Observations : _____

Calculated compressibility factor (CF) (**show your work!**):

Critical Thinking Questions

1. You have just assembled a volume ventilator and performed a leak test. The cycling pressure achieved when the wye was occluded was only 55 cm H_2O. Describe the step-by-step procedure you would use to rectify the problem.

2. You have successfully rectified the problem in Critical Thinking Question 1. How would you communicate to the incoming shift that this ventilator is ready for patient use?

3. Given the following data, calculate the compressible volume loss and actual V_T. **Show your work!**

    A. V_T = 500 mL
        CF = 4 mL/cm H_2O
        Peak pressure = 20 cm H_2O
        Lost volume = _____ mL
        Actual V_T = _____ mL

    B. V_T = 800 mL
        CF = 2 mL/cm H_2O
        Peak pressure = 30 cm H_2O
        Lost volume = _____ mL
        Actual V_T = _____ mL

    C. V_T = 700 mL
        CF = 3.5 mL/cm H_2O
        Peak pressure = 40 cm H_2O
        Lost volume = _____ mL
        Actual V_T = _____ mL

D. V_T = 200 mL
    CF = 2 mL/cm H_2O
    Peak pressure = 50 cm H_2O
    Lost volume = _____ mL
    Actual V_T = _____ mL

40

Ventilator Modes

INTRODUCTION

Technological advances and new microprocessors have increased the sophistication and variety of ways that a patient can be mechanically ventilated. Each method has a different goal. Is the goal to rest the patient's respiratory muscles, or do we allow the patient to do some work? Will we allow the patient to breathe spontaneously as a supplement to machine breaths or as the sole method of ventilation? Do we need to **augment** the patient's spontaneous breaths or increase the functional residual capacity (FRC)? Does the patient have difficulty primarily with oxygenation, ventilation, or both? What is the condition of the patient's airways and lung–thorax relationship? Is the patient "fighting the ventilator" or ready to be weaned? How familiar is the staff with the mode under consideration?[1] Different ventilator modes may potentially answer all these questions. The ventilator mode determines how the patient and machine function in harmony. The practitioner must recognize the different modes available with specific ventilators as well as understand the intricacies of each mode to optimize the patient's outcome.

Once the appropriate mode is selected, the practitioner must, in concert with the attending physician or through the use of protocol, determine the most appropriate values for the ventilator parameters, which include F_IO_2, tidal volume and respiratory rate (or minute ventilation), flow rate and pattern, inspiratory-to-expiratory ratios, inspiratory or expiratory pauses, sighs, and any pressure adjuncts.

This chapter explores common modes of mechanical ventilation and ventilator capabilities. Guidelines for initiation of ventilation and parameter selection, alarm settings, monitoring, and discontinuance of mechanical ventilation are addressed in Chapters 41, 42, and 43.

OBJECTIVES

Upon completion of this chapter, the student will be able to:

1. Differentiate the various modes of mechanical ventilation: control, assist/control, synchronized intermittent **mandatory** ventilation (SIMV), pressure control and **inverse** I:E ratio ventilation, pressure support, positive end-expiratory pressure (PEEP), and continuous positive airway pressure (CPAP).
2. Given any mechanical ventilator, locate and identify each mode and adjunct parameter available and determine how to use it.
3. Assess the limitations of each ventilator.
4. Evaluate the effects of manipulation of the various interdependent modes and adjunct parameters.
5. Compare and contrast the capabilities of critical care ventilators with home care ventilators.

KEY TERMS

augment   mandatory
inverse   synchrony

Exercises

EQUIPMENT REQUIRED

- [ ] Adult breathing circuits for ventilators available (needed for critical care and home care ventilators)
- [ ] HEPA bacteria filters
- [ ] Manufacturer's operation and maintenance manuals (videos if available)
- [ ] Water traps
- [ ] Humidifiers [heat and moisture exchanger (HME) and heated humidifier system]
- [ ] Sterile water
- [ ] Volume ventilators
- [ ] 50-psi oxygen source
- [ ] 50-psig regulator
- [ ] Bourdon gauge and Thorpe tube flowmeters
- [ ] High-pressure hoses
- [ ] Air compressor
- [ ] Blender
- [ ] Wrench
- [ ] T-adaptor with small-bore tubing connection and cap
- [ ] Test lungs and lung simulator (if available)
- [ ] Watch with a second hand
- [ ] Respirometer
- [ ] Oxygen analyzer and in-line adaptor
- [ ] Spring-loaded PEEP valve
- [ ] Self-contained (or sealed marine) 12-volt battery with connecting cables
- [ ] Metric ruler

It is suggested that the following exercises be performed with the ventilator alarms set on minimum/maximum settings so that students will not be intimidated by the noise and confusion during the initial learning experience (and so that instructors will not be unnerved). Once students gain comfort with the operation of the various ventilator controls, it would be valuable for the exercises to be repeated with the alarms set appropriately for clinical situations. Students can then observe the relationship between the machine settings, alarms, and patient care implications. The goals of the various modes of mechanical ventilation are outlined in Table 40.1. Most modern ventilators can achieve all of these modes. The student should perform all the exercises on a selected ventilator and then repeat the entire set of exercises on any other available brands, taking particular notice of the differences between the brands of ventilators used.

Table 40.1 Goals of Mechanical Ventilation Modes

Mode	Goal
Control	Precise V_E; patient's ventilatory drive controlled with medication
Assist/control	Ventilator does almost all work; ventilatory muscles rested
SIMV	Patient breathes spontaneously between mandatory ventilator breaths; ventilatory muscles used; also can be used as weaning technique or to help stabilize a patient fighting assist/control mode
Pressure support	Augments the V_T with a preselected amount of positive pressure; decreases work of breathing, including that superimposed by the artificial airway and circuitry
CPAP	Patient breathes spontaneously; continuous positive pressure gradient aids in oxygenation by increasing FRC
PEEP	Not a true mode but an adjunct to exhalation; aids oxygenation by increasing FRC
Pressure control	Used when one needs to reduce the mean airway pressure when high pressures are being used in volume ventilation
Inverse I:E	Aids in oxygenation
Airway pressure release ventilation (APRV) and bi-level ventilation	Strategies to improve oxygenation and lower mean airway pressure

EXERCISE 40.1 CONTROL AND ASSIST/CONTROL

1. Assemble a volume ventilator and verify its proper function as performed in Chapter 39. **Record the type/brand of ventilator used on your laboratory report.**
2. Adjust the settings to the following:
   Mode: Assist/Control (CMV)

   V_T = 600 mL

   f = 15/minute

   Peak flow = 30 Lpm (or percent inspiratory time = 33%)

   F_IO_2 = 0.21

   Make sure that all the alarms are set to the minimum/maximum settings.
3. Adjust the sensitivity to -10 cm H_2O.
4. Attach the test lung to the patient wye connection.
5. Count the respiratory rate and compare it with the rate set on the machine. **Record the result on your laboratory report.**
6. Observe the exhaled tidal volume and **record the result on your laboratory report.**
7. Squeeze the test lung several times to simulate an inspiratory effort. Observe the manometer. Count the rate at which you are squeezing the test lung and compare it with the displayed rate on the machine. **Record the results on your laboratory report. Explain on your laboratory report why the ventilator responded in this manner.**
8. Adjust the sensitivity to -2 cm H_2O.
9. Squeeze the test lung several times to simulate an inspiratory effort. Listen to the sound of the machine. Observe the manometer. Count the rate at which you are squeezing the test lung and compare it with the displayed rate on the machine. **Record the results and observations on your laboratory report.**
10. Observe the exhaled tidal volume and compare it with the displayed machine volume. **Record the result on your laboratory report.**
11. Adjust the rate to 4/minute. Squeeze the test lung at a minimum rate of 15/minute. Listen to the sound of the machine. Observe the manometer. Count the rate at which you are squeezing the test lung and compare it with the displayed rate on the machine. **Record the results and observations on your laboratory report.**
12. Observe the exhaled tidal volume and compare it with the displayed machine volume. **Record the result on your laboratory report.**
13. Stop squeezing the test lung. Wait 1 minute and observe the ventilator response. Count the ventilator rate. **Record your results and observations on your laboratory report.**
14. Repeat the exercise with a second ventilator.

EXERCISE 40.2 SYNCHRONIZED INTERMITTENT MANDATORY VENTILATION

1. Using the same equipment, change the mode to IMV or SIMV. **Record the type/brand of ventilator on your laboratory report.**
2. Maintain the settings as follows:
   V_T = 600 mL

   f = 15/minute

   Peak flow = 30 Lpm (or percent inspiratory time = 33%)

   F_IO_2 = 0.21

   Make sure all the alarms are set to the minimum/maximum settings.
3. Adjust the sensitivity to -2 cm H_2O.
4. Count the respiratory rate and observe the tidal volume, and **record them on your laboratory report.**
5. Squeeze the test lung several times to simulate an inspiratory effort. Observe the manometer. Count the rate at which you are squeezing the test lung and compare it with the displayed rate on the machine. **Record the results on your laboratory report.**

6. Continue to squeeze the lung. Listen to the sound of the machine and compare it with the assist/control mode. Observe the tidal volume for your manual squeezes and machine-delivered breaths. **Record the result and your observations on your laboratory report. Determine whether the machine is using IMV or SIMV.**

7. Decrease the set respiratory rate to 4/minute.

8. Squeeze the test lung to simulate an inspiratory effort.

9. Continue to squeeze the lung and count the rate at which you are squeezing. Listen to the sound of the machine and compare it with step 6. Observe and compare the spontaneous rate with the machine rate displayed. Observe and compare the tidal volume for your manual squeezes and machine-delivered breaths. **Record the results on your laboratory report.**

10. Stop squeezing the test lung. Wait 1 minute, listen to the sound of the machine, and observe the machine response. **Record your observations on the laboratory report.**

11. Reset any alarms if necessary. Resume squeezing the test lung. Observe the machine response and **record your observations on the laboratory report.**

12. Compare the ventilator responses in the SIMV mode to the assist/control mode. **Explain why these differences occur on your laboratory report.**

EXERCISE 40.3 POSITIVE END-EXPIRATORY PRESSURE/CONTINUOUS POSITIVE AIRWAY PRESSURE

1. Using the same equipment, set the mode to assist/control. **Record the type/brand of ventilator used on your laboratory report.**

2. Adjust the settings to the following:

   V_T = 500 mL

   f = 15/minute

   Peak flow = 30 Lpm (or percent inspiratory time = 25%)

   F_IO_2 = 0.21

   Make sure that all the alarms are set to the minimum/maximum settings.

3. Adjust the sensitivity to -3 cm H_2O.

4. Attach the test lung and turn on the ventilator.

5. Observe and compare the pressure manometer and the filling of the test lung at the end of inspiration and at the end of expiration. **Record the pressure readings at end inspiration and end expiration and your observations on your laboratory report.**

6. Adjust the PEEP to 5 cm H_2O.

7. Observe and compare the pressure manometer and the filling of the test lung at the end of inspiration and at the end of expiration. **Record the pressure readings at end inspiration and end expiration and your observations on your laboratory report.** Did the sensitivity need to be adjusted?

8. Adjust the PEEP to 8 cm H_2O.

9. Observe and compare the pressure manometer and the filling of the test lung at the end of inspiration and at the end of expiration. **Record the pressure readings at end inspiration and end expiration and your observations on your laboratory report.** Did the sensitivity need to be adjusted?

10. Decrease the PEEP setting to 0.

11. Change the mode to CPAP.

12. Adjust the CPAP pressure to 5 cm H_2O.

13. Squeeze the test lung to simulate a spontaneous breath.

14. Observe the pressure manometer and the filling of the test lung. **Record the pressure reading and your observations on your laboratory report.**

15. Adjust the CPAP to 10 cm H_2O.

16. Squeeze the test lung to simulate a spontaneous breath. Count the respiratory rate and **record it on your laboratory report.**

17. Observe and compare the pressure manometer and the filling of the test lung at the end of inspiration and at the end of expiration. **Record the pressure readings at end inspiration and end expiration and your observations on your laboratory report.**

18. Stop squeezing the test lung. Wait 1 minute and observe the machine response, rate, and tidal volume. **Record your results and observations on your laboratory report. Explain on your laboratory report why the ventilator responded as it did.**

19. Repeat the exercise with a second ventilator.

EXERCISE 40.4 PRESSURE SUPPORT MODE

EXERCISE 40.4.1 SYNCHRONIZED INTERMITTENT MANDATORY VENTILATION WITH PRESSURE SUPPORT

1. Using the same equipment, modify the mode to activate pressure support with the SIMV mode. **Record the type/brand of ventilator used on your laboratory report.**

2. Maintain the settings as at the end of Exercise 40.3:

   V_T = 600 mL

   f = 4/minute

   Peak flow = 30 Lpm (or percent inspiratory time = 33%)

   F_IO_2 = 0.21

   Make sure that all the alarms are set to the minimum/maximum settings.

3. Adjust the sensitivity to −2 cm H_2O.

4. Adjust the pressure support level to 5 cm H_2O.

5. Squeeze the test lung to simulate an inspiratory effort.

6. Continue to squeeze the lung and count the respiratory rate. Observe the tidal volume and manometer pressure readings for your manual squeezes and machine-delivered breaths. **Record the results on your laboratory report.**

7. While still squeezing the test lung, observe the pressure manometer. Listen to the sound of the machine. Compare the sound of the machine during a spontaneous breath in SIMV with pressure support with a spontaneous breath in SIMV without pressure support. **Record the pressure reading and your observations on your laboratory report.**

8. Increase the pressure support to 10 cm H_2O.

9. Squeeze the test lung to simulate an inspiratory effort.

10. Continue to squeeze the lung and count the respiratory rate. Listen to the sound of the machine and compare it with step 7. Observe the tidal volume for your manual squeezes and machine-delivered breaths. **Record the results and your observations on your laboratory report.**

EXERCISE 40.4.2 PRESSURE SUPPORT

1. Using the same equipment, modify the mode to activate pressure support without SIMV. This may require you to consult the operation manual to determine how this is achieved on a given ventilator. It may require the use of the CPAP mode.

2. Adjust the pressure support level to 0 cm H_2O. If the CPAP mode is required, make sure that the CPAP or PEEP pressure is set at zero.

3. Squeeze the test lung to simulate an inspiratory effort.

4. Continue to squeeze the lung. Observe the rate and tidal volume for your manual squeezes and machine-delivered breaths. **Record the results and observations on your laboratory report.**

5. While still squeezing the test lung, observe the pressure manometer. Listen to the sound of the machine. **Record the pressure reading and your observations on your laboratory report.**

6. Increase the pressure support to 5 cm H_2O.

7. Squeeze the test lung to simulate an inspiratory effort.

8. Continue to squeeze the lung. Listen to the sound of the machine and compare it with step 6. Observe the rate and tidal volume for your manual squeezes. **Record the results and your observations on your laboratory report.**

9. Increase the pressure support to 10 cm H_2O.

10. Squeeze the test lung to simulate an inspiratory effort.

11. Continue to squeeze the lung. Listen to the sound of the machine and compare it with step 6. Observe the rate and tidal volume for your manual squeezes. **Record the results and your observations on your laboratory report.**

12. Stop squeezing the test lung. Wait 1 minute and observe the rate and tidal volume. Observe the machine response. **Record your results and observations on your laboratory report.**

13. Repeat the exercise with a second ventilator.

EXERCISE 40.4.3 PRESSURE SUPPORT WITH CONTINUOUS POSITIVE AIRWAY PRESSURE

1. Maintain the ventilator in the pressure support mode as in Exercise 40.4.2. Set the pressure support to 10 cm H_2O. **Record the type/brand of ventilator used on your laboratory report.**

2. Squeeze the test lung to simulate an inspiratory effort.

3. Continue to squeeze the lung. Listen to the sound of the machine. Observe the rate, tidal volume, and filling of the test lung for your manual squeezes. **Record the results and your observations on your laboratory report.**

4. Add CPAP of 5 cm H_2O.

5. Continue to squeeze the lung. Listen to the sound of the machine and compare it with step 3. Observe the rate, tidal volume, and filling of the test lung for your manual squeezes. **Record the results and your observations on your laboratory report.**

EXERCISE 40.5 INVERSE I:E RATIO, PRESSURE CONTROL VENTILATION

EXERCISE 40.5.1 PRESSURE CONTROL

1. Using the same ventilator, set the mode control to pressure control, if available.

2. Connect the test lung or lung simulator to the patient wye. If you are using a lung simulator, set the compliance at 0.15 L/cm H_2O, the most compliant setting.

3. Set the controls to the following:

Inspiratory pressure = 10 cm H_2O

f = 15/minute

Peak flow = 30 Lpm (or percent inspiratory time = 33%)

4. Monitor the exhaled tidal volume and **record it on your laboratory report.**

5. Measure the I:E ratio and **record it on your laboratory report.**

6. Adjust the compliance to 0.05 L/cm H_2O.

7. Observe the exhaled tidal volume and **record it on your laboratory report.**

8. Measure the I:E ratio and **record it on your laboratory report.**

9. Repeat the exercise with a second ventilator.

EXERCISE 40.5.2 INVERSE I:E RATIO VENTILATION

1. Using the same ventilator, set the mode control to pressure control, if available.

2. Connect the test lung or lung simulator to the patient wye.

3. Set the controls to the following:

Inspiratory pressure = 15 cm H_2O

f = 15/minute

Compliance = 0.05 L/cm H_2O (decreased compliance)

4. Adjust the ventilator to inverse I:E ratio of 2:1 (if using the Siemens Servo 900C, adjust the percent inspiratory time to 67%).

5. Observe the exhaled tidal volume and **record it on your laboratory report.**

6. Measure the I:E ratio and **record it on your laboratory report.**

7. Calculate or determine the peak flow rate and **record it on your laboratory report.**

REFERENCES
1. Pilbeam, SP and Cairo, JM: Mechanical Ventilation: Physiological and Clinical Applications, ed 4. Mosby, St. Louis, 2006.

Laboratory Report

CHAPTER 40: VENTILATOR MODES

Name _____ Date _____

Course/Section _____ Instructor _____

Data Collection

EXERCISE 40.1 Control and Assist/Control

Type/brand of ventilator 1: _____

ASSIST/CONTROL RATE OF 15

SENSITIVITY: -10 cm H_2O

$V_T = 600$; $f = 15$/minute; Peak flow $= 30$ Lpm

Respiratory rate: _____

Exhaled V_T: _____

SIMULATED SPONTANEOUS BREATHING

Manometer observation and respiratory rate: _____

_____

_____

Exhaled V_T _____

Explain why the ventilator responded in this manner: _____

SENSITIVITY: -2 cm H_2O

Manometer observation and respiratory rate: _____

_____

_____

Exhaled V_T: _____

ASSIST/CONTROL RATE OF 4 WITH SPONTANEOUS RATE

Respiratory rate: _____

Exhaled V_T: _____

Manometer observation: _____

_____

_____

STOP SQUEEZING

Exhaled V_T: _____

Observations and rate: _____

_____

_____

Type/brand of ventilator 2: _____

ASSIST/CONTROL RATE OF 15

SENSITIVITY: -10 cm H_2O

Respiratory rate: _____

Exhaled V_T: _____

SIMULATED SPONTANEOUS BREATHING

Manometer observation and respiratory rate: _____

_____

_____

Exhaled V_T: _____

SENSITIVITY: -2 cm H_2O

Manometer observation and respiratory rate: _____

_____

_____

Exhaled V_T: _____

ASSIST/CONTROL RATE OF 4

Respiratory rate: _____

Exhaled V_T: _____

Manometer observation: _____

_____

_____

STOP SQUEEZING

Exhaled V_T: _____

Observations and rate: _____

_____

_____

Attach separate paper if additional ventilators are used.

EXERCISE 40.2 Synchronized Intermittent Mandatory Ventilation

Type/brand of ventilator 1: _____

SENSITIVITY: −2 cm H_2O

Machine rate: _____

Machine exhaled V_T: _____

Spontaneous respiratory rate: _____

Spontaneous exhaled V_T: _____

SIMV RATE 4/MINUTE

Machine rate: _____

Machine V_T: _____

Spontaneous respiratory rate: _____

Spontaneous exhaled V_T: _____

STOP SQUEEZING

Observations: _____

_____

RESUME SQUEEZING

Observations: _____

_____

Type/brand of ventilator 2: _____

SENSITIVITY: −2 cm H_2O

Machine rate: _____

Machine exhaled V_T: _____

Spontaneous respiratory rate: _____

Spontaneous exhaled V_T: _____

SIMV RATE 4/MINUTE

Machine rate: _____

Machine V_T: _____

Spontaneous respiratory rate: _____

Spontaneous exhaled V_T: _____

STOP SQUEEZING

Observations: _____

_____

RESUME SQUEEZING

Observations: _____

_____

Compare the ventilator response and your observations in the assist/control mode to the SIMV mode with spontaneous ventilations. Explain why these differences occur: _____

_____

_____

_____

Attach separate paper if additional ventilators are used.

EXERCISE 40.3 Positive End-Expiratory Pressure/Continuous Positive Airway Pressure

Type/brand of ventilator 1: _____

Initial pressure readings and observations: _____

_____

_____

5 cm H_2O pressure reading and observations: _____

_____

_____

Did the sensitivity need to be adjusted? _____

8 cm H_2O pressure reading and observations: _____

_____

_____

Did the sensitivity need to be adjusted? _____

CPAP 5 cm H_2O pressure reading and observations: _____

_____

_____

CPAP 10 cm H_2O pressure reading and observations: _____

_____

_____

Respiratory rate: _____

STOP SQUEEZING

Pressure reading and observations: _____

_____

_____

_____

Respiratory rate: _____ V_T: _____

Identify what clinical condition this exercise is supposed to simulate. Explain why the ventilator responded as it did:

_____

_____

_____

_____

Type/brand of ventilator 2: _____

Initial pressure readings and observations: _____

_____

_____

5 cm H_2O pressure reading and observations: _____

_____

_____

Did the sensitivity need to be adjusted? _____

8 cm H_2O pressure reading and observations: _____

_____

_____

Did the sensitivity need to be adjusted? _____

CPAP 5 cm H_2O pressure reading and observations: _____

_____

_____

CPAP 10 cm H_2O pressure reading and observations: _____

_____

_____

Respiratory rate: _____

STOP SQUEEZING

Pressure readings and observations: _____

_____

_____

Rate: _____ V_T: _____

Compare this ventilator's response with that of ventilator 1: _____

_____

_____

Attach separate paper if additional ventilators are used.

EXERCISE 40.4 Pressure Support Mode

EXERCISE 40.4.1 SYNCHRONIZED INTERMITTENT MANDATORY VENTILATION WITH PRESSURE SUPPORT

Type/brand of ventilator 1: _____

PRESSURE SUPPORT: 5 cm H_2O

SIMV respiratory *f*: _____

Exhaled machine V_T: _____

Machine peak pressure: _____

Spontaneous respiratory *f*: _____

Spontaneous exhaled V_T: _____

Spontaneous peak pressure: _____

Observations: _____

_____

PRESSURE SUPPORT: 10 cm H_2O

SIMV *f*: _____

Exhaled machine V_T: _____

Machine peak pressure: _____

Spontaneous *f*: _____

Spontaneous exhaled V_T: _____

Spontaneous peak pressure: _____

Observations: _____

_____

Type/brand of ventilator 2: _____

PRESSURE SUPPORT: 5 cm H_2O

SIMV *f*: _____

Exhaled machine V_T: _____

Machine peak pressure: _____

Spontaneous *f*: _____

Spontaneous exhaled V_T: _____

Spontaneous peak pressure: _____

Observations:_____

_____

PRESSURE SUPPORT: 10 cm H_2O

SIMV *f*: _____

Exhaled machine V_T: _____

Machine peak pressure: _____

Spontaneous *f*: _____

Spontaneous exhaled V_T: _____

Spontaneous peak pressure: _____

Observations: _____

_____

Attach separate paper if additional ventilators are used.

EXERCISE 40.4.2 PRESSURE SUPPORT

Type/brand of ventilator 1: _____

PRESSURE SUPPORT: 0 cm H_2O

f: _____

V_T: _____

Pressure reading: _____

Observations: _____

PRESSURE SUPPORT: 5 cm H_2O

f: _____

V_T: _____

Pressure reading: _____

Observations: _____

PRESSURE SUPPORT: 10 cm H_2O

f: _____

V_T: _____

Pressure reading: _____

Observations: _____

STOP SQUEEZING

f: _____

V_T: _____

Observations: _____

Type/brand of ventilator 2: _____

PRESSURE SUPPORT: 0 cm H_2O

f: _____

V_T: _____

Pressure reading: _____

Observations: _____

PRESSURE SUPPORT: 5 cm H_2O

f: _____

V_T: _____

Pressure reading: _____

Observations: _____

PRESSURE SUPPORT: 10 cm H_2O

f: _____

V_T: _____

Pressure reading: _____

Observations: _____

STOP SQUEEZING

f: _____

V_T: _____

Observations: _____

Attach separate paper if additional ventilators are used.

EXERCISE 40.4.3 PRESSURE SUPPORT WITH CONTINUOUS POSITIVE AIRWAY PRESSURE

Type/brand of ventilator 1: _____

CPAP: 0 cm H_2O, PRESSURE SUPPORT: 10 cm H_2O

f: _____

Observation of test lung: _____

_____

CPAP: 5 cm H_2O, PRESSURE SUPPORT: 10 cm H_2O

f: _____

V_T: _____

Observation of test lung: _____

_____

Type/brand of ventilator 2: _____

CPAP: 0 cm H_2O, PRESSURE SUPPORT: 10 cm H_2O

f: _____

V_T: _____

Observation of test lung: _____

_____

CPAP: 5 cm H_2O, PRESSURE SUPPORT: 10 cm H_2O

f: _____

V_T: _____

Observation of test lung: _____

_____

Attach separate paper if additional ventilators are used.

What is the effect of pressure support on the spontaneous exhaled volumes as compared with SIMV without pressure support

or CPAP without pressure support? _____

What is the best way to determine the ideal pressure support setting? _____

_____

_____

EXERCISE 40.5 Inverse I:E Ratio, Pressure Control Ventilation

EXERCISE 40.5.1 PRESSURE CONTROL

Type/brand of ventilator 1: _____

Exhaled V_T (most compliant): _____

Exhaled V_T (least compliant): _____

I:E ratio: _____

Type/brand of ventilator 2: _____

Exhaled V_T (most compliant): _____

Exhaled V_T (least compliant): _____

I:E ratio: _____

Attach separate paper if additional ventilators are used.

What type of patient conditions would be simulated by the most compliant setting? _____

What type of patient conditions would be simulated by the least compliant settings? _____

How does the lung compliance affect the I:E ratio? Why? _____

_____

_____

EXERCISE 40.5.2 INVERSE I:E RATIO VENTILATION

Type/brand of ventilator 1: _____

Exhaled V_T: _____

I:E ratio: _____

Peak flow rate: _____

Type/brand of ventilator 2: _____

Exhaled V_T: _____

I:E ratio: _____

Peak flow rate: _____

Attach separate paper if additional ventilators are used.

What precautions must be taken when using this mode of ventilation? Why? _____

_____

_____

_____

Critical Thinking Questions

1. Based on the data you collected during the laboratory exercises, do the following:

   A. Contrast the major differences of each brand of ventilator utilized.

   B. Discuss possible advantages and disadvantages of these differences. Relate these to effects on quality of patient care and patient comfort, ease of use for the practitioner, and cost-effectiveness (may require additional investigation and a literature search).

41 Ventilator Initiation

INTRODUCTION

With a better understanding of the types of ventilators, available parameters, and their interrelationships, the art of ventilator initiation can be explored. Although guidelines have been established for initial settings, each patient must be assessed individually and the ventilator parameters selected to achieve the optimal patient outcomes. This requires a prerequisite and comprehensive understanding of anatomy, physiology, pathophysiology, and fundamentals of respiratory care such as gas administration and airway management.

Once the initial ventilator settings have been determined, the corresponding alarm parameters must be selected to ensure patient safety. It is extremely important that the student be able to set these parameters appropriately and understand the implications of the alarm limits. Although different ventilators have different alarm systems, there are certain alarms that are basic to any ventilator.[1,2] Although some professionals consider that the new generation of ventilators may be overalarmed, which can lead to an ignoring of nuisance or false alarms, it is extremely important to recognize them. Mechanical ventilation has many hazards and complications. By appropriately adjusting ventilator settings and alarm parameters to meet individual patient needs, **iatrogenic** complications can be minimized.

OBJECTIVES

Upon completion of this chapter, the student will be able to:

1. Practice communication skills needed for the initiation of mechanical ventilation.
2. Determine the location and proper setting of available alarms on critical care and home care ventilators.
3. Given patient scenarios, determine the most appropriate mode of ventilation, tidal volume, respiratory rate, F_IO_2, peak flow rate or percent inspiratory time, I:E ratio, and pressure adjuncts, and initiate ventilation using critical care and home care ventilators.
4. Given the parameters selected in the scenarios, appropriately set the alarms.
5. Make recommendations and modifications to the ventilator settings based on patient assessment and data collection.
6. Apply infection control guidelines and standards associated with equipment and procedures, according to OSHA regulations and CDC guidelines.
7. Change the ventilator circuit, ensuring physical integrity and proper function with minimal risk or harm to the patient and healthcare provider.[2]

KEY TERMS

iatrogenic

Exercises

EQUIPMENT REQUIRED

- [ ] Adult breathing circuits for ventilators available
- [ ] HEPA bacteria filters
- [ ] Manufacturer's operation and maintenance manuals (videos if available)
- [ ] Water traps
- [ ] Humidifiers [heat and moisture exchanger (HME) and heated systems]
- [ ] Sterile water
- [ ] Volume ventilators
- [ ] 50-psi oxygen source
- [ ] 50-psig regulator
- [ ] Bourdon gauge and Thorpe tube flowmeters
- [ ] High-pressure hoses
- [ ] Air compressor

- [ ] Blender
- [ ] Wrench
- [ ] T-adaptor with small-bore tubing connection and cap
- [ ] Test lungs and lung simulator (if available)
- [ ] Watch with a second hand
- [ ] Respirometer
- [ ] Oxygen analyzer and in-line adaptor
- [ ] Spring-loaded PEEP valve
- [ ] Self-contained (or sealed marine) 12-volt battery with connecting cables
- [ ] Intubated or tracheostomized airway management trainer
- [ ] Hospital bed

EXERCISE 41.1 SETTING ALARM PARAMETERS

Not all ventilators have the same number and types of alarms. **Record the manufacturer, model of the available ventilator, and the alarm parameters on your laboratory report.**

EXERCISE 41.1.1 F_IO_2 OR GAS PRESSURE ALARMS

Obtain a critical care ventilator. Assemble the ventilator as in previous exercises. Be sure to check the unit for proper function and correct any malfunctions before use.

1. Observe the ventilator panel and determine what type of ventilator F_IO_2 alarm or gas pressure alarm is present. You may have to consult the manufacturer's manual. **Record the available alarms on your laboratory report.**

2. Connect the oxygen high-pressure hose to a Bourdon gauge or Thorpe tube flowmeter instead of a 50-psig oxygen source. Adjust the flow rate to 8 Lpm.

3. Set the ventilator parameters as follows:
   Mode = A/C
   f = 10/minute
   V_T = 500 mL
   F_IO_2 = 0.50
   Peak flow = 40 Lpm (or percent inspiratory time = 33%)
   Make sure that all alarm parameters are still set at minimum/maximum.

4. Turn on the ventilator and connect it to a test lung or lung simulator.

5. If the ventilator does not have a built-in oxygen analyzer, place one in-line.

6. Set the F_IO_2 alarm 5% lower than the F_IO_2 set on the ventilator.

7. Analyze the F_IO_2 and observe the ventilator for any activated alarms. **Record the F_IO_2 analyzed and observations of alarm status on your laboratory report.**

8. Adjust the flow rate to 15 Lpm.

9. Set the ventilator parameters as follows:
   Mode = A/C
   f = 20/minute
   V_T = 700 mL
   F_IO_2 = 1.0
   Peak flow = 70 Lpm (or percent inspiratory time = 20%)
   Make sure that all alarm parameters are still set at minimum/maximum.

10. Analyze the F_IO_2 and observe the ventilator for any activated alarms. **Record the F_IO_2 analyzed and observations of alarm status on your laboratory report.**

11. Turn the ventilator off. Disconnect the high-pressure hose and connect it to a 50-psig gas source.

12. Turn the ventilator on. Analyze the F_IO_2 and observe the ventilator for any activated alarms. **Record the F_IO_2 analyzed and observations of alarm status on your laboratory report.**

EXERCISE 41.1.2 HIGH-PRESSURE/LOW-PRESSURE ALARMS

1. Using the same ventilator as in Exercise 41.1.1, set the ventilator parameters as follows:
   Mode = A/C
   f = 12/minute
   V_T = 700 mL
   F_IO_2 = 0.21
   Peak flow = 35 Lpm (or percent inspiratory time = 25%)

2. Turn on the ventilator and connect it to a test lung or lung simulator.

3. Observe the system pressure on the manometer or digital display and the exhaled tidal volume, and **record the pressure and exhaled tidal volume on your laboratory report.**

4. Set the high-pressure limit 10 cm H_2O above the observed system pressure[1] and **record the setting on your laboratory report.**

5. If available, set the low-pressure limit 10 cm H_2O below the observed system pressure[1] and **record the setting on your laboratory report.**

6. Completely occlude the wye with your finger. Observe the pressure manometer and exhaled tidal volume, and **record your observations and the alarms activated on your laboratory report.**

7. Remove your finger and leave the circuit wye open. Observe the pressure manometer and exhaled tidal volume, and **record your observations and the alarms activated on your laboratory report.**

8. Reconnect the ventilator to the test lung.

EXERCISE 41.1.3 LOW EXHALED VOLUME ALARMS

1. Using the same ventilator, set the exhaled tidal volume alarm 100 to 150 mL lower than the exhaled tidal volume. If a low exhaled minute volume is available, set it by calculating a minute ventilation that has tidal volumes 100 to 150 mL less than the delivered tidal volume. **Record these settings on your laboratory report.**

2. Completely occlude the wye with your finger. Observe the pressure manometer and exhaled tidal volume, and **record your observations and the alarms activated on your laboratory report.**

3. Remove your finger and leave circuit wye open. Observe the pressure manometer and exhaled tidal volume, and **record your observations and the alarms activated on your laboratory report.**

4. Reconnect the ventilator to the test lung.

5. Change the following parameters:
   Mode = SIMV
   f = 6/minute

6. Squeeze the test lung to simulate spontaneous breathing at a rate of 6/minute, for a total rate of 12/minute.

7. Observe the ventilator and **record your observations and the alarms activated on your laboratory report.**

8. Readjust the alarms appropriately, if needed, and **record the adjusted alarm settings on your laboratory report.**

EXERCISE 41.1.4 OTHER VENTILATOR ALARMS

From the information gathered at the start of the exercises, set any of the other available alarm parameters and **record them on your laboratory report.** Remember that some of these choices will depend on the patient's clinical condition. Be prepared to defend the rationale used to determine your selections.

EXERCISE 41.2 VENTILATOR INITIATION

Given the following scenarios, select the mode and initial ventilator settings that you feel are appropriate. Be sure to set the alarms as well. Refer to Table 41.1 to aid in your selection. Each scenario should be performed on all critical care ventilators available in the laboratory.

Table 41.1 Guidelines for Initial Ventilator Setting Selection

Patient Type	Rate	V_T
Adults		
Normal lungs	10–12	10–12 mL/kg
Neuromuscular disease	6–10	12–15 mL/kg
Obstructive lung disease	8–10	10–12 mL/kg
Acute restrictive disease	12–20	8–10 mL/kg
Children		
8–16 yr	20–30	8–10 mL/kg
0–8 yr	25–35	6–8 mL/kg

Adapted from Wilkins, R et al. (eds): Egan's Fundamentals of Respiratory Care, ed 8. Mosby, St. Louis, 2003, p. 1023.

SCENARIO 1

You have been called to the trauma room. Mr. Scott is a 20-year-old, 150-lb, 5 ft. 6 inch, unrestrained driver of an automobile involved in a motor vehicle accident (MVA). He is unconscious and apneic with multiple rib fractures. He is already intubated with an 8.0-mm-ID endotracheal (ET) tube. The resident asks you to determine the initial ventilator settings.

1. Select the initial ventilator settings and **record them on your laboratory report.**
2. Evaluate the patient by performing the following:
    Vital signs
    Physical assessment of the chest
    Auscultation
    Suctioning
    Record what you would expect to find for the above parameters on your laboratory report.
3. Set the alarm parameters and **record them on your laboratory report.**

SCENARIO 2

Ms. Fumo is a 70-year-old, 100-lb, 5 ft. 2 inch, well-known COPD patient. She was admitted to the ER with fever, dyspnea, and productive cough. Over the past several hours her dyspnea has worsened and she has become lethargic. Her arterial blood gases (ABGs) on 2 L of nasal oxygen reveal the following:

pH = 7.18
$PaCO_2$ = 77 mm Hg
PaO_2 = 52 mm Hg

Her attending physician orders her intubated and asks for your recommendations for ventilator settings.

1. Select the initial ventilator settings and **record them on your laboratory report.**
2. Evaluate the patient by performing the following:
    Vital signs
    Physical assessment of the chest
    Auscultation
    Suctioning
    Record what you would expect to find for the above parameters on your laboratory report.
3. Set the alarm parameters, and **record them on your laboratory report.**

SCENARIO 3

Ms. Hoey is a 27-year-old, 90-lb, 5 ft. 4 inch, HIV-positive patient admitted with fever, dyspnea, and cough. A chest x-ray reveals bilateral pneumonia. Stat ABGs are drawn on a nonrebreather mask:

pH = 7.48
$PaCO_2$ = 32 mm Hg
PaO_2 = 48 mm Hg

Her vital signs are as follows:

Pulse = 120/minute
Respiratory rate = 32/minute and labored
Blood pressure = 110/60

1. Select the initial ventilator settings and **record them on your laboratory report.**
2. Evaluate the patient by performing the following:
   Vital signs
   Physical assessment of the chest
   Auscultation
   Suctioning
   Record what you would expect to find for the above parameters on your laboratory report.
3. Set the alarm parameters and **record them on your laboratory report.**

SCENARIO 4

You are the only therapist on duty. There was a cardiac arrest in the ER and the patient must be placed on a ventilator. Mrs. Raju is 65 years old, weighs 195 lb, is 5 ft. 7 inches, and has an extensive cardiac history. She is intubated with an 8.0-mm-ID ET tube. She is currently apneic. Her ABGs are as follows:

pH = 7.32
$PaCO_2$ = 33 mm Hg
PaO_2 = 122 mm Hg

These were drawn during the code while being manually ventilated with 1.0 F_IO_2:

1. Select the initial ventilator settings and **record them on your laboratory report.**
2. Evaluate the patient by performing the following:
   Vital signs
   Physical assessment of the chest
   Auscultation
   Suctioning
   Record what you would expect to find for the above parameters on your laboratory report.
3. Set the alarm parameters and record **them on your laboratory report.** Repeat the scenarios for each available critical care ventilator and **record all parameters on your laboratory report.**

EXERCISE 41.3 CIRCUIT CHANGES[3]

To simulate the conditions in the clinical setting, an intubated or tracheostomized airway management trainer should be positioned in a hospital bed if available. Have your laboratory partner count how many breaths are missed during the circuit change.

1. Set the ventilator to the following parameters:

   Mode = Control

   $f = 15$

   $V_T = 600$ mL

   $F_IO_2 = 0.40$

2. Gather the necessary equipment to perform a complete ventilator circuit change.

3. Assemble the equipment as completely as possible.

4. Place the assembled circuit on the bed with the wye placed aseptically proximal to the "patient." Place the other ends proximal to their corresponding connections on the ventilator as shown in Figure 41.1.

5. Silence the alarms.

6. Adjust the F_IO_2 on the ventilator to hyperoxygenate the "patient" before disconnection.

7. Instruct your partner to hold his or her breath beginning simultaneously from the time of "patient" disconnection and to continue breath holding until the "patient" is reconnected.

8. Quickly disconnect the circuit from the patient wye.

9. Quickly disconnect the other circuit connections from the ventilator.

10. Quickly attach the ends of the new circuit to the corresponding connections on the ventilator.

11. Rapidly assess the circuit for leaks and ensure ventilator function.

12. Reconnect the "patient" to the ventilator circuit. **Instruct your partner to resume breathing.**

13. Observe the pressure manometer and exhaled volumes.

14. Readjust the F_IO_2 and reset the alarms.

15. Determine the number of breaths lost by the "patient" and the total time to complete the circuit change. **Record the number of breaths and time taken on your laboratory report. Record your partner's impressions of his or her breath-holding experience.**

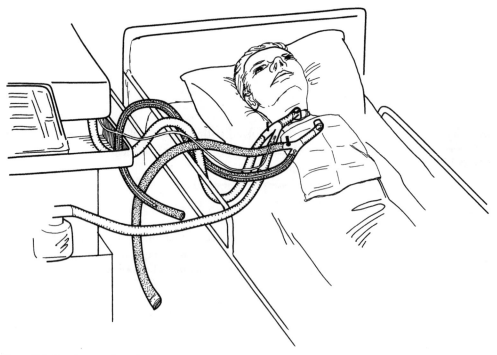

Figure 41.1. Changing a ventilator circuit.

REFERENCES

1. Chang, DW: Clinical Application of Mechanical Ventilation, ed 2. Delmar, Albany, 2001, p. 185.
2. Pilbeam, S: Mechanical Ventilation: Physiological and Clinical Applications, ed 4. Mosby, St. Louis, 2006, p. 106.
3. American Association for Respiratory Care: The AARC clinical practice guideline: Care of the ventilator circuit and its relation to ventilator-associated pneumonia. Respir Care 48:869–879, 2003.

Laboratory Report

CHAPTER 41: VENTILATOR INITIATION

Name _____   Date _____

Course/Section _____   Instructor _____

Data Collection

EXERCISE 41.1 Setting Alarm Parameters

Type/brand of ventilator 1: _____

Alarm parameters available: _____

_____

_____

_____

Type/brand of ventilator 2: _____

Alarm parameters available: _____

_____

_____

_____

EXERCISE 41.1.1 F_IO_2 OR GAS PRESSURE ALARMS

Type/brand of ventilator 1: _____

F_IO_2 or gas pressure alarms available: _____

_____

Type/brand of ventilator 2: _____

F_IO_2 or gas pressure alarms available: _____

_____

CONNECTION TO A FLOWMETER

Type/brand of ventilator 1: _____

Flow = 8 Lpm; f = 10; V_T = 500 mL; F_IO_2 = 0.50; PEFR = 40 Lpm

F_IO_2 analyzed: _____

Observations: _____

_____

_____

Flow = 15 Lpm; f = 20; V_T = 700 mL; F_IO_2 = 1.0; PEFR = 70 Lpm

F_IO_2 analyzed: _____

Observations: _____

_____

_____

CONNECTION TO 50-PSIG SOURCE

F_IO_2 analyzed: _____

Observations: _____

_____

_____

Type/brand of ventilator 2: _____

Flow = 8 Lpm; f = 10; V_T = 500 mL; F_IO_2 = 0.50; PEFR = 40 Lpm

F_IO_2 analyzed: _____

Observations: _____

_____

_____

Flow = 15 Lpm; f = 20; V_T = 700 mL; F_IO_2 = 1.0; PEFR = 70 Lpm

F_IO_2 analyzed: _____

Observations: _____

_____

_____

CONNECTION TO 50-PSIG SOURCE

F_IO_2 analyzed: _____

Observations: _____

_____

_____

Explain why the observations made in this exercise occurred.

_____

_____

What can you conclude regarding the relationships between pressures, flows, and F_IO_2? _____

_____

_____

How does this affect the ventilator setup? _____

_____

_____

EXERCISE 41.1.2 HIGH-PRESSURE/LOW-PRESSURE ALARMS

Type/brand of ventilator 1: _____

$f = 12$; $V_T = 700$ mL; $F_IO_2 = 0.21$; PEFR $= 35$ Lpm

Initial pressure observed: _____

Initial exhaled tidal volume: _____

High-pressure limit setting: _____

Low-pressure limit setting: _____

WYE OCCLUDED

Pressure observed: _____

Exhaled tidal volume: _____

Alarms activated: _____

WYE OPEN (UNOBSTRUCTED)

Pressure observed: _____

Exhaled tidal volume: _____

Alarms activated: _____

Type/brand of ventilator 2: _____

$f = 12$; $V_T = 700$ mL; $F_IO_2 = 0.21$; PEFR $= 35$ Lpm

Initial pressure observed: _____

Initial exhaled tidal volume: _____

High-pressure limit setting: _____

Low-pressure limit setting: _____

WYE OCCLUDED

Pressure observed: _____

Exhaled tidal volume: _____

Alarms activated: _____

WYE OPEN (UNOBSTRUCTED)

Pressure observed: _____

Exhaled tidal volume: _____

Alarms activated: _____

EXERCISE 41.1.3 LOW EXHALED VOLUME ALARMS

Type/brand of ventilator 1: _____

Low exhaled tidal volume alarm setting: _____

Low exhaled minute volume setting: _____

WYE OCCLUDED

Pressure observed: _____

Exhaled tidal volume: _____

Alarms activated: _____

WYE OPEN (UNOBSTRUCTED)

Pressure observed: _____

Exhaled tidal volume: _____

Alarms activated: _____

SIMV 6/SPONTANEOUS RATE 6

Alarms activated: _____

Alarms readjustment: _____

Type/brand of ventilator 2: _____

Low exhaled tidal volume alarm setting: _____

Low exhaled minute volume setting: _____

WYE OCCLUDED

Pressure observed: _____

Exhaled tidal volume: _____

Alarms activated: _____

WYE OPEN (UNOBSTRUCTED)

Pressure observed: _____

Exhaled tidal volume: _____

Alarms activated: _____

SIMV 6/SPONTANEOUS RATE 6

Alarms activated: _____

Alarm readjustment: _____

EXERCISE 41.1.4 OTHER VENTILATOR ALARMS

Type/brand of ventilator 1: _____

Alarms Available	Setting Determination	Rationale
_____	_____	_____
_____	_____	_____
_____	_____	_____
_____	_____	_____
_____	_____	_____
_____	_____	_____
_____	_____	_____

Type/brand of ventilator 2: _____

Alarms Available	Setting Determination	Rationale
_____	_____	_____
_____	_____	_____
_____	_____	_____
_____	_____	_____
_____	_____	_____
_____	_____	_____
_____	_____	_____

EXERCISE 41.2 Ventilator Initiation

SCENARIO 1

Type/brand of ventilator 1: _____

Mode: _____

V_T: _____

f: _____

Flow or percent inspiratory time: _____

F_IO_2: _____

Patient assessment:

    Vital signs: _____

    Physical assessment of the chest: _____

    Auscultation: _____

    Suctioning: _____

Alarm settings: _____

_____

_____

Type/brand of ventilator 2: _____

Mode: _____

V_T: _____

f: _____

Flow or percent inspiratory time: _____

F_IO_2: _____

Patient assessment:

    Vital signs: _____

    Physical assessment of the chest: _____

    Auscultation: _____

    Suctioning: _____

Alarm settings: _____

_____

_____

SCENARIO 2

Type/brand of ventilator 1: _____

Mode: _____

V_T: _____

f: _____

Flow or percent inspiratory time: _____

F_IO_2: _____

Patient assessment:

    Vital signs: _____

    Physical assessment of the chest: _____

    Auscultation: _____

    Suctioning: _____

Alarm settings: _____

_____

_____

Type/brand of ventilator 2: _____

Mode: _____

V_T: _____

f: _____

Flow or percent inspiratory time: _____

F_IO_2: _____

Patient assessment:

    Vital signs: _____

    Physical assessment of the chest: _____

    Auscultation: _____

    Suctioning: _____

Alarm settings: _____

_____

_____

SCENARIO 3

Type/brand of ventilator 1: _____

Mode: _____

V_T: _____

f: _____

Flow or percent inspiratory time: _____

F_IO_2: _____

Patient assessment:

    Vital signs: _____

    Physical assessment of the chest: _____

    Auscultation: _____

    Suctioning: _____

Alarm settings: _____

_____

_____

Type/brand of ventilator 2: _____

Mode: _____

V_T: _____

f: _____

Flow or percent inspiratory time: _____

F_IO_2: _____

Patient assessment:

    Vital signs: _____

    Physical assessment of the chest: _____

    Auscultation: _____

    Suctioning: _____

Alarm settings: _____

_____

_____

SCENARIO 4

Type/brand of ventilator 1: _____

Mode: _____

V_T: _____

f: _____

Flow or percent inspiratory time: _____

F_IO_2: _____

Patient assessment:

    Vital signs: _____

    Physical assessment of the chest: _____

    Auscultation: _____

    Suctioning: _____

Alarm settings: _____

_____

_____

Type/brand of ventilator 2: _____

Mode: _____

V_T: _____

f: _____

Flow or percent inspiratory time: _____

F_IO_2: _____

Patient assessment:

    Vital signs: _____

    Physical assessment of the chest: _____

    Auscultation: _____

    Suctioning: _____

Alarm settings: _____

_____

_____

EXERCISE 41.3 Circuit Changes

Type/brand of ventilator 1: _____

Breaths lost: _____

Time taken: _____

Breath-holding impressions: _____

_____

Type/brand of ventilator 2: _____

Breaths lost: _____

Time taken: _____

Breath-holding impressions: _____

Critical Thinking Questions

1. What are the purposes of alarms?

2. How can nuisance alarms be avoided?

3. The physicians in the scenarios want you to justify your initial ventilator settings in scenarios 1, 2, 3, and 4. How would you respond? Remember to include your rationale for machine and mode selection. (This question can also be done as an oral exercise with a fellow student or lab instructor acting as the physician.)

   Scenario 1:

   Scenario 2:

   Scenario 3:

   Scenario 4:

4. What safety precautions should be taken when performing a ventilator circuit change?

Procedural Competency Evaluation

STUDENT: _____   DATE: _____

ADULT VENTILATOR INITIATION

		PERFORMANCE RATING	PERFORMANCE LEVEL
Evaluator: ☐ Peer ☐ Instructor **Setting:** ☐ Lab ☐ Clinical Simulation			
Equipment Utilized: **Conditions (Describe):**			
Performance Level: S or ✓ = Satisfactory, no errors of omission or commission U = Unsatisfactory Error of Omission or Commission NA = Not applicable			
Performance Rating:			
5 **Independent:** Near flawless performance; minimal errors; able to perform without supervision; seeks out new learning; shows initiative; A = 4.7–5.0 average			
4 **Minimally Supervised:** Few errors, able to self-correct; seeks guidance when appropriate; B = 3.7–4.65			
3 **Competent:** Minimal required level; no critical errors; able to correct with coaching; meets expectations; safe; C = 3.0–3.65			
2 **Marginal:** Below average; critical errors or problem areas noted; would benefit from remediation; D = 2.0–2.99			
1 **Dependent:** Poor; unacceptable performance; unsafe; gross inaccuracies; potentially harmful; F = < 2.0			
Two or more errors of commission or omission of mandatory or essential performance elements will terminate the procedure, and require additional practice and/or remediation and reevaluation. Student is responsible for obtaining additional evaluation forms as needed from the Director of Clinical Education (DCE).			

PATIENT AND EQUIPMENT PREPARATION

1. Common Performance Elements Steps 1–8		
2. Connects the ventilator to the appropriate emergency electrical outlets		
3. Connects the high-pressure hoses to the appropriate 50-psi gas source outlets		
4. Attaches circuit, filters, and humidification systems as needed		
5. Turns on the ventilator and performs any required tests		
6. Performs any additional leak tests; corrects and verifies ventilator function		

ASSESSMENT AND IMPLEMENTATION

7. Common Performance Elements Steps 9 and 10		
8. Assesses indications for mechanical ventilation; evaluates the patient by performing: A. Vital signs, color, WOB, pulse oximetry, capnography B. Physical assessment of the chest C. Auscultation D. Airway size, type, placement, and patency E. Suctioning		
9. Selects the initial ventilator settings according to order or protocol		
10. Sets initial alarm parameters		
11. Connects the patient to the ventilator and adjusts the following as needed: A. Ventilator parameters and alarms B. Sensitivity (pressure or flow trigger) C. Mode D. Rate/frequency E. V_T/V_E F. PIP/ pressure support G. Flow rate/I-time%/Flow Pattern/I:E ratio		
12. Analyzes and adjusts F_IO_2 as indicated		
13. Adjusts circuit humidification system		
14. Notes LOC, use of sedation, and paralytics		
15. Observes and interprets ventilator graphics		
16. Completes patient-system ventilator check		

FOLLOW-UP

17. Common Performance Elements Steps 11–16		

SIGNATURES Student: _____ Evaluator: _____ Date: _____

Clinical Performance Evaluation

PERFORMANCE RATING:

5 **Independent:** Near flawless performance; minimal errors; able to perform without supervision; seeks out new learning; shows initiative; A = 4.7–5.0 average

4 **Minimally Supervised:** Few errors, able to self-correct; seeks guidance when appropriate; B = 3.7–4.65

3 **Competent:** Minimal required level; no critical errors; able to correct with coaching; meets expectations; safe; C = 3.0–3.65

2 **Marginal:** Below average; critical errors or problem areas noted; would benefit from remediation; D = 2.0–2.99

1 **Dependent:** Poor; unacceptable performance; unsafe; gross inaccuracies; potentially harmful; F = < 2.0

Circle the appropriate response below. Please be consistent, objective, and honest in your assessment of the student's clinical performance and ability.

PERFORMANCE CRITERIA	SCORE				
COGNITIVE DOMAIN					
1. Consistently displays knowledge, comprehension, and command of essential concepts	5	4	3	2	1
2. Demonstrates the relationship between theory and clinical practice	5	4	3	2	1
3. Able to select, review, apply, analyze, synthesize, interpret, and evaluate information; makes recommendations to modify care plan	5	4	3	2	1
PSYCHOMOTOR DOMAIN					
4. Minimal errors, no critical errors; able to self-correct; performs all steps safely and accurately	5	4	3	2	1
5. Selects, assembles, and verifies proper function and cleanliness of equipment; assures operation and corrects malfunctions; provides adequate care and maintenance	5	4	3	2	1
6. Exhibits the required manual dexterity	5	4	3	2	1
7. Performs procedure in a reasonable time frame for clinical level	5	4	3	2	1
8. Applies and maintains aseptic technique and PPE as required	5	4	3	2	1
9. Maintains concise and accurate patient and clinical records	5	4	3	2	1
10. Reports promptly on patient status/needs to appropriate personnel	5	4	3	2	1
AFFECTIVE DOMAIN					
11. Exhibits courteous and pleasant demeanor; shows consideration and respect, honesty, and integrity	5	4	3	2	1
12. Communicates verbally and in writing clearly and concisely	5	4	3	2	1
13. Preserves confidentiality and adheres to all policies	5	4	3	2	1
14. Follows directions, exhibits sound judgment, and seeks help when required	5	4	3	2	1
15. Demonstrates initiative, self-direction, responsibility, and accountability	5	4	3	2	1

TOTAL POINTS = _____ /15 = AVERAGE GRADE = _____

ADDITIONAL COMMENTS: IDENTIFY AREAS OF EXCELLENCE; LIST ERRORS OF OMISSION OR COMMISSION, CRITICAL ERRORS

SUMMARY PERFORMANCE EVALUATION AND RECOMMENDATIONS

☐ PASS: Satisfactory Performance

    ☐ Minimal supervision needed, may progress to next level provided specific skills, clinical time completed

    ☐ Minimal supervision needed, able to progress to next level without remediation

☐ FAIL: Unsatisfactory Performance (check all that apply)

    ☐ Minor reevaluation only

    ☐ Needs additional clinical practice before reevaluation

    ☐ Needs additional laboratory practice before skills performed in clinical area

    ☐ Recommend clinical probation

SIGNATURES

Evaluator (print name):   Evaluator signature: Date:

Student Signature: Date:

Student Comments:

Procedural Competency Evaluation

STUDENT: DATE:

VENTILATOR CIRCUIT CHANGE

Evaluator: ☐ Peer ☐ Instructor	**Setting:** ☐ Lab ☐ Clinical Simulation	PERFORMANCE RATING / PERFORMANCE LEVEL
Equipment Utilized:	**Conditions (Describe):**	

Performance Level:

S or ✓ = Satisfactory, no errors of omission or commission
U = Unsatisfactory Error of Omission or Commission
NA = Not applicable

Performance Rating:

5   **Independent:** Near flawless performance; minimal errors; able to perform without supervision; seeks out new learning; shows initiative; A = 4.7–5.0 average

4   **Minimally Supervised:** Few errors, able to self-correct; seeks guidance when appropriate; B = 3.7–4.65

3   **Competent:** Minimal required level; no critical errors; able to correct with coaching; meets expectations; safe; C = 3.0–3.65

2   **Marginal:** Below average; critical errors or problem areas noted; would benefit from remediation; D = 2.0–2.99

1   **Dependent:** Poor; unacceptable performance; unsafe; gross inaccuracies; potentially harmful; F = < 2.0

Two or more errors of commission or omission of mandatory or essential performance elements will terminate the procedure, and require additional practice and/or remediation and reevaluation. Student is responsible for obtaining additional evaluation forms as needed from the Director of Clinical Education (DCE).

PATIENT AND EQUIPMENT PREPARATION

1. Common Performance Elements Steps 1–8

ASSESSMENT AND IMPLEMENTATION

2. Common Performance Elements Steps 9 and 10

3. Assesses the patient and ventilator system prior to performing the circuit change

4. Ensures emergency equipment is available

5. Cleans outside surface of ventilator of dust and debris

6. Changes filters if needed

7. Has assistant, if available, manually ventilate the patient

8. Assembles the equipment as completely as possible

9. Places the assembled circuit on the bed with the wye positioned aseptically proximal to the patient

10. Places the other ends proximal to their corresponding connections on the ventilator

11. Silences the alarms

12. Adjusts the F_IO_2 on the ventilator to hyperoxygenate the patient prior to disconnection (or manually hyperinflates as appropriate)

13. Quickly disconnects the circuit from the patient wye

14. Quickly disconnects the other circuit connections from the ventilator

15. Quickly attaches the ends of the new circuit to the corresponding connections on the ventilator

16. Rapidly assesses the circuit for leaks and assures ventilator function

17. Reconnects the patient to the ventilator circuit

18. Changes any ancillary equipment as indicated (HME, MDI, or SVN in-line adapter, in-line suction catheter)

19. Observes the pressure and exhaled volume readings; corrects for leaks if needed

20. Verifies alarm function

21. Readjusts the F_IO_2 and resets the alarms

FOLLOW-UP

22. Common Performance Elements Steps 11–16

SIGNATURES   Student: Evaluator: Date:

Clinical Performance Evaluation

PERFORMANCE RATING:

5 **Independent:** Near flawless performance; minimal errors; able to perform without supervision; seeks out new learning; shows initiative; A = 4.7–5.0 average

4 **Minimally Supervised:** Few errors, able to self-correct; seeks guidance when appropriate; B = 3.7–4.65

3 **Competent:** Minimal required level; no critical errors; able to correct with coaching; meets expectations; safe; C = 3.0–3.65

2 **Marginal:** Below average; critical errors or problem areas noted; would benefit from remediation; D = 2.0–2.99

1 **Dependent:** Poor; unacceptable performance; unsafe; gross inaccuracies; potentially harmful; F = < 2.0

Circle the appropriate response below. Please be consistent, objective, and honest in your assessment of the student's clinical performance and ability.

PERFORMANCE CRITERIA	SCORE				
COGNITIVE DOMAIN					
1. Consistently displays knowledge, comprehension, and command of essential concepts	5	4	3	2	1
2. Demonstrates the relationship between theory and clinical practice	5	4	3	2	1
3. Able to select, review, apply, analyze, synthesize, interpret, and evaluate information; makes recommendations to modify care plan	5	4	3	2	1
PSYCHOMOTOR DOMAIN					
4. Minimal errors, no critical errors; able to self-correct; performs all steps safely and accurately	5	4	3	2	1
5. Selects, assembles, and verifies proper function and cleanliness of equipment; assures operation and corrects malfunctions; provides adequate care and maintenance	5	4	3	2	1
6. Exhibits the required manual dexterity	5	4	3	2	1
7. Performs procedure in a reasonable time frame for clinical level	5	4	3	2	1
8. Applies and maintains aseptic technique and PPE as required	5	4	3	2	1
9. Maintains concise and accurate patient and clinical records	5	4	3	2	1
10. Reports promptly on patient status/needs to appropriate personnel	5	4	3	2	1
AFFECTIVE DOMAIN					
11. Exhibits courteous and pleasant demeanor; shows consideration and respect, honesty, and integrity	5	4	3	2	1
12. Communicates verbally and in writing clearly and concisely	5	4	3	2	1
13. Preserves confidentiality and adheres to all policies	5	4	3	2	1
14. Follows directions, exhibits sound judgment, and seeks help when required	5	4	3	2	1
15. Demonstrates initiative, self-direction, responsibility, and accountability	5	4	3	2	1

TOTAL POINTS = _____ /15 = AVERAGE GRADE = _____

ADDITIONAL COMMENTS: IDENTIFY AREAS OF EXCELLENCE; LIST ERRORS OF OMISSION OR COMMISSION, CRITICAL ERRORS

SUMMARY PERFORMANCE EVALUATION AND RECOMMENDATIONS

☐ PASS: Satisfactory Performance

  ☐ Minimal supervision needed, may progress to next level provided specific skills, clinical time completed

  ☐ Minimal supervision needed, able to progress to next level without remediation

☐ FAIL: Unsatisfactory Performance (check all that apply)

  ☐ Minor reevaluation only

  ☐ Needs additional clinical practice before reevaluation

  ☐ Needs additional laboratory practice before skills performed in clinical area

  ☐ Recommend clinical probation

SIGNATURES

Evaluator (print name): _____ Evaluator signature: _____ Date: _____

Student Signature: _____ Date: _____

Student Comments:

42

Patient-Ventilator System Care and Maintenance

INTRODUCTION

From the initial application to the discontinuance of mechanical ventilation, respiratory care practitioners must be able to assess the integrity and effectiveness of the patient-ventilator system in order to make appropriate modifications to the care plan. The AARC clinical practice guideline is specific in defining the patient-ventilator system check. Although this evaluation has been frequently referred as a "vent check," it is the documented *evaluation* of a mechanical ventilator's function *and* of the patient's response to ventilatory support.[1] This routine evaluation must always begin with a complete assessment of the patient before proceeding to the functional evaluation of the machine. This assessment should include (but not be limited to) obtaining vital signs, cardiopulmonary auscultation, airway care, and evaluation for the presence of barotrauma or volutrauma.

Once the patient's response to ventilatory support has been evaluated, proper functioning of the equipment should be verified. This part of the evaluation should always include a correlation of the settings with the parameters or protocol ordered by the attending physician, setting and functioning of alarms, measurement of the inspired gas temperature, and analysis of the F_IO_2. As always, if the work is not documented, the work was not done. Accurate and timely documentation or charting is critical. It is the legal evidence that patient-ventilator system check was done in a timely and proper manner.

The goals of mechanical ventilation must be clearly established and continually refined so that monitoring of the patient-ventilator system leads to the desired outcomes.

OBJECTIVES

Upon completion of this chapter, the student will be able to:

1. Apply infection control guidelines and standards associated with equipment and procedures, according to OSHA regulations and CDC guidelines.
2. Perform patient assessment techniques.
3. Properly verify and document the function of the ventilator.
4. Perform calculations to verify and document the patient's response to mechanical ventilation. These calculations specifically include effective **dynamic** compliance (EDC), effective **static** compliance (C_{ST}), resistance, and auto-PEEP or intrinsic PEEP.
5. Analyze and interpret waveforms and data generated by the patient-ventilator system.
6. Practice the documentation skills required for a patient-ventilator system check on a ventilator flow sheet and the skills necessary to generate a narrative or shift note.
7. Practice communication skills needed for the reporting of clinically significant data to the members of the healthcare team.

KEY TERMS

dynamic   intrinsic   static   weaning

Exercises

EQUIPMENT REQUIRED

- ☐ Adult breathing circuits for ventilators available
- ☐ HEPA bacteria filters
- ☐ Manufacturer's operation and maintenance manuals
- ☐ Water traps
- ☐ Humidifiers [heat and moisture exchanger (HME) and heated system]
- ☐ Sterile water
- ☐ Volume ventilators
- ☐ Home care ventilators
- ☐ 50-psi oxygen source
- ☐ 50-psig regulator
- ☐ Blender
- ☐ Bourdon gauge and Thorpe tube flowmeters

- ☐ High-pressure hoses
- ☐ Air compressor
- ☐ Wrench
- ☐ T-adaptor with small-bore tubing connection and cap
- ☐ Test lungs and lung simulator (if available)
- ☐ Watch with second hand
- ☐ Respirometer
- ☐ Oxygen analyzer and in-line adaptor
- ☐ Spring-loaded PEEP valve
- ☐ Stethoscope
- ☐ Intubated or tracheostomized airway management trainer
- ☐ Hospital bed

EXERCISE 42.1 BASIC VENTILATOR MONITORING

These exercises require the initiation of mechanical ventilation for various patient scenarios, as in Chapter 41, followed by the simulation of a complete patient-ventilator system check and documentation as on a legal medical document. The ventilator system must be assembled completely (including gas and electrical sources) and its function must be verified before initiation. Components needed for each setup must be selected and obtained by each student. It is recommended that each scenario be repeated for each available ventilator, and students should completely disassemble the ventilator setup after completion of each scenario.

SCENARIO 1

1. Set up a volume ventilator with an adult setup and HME.
2. Initiate ventilation. Mr. Lisanti is a 21-year-old, 150-lb man who has just come from the operating room (OR) after a craniotomy and evacuation of a subdural hematoma. He is orally intubated, has no documented lung pathology, and is not a smoker. Initiate ventilation with the following settings: mode = A/C, V_T = 800 mL, f = 12/minute, and F_IO_2 = 0.35. All other settings and alarms are to be selected by you.
3. Perform a patient-ventilator system check, including patient assessment. Include oxygen analysis, cuff pressures, and airway care. **Record all pertinent data on the ventilator flow sheet provided in your laboratory report.**
4. Write a narrative note documenting your patient's status and any other data required to write a comprehensive shift note. **Record it on your laboratory report.** This will require you to use your imagination to create clinically relevant assessment data.

SCENARIO 2

1. Set up the ventilator with an adult setup and humidifier.
2. Initiate ventilation. Mrs. Kay is a 30-year-old, 110-lb woman who is in status asthmaticus. She is in severe acute respiratory acidosis with moderate hypoxemia and has just been nasally intubated. Initiate ventilation with the following settings: mode = A/C, V_T = 600 mL, f = 10/minute, and F_IO_2 = 0.50.
3. Perform a patient-ventilator system check, including patient assessment. Include oxygen analysis, cuff pressures, and airway care. **Record all pertinent data on the ventilator flow sheet provided in your laboratory report.**
4. Write a narrative note documenting your patient's status and any other data required to write a comprehensive shift note. **Record it on your laboratory report.** This will require you to use your imagination to create clinically relevant assessment data.

SCENARIO 3

1. Set up the ventilator with an adult setup and humidifier.
2. Initiate ventilation. Miss Aswama is a 38-year-old, 100-lb woman who has myasthenia gravis. She has been on the ventilator for several weeks with a tracheostomy. Adjust her settings as follows: mode = SIMV, V_T = 500 mL, f = 12/minute, F_IO_2 = 0.30, pressure support = 5 cm H_2O, and PEEP = 5 cm H_2O.
3. Perform a patient-ventilator system check, including patient assessment. Include oxygen analysis, cuff pressures, and airway care. **Record all pertinent data on the ventilator flow sheet provided in your laboratory report.**
4. Write a narrative note documenting your patient's status and any other data required to write a comprehensive shift note. **Record it on your laboratory report.** This will require you to use your imagination to create clinically relevant assessment data.

SCENARIO 4

1. Set up the ventilator with an adult setup. The type of humidification should be selected by you.
2. Initiate ventilation. Mr. Lagoudakis is a 60-year-old, 160-lb, 5 ft. 6 inch man who is a known COPD patient with a superimposed respiratory infection, possibly pneumonia. His ABGs are pH = 7.16, $PaCO_2$ = 77 mm Hg, and PaO_2 = 49 torr on a 0.40 air-entrainment mask. The attending physician requests your recommendations for ventilator mode and settings. Initiate ventilation as you see fit. Orally justify to your laboratory partner the rationale for your choices, and **document the rationale on your laboratory report.**
3. Perform a patient-ventilator system check, including patient assessment. Include oxygen analysis, cuff pressures, and airway care. **Record all pertinent data on the ventilator flow sheet provided in your laboratory report.**
4. Write a narrative note documenting your patient's status and any other data required to write a comprehensive shift note. **Record it on your laboratory report.** This will require you to use your imagination to create clinically relevant assessment data.

EXERCISE 42.2 DATA GENERATION FOR EVALUATION OF PATIENT STATUS

EXERCISE 42.2.1 EFFECTIVE DYNAMIC AND STATIC COMPLIANCE AND RESISTANCE CALCULATIONS

1. Using the equipment and settings in the preceding four scenarios, calculate the effective dynamic compliance (EDC) using the following formula. **Record the results on the ventilator flow sheet provided in your laboratory report.**

    V_T / Peak pressure − PEEP
2. Using the same four scenarios, calculate the effective static compliance (C_{ST}) using the following formula. **Record the results on your laboratory report.**

    V_T / Plateau pressure − PEEP

Remember that you have to obtain a plateau pressure by instituting an inspiratory pause or hold. This value is obtained in different ways depending on the brand of ventilator. Ventilators with external exhalation valves, such as home care ventilators or earlier models, may require that the exhalation valve tubing be kinked or pinched closed at peak inspiration to obtain an inspiratory hold until the plateau pressure is achieved. The tubing should then be released so exhalation can be completed.

3. From the preceding data, calculate resistance by using the following formula. **Record the results on your laboratory report.**

$$\text{Peak pressure} - \text{Plateau pressure} / \text{Flow rate}$$

EXERCISE 42.2.2 DETERMINATION OF AUTO-PEEP

To measure auto-PEEP, an expiratory hold must be implemented. How this is done depends on the type of ventilator used.

1. Consult the manufacturer's manual to determine the method of measuring auto-PEEP or implementing an expiratory hold.
2. Set up an adult ventilator on the following settings: mode = A/C, V_T = 700 mL, f = 24/minute, F_IO_2 = 0.21, PEEP = 3 cm H_2O, and peak flow = 40 Lpm (or percent inspiratory time = 20%).
3. Attach a test lung to the patient wye.
4. Initiate the expiratory hold or auto-PEEP measurement procedure.
5. Observe the pressure manometer or digital display for the final pressure reading once the pressure has equilibrated. If auto-PEEP is present the reading will be above the baseline PEEP value set. **Record the end-expiratory pressure observed on your laboratory report.**
6. Calculate auto-PEEP as follows, and **record on your laboratory report:** Auto-PEEP = End expiratory pressure − Baseline PEEP pressure.
7. Determine which ventilator parameters must be adjusted to eliminate the auto-PEEP. **Record on your laboratory report any recommendations you would make to a physician to change the ventilator orders.**

EXERCISE 42.3 WAVEFORM IDENTIFICATION AND INTERPRETATION

EXERCISE 42.3.1 IDENTIFICATION OF PRESSURE–TIME CURVES

Figure 42.1 shows a typical pressure–time curve. The horizontal (x) axis represents time; the vertical (y) axis represents pressure. Positive pressure inspiration is shown as a rise in pressure. The peak inspiratory pressure appears as the highest point of the curve. Exhalation is shown immediately after PIP and continues until the next inspiration. The beginning pressure is referred to as the baseline, which appears above zero when PEEP/CPAP modes are in use. The average mean airway pressure is calculated from the shaded area under the curve. A negative deflection immediately before a rise in pressure indicates the patient's effort in patient-initiated mandatory breaths (Fig. 42.2).

Small fluctuations in pressure represent a patient's spontaneous breathing efforts (Fig. 42.3).

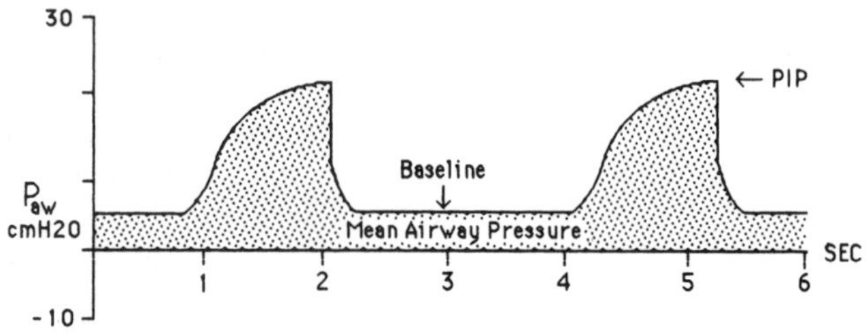

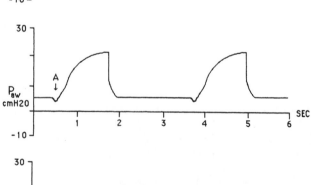

Figure 42.1. Typical pressure–time curve.

Figure 42.2. Patient-initiated mandatory (PIM) breaths.

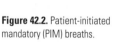

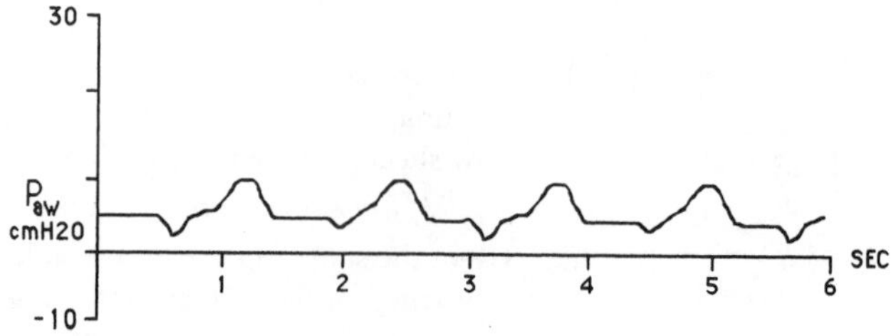

Figure 42.3. Spontaneous breathing.

Breaths that rise to a plateau and display varying inspiratory times indicate pressure-supported breaths (Fig. 42.4).

Breaths that rise to a plateau and display constant inspiratory time indicate pressure-controlled breaths (Fig. 42.5).

In some cases, a ventilator may not be able to meet the required patient inspiratory demand or the inspiratory flow may be set too low (Fig. 42.6).

A stable, static plateau pressure measurement is needed to accurately calculate resistance and compliance (Fig. 42.7).

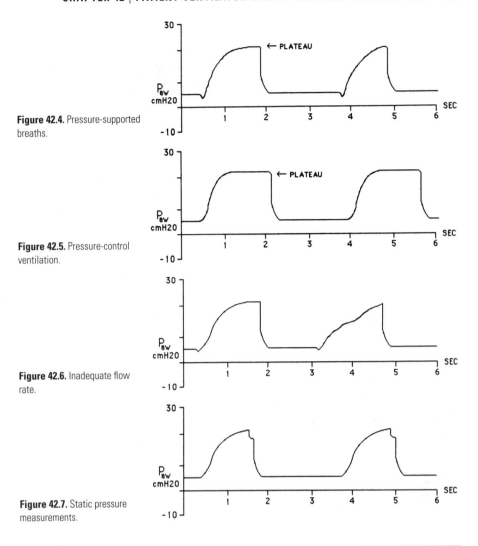

Figure 42.4. Pressure-supported breaths.

Figure 42.5. Pressure-control ventilation.

Figure 42.6. Inadequate flow rate.

Figure 42.7. Static pressure measurements.

EXERCISE 42.3.2 IDENTIFICATION OF FLOW–TIME CURVES

In this type of graphical representation, expiration is typically plotted below the baseline.

Figure 42.8 represents a typical flow–time curve in which inspiration is shown from **A** to **B** and expiration is shown from **B** to **C**. The peak inspiratory flow is the highest flow rate achieved during inspiration (**D**). The peak expiratory flow rate is shown as **E**.

Figure 42.9 illustrates various breath types.

Figure 42.10 shows a flow–time curve indicating auto-PEEP. Note that the expiratory flow does not return to baseline before the next breath is initiated.

Figure 42.11 shows inspiratory flow patterns that can be selected for mandatory, volume-based breaths on most ventilators.

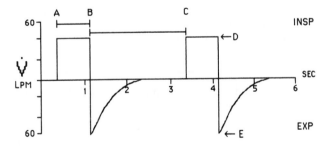

Figure 42.8. Typical flow–time curve.

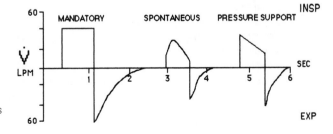

Figure 42.9. Flow–time curves indicating breath types.

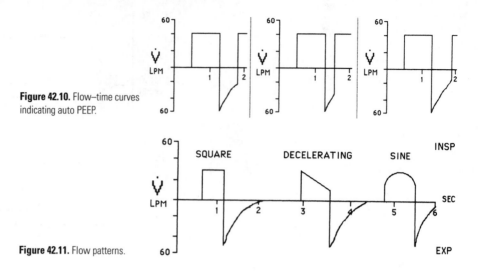

Figure 42.10. Flow–time curves indicating auto PEEP.

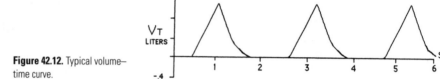

Figure 42.11. Flow patterns.

EXERCISE 42.3.3 IDENTIFICATION OF VOLUME–TIME CURVES

Figure 42.12 shows a typical volume–time curve in which the upslope indicates inspiratory volume and the downslope indicates expiratory volume. Inspiratory time is measured from the beginning of inspiration to the beginning of expiration. Expiratory time is measured from the beginning of exhalation to the beginning of the subsequent inspiration. In this figure, the patient has exhaled fully before the next breath. An increase in respiratory rate would be acceptable and would not cause air trapping.

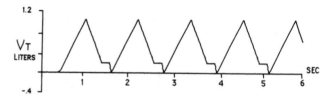

Figure 42.12. Typical volume–time curve.

Figure 42.13. Detecting air trapping or leaks.

Figure 42.13 indicates an exhalation that does not return to zero. Volume in and volume out are not always equal.

EXERCISE 42.3.4 PRESSURE–VOLUME LOOP

Figure 42.14 shows a typical pressure–volume loop for a mandatory breath. Pressure is plotted on the horizontal axis and volume on the vertical axis. The lower segment of the curve represents inspiration, the upper portion expiration. Inspiration is plotted first and the loop moves counterclockwise.

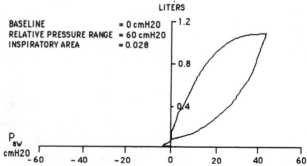

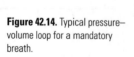

Figure 42.14. Typical pressure–volume loop for a mandatory breath.

BASELINE = 0 cmH20
RELATIVE PRESSURE RANGE = 60 cmH20
INSPIRATORY AREA = 0.028

*Figure 42.15 shows a pressure-triggered spontaneous breath with inspiration indicated by **A** and exhalation indicated by **B**. The entire inspiratory area appears to the left of the y axis and is plotted first so the entire loop moves clockwise.*

Figure 42.16 shows a pressure–volume loop for an assisted breath. The patient initiates the breath and inspiration begins plotting clockwise to the left of the y axis, but when the ventilator takes over, the plot direction shifts to counterclockwise to the right of the y axis.

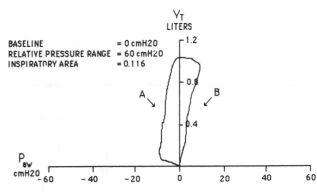

Figure 42.15. Pressure–volume loop for a spontaneous breath.

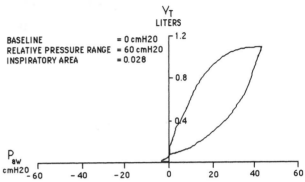

Figure 42.16. Pressure–volume loop for an assisted breath.

EXERCISE 42.3.5 INTERPRETATION OF WAVEFORMS

For Figures 42.17 through 42.23, identify the data indicated and **record your interpretations on the laboratory report.**

1. Figure 42.17:
   A. Mode of ventilation
   B. Inspiratory time for the first curve
   C. Line **A–B**
   D. What is occurring at point **C**?
   E. Suggested correction for point **C**

2. Figure 42.18:
   A. Mode of ventilation
   B. Explain the difference between curves **A** and **B**. What adjustment was made to correct curve **A**?

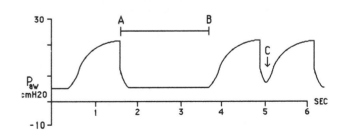

Figure 42.17. Evaluating respiratory events I.

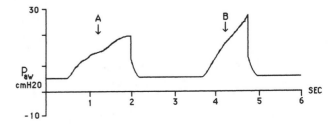

Figure 42.18. Evaluating respiratory events II.

3. Figure 42.19:
    A. Explain the difference in **A** for curves 1 and 2.
    B. What possible treatment interventions would have caused this change?
4. Figure 42.20:
    A. Mode of ventilation
    B. Respiratory rate
    C. Events at points **A** and **B**
5. Figure 42.21:
    A. Mode of ventilation
    B. Respiratory rate
    C. Events at points **A** and **B**
6. Figures 42.22 and 42.23:
    A. Which curve illustrates the greater work of breathing?
    B. What modalities could be implemented to result in the change from curve VI to curve VII?

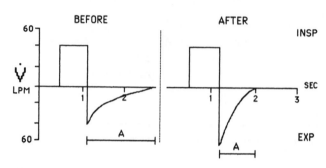

Figure 42.19. Evaluating respiratory events III.

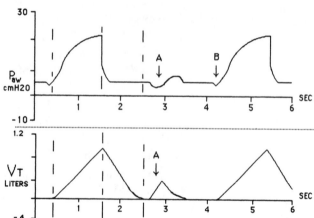

Figure 42.20. Evaluating respiratory events IV.

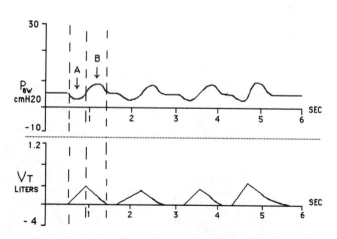

Figure 42.21. Evaluating respiratory events V.

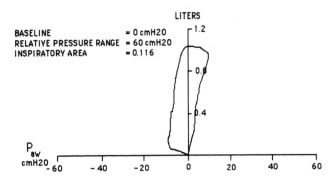

Figure 42.22. Evaluating respiratory events VI.

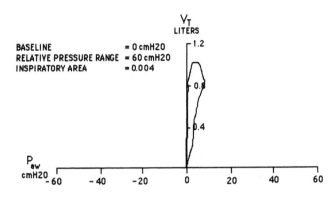

Figure 42.23. Evaluating respiratory events VII.

EXERCISE 42.4 SETTING MODIFICATION AND DOCUMENTATION

The following scenarios are continuations from the scenarios introduced in Exercise 42.1.

SCENARIO 1

Mr. Lisanti is a 21-year-old, 150-lb man who has just come from the OR after a craniotomy and evacuation of a subdural hematoma. He is orally intubated, has no documented lung pathology, and is not a smoker. Ventilation was initiated with the following settings: mode = A/C, V_T = 800 mL, f = 12/minute, and F_iO_2 = 0.35. An arterial blood gas was drawn 30 minutes later with the following results: pH = 7.29, $PaCO_2$ = 45 mm Hg, HCO_3 = 21, and PaO_2 = 110. The physician has requested that you adjust the ventilator to hyperventilate the patient for the first 24 hours and maintain the PaO_2 at 80 to 90 mm Hg.

1. Formulate the clinical data required to make recommendations for changes in the ventilator settings and **record them on your laboratory report.** Use any formulas or rules of thumb (see the Appendix) that are applicable to the situation.
2. With your lab partner acting as the physician, present your rationale orally.
3. The physician agrees with your recommendations. Implement the changes and **record them on your laboratory report.**

The next day, the patient has regained consciousness. You have measured bedside **weaning** *parameters and have decided that the patient is ready to be weaned*

1. Identify what the minimal acceptable values would be for VC, MIP, MVV, and V_T in this "patient" and **record them on your laboratory report.**

2. State what method of weaning you would recommend and **justify your answer on your laboratory report.**

SCENARIO 2

Mrs. Kay is a 30-year-old, 110-lb woman who is in status asthmaticus. She is in severe acute respiratory acidosis with moderate hypoxemia and has just been nasally intubated. Ventilation was initiated with the following settings: mode = A/C, V_T = 600 mL, f = 10/minute, and F_IO_2 = 0.50. Before taking the initial blood gas on the ventilator, you observe that the high-pressure alarm is continually sounding with each breath and only 480 mL of exhaled volume is measured. Auscultation reveals markedly diminished breath sounds bilaterally.

Identify the two most likely causes of this situation and make recommendations to correct these problems. **Record your answers on the laboratory report.**

Two days later, Mrs. Kay is stable and ready to be weaned. She is currently on SIMV 8/minute, V_T 600 mL, and F_IO_2 = 40%. Total breath rate is 28/minute and spontaneous V_T = 200 to 250 mL. Blood gases reveal pH = 7.48, $PaCO_2$ = 32 mm Hg, HCO_3 = 25, and PaO_2 = 135 mm Hg.

What changes would you recommend to commence weaning at this time? **Record your suggestions and rationale on the laboratory report.**

SCENARIO 3

Miss Aswama is a 38-year-old, 100-lb woman who has myasthenia gravis. She has been on the ventilator for several weeks with a tracheostomy: mode = SIMV, V_T = 500 mL, f = 12/minute, F_IO_2 = 0.30, pressure support = 5 cm H_2O, and PEEP = 5 cm H_2O. The capnometry reading has been stable at 38 mm Hg and SpO_2 = 94%, VC = 800 mL, and MIP = −30 cm H_2O. Weaning has begun on pressure support of 10 cm H_2O, CPAP = 3, and F_IO_2 = 0.30. One hour later, the capnometry reading is 45 mm Hg and SpO_2 = 88%.

What changes in vital signs and symptoms would you expect based on these values? What recommended changes would you make at this time? **Record your answers and rationale on the laboratory report.**

REFERENCES

1. AARC Clinical Practice Guideline. Patient-ventilator system checks. Respir Care 37(8):882–886, 1992.

Laboratory Report

CHAPTER 42: PATIENT-VENTILATOR SYSTEM CARE

Name _____   Date _____

Course/Section _____   Instructor _____

Data Collection

EXERCISE 42.1 Basic Ventilator Monitoring

SCENARIO 1

Mode = A/C, V_T = 800 mL, f = 12/minute, F_IO_2 = 0.35.

Use the patient-ventilator system check flow sheet and progress note forms to document your settings.

SCENARIO 2

Mode = A/C, V_T = 600 mL, f = 10/minute, F_IO_2 = 0.50.

Use the patient-ventilator system check flow sheet and progress note forms to document your settings.

SCENARIO 3

Mode = SIMV, V_T = 500 mL, f = 12/minute, F_IO_2 = 0.30, pressure support = 5 cm H_2O, PEEP = 5 cm H_2O.

Use the patient-ventilator system check flow sheet and progress note forms to document your settings.

SCENARIO 4

Use the patient-ventilator system check flow sheet and progress note forms to document your settings.

Rationale: _____

_____

EXERCISE 42.2 Data Generation for Evaluation of Patient Status

EXERCISE 42.2.1 EFFECTIVE DYNAMIC AND STATIC COMPLIANCE AND RESISTANCE CALCULATIONS

Show your work!

SCENARIO 1

EDC = _____

C_{ST} = _____

R_{AW} = _____

SCENARIO 2

EDC = _____

C_{ST} = _____

R_{AW} = _____

SCENARIO 3

EDC = _____

C_{ST} = _____

R_{AW} = _____

SCENARIO 4

EDC = _____

C_{ST} = _____

R_{AW} = _____

EXERCISE 42.2.2 DETERMINATION OF AUTO-PEEP

End-expiratory pressure = _____

Calculated auto-PEEP (**show your work!**) = _____

Recommendations and adjustments: _____

_____

_____

_____

EXERCISE 42.3 Waveform Identification and Interpretation

EXERCISE 42.3.5 INTERPRETATION OF WAVEFORMS

Figure 42.17

Mode of ventilation = _____

Inspiratory time for the first curve = _____

Line A–B = _____

What is occurring at point C? _____

_____

Suggested correction for point C: _____

_____

Figure 42.18

Mode of ventilation = _____

Explain the difference between curves **A** and **B**. What adjustment was made to correct curve **A**? _____

_____

_____

_____

Figure 42.19

Explain the difference in **A** for curves 1 and 2: _____

_____

_____

What possible treatment interventions would have caused this change? _____

_____

_____

Figure 42.20

Mode of ventilation = _____

Respiratory rate = _____

Event at point **A** = _____

Event at point **B** = _____

Figure 42.21

Mode of ventilation = _____

Respiratory rate = _____

Events at points **A** and **B** = _____

Figures 42.22 and 42.23

Which curve illustrates the greater work of breathing? What modalities could be implemented to result in a change from

curve VI and curve VII? _____

_____

_____

_____

_____

EXERCISE 42.4 Setting Modification and Documentation

SCENARIO 1

Clinical data required:

_____

_____

_____

_____

Formulas, rules of thumb used: _____

_____

_____

_____

_____

Changes implemented: _____

_____

_____

_____

_____

Minimal acceptable values:

VC _____

MIP _____

MVV _____

V_T _____

Method of weaning recommended and rationale: _____

_____

_____

_____

_____

_____

_____

SCENARIO 2

Identify the two most likely causes: _____

_____

_____

Recommendation to correct these problems: _____

_____

_____

_____

_____

What changes would you recommend two days later? _____

_____

_____

_____

_____

SCENARIO 3

What changes in vital signs and symptoms would you expect based on these values? What recommended changes would

you make at this time? _____

_____

_____

_____

_____

	PATIENT-VENTILATOR SYSTEM CHECK								PT ID:	
DATE										
TIME										
MODE										
SET RATE										
TOTAL RATE										
SET V_T/V_E										
EXH. V_T/V_E										
SPONT. V_T										
SET F_IO_2										
ANALYZED F_IO_2										
PSV										
PEEP/CPAP										
FLOW/%I-TIME										
FLOW PATTERN										
I:E RATIO										
SENSITIVITY										
PIP										
PLATEAU										
MAP										
HME/GAS TEMP										
HIGH P										
LOW P										
LOW V_T/V_E										
HI/LOW O_2										
LOW PEEP/CPAP										
TEMP ALARM										
AUTO-PEEP										
EDC										
CST										
RAW										
TUBE SIZE/TYPE										
TUBE PLACEMENT										
CUFF PRESS										
SpO_2										
$PECO_2$										
BP										
HR										
ECG										

	PATIENT-VENTILATOR SYSTEM CHECK										PT ID:	
TEMP												
pH												
$PaCO_2$												
COHB/METHB												
C.O.												
PAP												
PWP												
PvO_2												
SvO_2												
$CavO_2$												
SIGNATURE												

DATE	TIME	RESPIRATORY CARE PROGRESS NOTES

DATE	TIME	RESPIRATORY CARE PROGRESS NOTES
DATE	TIME	RESPIRATORY CARE PROGRESS NOTES

Procedural Competency Evaluation

STUDENT: **DATE:**

ADULT PATIENT-VENTILATOR SYSTEM CARE

	PERFORMANCE RATING	PERFORMANCE LEVEL
Evaluator: ☐ Peer ☐ Instructor **Setting:** ☐ Lab ☐ Clinical Simulation		
Equipment Utilized: **Conditions (Describe):**		

Performance Level:
 	
    S or ✓ = Satisfactory, no errors of omission or commission
    U = Unsatisfactory Error of Omission or Commission
    NA = Not applicable		

Performance Rating: **5** **Independent:** Near flawless performance; minimal errors; able to perform without supervision; seeks out new learning; shows initiative; A = 4.7–5.0 average **4** **Minimally Supervised:** Few errors, able to self-correct; seeks guidance when appropriate; B = 3.7–4.65 **3** **Competent:** Minimal required level; no critical errors; able to correct with coaching; meets expectations; safe; C = 3.0–3.65 **2** **Marginal:** Below average; critical errors or problem areas noted; would benefit from remediation; D = 2.0–2.99 **1** **Dependent:** Poor; unacceptable performance; unsafe; gross inaccuracies; potentially harmful; F = < 2.0 *Two or more errors of commission or omission of mandatory or essential performance elements will terminate the procedure, and require additional practice and/or remediation and reevaluation. Student is responsible for obtaining additional evaluation forms as needed from the Director of Clinical Education (DCE).*		
EQUIPMENT AND PATIENT PREPARATION		
1. Common Performance Elements Steps 1–8		
ASSESSMENT AND IMPLEMENTATION		
2. Common Performance Elements Steps 9 and 10		
3. Assesses patient by performing/observing:		
A. Vital signs		
B. Physical examination of the chest		
C. Auscultation		
D. Airway placement and patency		
E. Pulse oximetry		
F. E_tCO_2		
G. Hemodynamic stability parameters		
H. Subjective comfort level		
4. Assesses cuff inflation and adjusts if necessary		
5. Performs humidifier maintenance		
6. Analyzes F_IO_2		
7. Verifies all ventilator settings and adjusts if necessary		
8. Verifies all alarm settings and adjusts if necessary		
9. Assesses for weaning potential		
10. Measures spontaneous respiratory rate and volume, if indicated		
11. Calculates EDC, C_{st}, and R_{aw}		
12. Measures auto-PEEP and adjusts if necessary		
13. Analyzes and interprets waveforms and adjusts ventilator if necessary		
FOLLOW-UP		
14. Common Performance Elements Steps 11–16		

SIGNATURES   Student: Evaluator: Date:

Clinical Performance Evaluation

PERFORMANCE RATING:

5 **Independent:** Near flawless performance; minimal errors; able to perform without supervision; seeks out new learning; shows initiative; A = 4.7–5.0 average

4 **Minimally Supervised:** Few errors, able to self-correct; seeks guidance when appropriate; B = 3.7–4.65

3 **Competent:** Minimal required level; no critical errors; able to correct with coaching; meets expectations; safe; C = 3.0–3.65

2 **Marginal:** Below average; critical errors or problem areas noted; would benefit from remediation; D = 2.0–2.99

1 **Dependent:** Poor; unacceptable performance; unsafe; gross inaccuracies; potentially harmful; F = < 2.0

Circle the appropriate response below. Please be consistent, objective, and honest in your assessment of the student's clinical performance and ability.

PERFORMANCE CRITERIA	SCORE				
COGNITIVE DOMAIN					
1. Consistently displays knowledge, comprehension, and command of essential concepts	5	4	3	2	1
2. Demonstrates the relationship between theory and clinical practice	5	4	3	2	1
3. Able to select, review, apply, analyze, synthesize, interpret, and evaluate information; makes recommendations to modify care plan	5	4	3	2	1
PSYCHOMOTOR DOMAIN					
4. Minimal errors, no critical errors; able to self-correct; performs all steps safely and accurately	5	4	3	2	1
5. Selects, assembles, and verifies proper function and cleanliness of equipment; assures operation and corrects malfunctions; provides adequate care and maintenance	5	4	3	2	1
6. Exhibits the required manual dexterity	5	4	3	2	1
7. Performs procedure in a reasonable time frame for clinical level	5	4	3	2	1
8. Applies and maintains aseptic technique and PPE as required	5	4	3	2	1
9. Maintains concise and accurate patient and clinical records	5	4	3	2	1
10. Reports promptly on patient status/needs to appropriate personnel	5	4	3	2	1
AFFECTIVE DOMAIN					
11. Exhibits courteous and pleasant demeanor; shows consideration and respect, honesty, and integrity	5	4	3	2	1
12. Communicates verbally and in writing clearly and concisely	5	4	3	2	1
13. Preserves confidentiality and adheres to all policies	5	4	3	2	1
14. Follows directions, exhibits sound judgment, and seeks help when required	5	4	3	2	1
15. Demonstrates initiative, self-direction, responsibility, and accountability	5	4	3	2	1

TOTAL POINTS = _____ /15 = AVERAGE GRADE = _____

ADDITIONAL COMMENTS: IDENTIFY AREAS OF EXCELLENCE; LIST ERRORS OF OMISSION OR COMMISSION, CRITICAL ERRORS

SUMMARY PERFORMANCE EVALUATION AND RECOMMENDATIONS

☐ PASS: Satisfactory Performance

    ☐ Minimal supervision needed, may progress to next level provided specific skills, clinical time completed

    ☐ Minimal supervision needed, able to progress to next level without remediation

☐ FAIL: Unsatisfactory Performance (check all that apply)

    ☐ Minor reevaluation only

    ☐ Needs additional clinical practice before reevaluation

    ☐ Needs additional laboratory practice before skills performed in clinical area

    ☐ Recommend clinical probation

SIGNATURES

Evaluator (print name): _____   Evaluator signature: _____   Date: _____

Student Signature: _____   Date: _____

Student Comments:

43 Discontinuation of Mechanical Ventilation

INTRODUCTION

The initiation of invasive mechanical ventilation is an important decision. After ventilator initiation, the adequacy of the ventilatory strategies is constantly being assessed by the members of the healthcare team. However, prolonged invasive mechanical ventilation has serious complications and is extremely costly.[1] Therefore, once the patient's clinical condition has stabilized, the patient-ventilator care plan must be revised to develop a successful strategy for the discontinuation of mechanical ventilation. Often termed **weaning**, the process begins with the assessment of weaning readiness because it is important that the discontinuation effort not be premature.[2] The tolerance of a **spontaneous breathing test (SBT)**, coupled with other pertinent data, will help determine weaning readiness as well as the development of a weaning plan. These strategies include the complete removal of mechanical ventilation and allowing the patient to breath spontaneously, or the gradual removal of ventilatory support. More recently, the use of weaning **protocols** has been implemented to improve patient outcomes.[2,3] Respiratory care practitioners play a key role in the assessment of weaning readiness as well as in the implementation of weaning protocols and extubation as described in Chapter 24, Artificial Airway Care and Maintenance. Unfortunately, not every weaning attempt is successful. **Ventilator dependence** due to a failure to wean may result in the patient being transferred to a long-term ventilator or subacute care setting and generally means an overall reduction in the quality of life for the patient.

OBJECTIVES

Upon completion of this chapter, the student will be able to:

1. Identify the various weaning modalities found on commercially available ventilators.
2. Discuss the clinical considerations, including contraindications, for determining weaning readiness.
3. Evaluate the objective measurements required for determining weaning readiness.
4. Evaluate and implement a weaning protocol.

KEY TERMS

protocol

spontaneous breathing test (SBT)

ventilator dependence

weaning

Exercises

EQUIPMENT REQUIRED

- ☐ Adult breathing circuits for ventilators available
- ☐ HEPA bacteria filters
- ☐ Manufacturer's operation and maintenance manuals (videos if available)
- ☐ Water traps
- ☐ Humidifiers [heat and moisture exchanger (HME) and heated humidifier system]
- ☐ Sterile water
- ☐ Volume ventilators
- ☐ 50-psi oxygen source
- ☐ 50-psig regulator
- ☐ Bourdon gauge and Thorpe tube flowmeters
- ☐ High-pressure hoses
- ☐ Air compressor
- ☐ Blender
- ☐ Negative inspiratory force (NIF) meter/manometer
- ☐ Wrench
- ☐ T-adaptor with small-bore tubing connection and cap
- ☐ Test lungs and lung simulator (if available)
- ☐ Watch with a second hand
- ☐ Respirometer
- ☐ Oxygen analyzer and in-line adaptor

EXERCISE 43.1 WEANING MODALITIES

1. Review Table 40.1 Goals of Mechanical Ventilation Modes.
2. Review or repeat, if instructed, Exercises 40.2, 40.4.1, 40.4.2, and 40.4.3.
3. Identify the modes used for weaning. **Record the modes on your laboratory report.**
4. Identify the modes that can be used in combination during weaning. **Record the modes on your laboratory report.**

EXERCISE 43.2 ASSESSMENT DURING WEANING

Using your textbooks as well as other resources, complete Table 43.1 of weaning parameters. **Record the competed table on your laboratory report.**

Table 43.1 Patient Assessment Weaning Parameters

Parameter	Minimally Acceptable Value for Weaning
pH	
$PaCO_2$	
PaO_2	
F_IO_2	
PEEP	
PaO_2/F_IO_2	
Systolic BP	
Heart rate	
Hgb	
Chest x-ray	
CVP	
Pulmonary wedge pressure	
Urinary output	
Vital capacity	
Minute ventilation	
Negative inspiratory force (NIF)	
Maximum inspiratory pressure (MIP)	
Rapid shallow breathing index (RSBI)	
Mentation	
Sedation	

EXERCISE 43.3 WEANING PROTOCOLS

Your instructor will provide you with various weaning protocols from clinical sites, the AARC web site, or other sources. Read the protocols and **record the answers to the following questions on your laboratory report.**

1.   What is the first step in each protocol?
2.   List at least three contraindications to weaning.
3.   What parameters are measured in the protocols?
4.   How do the values compare to the values recorded in Exercise 43.2?
5.   If the criteria for weaning are met, is the patient given a spontaneous breathing trial?
6.   What measurements are made to document patient tolerance?
7.   What is the procedure if the patient does not tolerate the weaning effort?
8.   At what point is the physician notified of the patient's status?

REFERENCES
1. Marelich, GP, Murin, S, Battistella, F, Inciardi, J, Vierra, T, Roby, M: Protocol weaning of mechanical ventilation in medical and surgical patients by respiratory care practitioners and nurses. Chest 118:459–467, 2000.
2. McIntyre, NR, Cook, DJ, Ely, EW et al.: Evidence-based guidelines for weaning and discontinuing ventilator support. Chest 120(6):375–395, 2001.
3. Marx, WH, DeMaintenon, NL, Mooney, KF et al.: Cost reduction and outcome improvement in the intensive care unit. J Trauma 46:625–629, 1999.

Laboratory Report

CHAPTER 43: DISCONTINUATION OF MECHANICAL VENTILATION

Name _____ Date _____

Course/Section _____ Instructor _____

Data Collection

EXERCISE 43.1 Weaning Modalities

Modes used for weaning:

_____

_____

_____

_____

_____

_____

Modes used in combination:

_____

_____

_____

_____

_____

_____

EXERCISE 43.2 Assessment during Weaning

Parameter	Minimally Acceptable Value for Weaning
pH	
$PaCO_2$	
PaO_2	
F_IO_2	
PEEP	
PaO_2/F_IO_2	
Systolic BP	
Heart rate	
Hgb	
Chest x-ray	
CVP	
Pulmonary wedge pressure	
Urinary output	
Vital capacity	
Minute ventilation	
Negative inspiratory force (NIF)	
Maximum inspiratory pressure (MIP)	
Rapid shallow breathing index (RSBI)	
Mentation	
Sedation	

Exercise 43.3 Weaning Protocols

What is the first step in each protocol?

_____

_____

_____

_____

List at least three contraindications to weaning:

_____

_____

_____

_____

_____

What parameters are measured in the protocols?

_____

_____

_____

_____

_____

How do the values compare to the values recorded in Exercise 43.2?

_____

_____

_____

If the criteria for weaning are met, is the patient given a spontaneous breathing trial?

_____

_____

_____

_____

_____

_____

What measurements are made to document patient tolerance?

_____

_____

_____

_____

What is the procedure if the patient does not tolerate the weaning effort?

_____

_____

_____

_____

_____

_____

At what point is the physician notified of the patient's status?

_____

_____

_____

_____

_____

_____

Critical Thinking Questions

1. Can there be a psychological component to ventilator dependence? If so, what factors contribute to the dependence?

2. After several failed attempts at weaning, Mr. Smokes, a 65-year-old male with COPD, has been transferred to a ventilator-dependent care unit. What are some of the factors that might have contributed to the weaning failure? Include both subjective and objective assessments in your answer.

3. Based on the protocols used in Exercise 43.3, can you suggest any changes or additions that might improve the effectiveness of the protocol?

Procedural Competency Evaluation

STUDENT: **DATE:**

VENTILATOR WEANING PROTOCOLS

					PERFORMANCE RATING	PERFORMANCE LEVEL
Evaluator: ☐ Peer ☐ Instructor			**Setting:** ☐ Lab	☐ Clinical Simulation		
Equipment Utilized:			**Conditions (Describe):**			

Performance Level:

S or ✓ = Satisfactory, no errors of omission or commission
U = Unsatisfactory Error of Omission or Commission
NA = Not applicable

Performance Rating:

5 — **Independent:** Near flawless performance; minimal errors; able to perform without supervision; seeks out new learning; shows initiative; A = 4.7–5.0 average

4 — **Minimally Supervised:** Few errors, able to self-correct; seeks guidance when appropriate; B = 3.7–4.65

3 — **Competent:** Minimal required level; no critical errors; able to correct with coaching; meets expectations; safe; C = 3.0–3.65

2 — **Marginal:** Below average; critical errors or problem areas noted; would benefit from remediation; D = 2.0–2.99

1 — **Dependent:** Poor; unacceptable performance; unsafe; gross inaccuracies; potentially harmful; F = < 2.0

Two or more errors of commission or omission of mandatory or essential performance elements will terminate the procedure, and require additional practice and/or remediation and reevaluation. Student is responsible for obtaining additional evaluation forms as needed from the Director of Clinical Education (DCE).

	PERFORMANCE RATING	PERFORMANCE LEVEL
EQUIPMENT AND PATIENT PREPARATION		
1. Common Performance Elements Steps 1–8		
ASSESSMENT AND IMPLEMENTATION		
2. Common Performance Elements Steps 9 and 10		
3. Assesses patient for weaning readiness including mentation		
4. Checks chart for:		
A. Recent chest x-ray		
B. Recent ABG		
C. Laboratory results of CBC and hematology		
D. Adequate urinary output		
E. Discontinuance of sedation		
5. Assesses the following parameters:		
A. Hemodynamic stability		
B. Vital signs		
C. Vital capacity, negative inspiratory force (NIF), or maximal inspiratory pressure (MIP)		
6. Selects the proper mode for weaning		
7. Adjusts ventilator to proper modes and settings		
8. Explains the procedure to the patient if applicable		
9. Implements weaning protocol based on facility policy		
10. Monitors patient tolerance of the weaning procedure:		
A. Adequacy of oxygenation		
B. Adequacy of ventilation		
C. Hemodynamic stability		
11. Assesses subjective tolerance		
12. Readjusts ventilator settings as indicated by protocol		
13. Discontinues weaning if not tolerated and notifies RN and MD		
FOLLOW-UP		
14. Common Performance Elements Steps 11–16		

SIGNATURES   Student: Evaluator: Date:

Clinical Performance Evaluation

PERFORMANCE RATING:

5 **Independent:** Near flawless performance; minimal errors; able to perform without supervision; seeks out new learning; shows initiative; A = 4.7–5.0 average

4 **Minimally Supervised:** Few errors, able to self-correct; seeks guidance when appropriate; B = 3.7–4.65

3 **Competent:** Minimal required level; no critical errors; able to correct with coaching; meets expectations; safe; C = 3.0–3.65

2 **Marginal:** Below average; critical errors or problem areas noted; would benefit from remediation; D = 2.0–2.99

1 **Dependent:** Poor; unacceptable performance; unsafe; gross inaccuracies; potentially harmful; F = < 2.0

Circle the appropriate response below. Please be consistent, objective, and honest in your assessment of the student's clinical performance and ability.

PERFORMANCE CRITERIA	SCORE				
COGNITIVE DOMAIN					
1. Consistently displays knowledge, comprehension, and command of essential concepts	5	4	3	2	1
2. Demonstrates the relationship between theory and clinical practice	5	4	3	2	1
3. Able to select, review, apply, analyze, synthesize, interpret, and evaluate information; makes recommendations to modify care plan	5	4	3	2	1
PSYCHOMOTOR DOMAIN					
4. Minimal errors, no critical errors; able to self-correct; performs all steps safely and accurately	5	4	3	2	1
5. Selects, assembles, and verifies proper function and cleanliness of equipment; assures operation and corrects malfunctions; provides adequate care and maintenance	5	4	3	2	1
6. Exhibits the required manual dexterity	5	4	3	2	1
7. Performs procedure in a reasonable time frame for clinical level	5	4	3	2	1
8. Applies and maintains aseptic technique and PPE as required	5	4	3	2	1
9. Maintains concise and accurate patient and clinical records	5	4	3	2	1
10. Reports promptly on patient status/needs to appropriate personnel	5	4	3	2	1
AFFECTIVE DOMAIN					
11. Exhibits courteous and pleasant demeanor; shows consideration and respect, honesty, and integrity	5	4	3	2	1
12. Communicates verbally and in writing clearly and concisely	5	4	3	2	1
13. Preserves confidentiality and adheres to all policies	5	4	3	2	1
14. Follows directions, exhibits sound judgment, and seeks help when required	5	4	3	2	1
15. Demonstrates initiative, self-direction, responsibility, and accountability	5	4	3	2	1

TOTAL POINTS = _____ /15 = AVERAGE GRADE = _____

ADDITIONAL COMMENTS: IDENTIFY AREAS OF EXCELLENCE; LIST ERRORS OF OMISSION OR COMMISSION, CRITICAL ERRORS

SUMMARY PERFORMANCE EVALUATION AND RECOMMENDATIONS

☐ PASS: Satisfactory Performance

    ☐ Minimal supervision needed, may progress to next level provided specific skills, clinical time completed

    ☐ Minimal supervision needed, able to progress to next level without remediation

☐ FAIL: Unsatisfactory Performance (check all that apply)

    ☐ Minor reevaluation only

    ☐ Needs additional clinical practice before reevaluation

    ☐ Needs additional laboratory practice before skills performed in clinical area

    ☐ Recommend clinical probation

SIGNATURES

Evaluator (print name): _____ Evaluator signature: _____ Date: _____

Student Signature: _____ Date: _____

Student Comments:

CHAPTER 44

Neonatal/Pediatric Respiratory Care

INTRODUCTION

The respiratory system is very frequently the primary target in many infant and pediatric diseases. Therapeutic and technological advances in medicine have dramatically improved the survival of newborns. The high incidence of pediatric asthma and long-term survival of children with genetic disorders such as cystic fibrosis have contributed to the significant demand for perinatal/pediatric respiratory care specialists.

Since a family-centered approach to patient care is essential to cope with the additional psychological and emotional stress encountered when a child is sick,[1] the respiratory care student must learn how to interact and communicate with families in these difficult times.

Although basic concepts of quality patient care are similar in adults and children, the indications, goals, and hazards associated with respiratory care must be modified to meet the special needs of this patient population. Techniques, procedures, equipment, and expected outcomes are frequently significantly altered from the adult population.[2,3]

OBJECTIVES

Upon completion of this chapter, the student will be able to:

1. Practice communication skills needed for the instruction of patients and family members in respiratory care of neonatal and pediatric patients.
2. Apply patient assessment techniques to a neonatal or pediatric patient.
3. Modify respiratory care procedures to meet the special needs of the neonatal or pediatric patient.
4. Apply infection control guidelines and standards associated with equipment and procedures, according to OSHA regulations and CDC guidelines.
5. Demonstrate the required steps to resuscitate a newborn according to the current neonatal resuscitation program guidelines.
6. Select, assemble, verify, and document the function of a neonatal CPAP.
7. Practice communication skills needed for the reporting of clinically significant data to the members of the healthcare team.

KEY TERMS

acrocyanosis
amniotic fluid
Apgar score
breech

eclampsia
gestation
gravida

meconium
neonate
oligohydramnios

para
polyhydramnios
pre-eclampsia

Exercises

EQUIPMENT REQUIRED

- [ ] Infant airway management trainer
- [ ] Infant mannequin
- [ ] Pediatric care doll or mannequin
- [ ] Small-volume nebulizers
- [ ] Large-volume nebulizers
- [ ] Endotracheal tube connector
- [ ] HEPA bacteria filters
- [ ] Manufacturers' operation and maintenance manuals (videos if available)
- [ ] 50-psi oxygen source
- [ ] Infant ventilator circuits
- [ ] 50-psig regulator
- [ ] Bourdon gauge and Thorpe tube flowmeters
- [ ] High-pressure hoses
- [ ] Air compressor
- [ ] Blender
- [ ] Wrenches
- [ ] T-adaptor with small-bore tubing connection and cap
- [ ] Watch with second hand
- [ ] Respirometer
- [ ] Respiratory transfer set (continuous feed system)

- [ ] Sterile water
- [ ] Humidifiers
- [ ] Water traps
- [ ] Temperature probes
- [ ] Oxygen analyzers
- [ ] Cloth tape
- [ ] Neonatal and pediatric sizes of the following:
  - [ ] Nasal cannula
  - [ ] Oxygen masks
  - [ ] Aerosol masks
  - [ ] Spacers with masks
- [ ] Bulb syringe
- [ ] Suction catheters
- [ ] Infant nasal CPAP setup
- [ ] Percussion cups
- [ ] Ventilator circuits (heated-wire circuits if available)
- [ ] Stethoscopes
- [ ] Blood pressure cuffs
- [ ] Endotracheal tubes
- [ ] Miller laryngoscope blades and handles
- [ ] Infant manual resuscitators with masks

EXERCISE 44.1 PATIENT ASSESSMENT IN THE NEWBORN

EXERCISE 44.1.1 MATERNAL ASSESSMENT

For this exercise, students either independently or as a group will need to get permission from a pregnant woman or any woman who has given birth to perform a "prenatal" history and interview.

1. Introduce yourself and your department to the mother.
2. Explain the purpose of the interview.
3. Interview the mother and take a history with special emphasis on the following:

   Date of birth

   Date of last menses

   Number of pregnancies (**gravida**) and number carried to term (**para**)

   Multiple **gestations**

   Any medications taken during pregnancy

   History of diabetes, hypertension, toxemia, **pre-eclampsia,** maternal hypertension, **eclampsia,** previous fetal loss, smoking, pulmonary disease, previous **breech** births, rH factors, **oligohydramnios, polyhydramnios,** previous **meconium** stains, previous placental problems, maternal sepsis, in utero infections, cardiac disease, drug use, alcohol use, sexually transmitted diseases.

4. **Chart the history on your laboratory report.**

EXERCISE 44.1.2 PREPARATION FOR RESUSCITATION OF THE NEWBORN

Table 44.1 shows the equipment and supplies needed for resuscitation of the **neonate.** Prepare a cart or table with all the equipment and supplies needed before performing the following exercises.

Table 44.1 Neonatal Resuscitation Equipment

Radiant warmer
Suction equipment
Bulb syringe
Vacuum
Suction catheter
DeLee trap
Ventilation equipment
Resuscitation bag
Masks
Pressure manometer
Oxygen tubing
Oxygen source
Laryngoscope
Handles
Batteries
Blades
Endotracheal tubes (sizes 2.5 to 4 mm)
Nasogastric tubes
Umbilical vessel catheter equipment
Syringes
Blood gas analysis equipment

EXERCISE 44.1.3 RESUSCITATION OF THE NEWBORN

In the following scenarios the initiation of basic life support will be required. It is expected that the student will have already had instruction in basic life support for healthcare providers before this laboratory. Refer to current American Heart Association (AHA)[4] or American Red Cross (ARC) cardiopulmonary resuscitation (CPR) guidelines for specific details.

Table 44.2 shows the Apgar scoring system.

Using the algorithm shown in Figure 44.1, simulate on an infant mannequin what would need to be done in the following scenarios.

Table 44.2 Apgar Scoring System

	0	1	2
Heart rate	None	<100	>100
Respiratory rate	None	Weak, irregular	Strong cry
Color	Pale blue	Acrocyanosis	Pink
Reflex irritability	No response	Grimace	Cry, cough, or sneeze
Muscle tone	Limp	Some flexion	Well-flexed

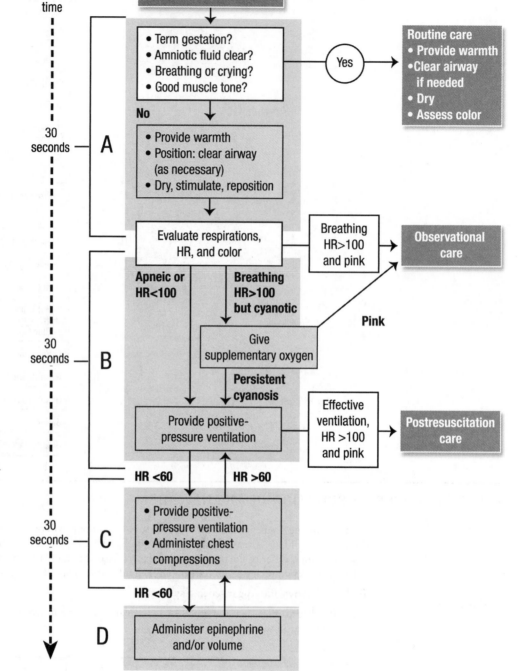

Figure 44.1. Overview of resuscitation in the delivery room. HR indicates heart rate (shown in bpm). Endotracheal intubation may be considered at several steps. (From American Heart Association, American Academy of Pediatrics. 2005 American Heart Association (AHA) Guidelines for Cardiopulmonary Resuscitation (CPR) and Emergency Cardiovascular Care (ECC) of Pediatric and Neonatal Patients: Neonatal Resuscitation Guidelines. Pediatrics 117(5): e1029–e1038, 2006, with permission.)

Scenario 1: Baby Boy Marcos

*You are present for the delivery of a 42-week-gestation neonate. The mother has been in labor for 30 hours and has evidence of meconium staining in the **amniotic fluid**.*

The following is noted in the initial assessment of Baby Boy Marcos:

Weight 8.0 lb

Central cyanosis

Grimaces noted when bulb suction of nares performed

Heart rate 90

Respiratory rate 40 with periods of apnea, retractions noted

Extremities some flexion

1. Perform an **Apgar score** for this scenario, and **record the score on your laboratory report.**
2. Referring to the resuscitation algorithm, perform the required resuscitation procedures.
3. **"Chart"** the event on your laboratory report.

Scenario 2: Baby Girl A and Baby Girl B Williams

You have been called to the delivery room in anticipation of the delivery of 30-week-gestation twins.

The following is noted in the initial assessment of Baby Girl A:

Weight 3.5 lb

Complete cyanosis

No grimaces noted when bulb suction of nares performed

Heart rate 60

Respiratory rate none

Limp

The following is noted in the initial assessment of Baby Girl B:

Weight 4.0 lb

Acrocyanosis

Crying and sneeze stimulated with bulb suction of nares

Heart rate 130

Respiratory rate 60 and irregular

Well-flexed

1. Perform an Apgar score for each twin and **record the scores on your laboratory report.**
2. Referring to the resuscitation algorithm, perform the required resuscitation procedures for each twin.
3. **Chart the events on your laboratory report.**

EXERCISE 44.2 NASAL CONTINUOUS POSITIVE AIRWAY PRESSURE FOR THE INFANT[3]

1. For Baby Boy Marcos in Scenario 1, Exercise 44.1.3: After a successful resuscitation, the baby is placed on nasal CPAP of 5 cm H_2O and an F_IO_2 of 0.80. Set up the equipment needed as shown in Figure 44.2.
2. Initiate CPAP using a mannequin. "Chart" the procedure, documenting your "patient" assessment and any other data required to write a comprehensive note, and **record it on your laboratory report.** This will require you to use your imagination to create clinically relevant assessment data. Include expected capillary blood gases and noninvasive monitoring results.

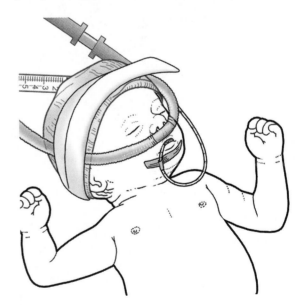

Figure 44.2. Infant nasal continuous positive airway pressure (CPAP) setup.

REFERENCES

1. Barnhart, SL and Czervinske, MP: Clinical Handbook of Perinatal and Pediatric Respiratory Care. WB Saunders, Philadelphia, 2002.
2. American Association for Respiratory Care: AARC clinical practice guideline: Selection of an oxygen delivery device for neonatal and pediatric patients. Revision and update. Respir Care 4(47):707–716, 2002.
3. American Association for Respiratory Care: AARC clinical practice guideline: Application of continuous positive pressure to neonates via nasal prongs, nasopharyngeal tube, or nasal mask. Revision and update. Respir Care 49(9):1100–1108, 2004.
4. 2005 American Heart Association (AHA) Guidelines for Cardiopulmonary Resuscitation (CPR) and Emergency Cardiovascular Care (ECC) of Pediatric and Neonatal Patients: Neonatal resuscitation guidelines. Pediatrics 117:1029–1038, 2006.

Laboratory Report

CHAPTER 44: NEONATAL/PEDIATRIC RESPIRATORY CARE

Name _____   Date _____

Course/Section _____   Instructor _____

Data Collection

EXERCISE 44.1 Patient Assessment in the Newborn

EXERCISE 44.1.1 MATERNAL ASSESSMENT

_____
_____
_____
_____
_____
_____
_____
_____
_____

EXERCISE 44.1.3 RESUSCITATION OF THE NEWBORN

Scenario 1: Baby Boy Marcos

Apgar score: _____

Charting: _____
_____
_____
_____
_____
_____
_____
_____

Scenario 2: Baby Girl A and Baby Girl B Williams

BABY GIRL A

Apgar score: _____

Charting: _____

_____

_____

_____

_____

_____

_____

_____

_____

_____

BABY GIRL B

Apgar score: _____

Charting: _____

_____

_____

_____

_____

_____

_____

_____

_____

_____

EXERCISE 44.2 Nasal Continuous Positive Airway Pressure for the Infant

BABY BOY MARCOS

Charting: _____

_____

_____

_____

_____

_____

_____

_____

Critical Thinking Questions

1. For the following respiratory care procedures, identify the major differences between adult and pediatric care and explain the rationale for the differences:

    A.   Oxygen therapy

    B.   Aerosol delivery

    C.   Suctioning

    D.   Airway care

    E.   Chest physiotherapy

    F.   Noninvasive monitoring

    G.   Blood gas analysis

2. Compare the procedures for basic life support in infants, children, and adults for the following:

    A.   Age criteria

    B.   Head position

    C.   Location for pulse check

    D.   Rate of compression for single rescuer

    E.   Rate of compression for double rescuer

F.   Ratio of compression to ventilations for single rescuer

G.   Ratio of compression to ventilations for double rescuer

H.   Depth of compression

I.   Rate of rescue breathing

J.   Hand position

K.   Obstructed airway maneuvers

L.   Timing for activation of EMS

Procedural Competency Evaluation

STUDENT: _____ DATE: _____

NASAL CPAP INITIATION

	PERFORMANCE RATING	PERFORMANCE LEVEL
Evaluator: ☐ Peer ☐ Instructor **Setting:** ☐ Lab ☐ Clinical Simulation		
Equipment Utilized: _____ **Conditions (Describe):** _____		

Performance Level:

S or ✓ = Satisfactory, no errors of omission or commission
U = Unsatisfactory Error of Omission or Commission
NA = Not applicable

Performance Rating:

5 **Independent:** Near flawless performance; minimal errors; able to perform without supervision; seeks out new learning; shows initiative; A = 4.7–5.0 average

4 **Minimally Supervised:** Few errors, able to self-correct; seeks guidance when appropriate; B = 3.7–4.65

3 **Competent:** Minimal required level; no critical errors; able to correct with coaching; meets expectations; safe; C = 3.0–3.65

2 **Marginal:** Below average; critical errors or problem areas noted; would benefit from remediation; D = 2.0–2.99

1 **Dependent:** Poor; unacceptable performance; unsafe; gross inaccuracies; potentially harmful; F = < 2.0

Two or more errors of commission or omission of mandatory or essential performance elements will terminate the procedure, and require additional practice and/or remediation and reevaluation. Student is responsible for obtaining additional evaluation forms as needed from the Director of Clinical Education (DCE).

	PERFORMANCE RATING	PERFORMANCE LEVEL
PATIENT AND EQUIPMENT PREPARATION		
1. Common Performance Elements Steps 1–8		
2. Identifies the circuit components of a continuous flow CPAP circuit and assembles properly		
3. Performs required leak test (if applicable)		
ASSESSMENT AND IMPLEMENTATION		
4. Common Performance Elements Steps 9 and 10		
5. Turns the unit or system on and selects proper mode, pressures, ramp or rise time, F_IO_2, and timed inspiration		
6. Checks alarm function and sets alarms		
7. Positions patient and applies the nasal prongs		
8. Attaches the tubing to supports and confirms proper fit and comfort		
9. Evaluates waveforms to identify tidal volume, rate, pressures and flow, air trapping, or auto-PEEP		
10. Adjusts the CPAP pressure to conform with the physician's order		
11. Reassess vital signs, SpO_2, breath sounds, respiratory rate, and ventilatory status		
12. Determines how patient is tolerating the procedure, including effectiveness		
FOLLOW-UP		
13. Common Performance Elements Steps 11–16		

SIGNATURES Student: _____ Evaluator: _____ Date: _____

Clinical Performance Evaluation

PERFORMANCE RATING:

5   **Independent:** Near flawless performance; minimal errors; able to perform without supervision; seeks out new learning; shows initiative; A = 4.7–5.0 average

4   **Minimally Supervised:** Few errors, able to self-correct; seeks guidance when appropriate; B = 3.7–4.65

3   **Competent:** Minimal required level; no critical errors; able to correct with coaching; meets expectations; safe; C = 3.0–3.65

2   **Marginal:** Below average; critical errors or problem areas noted; would benefit from remediation; D = 2.0–2.99

1   **Dependent:** Poor; unacceptable performance; unsafe; gross inaccuracies; potentially harmful; F = < 2.0

Circle the appropriate response below. Please be consistent, objective, and honest in your assessment of the student's clinical performance and ability.

PERFORMANCE CRITERIA	SCORE				
COGNITIVE DOMAIN					
1. Consistently displays knowledge, comprehension, and command of essential concepts	5	4	3	2	1
2. Demonstrates the relationship between theory and clinical practice	5	4	3	2	1
3. Able to select, review, apply, analyze, synthesize, interpret, and evaluate information; makes recommendations to modify care plan	5	4	3	2	1
PSYCHOMOTOR DOMAIN					
4. Minimal errors, no critical errors; able to self-correct; performs all steps safely and accurately	5	4	3	2	1
5. Selects, assembles, and verifies proper function and cleanliness of equipment; assures operation and corrects malfunctions; provides adequate care and maintenance	5	4	3	2	1
6. Exhibits the required manual dexterity	5	4	3	2	1
7. Performs procedure in a reasonable time frame for clinical level	5	4	3	2	1
8. Applies and maintains aseptic technique and PPE as required	5	4	3	2	1
9. Maintains concise and accurate patient and clinical records	5	4	3	2	1
10. Reports promptly on patient status/needs to appropriate personnel	5	4	3	2	1
AFFECTIVE DOMAIN					
11. Exhibits courteous and pleasant demeanor; shows consideration and respect, honesty, and integrity	5	4	3	2	1
12. Communicates verbally and in writing clearly and concisely	5	4	3	2	1
13. Preserves confidentiality and adheres to all policies	5	4	3	2	1
14. Follows directions, exhibits sound judgment, and seeks help when required	5	4	3	2	1
15. Demonstrates initiative, self-direction, responsibility, and accountability	5	4	3	2	1

TOTAL POINTS =   /15 = AVERAGE GRADE =

ADDITIONAL COMMENTS: IDENTIFY AREAS OF EXCELLENCE; LIST ERRORS OF OMISSION OR COMMISSION, CRITICAL ERRORS

SUMMARY PERFORMANCE EVALUATION AND RECOMMENDATIONS

☐ PASS: Satisfactory Performance

     ☐ Minimal supervision needed, may progress to next level provided specific skills, clinical time completed

     ☐ Minimal supervision needed, able to progress to next level without remediation

☐ FAIL: Unsatisfactory Performance (check all that apply)

     ☐ Minor reevaluation only

     ☐ Needs additional clinical practice before reevaluation

     ☐ Needs additional laboratory practice before skills performed in clinical area

     ☐ Recommend clinical probation

SIGNATURES

Evaluator (print name):   Evaluator signature: Date:

Student Signature: Date:

Student Comments:

Procedural Competency Evaluation

STUDENT: _____   DATE: _____

OXYGEN HOOD

					PERFORMANCE RATING	PERFORMANCE LEVEL
Evaluator: ☐ Peer ☐ Instructor		**Setting:** ☐ Lab		☐ Clinical Simulation		
Equipment Utilized:		**Conditions (Describe):**				

Performance Level:

S or ✓ = Satisfactory, no errors of omission or commission
U = Unsatisfactory Error of Omission or Commission
NA = Not applicable

Performance Rating:

5   **Independent:** Near flawless performance; minimal errors; able to perform without supervision; seeks out new learning; shows initiative; A = 4.7–5.0 average

4   **Minimally Supervised:** Few errors, able to self-correct; seeks guidance when appropriate; B = 3.7–4.65

3   **Competent:** Minimal required level; no critical errors; able to correct with coaching; meets expectations; safe; C = 3.0–3.65

2   **Marginal:** Below average; critical errors or problem areas noted; would benefit from remediation; D = 2.0–2.99

1   **Dependent:** Poor; unacceptable performance; unsafe; gross inaccuracies; potentially harmful; F = < 2.0

Two or more errors of commission or omission of mandatory or essential performance elements will terminate the procedure, and require additional practice and/or remediation and reevaluation. Student is responsible for obtaining additional evaluation forms as needed from the Director of Clinical Education (DCE).

EQUIPMENT AND PATIENT PREPARATION

1. Common Performance Elements Steps 1–8

ASSESSMENT AND IMPLEMENTATION

2. Common Performance Elements Steps 9 and 10

3. Connects blender or air and oxygen flowmeters

4. Attaches nebulizer or humidifier to blender or flowmeters

5. Fills with sterile water if not prefilled or sets up continuous feed system

6. Attaches servo-controlled heater and plugs into electrical outlet; sets temperature to 32–37°C

7. Adjusts blender or nebulizer to prescribed F_iO_2 or adjusts liter flow >7 Lpm

8. Attaches large-bore tubing to nebulizer outlet and oxygen hood inlet; uses water drainage bag

9. Inserts temperature probe in appropriate location

10. Places infant in the oxygen hood and loosely seals around the neck

11. Analyzes F_iO_2 at infant mouth

12. Allows for warm-up time and adjusts heater if necessary to ensure neutral thermal environment

13. Assesses oxygenation and ventilation

FOLLOW-UP

14. Places cap or unplugs analyzer when not in use

15. Common Performance Elements Steps 11–16

SIGNATURES   Student: _____   Evaluator: _____   Date: _____

Clinical Performance Evaluation

PERFORMANCE RATING:

5 **Independent:** Near flawless performance; minimal errors; able to perform without supervision; seeks out new learning; shows initiative; A = 4.7–5.0 average

4 **Minimally Supervised:** Few errors, able to self-correct; seeks guidance when appropriate; B = 3.7–4.65

3 **Competent:** Minimal required level; no critical errors; able to correct with coaching; meets expectations; safe; C = 3.0–3.65

2 **Marginal:** Below average; critical errors or problem areas noted; would benefit from remediation; D = 2.0–2.99

1 **Dependent:** Poor; unacceptable performance; unsafe; gross inaccuracies; potentially harmful; F = < 2.0

Circle the appropriate response below. Please be consistent, objective, and honest in your assessment of the student's clinical performance and ability.

PERFORMANCE CRITERIA	SCORE				
COGNITIVE DOMAIN					
1. Consistently displays knowledge, comprehension, and command of essential concepts	5	4	3	2	1
2. Demonstrates the relationship between theory and clinical practice	5	4	3	2	1
3. Able to select, review, apply, analyze, synthesize, interpret, and evaluate information; makes recommendations to modify care plan	5	4	3	2	1
PSYCHOMOTOR DOMAIN					
4. Minimal errors, no critical errors; able to self-correct; performs all steps safely and accurately	5	4	3	2	1
5. Selects, assembles, and verifies proper function and cleanliness of equipment; assures operation and corrects malfunctions; provides adequate care and maintenance	5	4	3	2	1
6. Exhibits the required manual dexterity	5	4	3	2	1
7. Performs procedure in a reasonable time frame for clinical level	5	4	3	2	1
8. Applies and maintains aseptic technique and PPE as required	5	4	3	2	1
9. Maintains concise and accurate patient and clinical records	5	4	3	2	1
10. Reports promptly on patient status/needs to appropriate personnel	5	4	3	2	1
AFFECTIVE DOMAIN					
11. Exhibits courteous and pleasant demeanor; shows consideration and respect, honesty, and integrity	5	4	3	2	1
12. Communicates verbally and in writing clearly and concisely	5	4	3	2	1
13. Preserves confidentiality and adheres to all policies	5	4	3	2	1
14. Follows directions, exhibits sound judgment, and seeks help when required	5	4	3	2	1
15. Demonstrates initiative, self-direction, responsibility, and accountability	5	4	3	2	1

TOTAL POINTS =   /15 = AVERAGE GRADE =

ADDITIONAL COMMENTS: IDENTIFY AREAS OF EXCELLENCE; LIST ERRORS OF OMISSION OR COMMISSION, CRITICAL ERRORS

SUMMARY PERFORMANCE EVALUATION AND RECOMMENDATIONS

☐ PASS: Satisfactory Performance

  ☐ Minimal supervision needed, may progress to next level provided specific skills, clinical time completed

  ☐ Minimal supervision needed, able to progress to next level without remediation

☐ FAIL: Unsatisfactory Performance (check all that apply)

  ☐ Minor reevaluation only

  ☐ Needs additional clinical practice before reevaluation

  ☐ Needs additional laboratory practice before skills performed in clinical area

  ☐ Recommend clinical probation

SIGNATURES

Evaluator (print name):   Evaluator signature: Date:

Student Signature: Date:

Student Comments:

Procedural Competency Evaluation

STUDENT: **DATE:**

OXYGEN TENT

Evaluator: ☐ Peer ☐ Instructor   **Setting:** ☐ Lab   ☐ Clinical Simulation

Equipment Utilized: **Conditions (Describe):**

Performance Level:

S or ✓ = Satisfactory, no errors of omission or commission
U = Unsatisfactory Error of Omission or Commission
NA = Not applicable

Performance Rating:

5   **Independent:** Near flawless performance; minimal errors; able to perform without supervision; seeks out new learning; shows initiative; A = 4.7–5.0 average

4   **Minimally Supervised:** Few errors, able to self-correct; seeks guidance when appropriate; B = 3.7–4.65

3   **Competent:** Minimal required level; no critical errors; able to correct with coaching; meets expectations; safe; C = 3.0–3.65

2   **Marginal:** Below average; critical errors or problem areas noted; would benefit from remediation; D = 2.0–2.99

1   **Dependent:** Poor; unacceptable performance; unsafe; gross inaccuracies; potentially harmful; F = < 2.0

Two or more errors of commission or omission of mandatory or essential performance elements will terminate the procedure, and require additional practice and/or remediation and reevaluation. Student is responsible for obtaining additional evaluation forms as needed from the Director of Clinical Education (DCE).

	PERFORMANCE RATING	PERFORMANCE LEVEL
EQUIPMENT AND PATIENT PREPARATION		
1. Common Performance Elements Steps 1–8		
2. Educates patient's family on oxygen safety		
ASSESSMENT AND IMPLEMENTATION		
3. Common Performance Elements Steps 9 and 10		
4. Attaches canopy to tent frame		
5. Connects gas inlet and outlet hoses to portholes of the canopy		
6. Assembles nebulizer and fills reservoir with sterile water		
7. Turns the unit on		
8. Attaches drain hose to collection bottle		
9. Attaches high pressure hose to oxygen flowmeter or 50 psi DISS outlet		
10. Verifies mist production		
11. Ensures no electrical hazards are present		
12. Places tent over the bed and flushes tent for 5 minutes		
13. Places infant or child in the tent		
14. Analyzes F_IO_2		
FOLLOW-UP		
15. Common Performance Elements Steps 11–16		

SIGNATURES   Student: Evaluator: Date:

Clinical Performance Evaluation

PERFORMANCE RATING:

5 **Independent:** Near flawless performance; minimal errors; able to perform without supervision; seeks out new learning; shows initiative; A = 4.7–5.0 average

4 **Minimally Supervised:** Few errors, able to self-correct; seeks guidance when appropriate; B = 3.7–4.65

3 **Competent:** Minimal required level; no critical errors; able to correct with coaching; meets expectations; safe; C = 3.0–3.65

2 **Marginal:** Below average; critical errors or problem areas noted; would benefit from remediation; D = 2.0–2.99

1 **Dependent:** Poor; unacceptable performance; unsafe; gross inaccuracies; potentially harmful; F = < 2.0

Circle the appropriate response below. Please be consistent, objective, and honest in your assessment of the student's clinical performance and ability.

PERFORMANCE CRITERIA | SCORE

PERFORMANCE CRITERIA					
COGNITIVE DOMAIN					
1. Consistently displays knowledge, comprehension, and command of essential concepts	5	4	3	2	1
2. Demonstrates the relationship between theory and clinical practice	5	4	3	2	1
3. Able to select, review, apply, analyze, synthesize, interpret, and evaluate information; makes recommendations to modify care plan	5	4	3	2	1
PSYCHOMOTOR DOMAIN					
4. Minimal errors, no critical errors; able to self-correct; performs all steps safely and accurately	5	4	3	2	1
5. Selects, assembles, and verifies proper function and cleanliness of equipment; assures operation and corrects malfunctions; provides adequate care and maintenance	5	4	3	2	1
6. Exhibits the required manual dexterity	5	4	3	2	1
7. Performs procedure in a reasonable time frame for clinical level	5	4	3	2	1
8. Applies and maintains aseptic technique and PPE as required	5	4	3	2	1
9. Maintains concise and accurate patient and clinical records	5	4	3	2	1
10. Reports promptly on patient status/needs to appropriate personnel	5	4	3	2	1
AFFECTIVE DOMAIN					
11. Exhibits courteous and pleasant demeanor; shows consideration and respect, honesty, and integrity	5	4	3	2	1
12. Communicates verbally and in writing clearly and concisely	5	4	3	2	1
13. Preserves confidentiality and adheres to all policies	5	4	3	2	1
14. Follows directions, exhibits sound judgment, and seeks help when required	5	4	3	2	1
15. Demonstrates initiative, self-direction, responsibility, and accountability	5	4	3	2	1

TOTAL POINTS = _____ /15 = AVERAGE GRADE = _____

ADDITIONAL COMMENTS: IDENTIFY AREAS OF EXCELLENCE; LIST ERRORS OF OMISSION OR COMMISSION, CRITICAL ERRORS

SUMMARY PERFORMANCE EVALUATION AND RECOMMENDATIONS

☐ PASS: Satisfactory Performance

    ☐ Minimal supervision needed, may progress to next level provided specific skills, clinical time completed

    ☐ Minimal supervision needed, able to progress to next level without remediation

☐ FAIL: Unsatisfactory Performance (check all that apply)

    ☐ Minor reevaluation only

    ☐ Needs additional clinical practice before reevaluation

    ☐ Needs additional laboratory practice before skills performed in clinical area

    ☐ Recommend clinical probation

SIGNATURES

Evaluator (print name): _____ Evaluator signature: _____ Date: _____

Student Signature: _____ Date: _____

Student Comments:

45 Neonatal/Pediatric Ventilation

INTRODUCTION

During the last decade many great advances have been made in perinatology, especially in the area of newborn pulmonary disorders and neonatal ventilation. Further refinements of conventional mechanical ventilation, along with a better understanding of high-frequency ventilation, have improved outcomes for neonates. It is therefore essential that the respiratory care student becomes familiar with these techniques and shows dexterity not only during the setup of mechanical ventilators but also during the adjustment of ventilator parameters.

Although the physiologic objectives for mechanical ventilation in the pediatric patient are basically the same as those in adult patients, the pediatric patient presents with some of the most clinical challenging situations in critical care.[1]

OBJECTIVES

Upon completion of this chapter, the student will be able to:

1. Select, assemble, verify, and document the function of a time-cycled, pressure-controlled ventilator.
2. Practice the documentation skills required for a neonatal or pediatric patient-ventilator system check on a ventilator flow sheet and the skills necessary to generate a narrative or shift note.
3. Practice communication skills needed for the reporting of clinically significant data to the members of the healthcare team.

KEY TERMS

amplitude
chest wiggle
circumoral

hertz (Hz)
high-frequency
ventilators

nasal continuous positive
airway pressure
(NCPAP)

Exercises

EQUIPMENT REQUIRED

- [ ] Pediatric care doll or mannequin
- [ ] Infant/pediatric ventilators
- [ ] High-frequency ventilator (optional)
- [ ] Endotracheal tube connector
- [ ] HEPA bacteria filters
- [ ] Manufacturers' operation and maintenance manuals (videos if available)
- [ ] 50-psi oxygen source
- [ ] Infant ventilator circuits
- [ ] 50-psig regulator
- [ ] Bourdon gauge and Thorpe tube flowmeters
- [ ] High-pressure hoses
- [ ] Air compressor
- [ ] Blender
- [ ] Wrenches
- [ ] T-adaptor with small-bore tubing connection and cap

- [ ] Watch with second hand
- [ ] Respirometer
- [ ] Respiratory transfer set (continuous feed system)
- [ ] Sterile water
- [ ] Wick humidifiers
- [ ] Water traps
- [ ] Infant test lungs
- [ ] Infant lung simulator (optional)
- [ ] Temperature probes
- [ ] Oxygen analyzers
- [ ] Suction catheters
- [ ] Ventilator circuits (heated-wire circuits if available)
- [ ] Endotracheal and tracheostomy tubes
- [ ] Miller laryngoscope blades and handles

EXERCISE 45.1 TIME-CYCLED/PRESSURE-LIMITED VENTILATORS

EXERCISE 45.1.1 VENTILATOR ASSEMBLY

1. Select an infant ventilator, water traps, bacteria filters, humidifier, and infant test lung or mannequin. **Record the ventilator make and model on your laboratory report.**
2. Obtain the maintenance manual for the ventilator selected. In the manual, find the manufacturer's recommendations for the following:

   Changing and cleaning of bacteria filters

   Fan filters

   Sterilization or disinfection instructions for internal and external parts and surfaces

   Requirements for routine maintenance

   Record this information on your laboratory report.
3. Locate the chronometer and **record the number of hours of use on your laboratory report.**
4. Assemble the ventilator as shown according to the manufacturer's instructions.
5. Repeat this exercise for each ventilator provided.

EXERCISE 45.1.2 IDENTIFICATION OF CONTROLS

1. On the same infant ventilator used in Exercise 45.1.1, identify the following controls. It is important to note that not all ventilators have the same controls, but they have several controls in common. Refer to Chapter 39 to review ventilator controls.

   High-pressure limit

   Rate

   F_IO_2

   Flow

   Inspiratory time

   Expiratory time

   Mode selection

Low inspiratory pressure

Low PEEP/CPAP

Low oxygen pressure

Low air pressure

Prolonged inspiratory pressure

Ventilator inoperative

Overpressure relief valve

2. **Record the controls identified on your laboratory report.**

3. Repeat this exercise for each ventilator provided.

EXERCISE 45.1.3 MANIPULATION OF CONTROLS

1. Adjust the settings to the following:

    Mode = IMV or SIMV

    PIP = 20 cm H_2O

    f = 20/minute

    Flow rate = 9 Lpm

    Inspiratory time = 0.4 second

    PEEP = 5 cm H_2O

    F_1O_2 = 1.0

    Make sure that all the alarms are set to the appropriate settings. **Record the alarm settings selected on your laboratory report.**

2. Attach the infant test lung to the patient wye connection.

3. Observe the inflation of the test lung and **record your observations on your laboratory report.**

4. Squeeze the test lung several times to simulate an inspiratory effort and rate of 40/minute. Observe the manometer. Count the rate at which you are squeezing the test lung and compare it with the displayed rate on the machine. **Record the results on your laboratory report.**

5. Observe the test lung expansion and compare it with step 3. **Record your observations on your laboratory report.**

6. Adjust the inspiratory time to 1 second. Squeeze the test lung at a minimum rate of 40/minute. Listen to the sound of the machine. Observe the manometer and alarms. **Record the results and observations on your laboratory report.**

7. Observe the test lung expansion and compare it with step 5. **Record the result on your laboratory report.**

8. Return the inspiratory time to 0.4 second. Decrease the rate to 5/minute.

9. Stop squeezing the test lung. Wait 1 minute and observe the ventilator response. Count the ventilator rate. **Record your results and observations on your laboratory report.**

10. Change the flow rate to 2 Lpm. Continue simulating spontaneous respirations at a rate of 40/minute. Observe the test lung expansion, manometer, and alarms. **Record your observations on your laboratory report.**

11. Change the flow rate to 12 Lpm. Continue simulating spontaneous respirations at a rate of 40/minute. Observe the test lung expansion, manometer, and alarms. **Record your observations on your laboratory report.**

12. Return the flow to 9 Lpm. Adjust the PIP to 10 cm H_2O. Continue simulating spontaneous respirations at a rate of 40/minute. Observe the test lung expansion, manometer, and alarms. **Record your observations on your laboratory report.**

13. Adjust the PIP to 30 cm H_2O. Continue simulating spontaneous respirations at a rate of 40/minute. Observe the test lung expansion, manometer, and alarms. **Record your observations on your laboratory report.**

EXERCISE 45.2 HIGH-FREQUENCY VENTILATORS

Audiovisual training videotapes are available from several high-frequency ventilator manufacturers. Your instructor may have these available in the laboratory.

Because of the complexity of this technology and the lack of availability of the equipment for many respiratory care schools, it is recommended that arrangements be made for a manufacturer's demonstration of the equipment. An observational experience in the clinical setting would also be useful.

1. Obtain a high-frequency ventilator, if available. Set up the ventilator as shown in Figure 45.1.
2. Attach a test lung to the circuit.
3. Initiate high-frequency ventilation (HFV) using Table 45.1 as a guide.
4. Indicators for adequate inflation during HFV include the following[1]:

   Chest x-ray findings
   Chest wiggle
   P_{TCO_2} and P_{TCCO_2} values
   SpO_2
   C_{ST}
   Hemodynamic status
   a/A ratio
   Alveolar ventilation is directly proportional to the amplitude setting.[2]

5. **"Chart" the initiation of high-frequency ventilation on Baby Girl A on your laboratory report.**
6. Adjust the amplitude to 11. Observe the test lung and **record your observations on your laboratory report.**
7. Adjust the amplitude to 51. Observe the test lung and **record your observations on your laboratory report.**
8. Return the **amplitude** to 24. Adjust the settings to 10 Hz (600 beats or cycles/minute). Determine the I:E ratio and **record your answer on your laboratory report.** Observe the test lung and **record your observations on your laboratory report.**
9. Adjust the settings to 22 Hz (1320 beats or cycles/minute). Observe the test lung and **record your observations on your laboratory report.**

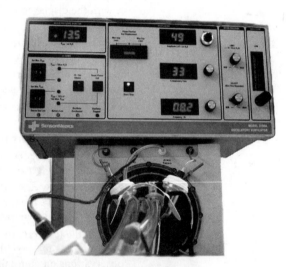

Figure 45.1. High-frequency oscillator ventilator.

Table 45.1 Initial HFV Settings[2]
(Premature Infants <2.5 kg)

Frequency	15 Hz (900 bpm); range 6–15 Hz
	6–12 Hz with air leaks
Inspiratory time	Fixed at 18 ms (0.018 sec)
I:E Ratio	Dependent on rate
	Amplitude 24 (11–51)
	Adjust until vigorous chest wall vibrations seen
	Titrate based on $PaCO_2$
	To change $PaCO_2$ ± 2–4mm Hg change amplitude 3 units
	To change $PaCO_2$ ± 5–9 mm Hg change amplitude 6 units
PEEP	Equal to MAP on CMV

bpm = beats per minute.

EXERCISE 45.3 INITIATING MECHANICAL VENTILATION IN AN INFANT

EXERCISE 45.3.1 SCENARIO 1

Baby Boy 1 is currently on NCPAP = 5 cm H_2O and an F_IO_2 = 0.80. The following data are obtained:

SpO_2 = 85%

$PTCCO_2$ = 75 mm Hg

Capillary stick pH = 7.20

1. The physician has asked you to initiate mechanical ventilation. Using Table 45.2 as a guide, adjust the ventilator and initiate mechanical ventilation.

2. Perform a patient-ventilator system check, including "patient" assessment. Include oxygen analysis and airway care. **Record all pertinent data on the ventilator flow sheet provided in your laboratory report.**

3. A blood gas is obtained after your initial settings:

   pH = 7.32

   PaO_2 = 120 mm Hg

   $PaCO_2$ = 60 mm Hg

   Adjust the ventilator settings according to Table 45.3. Perform a patient-ventilator system check, including "patient" assessment. Include oxygen analysis and airway care. **Record all pertinent data on the ventilator flow sheet provided in your laboratory report.**

4. Write a narrative note documenting your "patient's" status and any other data required to write a comprehensive shift note. **Record it on your laboratory report.** This will require you to use your imagination to create clinically relevant assessment data.

Table 45.2 Initial Ventilator Parameters

Suggested Initial Ventilator Settings for Newborn Infants*		
	With Normal Lungs	**With Noncompliant (Stiff) Lungs or RDS**
PIP	12–18 cm H_2O	20–25 cm H_2O
Respiratory rate	10–20 breaths/min	20–40 breaths/min
PEEP	2–3 cm H_2O	4–5 cm H_2O
Flow rate	4–10 L/min	4–10 L/min
Inspiratory time	0.4–0.8 sec	0.3–0.5 sec
I:E ratio	1:2–1:10	1:1–1:3
F_IO_2	To maintain PaO_2 >50 mm Hg	To maintain PaO_2 >50 mm Hg

*RDS = respiratory distress syndrome; PIP = peak inspiratory pressure; PEEP = positive end-expiratory pressure; I:E ratio = inspiratory-expiratory ratio; F_IO_2 = fractional concentration of oxygen in inspired gas; PaO_2 = partial pressure of arterial oxygen

From Whitaker, K: Comprehensive Perinatal and Pediatric Respiratory Care. Delmar, Albany, 2001, p. 508, with permission.

Table 45.3 Suggested Neonatal Ventilator Adjustments

Setting	Adjustment Increment	Anticipated Results
F_IO_2	2–5 (%)	Change in PaO_2
PIP	+1–2 (cm H_2O)	Increased PaO_2
		Decreased PaO_2
PEEP	+1–2 (cm H_2O)	Increased PaO_2
		Decreased PaO_2
T1	+0.1–0.2 (sec)	Increased PaO2
	−0.1–0.2 (sec)	Better synchronization
Rate	2–5 (breaths per minute)	Change in $PaCO_2$

From Czervinske, MP and Barnhart, SL: Perinatal and Pediatric Respiratory Care. WB Saunders, Philadelphia, 1995, p. 81, with permission.

EXERCISE 45.3.2 SCENARIO 2

Baby Girl B is presently in the NICU receiving an F_IO_2 = 0.40 via oxyhood. You have noticed increasing expiratory grunting, retractions, and periods of apnea and bradycardia over the last hour. As you are suctioning the patient, she has a complete respiratory arrest. The nurse is manually ventilating while you set up and initiate mechanical ventilation.

1. Select the appropriate size endotracheal tube and **record your selection on your laboratory report.**

2. Baby Girl B is now intubated. Determine the appropriate ventilatory parameters and initiate ventilation. Perform a patient-ventilator system check, including "patient" assessment. Include oxygen analysis and airway care. **Record all pertinent data on the ventilator flow sheet provided in your laboratory report.**

3. A blood gas is obtained after your initial settings:

   pH = 7.45
   $PaCO_2$ = 35 mm Hg
   PaO_2 = 45 mm Hg

   Adjust the ventilator settings according to Table 45.3. Perform a patient-ventilator system check, including "patient" assessment. Include oxygen analysis and airway care. **Record all pertinent data on the ventilator flow sheet provided in your laboratory report.**

4. Write a narrative note documenting your "patient's" status and any other data required to write a comprehensive shift note. **Record it on your laboratory report.** This will require you to use your imagination to create clinically relevant assessment data.

EXERCISE 45.4 PEDIATRIC VENTILATION

Obtain an appropriate ventilator for pediatric patients, set it up, and verify the function. **Record the make and model on your laboratory report.**

For each of the following scenarios, initiate mechanical ventilation according to the guidelines outlined in Table 41.1.

EXERCISE 45.4.1 SCENARIO 3

Amanda Chung is an 8-month-old infant admitted with respiratory syncytial virus (RSV) pneumonia. She weighs 16 lb. Initial blood gases reveal the following:

   pH = 7.15
   $PaCO_2$ = 65 mm Hg
   PaO_2 = 40 mm Hg

1. Select the appropriate size and type of airway, and **record your selection on your laboratory report.**

2. The physician asks you to determine the appropriate ventilatory mode and parameters and initiate ventilation. Perform a patient-ventilator system check, including "patient" assessment. Include oxygen analysis and airway care. **Record all pertinent data on the ventilator flow sheet provided in your laboratory report.**

3. Write a narrative note documenting your "patient's" status and any other data required to write a comprehensive shift note. **Record it on your laboratory report.** This will require you to use your imagination to create clinically relevant assessment data.

EXERCISE 45.4.2 SCENARIO 4

Chiam Goldfarb is a 3-year-old child brought to the emergency room unconscious after ingestion of an unknown quantity of paint thinner. Initial assessment reveals a 35-lb, well-nourished child with the following findings:

Pulse 140/minute

f = 45/minute with sternal retractions

Stridor

Nasal flaring

Breath sounds diminished with diffuse bilateral wheezes

Color pale with **circumoral** cyanosis

An attempt to intubate the child is unsuccessful due to severe glottic edema.

1. Select the appropriate size and type of airway, and **record your selection on your laboratory report.**

2. The physician asks you to determine the appropriate ventilatory mode and parameters and initiate ventilation. Perform a patient-ventilator system check, including "patient" assessment. Include oxygen analysis and airway care. **Record all pertinent data on the ventilator flow sheet provided in your laboratory report.**

3. Write a narrative note documenting your "patient's" status and any other data required to write a comprehensive shift note. **Record it on your laboratory report.** This will require you to use your imagination to create clinically relevant assessment data.

REFERENCES

1. Czervinske, MP and Barnhart, SL: Perinatal and Pediatric Respiratory Care. WB Saunders, Philadelphia, 2003, p. 310.

2. Klein, JM: Management Strategies with High Frequency Ventilation in Neonates: Infant Star Ventilator. Presented at 41st Annual AARC Convention, Orlando, FL, 1995.

Laboratory Report

CHAPTER 45: NEONATAL/PEDIATRIC VENTILATION

Name _____ Date _____

Course/Section _____ Instructor _____

Data Collection

EXERCISE 45.1 Time-Cycled/Pressure-Limited Ventilators

EXERCISE 45.1.1 VENTILATOR ASSEMBLY

Ventilator make and model: _____

_____

Manufacturer's recommendations:

1. Changing and cleaning of bacteria filters: _____

_____

2. Fan filters: _____

_____

3. Sterilization or disinfection instructions for internal and external parts and surfaces: _____

_____

4. Requirements for routine maintenance: _____

_____

Number of hours of use: _____

EXERCISE 45.1.2 IDENTIFICATION OF CONTROLS

_____

_____

_____

_____

_____

_____

_____

_____

_____

_____

EXERCISE 45.1.3 MANIPULATION OF CONTROLS

Mode = IMV or SIMV

PIP = 20 cm H_2O

f = 20/minute

Flow rate = 9 Lpm

Inspiratory time = 0.4 second

PEEP = 5 cm H_2O

F_IO_2 = 1.0

Alarm settings: _____

_____

_____

_____

_____

_____

Observation of the inflation of the test lung: _____

_____

_____

_____

_____

Spontaneous rate = 40/minute: _____

_____

_____

_____

Observation of the manometer: _____

_____

_____

_____

Rate comparison: _____

_____

_____

Comparison of test lung expansion with step 3: _____

_____

_____

Inspiratory time = 1 second, spontaneous rate = 40/minute: _____

Observation of the manometer and alarms: _____

_____

_____

_____

_____

Comparison of the test lung expansion with step 5: _____

_____

_____

_____

_____

Inspiratory time = 0.4 second, rate = 5/minute, spontaneous rate = 0: _____

Observation of ventilator response: _____

_____

_____

_____

_____

Flow rate = 2 Lpm, spontaneous rate = 40/minute: _____

Observation of the test lung expansion, manometer, and alarms:

_____

_____

_____

_____

_____

Flow rate = 12 Lpm: _____

Observation of the test lung expansion, manometer, and alarms:

_____

_____

_____

_____

_____

Flow rate = 9 Lpm, PIP = 10 cm H_2O: _____

Observation of the test lung expansion, manometer, and alarms:

_____

_____

_____

_____

PIP = 30 cm H_2O: _____

Observation of the test lung expansion, manometer, and alarms:

_____

_____

_____

_____

EXERCISE 45.2 High-Frequency Ventilators

"Charting" of HFV on Baby Girl A: _____

_____

_____

_____

_____

_____

_____

_____

_____

Amplitude = 11. Observations: _____

_____

_____

_____

_____

Amplitude = 51. Observations: _____

_____

_____

_____

Amplitude = 24; Frequency = 10 Hz (600 bpm):

Observations: _____

_____

_____

_____

I:E ratio (**show your work!**): _____

Observations: _____

_____

_____

_____

Frequency = 22 Hz (1320 bpm): Observations: _____

_____

_____

_____

_____

EXERCISE 45.3 Initiating Mechanical Ventilation in an Infant

EXERCISE 45.3.1 SCENARIO 1

Baby Boy A is currently on NCPAP = 5 cm H_2O and an F_1O_2 = 0.80. The following data are obtained: SpO_2 = 85%, P_{TCCO_2} = 75 mm Hg, capillary stick pH = 7.20.

(**Insert ventilator flow sheet at end of laboratory report.**)

"Charting": _____

_____

_____

_____

_____

_____

_____

_____

EXERCISE 45.3.2 SCENARIO 2

Size endotracheal tube: _____

(**Insert ventilator flow sheet at end of laboratory report.**)

"Charting": _____

_____

_____

_____

_____

_____

_____

_____

_____

_____

_____

EXERCISE 45.4 Pediatric Ventilation

Make and model of ventilator: _____

EXERCISE 45.4.1 SCENARIO 3

Size and type of airway: _____

(Insert ventilator flow sheet at end of laboratory report.)

"Charting": _____

_____

_____

_____

_____

_____

_____

_____

_____

_____

_____

_____

EXERCISE 45.4.2 SCENARIO 4

Size and type of airway: _____

(Insert ventilator flow sheet at end of laboratory report.)

"Charting": _____

_____

_____

_____

_____

_____

_____

_____

_____

_____

Critical Thinking Questions

1. Explain how an incorrect flow rate setting (too high and too low) on a pressure-limited time-cycled ventilator affects the volume delivered.

2. Compare and contrast mechanical ventilation of an adult with mechanical ventilation of an infant. Be sure to include similarities and differences.

	PATIENT-VENTILATOR SYSTEM CHECK										PT ID:		
DATE													
TIME													
MODE													
SET RATE													
TOTAL RATE													
SET F_IO_2													
ANALYZED F_IO_2													
PEEP/CPAP													
FLOW/%I-TIME													
I:E RATIO													
SENSITIVITY													
PIP													
PLATEAU													
MAP													
GAS TEMP													
HIGH P													
LOW P													
LOW V_T/V_E													
HI/LOW O_2													
LOW PEEP/CPAP													
TEMP ALARM													
TUBE SIZE/TYPE													
TUBE PLACEMENT													
CUFF PRESS													
SpO_2													
$PECO_2$													
BP													
HR													
ECG													
TEMP													
pH													
$PaCO_2$													
COHB/METHB													
C.O.													
PAP													
PWP													
PvO_2													
SvO_2													
$CavO_2$													
SIGNATURE													

DATE	TIME	RESPIRATORY CARE PROGRESS NOTES

Procedural Competency Evaluation

STUDENT: **DATE:**

NEONATAL/PEDIATRIC VENTILATOR INITIATION

	PERFORMANCE RATING	PERFORMANCE LEVEL
Evaluator: ☐ Peer ☐ Instructor **Setting:** ☐ Lab ☐ Clinical Simulation		
Equipment Utilized: **Conditions (Describe):**		
Performance Level: S or ✓ = Satisfactory, no errors of omission or commission U = Unsatisfactory Error of Omission or Commission NA = Not applicable		
Performance Rating: **5** **Independent:** Near flawless performance; minimal errors; able to perform without supervision; seeks out new learning; shows initiative; A = 4.7–5.0 average **4** **Minimally Supervised:** Few errors, able to self-correct; seeks guidance when appropriate; B = 3.7–4.65 **3** **Competent:** Minimal required level; no critical errors; able to correct with coaching; meets expectations; safe; C = 3.0–3.65 **2** **Marginal:** Below average; critical errors or problem areas noted; would benefit from remediation; D = 2.0–2.99 **1** **Dependent:** Poor; unacceptable performance; unsafe; gross inaccuracies; potentially harmful; F = < 2.0 *Two or more errors of commission or omission of mandatory or essential performance elements will terminate the procedure, and require additional practice and/or remediation and reevaluation. Student is responsible for obtaining additional evaluation forms as needed from the Director of Clinical Education (DCE).*		
PATIENT AND EQUIPMENT PREPARATION		
1. Common Performance Elements Steps 1–8		
2. Connects the ventilator to the appropriate emergency electrical outlets		
3. Connects the high pressure hoses to the appropriate 50 psi gas source outlets		
4. Attaches circuit, filters, and humidification systems as needed		
5. Turns on the ventilator and performs any required tests		
6. Performs any additional leak tests; corrects and verifies ventilator function		
ASSESSMENT AND IMPLEMENTATION		
7. Common Performance Elements Steps 9 and 10		
8. Evaluates the patient by assessing: A. Vital signs, color, WOB, pulse oximetry, capnography, and transcutaneous monitoring B. Physical assessment of the chest C. Airway size, type, placement, and patency D. Auscultation E. Suctioning		
9. Selects initial ventilator settings according to order or protocol		
10. Sets initial alarm parameters		
11. Connects the patient to the ventilator and adjusts the following as needed: A. Ventilator parameters and alarms B. Sensitivity C. Mode D. Rate/Frequency E. VT/VE F. PIP G. Pressure support H. Flow rate/I-time% flow pattern /I:E ratio I. Analyzes and adjusts F_IO_2 as indicated J. Adjusts circuit humidification system K. Observes and interprets ventilator graphics L. Note LOC, use of sedation, and paralytics		
12. Completes patient-ventilator system check		
FOLLOW-UP		
13. Common Performance Elements Steps 11–16		

SIGNATURES   Student: Evaluator: Date:

Clinical Performance Evaluation

PERFORMANCE RATING:

5 **Independent:** Near flawless performance; minimal errors; able to perform without supervision; seeks out new learning; shows initiative; A = 4.7–5.0 average

4 **Minimally Supervised:** Few errors, able to self-correct; seeks guidance when appropriate; B = 3.7–4.65

3 **Competent:** Minimal required level; no critical errors; able to correct with coaching; meets expectations; safe; C = 3.0–3.65

2 **Marginal:** Below average; critical errors or problem areas noted; would benefit from remediation; D = 2.0–2.99

1 **Dependent:** Poor; unacceptable performance; unsafe; gross inaccuracies; potentially harmful; F = < 2.0

Circle the appropriate response below. Please be consistent, objective, and honest in your assessment of the student's clinical performance and ability.

PERFORMANCE CRITERIA	SCORE				
COGNITIVE DOMAIN					
1. Consistently displays knowledge, comprehension, and command of essential concepts	5	4	3	2	1
2. Demonstrates the relationship between theory and clinical practice	5	4	3	2	1
3. Able to select, review, apply, analyze, synthesize, interpret, and evaluate information; makes recommendations to modify care plan	5	4	3	2	1
PSYCHOMOTOR DOMAIN					
4. Minimal errors, no critical errors; able to self-correct; performs all steps safely and accurately	5	4	3	2	1
5. Selects, assembles, and verifies proper function and cleanliness of equipment; assures operation and corrects malfunctions; provides adequate care and maintenance	5	4	3	2	1
6. Exhibits the required manual dexterity	5	4	3	2	1
7. Performs procedure in a reasonable time frame for clinical level	5	4	3	2	1
8. Applies and maintains aseptic technique and PPE as required	5	4	3	2	1
9. Maintains concise and accurate patient and clinical records	5	4	3	2	1
10. Reports promptly on patient status/needs to appropriate personnel	5	4	3	2	1
AFFECTIVE DOMAIN					
11. Exhibits courteous and pleasant demeanor; shows consideration and respect, honesty, and integrity	5	4	3	2	1
12. Communicates verbally and in writing clearly and concisely	5	4	3	2	1
13. Preserves confidentiality and adheres to all policies	5	4	3	2	1
14. Follows directions, exhibits sound judgment, and seeks help when required	5	4	3	2	1
15. Demonstrates initiative, self-direction, responsibility, and accountability	5	4	3	2	1

TOTAL POINTS = ____ /15 = AVERAGE GRADE = ____

ADDITIONAL COMMENTS: IDENTIFY AREAS OF EXCELLENCE; LIST ERRORS OF OMISSION OR COMMISSION, CRITICAL ERRORS

SUMMARY PERFORMANCE EVALUATION AND RECOMMENDATIONS

☐ PASS: Satisfactory Performance

    ☐ Minimal supervision needed, may progress to next level provided specific skills, clinical time completed

    ☐ Minimal supervision needed, able to progress to next level without remediation

☐ FAIL: Unsatisfactory Performance (check all that apply)

    ☐ Minor reevaluation only

    ☐ Needs additional clinical practice before reevaluation

    ☐ Needs additional laboratory practice before skills performed in clinical area

    ☐ Recommend clinical probation

SIGNATURES

Evaluator (print name): _____   Evaluator signature: _____   Date: ____

Student Signature: _____   Date: ____

Student Comments: